Clinical Diabetes Research

Clinical Diabetes Research

Methods and Techniques

Edited by

Michael Roden

Medical Department, Hanusch Teaching Hospital,
Medical University of Vienna
Karl Landsteiner Institute for Endocrinology and Metabolism, Vienna

John Wiley & Sons, Ltd

Other Wiley Editorial Offices

John Wiley & Sons Inc., 111 River Street, Hoboken, NJ 07030, USA

Jossey-Bass, 989 Market Street, San Francisco, CA 94103-1741, USA

Wiley-VCH Verlag GmbH, Boschstr. 12, D-69469 Weinheim, Germany

John Wiley & Sons Australia Ltd, 33 Park Road, Milton, Queensland 4064, Australia

John Wiley & Sons (Asia) Pte Ltd, 2 Clementi Loop #02-01, Jin Xing Distripark, Singapore 129809

John Wily & Sons Canada Ltd, 6045 Freemont Blvd, Mississauga, Ontario, L5R 4J3

Wiley also publishes its books in a variety of electronic formats. Some content that appears in print may not be available in electronic books.

Anniversary Logo Design: Richard J. Pacifico

Library of Congress Cataloging in Publication Data

Clinical diabetes research : methods and techniques / edited by Michael Roden.
    p. ; cm.
Includes bibliographical references.
ISBN 978-0-470-01728-9 (cloth : alk. paper)
1. Diabetes. 2. Diabetes—Research. I. Roden, Michael, Dr.
[DNLM: 1. Diabetes Mellitus. 2. Clinical Trials. WK 810 C6413 2007]
RC660.C463 2007
616.4′620072—dc2   2007015950

British Library Cataloguing in Publication Data

A catalogue record for this book is available from the British Library

ISBN 978-0-470-01728-9

Typeset in 10/12pt Times by Integra Software Services Pvt. Ltd, Pondicherry, India
Printed and bound in Great Britain by CPI Antony Rowe, Chippenham and Eastbourne
This book is printed on acid-free paper responsibly manufactured from sustainable forestry
in which at least two trees are planted for each one used for paper production.
Cover images kindly provided by Dr Julia Szendrödi, Karl-Landsteiner Institute for Endocrinology and Metabolism, at the MR Center of Excellence, University of Vienna (the magnetic resonance picture) and Agnes Roden, Department of Internal Medicine III, Medical University of Vienna (the PET scan). The graph displays the suppression of endogenous glucose production during ingestion of a mixed meal in humans and was produced in the lab of Professor Roden.

Contents

List of Contributors

Stephanie A. Amiel BSc, MD, FRCP, RD Lawrence Professor of Diabetic Medicine, Gene and Cell Based Therapy, Diabetes Research Group, Diabetes, Endocrinology and Metabolism, King's College London School of Medicine, London, UK

Henning Beck-Nielsen MD, DMSc, Head of the Department of Endocrinology, Odense University Hospital, Professor of Endocrinology, University of Southern Denmark, and Head of the Danish PhD School of Molecular Metabolism, Odense, Denmark

Ayad Al-Bermani MD, Specialist Registrar in Medical Ophthalmology, Ophthalmology Department, Royal Victoria Infirmary, Newcastle upon Tyne, UK

Andrew J.M. Boulton MD, FRCP, DSc, Professor of Medicine, Medicine University of Manchester, Manchester, UK

Attila Brehm MD, Assistant, First Medical Department, Hanusch Hospital (Academic Teaching Hospital, Medical University of Vienna), Vienna, Austria

Pratik Choudhary MB, BS, Gene and Cell Based Therapy, Diabetes Research Group, Diabetes, Endocrinology and Metabolism, King's College London School of Medicine, London, UK

Carole Cull PhD, University Research Lecturer, Senior Medical Statistician, Diabetes Trials Unit, Oxford Centre for Diabetes, Endocrinology and Metabolism, Churchill Hospital, Headington, Oxford, UK

Michael Gaster MD, PhD, Specialist in General Medicine. Associated Professor at the Molecular Endocrinology Unit, Odense University Hospital, Odense, Denmark

Danielle A. Gilge PhD, Candidate, Nutrition, Case Western Reserve University, Cleveland, Ohio, USA

Leif Groop MD, PhD, Professor, Head, Lund University Diabetes Centre, Department of Clinical Sciences, Diabetes and Endocrinology, Lund University, Malmoe, Sweden

Kurt Højlund MD, PhD, Senior Registrar, Post Doc, Department of Endocrinology, Odense University, Odense, Denmark

Patricia Iozzo PhD, Turku PET Centre, University of Turku, Turku, Finland and PET Centre, Institute of Clinical Physiology, CNR National Research Council, Pisa, Italy

Christian Joukhadar MD, Lecturer, Department of Clinical Pharmacology, Medical University Vienna, Vienna General Hospital, Vienna, Austria

John Griffith Jones DSc, Senior Researcher and Invited Assistant Professor, Intermediary Metabolism, Center for Neurosciences and Cell Biology, Department of Biochemistry, University of Coimbra, Coimbra, Portugal

Juhani Knuuti, Professor, Turku PET Centre, University of Turku, Turku, Finland

Martin Kr̆s̆̆ák PhD, Departments of Radiodiagnostics and Internal Medicine III, Medical University Vienna, Vienna, Austria

Bernard Landau MD, PhD, Division of Clinical and Molecular Endocrinology, Case Western Reserve University, Cleveland, Ohio, USA

Charlotte Ling MSc, PhD, Associate Professor, Lund University Diabetes Centre, Department of Clinical Sciences, Diabetes and Endocrinology, Lund University, Malmoe, Sweden

Andrea Mari PhD Senior Research Scientist, Institute of Biomedical Engineering, National Research Council, Padova, Italy

Sally M. Marshall BSc, MD, FRCP, Professor of Diabetes, Diabetes Research Group, School of Clinical Sciences, Faculty of Medicine, University of Newcastle upon Tyne, Newcastle upon Tyne, UK

John M. Miles MD, Professor of Medicine, Endocrine Research Unit, Division of Endocrinology, Diabetes, Metabolism and Nutrition, Mayo Clinic, Rochester, Minnesota, USA

Markus Müller MD, Professor, Head, Department of Clinical Pharmacology, Medical University of Vienna, Vienna General Hospital, Vienna, Austria

Robert H. Nelson MD, Instructor, Endocrine Research Unit, Division of Endocrinology, Diabetes, Metabolism and Nutrition, Mayo Clinic, Rochester, Minnesota, USA

Pirjo Nuutila MD, Professor, Turku PET Centre and Department of Medicine, University of Turku, Finland

Giovanni Pacini DSC, Head, Metabolic Unit, Institute of Biomedical Engineering, Italian National Research Council, Padova, Italy

Johannes Pleiner MD, Lecturer in Clinical Pharmacology, Cardiovascular Pharmacology, Department of Clinical Pharmacology, Medical University Vienna, Vienna, Austria

Stephen F. Previs PhD, Assistant Professor, Nutrition, Case Western Reserve University, Cleveland, Ohio, USA

Susan Pye MSc, Research Associate, Diabetes and Metabolism Research Unit, Ottawa Hospital and Ottawa Health Research Unit, Ottawa, Canada

Nadia Rachdaoui PhD, Instructor, Division of Clinical and Molecular Endocrinology, Department of Medicine, Case Western Reserve University, Cleveland, Ohio, USA

Haris Rathur MRCP, Specialist Registrar, Diabetes and Endocrinology, Medicine, Manchester Royal Infirmary, Manchester, UK

Jerry Radziuk PhD, MD, CM, Professor, Departments of Medicine and of Physiology, Director, Diabetes and Metabolism Research Unit, University of Ottawa, Ottawa Hospital and Ottawa Health Research Unit, Ottawa, Canada

Michael Roden, MD, Head/Director, Medical Department, Hanusch Teaching Hospital, Medical University of Vienna and Karl Landsteiner Institute for Endocrinology and Metabolism, Vienna, Austria

Irene Stratton MSc, University Research Lecturer, Senior Medical Statistician, Diabetes Trials Unit, Oxford Centre for Diabetes, Endocrinology and Metabolism, Churchill Hospital, Oxford, UK

Roy Taylor MD, Professor of Medicine and Metabolism, Honorary Consultant Physician, School of Clinical Medical Sciences, Newcastle University and Diabetes Centre, Newcastle upon Tyne, UK

Ming Ming Teh MB, BS, Clinical Research Fellow, Gene and Cell Based Therapy, Diabetes Research Group, Diabetes, Endocrinology and Metabolism, King's College London School of Medicine, London, UK

Michael Wolzt MD, Consultant Physician, Associate Professor, Medical University of Vienna, Division of Cardiovascular Medicine, Department of Clinical Pharmacology, Medical University of Vienna, Vienna, Austria

Dan Ziegler MD, Professor of Internal Medicine, Consultant Physician, Institute of Clinical Diabetes Research, German Diabetes Center, Leibniz Center at the Heinrich Heine University, Düsseldorf, Germany

1

Basics of Clinical Metabolic Research

Michael Roden

Metabolic diseases, particularly obesity, dyslipidaemia and type 2 diabetes mellitus (T2DM), as well as conditions of increased risk for these diseases such as factors of the (dys)metabolic syndrome have become dramatically more prevalent over the last decade. Both in the industrialised world and, even more so, in developing regions and countries – which feature rapidly increasing economies and are adopting the so-called Western lifestyle – these diseases, particularly overweightness and obesity, are a growing health problem (Kopelman 2000). It is assumed that T2DM could be the largest epidemic in human history (Zimmet 2005) as more than 190 million people worldwide are diabetic and more than 300 million suffer from impaired glucose tolerance, the immediate pre-diabetic state. Recent calculations suggest that in the year 2025 more than 300 million people will have overt diabetes, mainly T2DM, with excessive growth in developing countries (King et al. 1998).

Diabetes mellitus is already the leading cause of blindness among working-age adults, of end-stage renal disease and of non-traumatic loss of limb (Ullbrecht et al. 2004; Williamson et al. 2004). The global mortality attributable to diabetes in the year 2000 was estimated to be 2.9 million deaths, which was 5.2 % of all death. Thus diabetes is the fifth leading cause of death globally. About 2–3 % of the population in low-economy countries and up to 8 % in the United States and Canada die because of diabetes (Roglic et al. 2005). The costs caused by diabetes are enormous.Currently diabetes care accounts for 2–7 % of the total national health care budgets in Western countries, amounting to $132 billion in the United States in 2002 (ADA 2003). These data underline the importance of understanding the cellular mechanisms of the causes and complications of type 2 diabetes mellitus in order to offer better targeted and more effective treatment or even prevention of the disease.

Over the last decades, we have learned a lot from *in vitro* experiments in isolated tissues and cell cultures, but especially from *in vivo* studies in mouse models of modified insulin secretion or action (Nandi et al. 2004). Nevertheless, the phenotypes resulting from the various tissue-specific knockout or overexpression mouse models of diabetes or metabolic diseases do not generally resemble the phenotypes of corresponding diseases in humans. In addition to species differences and technical limitations of metabolic studies in small animals,

Clinical Diabetes Research: Methods and Techniques   Edited by Michael Roden
© 2007 John Wiley & Sons, Ltd   ISBN 978-0-470-01728-9

this observation can likely be explained by gene-environment interactions influencing the human phenotypes of metabolic disorders. This makes detailed studies in humans under *in vivo* conditions mandatory.

Starting from simple endocrine and metabolic stimulation or suppression tests such as the insulin and glucagon administration or glucose tolerance tests, a series of more sophisticated tests has been developed over the last three decades. This development is mirrored by the near-exponential rise in original papers and reviews on the topics 'diabetes' and 'metabolic diseases' in peer-reviewed journals since 1970 (Figure 1.1). Among those publications, some key methodological papers speeded up the development of clinical metabolic research. These key papers include the description and validation of standardised insulin sensitivity and secretion tests such as the glucose clamp (Tobin et al. 1979) and minimal modeling of glucose and insulin concentrations during the intravenous glucose tolerance test (Bergman et al. 1981). Later on, tissue-specific metabolism became accessible by applying *in vivo* multinuclear magnetic resonance spectroscopy (MRS) (Shulman et al. 1990; Krssak et al. 1999) or positron emission tomography (PET) (Nuutila et al. 1993). Novel applications of stable isotopes as labels of molecules, e.g. ^2H_2O, later allowed quantification of complex metabolic fluxes such as rates of gluconeogenesis from different sources and glycogenolysis from one single blood sample (Landau et al. 1995) (NOTE: I would like to express my grief for my long-term mentor and friend, Professor Landau, an outstanding researcher and scientist in the field of metabolism, who passed away during the printing of this book). Combining the different techniques, e.g. MRS and ^2H_2O (Kunert et al. 2003), further stimulated research on human metabolism and detailed metabolic phenotyping of various populations is now widely used.

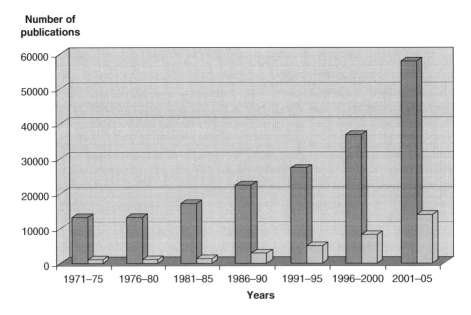

Figure 1.1 Number of original papers (dark columns) and reviews (light columns) in five-year intervals from 1970 to 2005 based on MEDLINE searching for the terms 'diabetes' or 'metabolic diseases'.

Despite the rising interest in clinical research, many basic questions regarding metabolism in humans are unanswered or have not been addressed in sufficient detail. A major issue is the role of aging in intermediary metabolism. which was studied in detail *in vivo* in humans only recently. Petersen et al. (2004) assessed glucose fluxes and ectopic lipid deposition as well as mitochondrial oxidation and phosphorylation under *in vivo* conditions and found ~40 % lower flux rates through the tricarboxylic acid cycle and adenosine-tris-phosphate synthesis, possibly explaining the reduced insulin sensitivity and elevated ectopic lipid content in elderly humans. Nevertheless, it remains unclear whether aging is generally associated with impaired insulin sensitivity; specific genetic or even acquired abnormalities could be responsible for reduced mitochondrial function not only during aging but also in other metabolic disorders (Stark & Roden 2007). Likewise, sex and ethnicity can variably affect metabolic characteristics including body fat and its distribution, lipid metabolism and insulin action, which further complicates interpretation of clinical metabolic studies (Woods et al. 2003; Carulli et al. 2005).

These aspects of human metabolism culminate in the recent discussions on definitions of metabolic disorders summarised by the term '(dys)metabolic syndrome' or 'syndrome X', which was introduced by Reaven about 20 years ago (Reaven 1988) and increasingly studied over the next decades (Figure 1.2). The World Health Organisation (WHO), the European Group for Insulin Resistance (EGIR), the Adult Treatment Panel (ATP III) and the International Diabetes Foundation (IDF) re-defined the metabolic syndrome, and more definitions are coming up due to different combinations and cut-off points of continuous variables, such as fasting plasma glucose, triglycerides or variable indices of body fat content (Table 1.1). The current discussion focuses on the relative importance of the compounds of the metabolic syndrome and the issue of whether it is a syndrome at all (Kahn et al. 2005). This controversy mostly results from different interpretations and understandings of this term, which can be used 1) to explain a series of factors by one underlying causal factor, be it insulin

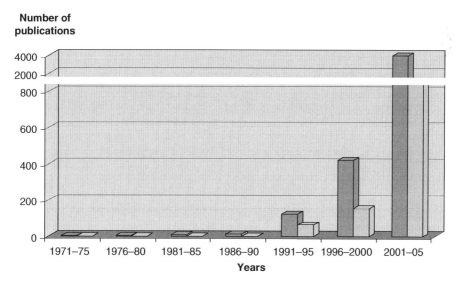

Figure 1.2 Number of original papers (dark columns) and reviews (light columns) in five-year intervals from 1970 to 2005 based on MEDLINE searching for the term 'metabolic syndrome'.

Table 1.1 Definitions of the metabolic syndrome by the World Health Organisation (WHO), the European Group for Insulin resistance (EGIR), the Adult Treatment Panel (ATP III) and the International Diabetes Foundation (IDF). Key: DM – Diabetes mellitus; IGT – impaired glucose tolerance; IFG – impaired fasting glucose

WHO (1999)	EGIR (1999)	ATPIII (2001)	IDF (2005)
Main criteria Insulin resistance *OR* DM / IGT / IFG	*Main criterion* Insulin resistance		*Main criterion* Abdominal obesity
Other components Hypertension ≥ 140/90 mmHg Dyslipidaemia Central obesity Microalbuminura *(two or more)*	*Other components* Hyperglycaemia Hypertension ≥ 140/90 mmHg Dyslipidaemia Central obesity *(two or more)*	Abdominal obesity High triglycerides Low HDL-C Hypertension ≥ 130/85 mmHg High fasting glucose/DM *(two or more)*	*PLUS* Hyper-triglyceridaemia Low HDL-C Hypertension ≥ 130/85 mmHg High fasting glucose/DM *(two or more)*

resistance or obesity; 2) to provide an easy cardiovascular risk cluster in addition to the known traditional risk makers such as cigarette smoking or LDL-cholesterol; or 3) to create a novel clinical syndrome or disease requiring specific treatment. We are currently lacking detailed knowledge of the interaction between numerous polygenic and environmental mediators, variation between populations and ethnic groups and time-dependent changes in these continuous variables. Above all, the physiological basis for the several metabolic disorders remains largely unknown at present.

In addition to its relevance for understanding human pathophysiology, clinical metabolic research is becoming important as a tool in clinical trials on non-pharmacological treatment and even more on drug treatment for today's major epidemiological threats. Of note, searching the MEDLINE detects 580 clinical trials in the 1970s, 1,464 in the 1980s, 5,236 in the 1990s – and already 7,568 between 2000 and 2006.

The sections of this book cover the relevant aspects of current clinical research in humans and are designed to address the researcher's need for theoretical and practical knowledge in this field.

References

Abate N, Chandalia M (2003) The impact of ethnicity on type 2 diabetes *J Diabetes Complications* **17**, 39–58

American Diabetes Association (ADA) (2003) Economic Costs of Diabetes in the US in 2002 *Diabetes Care* **26**, 917–32

Bergman RN, Phillips LS, Cobelli C (1981) Physiologic evaluation of factors controlling glucose tolerance in man: measurement of insulin sensitivity and beta-cell glucose sensitivity from the response to intravenous glucose *J Clin Invest* **68**, 1456–67

Carulli L, Rondinella S, Lombardini S, Canedi I, Loria P, Carulli N (2005) Review article: diabetes, genetics and ethnicity *Aliment Pharmacol Ther* **22**, Suppl 2, 16–9

DeFronzo RA, Tobin JD, Andres R (1979) Glucose clamp technique: a method for quantifying insulin secretion and resistance *Am J Physiol* **237**, E214–23

Kahn R, Buse J, Ferrannini E, Stern M (2005) The metabolic syndrome: time for a critical appraisal. Joint statement from the American Diabetes Association and the European Association for the Study of Diabetes *Diabetologia* **48**, 1684–99

King H, Aubert RE, Herman WH (1998) Global burden of diabetes, 1995–2025: prevalence, numerical estimates, and projections *Diabetes Care* **21**, 1414–31

Kopelman PG (2000) Obesity as a medical problem *Nature* **404**, 635–43

Krssak M, Falk Petersen K, Dresner A, DiPietro L, Vogel SM, Rothman DL et al. (1999) Intramyocellular lipid concentrations are correlated with insulin sensitivity in humans: a 1H NMR spectroscopy study *Diabetologia* **42**, 113–16, erratum on p. 386 and on p. 1269

Kunert O, Stingl H, Rosian E, Krssak M, Bernroider E, Seebacher W et al. (2003) Intramyocellular lipid concentrations are correlated with insulin sensitivity in humans: a 1H NMR spectroscopy study *Diabetes* **52**, 2475–82

Landau BR, Wahren J, Chandramouli V, Schumann WC, Ekberg K, Kalhan SC (1995) Use of 2H2O for estimating rates of gluconeogenesis: application to the fasted state *J Clin Invest* **95**, 172–8

Nandi A, Kitamura Y, Kahn CR, Accili D (2004) Mouse models of insulin resistance *Physiol Rev* **84**, 623–47

Nuutila P, Knuuti J, Ruotsalainen U, Koivisto VA, Eronen E, Teras M et al. (1993) Insulin resistance is localized to skeletal but not heart muscle in type 1 diabetes *Am J Physiol* **264**, E756–62

Petersen KF, Befroy D, Dufour S, Dziura J, Ariyan C, Rothman DL et al. (2003) Mitochondrial dysfunction in the elderly: possible role in insulin resistance *Science* **300**, 1140–2

Reaven GM (1988) Banting lecture 1988: role of insulin resistance in human disease *Diabetes* **37**, 1595–1601

Roglic G, Unwin N, Bennett PH, Mathers C, Tuomilehto J, Nag S et al. (2005) The burden of mortality attributable to diabetes: realistic estimates for the year 2000 *Diabetes Care* **28**, 2130–5

Shulman GI, Rothman DL, Jue T, Stein P, DeFronzo RA, Shulman RG (1990) *N Engl J Med* **322**, 223–8

Stark R, Roden M (2007) Mitochondrial function and endocrine diseases – ESCI Award 2006 *Europ J Clin Invest* (in press)

Ulbrecht JS, Cavanagh PR, Caputo GM (2004) Foot problems in diabetes: an overview *Clin Infect Dis* **39**, Suppl 2, 273–82

Williamson DF, Vinicor F, Bowman BA (2004) Primary prevention of type 2 diabetes mellitus by lifestyle intervention: implications for health policy *Ann Intern Med* **40**, 951–7

Woods SC, Gotoh K, Clegg DJ (2003) *Exp Biol Med* **228**, 1175–80

Zimmet P (2005) *Am J Med* **118**, Suppl 2, 3S–8S

2

Methods for the Assessment of β-Cell Function *In Vivo*

Andrea Mari and **Giovanni Pacini**

Introduction

The β cell plays a key role in the maintenance of glucose homeostasis and β-cell dysfunction is a characteristic feature of many states of glucose intolerance. Thus, the assessment of β-cell function is of fundamental importance in the study of metabolic disorders, particularly type 2 diabetes, and in the evaluation of drugs to treat β-cell dysfunction. At the present time, β-cell function continues to be very actively studied, as strategies for preventing the decline of β-cell function and design of drugs that may achieve this effect are a promise for the alleviation of the burden of diabetes.

The scope of this chapter is to provide a comparative and critical account of the most important methods for the assessment of β-cell function *in vivo*. We illustrate the basic technical aspects of the methodologies, referring the reader to the original publications for the details of test protocols. We also try to relate the characteristics of the *in vivo* tests to the β-cell molecular processes, knowledge of which has been greatly increased in the recent years. We hope that this attempt, though imperfect, will improve critical understanding of the methods. Other useful reviews of β-cell function assessment can be found in several journals (Hovorka & Jones 1994; Kahn 2003; Pacini & Mari 2003; Ferrannini & Mari 2004; Mari 2006) and textbooks (Porte et al. 2003; DeFronzo et al. 2004; LeRoith et al. 2004).

Methods for insulin secretion *in vivo*

The assessment of β-cell function requires the determination of the insulin secretory response to a given stimulus and, if the stimulus is not standardised, normalisation of the response to the stimulus. Thus, the evaluation of insulin secretion is a prerequisite for the assessment of β-cell function. The insulin secretory response can be simply determined from insulin concentration, or else from C-peptide levels using more complex methodologies.

Clinical Diabetes Research: Methods and Techniques   Edited by Michael Roden
© 2007 John Wiley & Sons, Ltd   ISBN 978-0-470-01728-9

Insulin concentration

Simple measurement of plasma insulin is a classic approach still employed in many studies. However, peripheral insulin concentration reflects pancreatic insulin secretion only partially. Insulin in fact undergoes a first pass hepatic removal of about 50 %, i.e. about half the insulin secretion never reaches the periphery. Most importantly, insulin clearance, of which hepatic extraction is a major determinant, may vary in different metabolic conditions (Duckworth et al. 1998). Differences in peripheral insulin may not only reflect differences in insulin secretion but also differences in insulin clearance (Ferrannini et al. 1997; Camastra et al. 2005). Nevertheless, the observed insulin concentration profile almost parallels that of insulin secretion, as insulin kinetics is fast. Rapid insulin release, such as that seen in first phase secretion, is clearly reflected in insulin concentration.

C-peptide methods

To avoid the problem of non-constant insulin clearance, an alternative approach based on the measurement of C-peptide was developed almost 30 years ago (Eaton et al. 1980). C-peptide

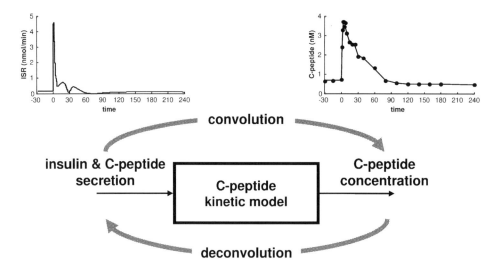

Figure 2.1 Illustration of deconvolution. The mathematical representation of the relationship between insulin secretion (ISR) and C-peptide concentration is based on *convolution*. The determinant of this relationship is the C-peptide concentration response to a C-peptide bolus injection, which quantitatively describes C-peptide kinetics. Convolution is the operation with which C-peptide concentration is calculated from ISR. If C-peptide kinetics is known (either by direct assessment or using the allometric formula of Van Cauter et al. (1992)), it is possible to reverse the convolution operator and calculate ISR from C-peptide concentration. This operation is called *deconvolution* and is illustrated in the graphs on the top (data from Figure 2.4). In this example, ISR is represented as a piecewise constant function over one-minute intervals (top left). For a given ISR time-course, the C-peptide kinetic model allows calculation (by convolution) of the corresponding C-peptide concentration. Thus, the ISR values can be determined by fitting the calculated C-peptide values to the measured ones. This is done using a modified least-squares method that ensures a smooth ISR profile. The graphs on top show measured (dots) and fitted (solid line) C-peptide values obtained with this procedure (right graph) and the calculated ISR (left graph).

is co-secreted with insulin in equimolar amounts, undergoes negligible hepatic extraction and has linear and relatively constant kinetics. Thus, C-peptide concentration reflects more precisely true pancreatic insulin secretion, although its time-course, compared to that of insulin concentration, is somewhat blunted and delayed with respect to insulin secretion. For this reason, a mathematical operation, called deconvolution, is used to reconstruct insulin secretion from C-peptide concentration. Deconvolution, illustrated in Figure 2.1, is the mathematical operation with which C-peptide (i.e. insulin) secretion is calculated from C-peptide concentration (see Hovorka & Jones 1994 for details).

To perform deconvolution, C-peptide kinetics must be known. In the original approach (Eaton et al. 1980), followed in several successive studies, C-peptide kinetics was determined by a bolus injection of biosynthetic C-peptide in each individual. In a later study (Van Cauter et al. 1992), the difficulty of the assessment of the individual C-peptide kinetics was circumvented by developing a method by which approximate C-peptide kinetic parameters could be derived from anthropometric measurements. This approach has made wide application of the C-peptide deconvolution methodology possible, and is currently one of the most common methods for insulin secretion.

C-peptide deconvolution remains unfortunately a rather specialised approach, as it requires specific software and technical expertise (Hovorka & Jones 1994). A publicly available (though rather old) program for deconvolution (Hovorka et al. 1996) can be found at http://www.soi.city.ac.uk/~sg331/software.html (web search keywords: isec,site:city.ac.uk).

β-cell response characteristics

in vivo β-cell response

Figure 2.2 summarises the most relevant characteristics of a normal β-cell response: 1) when glucose is raised gradually, insulin secretion is progressively stimulated (Figure 2.2A) and a dose-response relationship is observed between glucose concentration and insulin secretion (Figure 2.2B). 2) When glucose concentration is briskly increased and maintained at a suprabasal level, insulin secretion shows a biphasic pattern, with an initial burst (first phase insulin secretion) followed by a gradually increasing secretion that approaches a nearly constant level after about 1–2 h (second phase insulin secretion) (Figure 2.2C). The amplitude of both first and second phase response is a function of the glucose increment; the amplitude of the second phase depends on the β-cell dose-response. A biphasic response is also observed with the intravenous glucose tolerance test (IVGTT), in which a strong first phase secretion peak is followed by a slower and more blunted secretion rise. 3) Prolonged exposure to hyperglycaemia produces an increase of the insulin response (both first and second phase). This phenomenon, called potentiation, is clearly visible by repeating the same stimulus after a short rest period (Figure 2.2C). 4) The β-cell response to an oral glucose stimulus, such as an oral glucose tolerance test (OGTT), is considerably higher than that obtained with an intravenous glucose infusion at matched glucose levels (Figure 2.2D). This augmentation of the secretory response is mainly attributed to gut-secreted hormones called incretins, and in particular to glucose-dependent insulinotropic peptide (GIP) and glucagon-like peptide-1 (GLP-1). 5) The β-cell responds also to various non-glucose stimuli (e.g. some aminoacids, sulphonylureas and glucagon). An aminoacid frequently used in β-cell function testing is arginine, which is a powerful secretagogue. Injection of arginine produces a strong first phase insulin response, which is potentiated by hyperglycaemia (Figure 2.2E). 6) In the presence of insulin resistance, β-cell function is increased to cope with the increased insulin demand necessary to set resistant glucose uptake and production processes to adequate levels. This phenomenon is exemplified in Figure 2.2F for the acute insulin response (AIR),

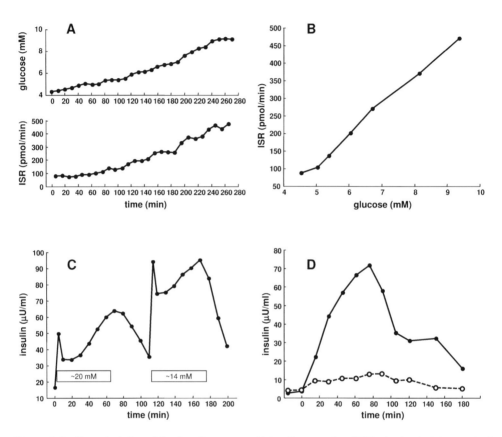

Figure 2.2 Characteristics of the β-cell response: A) insulin secretion (ISR) obtained with a gradual increase in glucose concentration; B) the corresponding dose-response relating glucose concentration to insulin secretion. Redrawn from Byrne et al. (1995); C) response to a repeated square wave of hyperglycaemia (mean glucose levels shown in the bars). Both glucose stimulations produce the typical biphasic secretory pattern. Potentiation of the secretory response is evident in the second stimulus. Redrawn from Cerasi (1981); D) Enhancement of the secretory response observed when glucose is administered orally. The insulin curves are obtained with an OGTT (closed circles and solid line) and with an intravenous glucose infusion reproducing the same glucose levels of the OGTT (open circles and dashed line). Redrawn from Nauck et al. (1986); E) response to arginine injection at different glucose levels. The four smaller peaks are relative to a basal glucose concentration of ~5 mM – glucose levels for the higher peaks are shown in the bars above the peaks. The response to arginine is potentiated by hyperglycaemia. Redrawn from Ward et al. (1984); F) inverse relationship between the minimal model parameter of insulin sensitivity (S_I) and the acute insulin response to an IVGTT (AIR). The solid line represents a hyperbolic interpolation in a group of 93 subjects (the dashed lines represent the dispersion, as percentiles of the disposition index). As a subject becomes insulin resistant (from point S to R), his secretion increases to maintain glucose tolerance normal. Redrawn from Kahn et al. (1993).

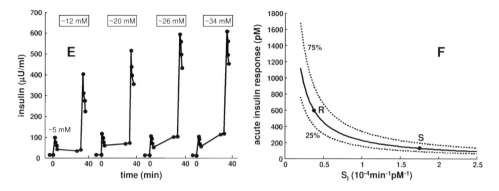

Figure 2.2 Continued.

a parameter of first phase secretion of the IVGTT (see below). Fasting insulin secretion exhibits a similar relationship with insulin sensitivity.

While the β-cell characteristics illustrated in Figure 2.2 are well known, the relative importance of the various response modes to glucose regulation and the pathophysiology of type 2 diabetes is still debated. The response modes are often but not always correlated (Ferrannini & Mari 2004). Therefore, although the use of a single β-cell function index may be a practical necessity, complete assessment of β-cell function requires multiple indices.

Cellular processes underlying the β-cell response

Some background on the relevant cellular processes is useful to shed light on the physiological meaning of the β-cell response characteristics observed in the various tests, although our understanding of the molecular aspects of insulin secretion is still largely incomplete. The molecular aspects of β-cell secretion are discussed in depth in several excellent reviews (Henquin 2000; Rorsman et al. 2000; Bratanova-Tochkova et al. 2002; Henquin et al. 2002; Straub & Sharp 2002).

Figure 2.3 is a simplified representation of the β-cell secretory machinery. Two pathways, denoted as *triggering* and *amplifying* (Henquin 2000), are shown. In the triggering pathway, glucose activates exocytosis by increasing cytosolic calcium concentration through a chain of events that ends with the opening of the calcium channels and an influx of extracellular calcium (see the legend to Figure 2.3). Through the amplifying pathway, glucose modulates insulin secretion independently of changes in calcium concentration. Both these pathways are important determinants of the β-cell response.

In the β cell, insulin is stored in granules. Only granules in a specific status (usually denoted as *immediately releasable*) can undergo exocytosis by activation of the triggering pathway. The translocation of granules from one status to another is an additional determinant of the phasic insulin response. According to some viewpoints, an immediately releasable pool of granules is responsible for first phase insulin release (Daniel et al. 1999), while the second phase involves the translocation of new granules to the plasma membrane (see the reviews cited above).

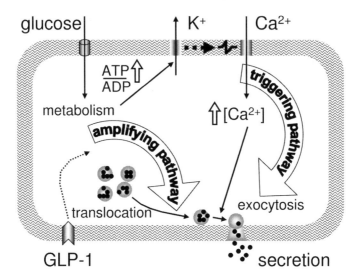

Figure 2.3 Simplified representation of the β cell. In the triggering pathway, glucose metabolism, which depends on glucose influx through the glucose transporters, modulates the ATP/ADP ratio, which increases (block arrow) when glucose concentration and metabolism increase. The increase in the ATP/ADP ratio closes the ATP-sensitive potassium channels; the closure of these channels produces a membrane depolarisation that opens the voltage-dependent calcium channels. Opening of the calcium channels increases the calcium influx and the cytosolic calcium concentration, which triggers exocytosis of the insulin granules that are ready for release. The amplifying pathway, which encompasses complex and incompletely understood phenomena depicted here very schematically, is responsible for increases in insulin secretion independent of changes in cytosolic calcium concentration. This pathway is also activated by glucose metabolism. The incretin hormones (GLP-1 in the figure) are thought to interact with the amplifying pathway to augment insulin secretion. Another key phenomenon in insulin release is the translocation of granules from pools inside the cell to the plasma membrane, as only granules in a particular state on the plasma membrane can be released by calcium-mediated exocytosis.

β-cell function tests

Intravenous vs. oral tests

An important distinction should be made between intravenous and oral β-cell function tests. In fact, ingestion of glucose stimulates the entero-insular axis, i.e. a complex hormonal and neural response that markedly potentiates insulin secretion (Figure 2.2D) (Unger & Eisentraut 1969; Fehmann et al. 1995; Creutzfeldt 2001). The magnitude of the potentiation response depends not only on the degree of neural activation and secretion of gut incretin hormones but also on intrinsic β-cell function, as incretin hormones bind to specific β-cell receptors and activate signalling for secretion (Figure 2.3). Thus, oral tests give a more comprehensive assessment of β-cell function, but they cannot distinguish the intrinsic β-cell defects from those of the entero-insular axis (e.g. a defective GLP-1 production or impaired neural stimulation). In addition, with oral tests the secretory stimulus (e.g. glucose concentration) cannot be standardised, and thus assessment of β-cell function requires appropriate methods for normalisation of insulin secretion to the stimulus.

Intravenous glucose tolerance test (IVGTT)

The IVGTT is the typical test for first phase insulin secretion, although a second phase is also present. For first phase assessment, a 10-min IVGTT is sufficient. However, the IVGTT is often also used to evaluate insulin sensitivity with the minimal model and possibly second phase secretion. Here the test format for the minimal model, which is the most widely used, will be described. More details can be found in Chapter 3.

The IVGTT minimal model protocol (Figure 2.4) is as follows: 1) a standardised glucose bolus (0.3 g/kg body weight) is injected after a baseline control period of about 20–30 min; 2) glucose, insulin and often C-peptide concentrations are measured at frequent intervals (12–30 samples) for 3–4 h. Frequent samples (at 1–2 min intervals) are collected in the initial 8–10 min for first phase assessment; 3) the typical first phase secretion index is the *acute insulin response* (AIR), i.e. the average incremental insulin concentration obtained in the first 5–10 min of the test; 4) second phase insulin secretion is calculated using empirical indices, usually computed from the areas under the insulin and glucose concentration curves, or by modeling (Toffolo et al. 1980; Toffolo et al. 1995; Toffolo et al. 1999), using both insulin and C-peptide; 5) In the insulin-modified IVGTT (shown in Figure 2.4), used to improve the minimal model insulin sensitivity estimate, a standardised insulin dose (0.03–0.05 U/kg) is administered 20 min after the glucose bolus. Exogenous insulin obviously masks the endogenous insulin response. However, if C-peptide concentration is measured, the second phase can be still determined (Toffolo et al. 1999) (with the proviso that exogenous insulin may interfere with endogenous secretion).

The IVGTT, together with the hyperglycaemic clamp, is the typical test for first phase insulin secretion, and AIR is the most widely used index. Assessment of second phase secretion is on the other hand made difficult by the necessity of accounting for glucose levels, which may vary considerably. Compared to AIR, the empirical and the model-based indices of second phase secretion have received limited attention. First phase insulin release depends on the amplitude of the glucose increment after the bolus. However, as the glucose dose is standardised, it is reputed that AIR does not require normalisation to the glucose peak. On the other hand, in normal subjects AIR is dependent on insulin sensitivity (Figure 2.2F). Thus, AIR per se may not be a good index of β-cell function, i.e. comparison of AIR in populations with different insulin sensitivity may lead to inappropriate conclusions. This important problem is discussed in a later section.

One drawback of the IVGTT is that first phase insulin secretion, though important, is only one of the modes of response of the β cell, and is thus insufficient to characterise β-cell function satisfactorily. As known since long time (Seltzer et al. 1967) and re-emphasized recently (Ferrannini & Mari 2004), diabetic subjects may totally lack first phase secretion but still respond to an OGTT.

First phase secretion quite likely represents the discharge of a pool of immediately releasable insulin granules through the activation of the triggering pathway (Daniel et al. 1999; Rorsman et al. 2000; Straub & Sharp 2002). As the magnitude of this pool depends on a complex equilibrium between exocytosis and refilling from a precursor pool, in which several cellular processes are involved, an observed defect of first phase insulin release may result from quite different causes. Therefore, while there is ample evidence that

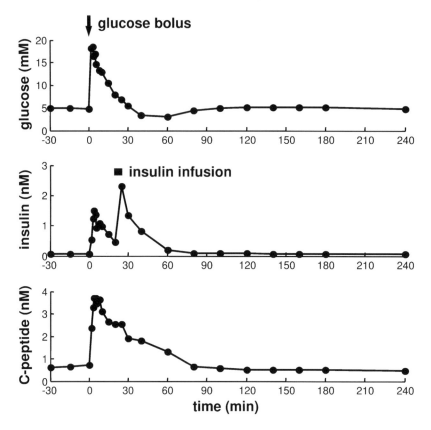

Figure 2.4 Illustration of the IVGTT protocol. The figure shows the insulin-modified frequently sampled IVGTT (23 samples), which is currently in use for assessing both insulin sensitivity (with the minimal model) and secretion. A 0.3 g/kg body weight glucose bolus is given at time 0, and a five-minute insulin infusion (0.03 U/kg) is administered after between 20 and 25 min. The regular IVGTT protocol is similar but does not include insulin infusion. Shorter and less frequently sampled protocols can be employed, in particular if only first phase secretion is needed. Measurement of C-peptide is optional, but allows calculation of insulin secretion by deconvolution during the whole test, avoiding the confounding effect of exogenous insulin (see Figure 2.1). Individual data from Mari (1998).

first phase secretion is a sensitive marker of β-cell function, impairment of this function may not be a primary β-cell defect (Mari 2006).

Hyperglycaemic glucose clamp

The hyperglycaemic glucose clamp (DeFronzo et al. 1979) assesses both first and second phase secretion. The protocol is as follows (see Figure 2.5): 1) after an initial baseline control period, an intravenous priming dose of glucose, followed by a variable glucose infusion, is administered to sharply raise glucose concentration to the desired hyperglycaemic value; 2) to keep glucose concentration constant in the successive period, glucose infusion rate is frequently adjusted based on quick bedside measurement of glucose concentration, similarly to the euglycemic clamp (see Chapter 4). An approximate equilibrium is reached after about

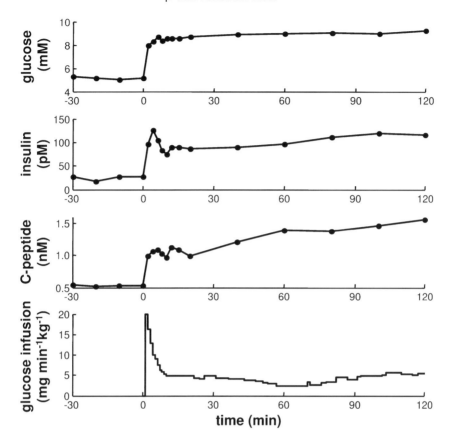

Figure 2.5 Illustration of the hyperglycaemic clamp protocol. A 4 mM step in glucose concentration (top panel) is generated by a primed glucose infusion (bottom panel), as described by DeFronzo et al. (1979). The priming is performed by increasing the glucose infusion rate in the initial 10 min (bottom panel). The glucose infusion rate is frequently adjusted based on quick bedside glucose concentration measurements to keep glucose constant. The typical biphasic insulin response is visible in the second panel. Individual data from Natali et al. (1998).

two hours; 3) glucose and insulin (and possibly C-peptide) are sampled in the basal period, frequently in the initial 8–10 min to assess first phase secretion, and successively during the final steady-state period to evaluate the second phase; 4) the secretory response can be evaluated from insulin concentration, using C-peptide deconvolution and also by modeling (Bonadonna et al. 2003). Several indices of first and second phase secretion can be calculated (e.g. AIR, absolute and incremental insulin or secretion values during the second phase); 5) because insulin secretion is available at two glucose levels (basal and hyperglycaemic), the test yields two points of the β-cell dose-response relating insulin secretion to glucose concentration; 6) diabetic subjects are usually not brought to euglycaemia by infusing insulin before the hyperglycaemic clamp is started, as typically done with the euglycemic clamp for insulin sensitivity, as this would confound the endogenous insulin response. Thus, the hyperglycaemic clamp typically evaluates the insulin secretion increment at a fixed glucose concentration increment, rather than absolute insulin secretion at standardised glucose levels (as is done with the graded glucose infusion test, discussed below).

The hyperglycaemic glucose clamp, though cumbersome, is the typical test for both first and second phase secretion. Because glucose levels are standardised, the hyperglycaemic clamp is a test of β-cell function, though comparison between subjects with different glucose levels (e.g. normal and diabetic subjects) may not be possible.

The hyperglycaemic clamp index of first phase secretion is similar to that obtained with the IVGTT and shares the same physiological interpretation. In contrast to the first phase, which is mainly dependent on the activation of the triggering pathway, the second phase response depends on the activation of the amplifying pathway (Figure 2.3).

Graded glucose infusion test

The graded glucose infusion test (Byrne et al. 1995) is an experimental determination of the β-cell dose-response relating insulin secretion to glucose concentration (Figure 2.2A and B). The procedure is as follows: 1) after a basal control period, glucose is infused in multiple 40-min steps at progressively increasing rates, so that glucose levels increase gradually (Figure 2.2A); 2) glucose and C-peptide concentrations are measured and insulin secretion is calculated by deconvolution; 3) the mean insulin secretion values at the end of each step are plotted against the corresponding mean glucose levels, thus obtaining an individual β-cell dose-response (Figure 2.2B); 4) to determine insulin secretion at glucose values below baseline, and in particular to test diabetic subjects at glucose concentrations comparable to normal fasting glucose values, glucose is lowered by an insulin bolus or infusion before the start of the graded glucose infusion. Because insulin secretion is computed from C-peptide, insulin infusion does not interfere with the calculations. Thus, the β-cell dose-response can be determined at standardised glucose levels in both normal and diabetic subjects.

The graded infusion test, though cumbersome (almost six hours), is a direct and standardised evaluation of the β-cell dose-response. The dose-response is an essential feature of the β cell, also observable at a cellular level (Henquin 2000), and clearly characterises the β-cell function impairment in various pathophysiological states (e.g. Byrne et al. 1996). As for second phase secretion from the hyperglycaemic clamp, the dose-response obtained with this test is in relation with the activation of the amplifying pathway (Figure 2.3). The graded infusion test does not assess first phase secretion.

Arginine tests

The injection of arginine produces a large burst in insulin secretion that is reputed to represent a form of maximal first phase insulin release. The secretory response to arginine is dependent on the prevailing glucose levels and is usually stronger than that elicited by glucose injection such as in the IVGTT. The basic arginine test requires measurement of insulin (and possibly C-peptide) concentration before the arginine injection and successively for about 10 min. The study protocol is similar to that employed with the IVGTT, with injection of arginine instead of glucose and about 10-min sampling. The secretory response is typically expressed as the mean incremental insulin (or C-peptide) level after arginine injection, similarly to the IVGTT AIR.

An important variant of the basic arginine test involves multiple injections of arginine at different glucose levels (Ward et al. 1984) (Figure 2.2E). The rationale of this approach is that exposure to hyperglycaemia for a short time potentiates the insulin response to arginine and the magnitude of the potentiation effect, in addition to the absolute response to arginine, is an index of β-cell function. An outline of this quite complex experimental test is the following (see Ward et al. 1984 for details): 1) arginine is injected in basal conditions and the response analysed as described above; 2) glucose is infused at a variable rate for about 30 min to raise glucose concentration to a fixed level (similarly to a hyperglycaemic clamp) and a second arginine bolus is given. The same procedure is repeated at multiple glucose levels. The maximal response to arginine is obtained at a glucose level of about 30 mmol/l; 3) a dose-response, relating the glucose levels at which arginine is injected and the corresponding secretory responses, is constructed (Figure 2.6). Beside the absolute responses, an index of β-cell function is the slope of this dose-response, evaluated between the first two glucose levels (classically denoted as *glucose potentiation slope*); 4) to study the arginine response in diabetic subjects at the same glucose levels as normal subjects, insulin is infused before the test to lower glucose concentration. Arginine activates the triggering pathway, though with mechanisms different from glucose (Smith et al. 1997; Henquin 2000). In comparison to the IVGTT, the arginine test releases a larger pool of insulin granules – the physiological significance of this is unclear – and elicits a first phase response in diabetic subjects.

The arginine test at multiple glucose levels is unique in its investigation of the potentiating effects of hyperglycaemia and their impairment. No other test for exploring this β-cell function has received a similarly wide application. Despite how interesting this mode of response of the β cell is, however, the complexity of the test is a serious drawback.

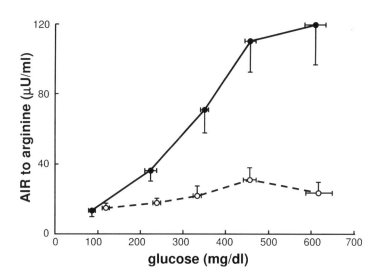

Figure 2.6 Dose-response relating the pre-arginine injection glucose levels and the acute insulin response to arginine (AIR, mean incremental insulin levels after injection). The glucose potentiation slope is the initial slope of the curves. The solid line is the dose-response in normal subjects; the broken line is that in type 2 diabetic subjects. Redrawn from Ward et al. (1984).

OGTT and meal tests

The OGTT methods are based on a standard 75 g OGTT and on measurement of glucose, insulin and possibly C-peptide in a variable number of blood samples, usually five or more, collected over 2–3 h (see e.g. Reinauer et al. 2003, available online at http://www.who.int/bookorders/anglais/catalog1.jsp?sesslan=1 (web search keywords: reinauer,site:www.who.int), for details on the protocol). A typical sampling schedule is 0 (pre-load), 30, 60, 90 and 120 min post glucose load. A standardised mixed meal is often used in place of the OGTT, with the same purpose and similar characteristics.

With the OGTT and meal tests, insulin concentration or secretion must be normalised to the prevailing glucose levels, which are clearly not standardised. This is achieved using empirical indices or modeling methods. The empirical indices are typically ratios between insulin and glucose levels. Perhaps the most widely used formula is the so-called *insulinogenic index*, calculated as the ratio between the supra-basal increments at 30 min of insulin and glucose concentration (see e.g. Pacini & Mari 2003). Similar indices based on the areas under the concentration curves have also been proposed. A recent alternative approach uses empirical formulas to provide estimates of the first and second phase insulin secretion as calculated using a hyperglycaemic clamp (Stumvoll et al. 2000, 2001). These formulas have been derived from a regression analysis of the OGTT indices against the hyperglycaemic clamp.

The modeling methods, discussed in the following section, have the conceptual advantage of being based on an explicit mathematical representation of the dynamic relationship between glucose concentration and insulin secretion. They provide an estimate of the β-cell dose-response relating insulin secretion to glucose concentration during the oral test. Some models also provide a parameter quantifying early insulin release during the oral test (Breda et al. 2001; Cretti et al. 2001; Mari et al. 2002a, 2002b), reputed to be a marker of first phase secretion. This parameter, however, may have limited reliability (Mari et al. 2002a; Steil et al. 2004). One model provides a potentiation parameter (Mari et al. 2002a, 2002b).

The OGTT and meal tests elicit a complex β-cell response. Not only the triggering and amplifying pathways involved in the intravenous tests are activated, but also the pathways stimulated by the activation of the entero-insular axis, such as the GLP-1 receptor signalling (Figure 2.3). Thus, oral tests give a more complete assessment of β-cell function. However, the relative roles of the various mechanisms involved in the response cannot be evaluated.

HOMA

As with the HOMA method for insulin resistance (see Chapter 3), the calculation of the HOMA β-cell function index (HOMA-B) requires only fasting glucose and insulin measurements. A model-based version of the method (HOMA2, http://www.dtu.ox.ac.uk/homa/ (web search keywords: homa calculator,site:dtu.ox.ac.uk) is recommended, although a formula is also available: HOMA-B = constant X fasting insulin/(fasting glucose − 3.5) (Matthews et al. 1985). The advantages of the HOMA2 computer index have not been demonstrated (Mari 2006).

HOMA-B is an empirical index that does not represent a specific β-cell characteristic. Its performance in comparison to the hyperglycaemic clamp is mediocre (Hanson et al. 2000). HOMA-B, being proportional to fasting insulin, is expected to be inversely related to insulin sensitivity in normotolerant subjects, as is AIR (see below). Thus adjustment for insulin sensitivity is necessary, but if only fasting measurements are available, the correction cannot be made (Mari et al. 2005a).

Modelling methods

Modeling methods deserve specific attention because they are often used not only with tests in which the glucose levels cannot be controlled, such as the OGTT, but also in standardised tests such as the IVGTT or the hyperglycaemic clamp. Furthermore, β-cell models have had an important historical role in the understanding of β-cell function (Bergman & Urquhart 1971; Grodsky 1972; Licko 1973; Cerasi et al. 1974). See Mari (2002) for a more comprehensive review. This section discusses only models used to determine β-cell function parameters; models for simple insulin secretion are discussed in previous reviews (Pacini 1994; Mari 2002).

The models currently used for β-cell function assessment are simplifications tailored for the clinical tests of historical β-cell models. Figure 2.7A shows the common paradigm of these models, which is based on the C-peptide methodology discussed previously. The leftmost block represents the β-cell model, which is a mathematical representation of the dynamic relationship between glucose concentration (the input to the model block) and insulin secretion (the output). The β-cell model contains parameters representing specific β-cell characteristics, such as the dose-response (see below). The β-cell model is coupled to a model of C-peptide kinetics (the rightmost block), which describes the dynamic relationship between insulin secretion and C-peptide concentration. The C-peptide model is assumed to be known, the typical model being that used for simple deconvolution (Van Cauter et al. 1992). Thus, the two blocks represent the dynamic relationship between glucose and C-peptide concentration, which are both measured variables. C-peptide concentration depends on glucose concentration (the input function) and on the parameters of the β-cell model. Once glucose and C-peptide concentration are obtained from a test, the β-cell model parameters are estimated by fitting the model to the data.

The most frequently used β-cell model variants have the structure depicted in Figures 2.7B and C. A common feature is the β-cell dose-response, which is the model estimate of the dose-response that can be obtained with the graded glucose infusion test (with the proviso that intravenous and oral tests do not yield the same dose-response). Some models include additional secretion components. In particular, some models provide parameters describing the anticipation of insulin release related to the first phase mechanisms (Breda et al. 2001; Cretti et al. 2001; Mari et al. 2002a, 2002b) (Figures 2.7B and C). These models, however, describe differently other aspects of the dynamic relationship between glucose concentration and insulin secretion, i.e. they include a delay between glucose concentration and secretion (Breda et al. 2001; Cretti et al. 2001) (Figure 2.7B) or a factor accounting for potentiation phenomena (Mari et al. 2002a, 2002b) (Figure 2.7C). See Mari (2002) and Ferrannini & Mari (2004) for a more comprehensive discussion.

The modeling methods are a valuable tool for interpreting tests that do not have standard-ised glucose levels, such as the oral tests, as they are based on a physiological representation of the β cell, though simplified. At least in principle, modeling approaches are preferable to empirical ones, in which normalisation to the glucose levels is not based on physio-logical principles. In addition, some models provide multiple parameters, with which a more complete characterisation of β-cell function can be achieved (Breda et al. 2001; Mari

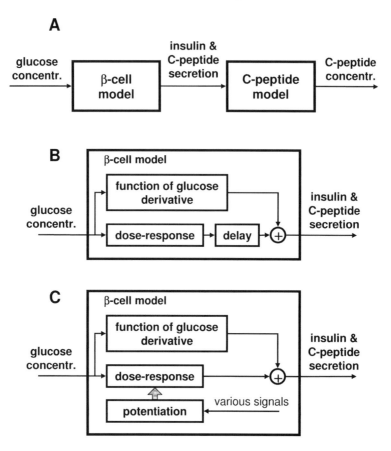

Figure 2.7 Illustration of modeling methods: A) the combination of a β-cell model (containing β-cell function parameters to be estimated) and a model of C-peptide kinetics (assumed to be known) provides a mathematical relationship between observed glucose and C-peptide concentrations. This mathematical relationship is used to estimate the β-cell function parameters from glucose and C-peptide data; B) β-cell model incorporating a dose-response, a description of the anticipation of insulin release related to the first phase mechanisms and a delay between glucose concentration and insulin secretion (Breda et al. 2001; Cretti et al. 2001). The model (Hovorka et al. 1998) has a similar structure but includes only the dose-response; C) β-cell model incorporating a dose-response, a description of the anticipation of insulin release related to the first phase mechanisms and a description of potentiation phenomena that modulate the dose-response (Mari et al. 2002a, 2002b).

et al. 2002a, 2002b). But the practical application of these methods requires specialised software and expertise.

β-cell function and insulin sensitivity

It is an old observation that β-cell function adapts to insulin resistance in order to maintain glucose tolerance normal (see Kahn 2003; Ahrén & Pacini 2004; Mari et al. 2005a for reviews). This observation led to the concept that β-cell function cannot be correctly assessed unless insulin sensitivity is also measured and the β-cell function parameters are adjusted for the degree of insulin resistance. Failure to account for insulin resistance may produce false results, as well illustrated in Bergman et al. (2002).

The most widely used approach to account for insulin resistance is the so-called *disposition index*, derived from the use of the IVGTT and the minimal model for insulin sensitivity. According to this approach, the index of β-cell function corrected for insulin sensitivity (the disposition index) is the product of AIR and the index of insulin sensitivity S_I.

The disposition index approach rests on the assumption that the β-cell adaptation to insulin resistance follows precisely a hyperbolic law. If β and σ denote the β-cell function and insulin sensitivity indices respectively, it is assumed that in a normal subject $\beta = k/\sigma$, where k is a constant for that individual. Thus, while β differs in different states of insulin resistance (because of β-cell adaptation), $\beta\sigma$, i.e. the disposition index, is a β-cell function index that does not change if the subject's insulin sensitivity changes. Quantitative support for this tenet has come from the analysis of the relationship between the acute insulin response in an IVGTT and the minimal model insulin sensitivity index S_I (Kahn et al. 1993) (Figure 2.2F).

This correct principle has however been subject to abuse, particularly because it has been applied indiscriminately to all β-cell function and insulin sensitivity indices without previous testing of the appropriateness of the assumptions. To ensure that this principle is correctly applied (see Mari et al. 2005a for more details) it is necessary that: 1) the insulin sensitivity and β-cell function tests yield indices that are substantially independent, i.e. are not intrinsically correlated. The HOMA indices are intrinsically dependent, but so also may be the indices resulting from the use of the hyperglycaemic clamp for assessment of second phase secretion and insulin sensitivity; 2) it must be verified that there is a relationship between the specific β-cell function and insulin sensitivity indices in a population of control subjects, because otherwise correction for insulin resistance is unjustified; 3) it must be verified that the relationship is precisely the hyperbola of equation $\beta = k/\sigma$; otherwise the disposition index calculated as the simple product is not valid. If the relationship is not a hyperbola, alternative formulations can be used (see Mari et al. 2005a for discussion); 4) caution should be used in the interpretation of the relationships between the disposition index and other physiological variables, as these may reflect relationships with insulin sensitivity, a component of the disposition index, rather than with β-cell function.

Comparative evaluation of methods

In contrast to the assessment of insulin sensitivity – for which the euglycemic hyperinsulinemic glucose clamp is commonly reputed the gold standard – for the evaluation of β-cell function no true gold standard exists. This is due to the complexity of β-cell response, which cannot be disclosed by a single test. In addition, the most informative tests are considerably complex and thus have limited applicability. Table 2.1 summarises the characteristics of the tests illustrated in this chapter, while Table 2.2 gives some general suggestions for their practical realisation.

Intravenous standardised tests have the advantage that they do not need normalisation of the secretory response to a variable stimulus, as do the oral tests, which may be difficult or imprecise. Among the intravenous tests, the hyperglycaemic clamp is possibly the most convenient compromise between experimental complexity and accuracy of outcome. The graded glucose infusion test gives a better assessment of the β-cell dose-response, but is

Table 2.1 Summary of Tests' Characteristics

test	β-cell function characteristics tested	specific equipment	insulin sensitivity[1]	C-peptide[2]	complexity[3]
IVGTT	first phase; empirical second phase indices; some index of the β-cell dose-response by modeling	infusion pump[4], modeling software[5]	yes	optional	+ + +[6]
Hyperglycaemic clamp	first and second phase indices	infusion pump, glucose analyser for bedside measurement	yes	optional	+ + + +
Graded glucose infusion test	β-cell dose-response	infusion pump	no	necessary	+ + + + +
Arginine, basic	'maximal' insulin response		no	optional	+ +
Arginine, glucose potentiation	'maximal' insulin response, potentiation of the insulin response with exposure to hyperglycaemia	infusion pump	no	optional	+ + + + +
OGTT + empirical indices	empirical β-cell function indices (typically the insulinogenic index); surrogate first and second phase indices		yes	optional	+ +
OGTT + modeling	first phase marker, β-cell dose-response, potentiation parameters	modeling software	yes	necessary	+ + +
HOMA	empirical β-cell function index		yes	optional	+

1. See Chapter 3 for a discussion of the indices.
2. Tests requiring C-peptide also require software for deconvolution. C-peptide deconvolution can be used with all tests.
3. Complexity ranking is somewhat subjective (+ = simplest; + + + + + = most complex).
4. The infusion pump is used for insulin infusion in insulin-modified IVGTT.
5. Modeling software to calculate additional β-cell function indices is optional.
6. The IVGTT complexity depends remarkably on the specific protocol used and on the data analysis procedures.

Table 2.2 Practical Considerations

- Select test considering:

  o Desired β-cell function indices;

  o Test complexity;

  o Availability of laboratory equipment and software for data analysis;

  o Possibility of also assessing insulin sensitivity.

- Use intravenous standardised tests if appropriate normalisation to glucose levels is difficult.

- Keep in mind that very simplified tests have limited reliability.

- Verify on the original references the protocol details, dosages and sampling schedule before planning experiments. Strict observance of the protocol is important for test quality.

- Use reliable insulin (and C-peptide) assays and perform measurements accurately.

- Use C-peptide to calculate insulin secretion by deconvolution when possible.

- If the test is used to compare groups, be sure that tests yield results that are comparable. For instance, hyperglycaemic clamps at different glucose levels are not comparable.

- Keep in mind that β-cell function may depend on insulin resistance. For instance, first phase secretion indices from the IVGTT cannot be compared if insulin sensitivity is different.

- Use caution with indices that express β-cell function in relation to insulin sensitivity (in particular with the disposition index). The assumptions under which these indices are valid must be verified.

experimentally very cumbersome. On the other hand, the IVGTT is only partially standardised: assessment of second phase secretion requires empirical or modeling procedures analogous to those of the oral tests.

Oral tests have the difficulty of requiring appropriate methods for normalisation of the secretory response to the stimulus. Empirical parameters, such as the insulinogenic index, do not have a clear physiological interpretation and sometimes exhibit outliers (very high or negative values). Modeling methods have the advantage of providing β-cell parameters with a better physiological basis and have proved to be quite effective for assessing the role of β-cell function in various pathophysiological states (e.g. Camastra et al. 2005; Ferrannini et al. 2005). In addition, with oral tests, in contrast to intravenous tests, β-cell function is evaluated in conditions that are closer to those of normal living. This has been of remarkable usefulness in the evaluation of drug efficacy (Mari et al. 2005b, 2005c). Thus, oral tests with modeling analysis are an interesting option to consider, although the practical difficulties of the modeling analysis may be an obstacle.

Oversimplified tests such as HOMA-B have a rather limited power and reliability. They should not be regarded as real option for β-cell function assessment when a study is designed, but rather as a last resort for the interpretation of already collected data. In this way, if the necessary caution is used in interpretation, such approaches may have some value.

A difficulty in the comparative evaluation of β-cell function tests is that our current understanding of the β cell is insufficient to envisage a single β-cell parameter (or a small number of indices) fully representative of the β-cell status. Although different β-cell function indices may be correlated, this is not necessarily always the case (Ferrannini & Mari 2004). Progress towards a better and simpler characterisation of β-cell function may be expected from our constant advancements in the understanding of the β cell. At present, however, assessment of β-cell function requires multiple indices, and thus is, in practice, inevitably incomplete and often approximate.

Conclusion

This review has shown that many methods for the assessment of β-cell function are available. The existence of several approaches is to a substantial extent dictated by the fact that the β-cell response is complex, and no single test is sufficient for a complete characterisation of β-cell function. Since every method has its inevitable limitations, the choice should be guided by a critical examination of test characteristics in relation to the investigator's needs and constraints. In addition, whatever approach is used, when the results are interpreted the nature and limitations of the test should be kept in mind in order to avoid overinterpretation. We hope that the present discussion has been helpful in achieving these goals.

References

Ahrén B, Pacini G (2004) Importance of quantifying insulin secretion in relation to insulin sensitivity to accurately assess beta cell function in clinical studies *Eur J Endocrinol* **150**, 97–104

Bergman RN, Ader M, Hücking K et al. (2002) Accurate assessment of beta-cell function: the hyperbolic correction *Diabetes* **51**, Suppl 1, S212–220

Bergman RN, Urquhart J (1971) The pilot gland approach to the study of insulin secretory dynamics *Recent Prog Horm Res* **27**, 583–605

Bonadonna RC, Stumvoll M, Fritsche A et al. (2003) Altered homeostatic adaptation of first- and second-phase beta-cell secretion in the offspring of patients with type 2 diabetes: studies with a minimal model to assess beta-cell function *Diabetes* **52**, 470–480

Bratanova-Tochkova TK, Cheng H, Daniel S et al. (2002) Triggering and augmentation mechanisms, granule pools, and biphasic insulin secretion *Diabetes* **51**, Suppl 1, S83–90

Breda E, Cavaghan MK, Toffolo G et al. (2001) Oral glucose tolerance test minimal model indexes of beta-cell function and insulin sensitivity *Diabetes* **50**, 150–158

Byrne MM, Sturis J, Polonsky KS (1995) Insulin secretion and clearance during low–dose graded glucose infusion *Am J Physiol* **268**, E21–E27

Byrne MM, Sturis J, Sobel RJ et al. (1996) Elevated plasma glucose 2 h postchallenge predicts defects in beta-cell function *Am J Physiol* **270**, E572–579

Camastra S, Manco M, Mari A et al. (2005) β-cell function in morbidly obese subjects during free living: long-term effects of weight loss *Diabetes* **54**, 2382–2389

Cerasi E (1981) Differential actions of glucose on insulin release: re-evaluation of a mathematical model In: Cobelli C, Bergman RN (Eds) *Carbohydrate Metabolism Quantitative Physiology and Mathematical Modelling*, Wiley, Chichester, pp. 3–22

Cerasi E, Fick G, Rudemo M (1974) A mathematical model for the glucose induced insulin release in man *Eur J Clin Invest* **4**, 267–278

Cretti A, Lehtovirta M, Bonora E et al. (2001) Assessment of beta-cell function during the oral glucose tolerance test by a minimal model of insulin secretion *Eur J Clin Invest* **31**, 405–416

Creutzfeldt, W (2001) The entero-insular axis in type 2 diabetes – incretins as therapeutic agents *Exp Clin Endocrinol Diabetes* **109** Suppl 2, S288–303

Daniel S, Noda M, Straub SG et al. (1999) Identification of the docked granule pool responsible for the first phase of glucose-stimulated insulin secretion *Diabetes* **48**, 1686–1690

DeFronzo RA, Ferrannini E, Keen H et al. (Eds) (2004) *International Textbook of Diabetes Mellitus*, Wiley, Chichester

DeFronzo RA, Tobin JD, Andres R (1979) Glucose clamp technique: a method for quantifying insulin secretion and resistance *Am J Physiol* **273**, E214–E223

Duckworth WC, Bennett RG, Hamel FG (1998) Insulin degradation: progress and potential *Endocr Rev* **19**, 608–624

Eaton RP, Allen RC, Schade DS et al. (1980) Prehepatic insulin production in man: kinetic analysis using peripheral connecting peptide behavior *J Clin Endocrinol Metab* **51**, 520–528

Fehmann HC, Goke R, Goke B (1995) Cell and molecular biology of the incretin hormones glucagon-like peptide-I and glucose-dependent insulin releasing polypeptide *Endocr Rev* **16**, 390–410

Ferrannini E, Gastaldelli A, Miyazaki Y et al. (2005) β-cell function in subjects spanning the range from normal glucose tolerance to overt diabetes: a new analysis *J Clin Endocrinol Metab* **90**, 493–500

Ferrannini E, Mari A (2004) Beta-cell function and its relation to insulin action in humans: a critical appraisal *Diabetologia* **47**, 943–956

Ferrannini E, Natali A, Bell P et al. (1997) Insulin resistance and hypersecretion in obesity European Group for the Study of Insulin Resistance (EGIR) *J Clin Invest* **100**, 1166–1173

Grodsky GM (1972) A threshold distribution hypothesis for packet storage of insulin and its mathematical modeling *J Clin Invest* **51**, 2047–2059

Hanson RL, Pratley RE, Bogardus C ct al. (2000) Evaluation of simple indices of insulin sensitivity and insulin secretion for use in epidemiologic studies *Am J Epidemiol* **151**, 190–198

Henquin JC (2000) Triggering and amplifying pathways of regulation of insulin secretion by glucose *Diabetes* **49**, 1751–1760

Henquin JC, Ishiyama N, Nenquin M et al. (2002) Signals and pools underlying biphasic insulin secretion *Diabetes* **51**, Suppl 1, S60–67

Hovorka R, Chassin L, Luzio SD et al. (1998) Pancreatic β-cell responsiveness during meal tolerance test: model assessment in normal subjects and subjects with newly diagnosed noninsulin-dependent diabetes mellitus *J Clin Endocrinol Metab* **83**, 744–750

Hovorka R, Jones RH (1994) How to measure insulin secretion *Diabetes Metab Rev* **10**, 91–117

Hovorka R, Soons PA, Young MA (1996) ISEC: a program to calculate insulin secretion *Comput Methods Programs Biomed* **50**, 253–264

Kahn SE (2003) The relative contributions of insulin resistance and beta-cell dysfunction to the pathophysiology of Type 2 diabetes *Diabetologia* **46**, 3–19

Kahn SE, Prigeon RL, McCulloch DK et al. (1993) Quantification of the relationship between insulin sensitivity and β-cell function in human subjects: evidence for a hyperbolic function *Diabetes* **42**, 1663–1672

LeRoith D, Taylor SI, Olefsky JM (Eds) (2004) *Diabetes Mellitus: a fundamental and clinical text*, Lippincott Williams & Wilkins, Philadelphia

Licko V (1973) Threshold secretory mechanism: a model of derivative element in biological control *Bull Math Biol* **35**, 51–58

Mari A (1998) Assessment of insulin sensitivity and secretion with the labeled intravenous glucose tolerance test: improved modeling analysis *Diabetologia* **41**, 1029–1039

Mari A (2002) Mathematical modeling in glucose metabolism and insulin secretion *Curr Opin Clin Nutr Metab Care* **5**, 495–501

Mari A (2006) Methods of assessment of insulin sensitivity and β-cell function *Immun Endoc & Metab Agents – Med Chem* **6**, 91–104

Mari A, Ahrén B, Pacini G (2005a) Assessment of insulin secretion in relation to insulin resistance *Curr Opin Clin Nutr Metab Care* **8**, 529–533

Mari A, Gastaldelli A, Foley JE et al. (2005b) Beta-cell function in mild type 2 diabetic patients: effects of 6-month glucose lowering with nateglinide *Diabetes Care* **28**, 1132–1138

Mari A, Sallas WM, He YL et al. (2005c) Vildagliptin, a dipeptidyl peptidase-IV inhibitor, improves model-assessed beta-cell function in patients with type 2 diabetes *J Clin Endocrinol Metab* **90**, 4888–4894

Mari A, Schmitz O, Gastaldelli A et al. (2002a) Meal and oral glucose tests for the assessment of β-cell function: modeling analysis in normal subjects *Am J Physiol Endocrinol Metab* **283**, E1159–E1166

Mari A, Tura A, Gastaldelli A et al. (2002b) Assessing insulin secretion by modeling in multiple–meal tests: role of potentiation *Diabetes* **51**, Suppl 1, S221–S226

Matthews DR, Hosker JP, Rudenski AS et al. (1985) Homeostasis model assessment: insulin resistance and β-cell function from fasting plasma glucose and insulin concentrations in man *Diabetologia* **28**, 412–419

Natali A, Gastaldelli A, Galvan AQ et al. (1998) Effects of acute alpha 2-blockade on insulin action and secretion in humans *Am J Physiol* **274**, E57–64

Nauck MA, Homberger E, Siegel EG et al. (1986) Incretin effects of increasing glucose loads in man calculated from venous insulin and C-peptide responses *J Clin Endocrinol Metab* **63**, 492–498

Pacini G (1994) Mathematical models of insulin secretion in physiological and clinical investigations *Comput Methods Programs Biomed* **41**, 269–285

Pacini G, Mari A (2003) Methods for clinical assessment of insulin sensitivity and beta-cell function *Best Pract Res Clin Endocrinol Metab* **17**, 305–322

Porte D, Sherwin RS, Baron A (Eds) (2003) *Ellenberg and Rifkin's Diabetes Mellitus*, McGraw-Hill, New York

Reinauer H, Home P, Kanagasabapathy A et al. (2003) Laboratory Diagnosis and Monitoring of Diabetes Mellitus WHO Department of Blood Safety & Clinical Technology

Rorsman P, Eliasson L, Renstrom E et al. (2000) The cell physiology of biphasic insulin secretion *News Physiol Sci* **15**, 72–77

Seltzer HS, Allen EW, Herron AL Jr et al. (1967) Insulin secretion in response to glycemic stimulus: relation of delayed initial release to carbohydrate intolerance in mild diabetes mellitus *J Clin Invest* **46**, 323–335

Smith PA, Sakura H, Coles B et al. (1997) Electrogenic arginine transport mediates stimulus-secretion coupling in mouse pancreatic beta-cells *J Physiol* **499**, 625–635

Steil GM, Hwu CM, Janowski R et al. (2004) Evaluation of insulin sensitivity and beta-cell function indexes obtained from minimal model analysis of a meal tolerance test *Diabetes* **53**, 1201–1207

Straub SG, Sharp GW (2002) Glucose-stimulated signaling pathways in biphasic insulin secretion *Diabetes Metab Res Rev* **18**, 451–463

Stumvoll M, Mitrakou A, Pimenta W et al. (2000) Use of the oral glucose tolerance test to assess insulin release and insulin sensitivity *Diabetes Care* **23**, 295–301

Stumvoll M, Van Haeften T, Fritsche A et al. (2001) Oral glucose tolerance test indexes for insulin sensitivity and secretion based on various availabilities of sampling times *Diabetes Care* **24**, 796–797

Toffolo G, Bergman RN, Finegood DT et al. (1980) Quantitative estimation of beta-cell sensitivity to glucose in the intact organism: a minimal model of insulin kinetics in the dog *Diabetes* **29**, 979–990

Toffolo G, Cefalu WT, Cobelli C (1999) Beta-cell function during insulin-modified intravenous glucose tolerance test successfully assessed by the C-peptide minimal model *Metabolism* **48**, 1162–1166

Toffolo G, De Grandi F, Cobelli C (1995) Estimation of beta-cell sensitivity from intravenuous glucose tolerance test C-peptide data *Diabetes* **44**, 845–854

Unger RH, Eisentraut AM (1969) Entero-insular axis *Arch Intern Med* **123**, 261–266

Van Cauter E, Mestrez F, Sturis J et al. (1992) Estimation of insulin secretion rates from C-peptide levels. Comparison of individual and standard kinetic parameters for C-peptide clearance *Diabetes* **41**, 368–377

Ward WK, Bolgiano DC, McKnight B et al. (1984) Diminished β-cell secretory capacity in patients with noninsulin-dependent diabetes mellitus *J Clin Invest* **74**, 1318–1328

3

Assessment of Insulin Sensitivity from Steady-State and Dynamic Tests

Giovanni Pacini and Andrea Mari

Introduction

Berson & Yalow (1970) defined insulin resistance as *'a state in which greater-than-normal amounts of insulin are required to elicit a quantitatively normal response'*. Several books cover all the biological, physiological and pathological aspects of impaired insulin action (e.g. Moller 1993, Reaven & Laws 1999, Krentz 2002, Porte et al. 2003, DeFronzo et al. 2004) and stress its possible role in the development of vascular diseases, which is the major clinical concern. Insulin resistance is also associated directly or indirectly with diabetes and a wide range of other diseases and may arise at any time during the course of life. A correct and reliable quantification of insulin resistance is clearly important for diagnosis, therapy, prognosis, monitoring of the follow-up and the evaluation of drugs.

Even if several factors influence insulin-mediated glucose uptake, such as lipid metabolism, ion transport, inflammatory processes, protein synthesis, endothelial function, gene transcription and so on, insulin remains the main regulator of glucose homeostasis. Thus the major processes controlled by insulin are the stimulation of glucose uptake, mainly by muscles and adipose tissue, and the inhibition of the hepatic glucose production. A schematic representation of the glucose-insulin system is shown in Figure 3.1. Measuring insulin sensitivity means assigning a value to the change of glucose disappearance from blood for a unit change of systemic insulin.

The glucose clamp is considered the gold standard for measuring insulin sensitivity. This technique is discussed in Chapter 4 and has been the subject of several excellent reviews (e.g. Bergman et al. 1985; Ferrannini & Mari 1998; DeFronzo et al. 2004). Direct measurements of uptake and production require the use of tracers (Wolfe 1992) (see Chapter 6). Here, we describe those tests that are simpler than the clamp and which can be performed more easily in a normal clinical setting and, for every test, the methods for its data analysis.

Clinical Diabetes Research: Methods and Techniques   Edited by Michael Roden
© 2007 John Wiley & Sons, Ltd   ISBN 978-0-470-01728-9

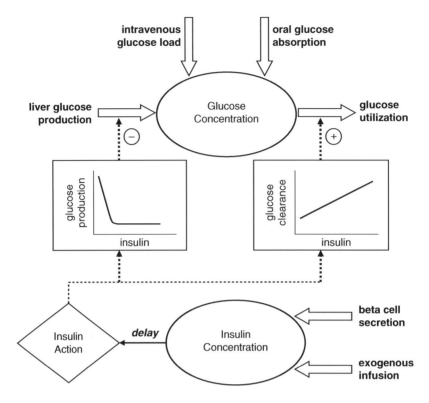

Figure 3.1 Schematic representation of the processes involved in glucose homeostasis. Input into the peripheral glucose space (where glucose measurements are performed) can occur from either intravenous injections (IVGTT, Clamp, IST) or oral load (OGTT) and endogenous glucose production (HOMA, QUICKI, IIT). Peripheral insulin (measured variable) either remains at its fasting level (HOMA, QUICKI) or changes because of exogenous infusion/injection (Clamp, ISI, IIT, insulin-modified-FSIGT) or for stimulated endogenous release (OGTT, IVGTT). Insulin action is delayed with respect to plasma concentration. Insulin increases peripheral glucose clearance and inhibits liver glucose output. Models for the assessment of insulin sensitivity (minimal model, OGIS, HOMA) consist of a mathematical representation of these processes with various assumptions and simplifications. All tests base the calculation of insulin sensitivity on evaluation of changes in glucose concentration in relation to peripheral insulin levels.

In the following sections, the test descriptions highlight specific protocol features. In addition to the specific test aspects, some general rules apply to all experimental settings. In particular, it is advisable that the subject maintains his/her usual lifestyle during the day(s) preceding the test, but with abstinence from alcohol and tobacco. If the experimental procedure is carried out in an outpatient setting, physical exercise should be avoided (no bicycling nor running to the place of the test) and it is prudent in any case to make the subject rest for some time before starting blood collection.

Insulin sensitivity from steady-state tests

When blood glucose levels are in dynamic equilibrium, the rate at which glucose is endogenously produced or exogenously administered is equal to the rate of glucose utilisation, mostly controlled by insulin. In basal conditions, glycaemia depends on the concomitant level of insulin. If glucose and insulin are exogenously given, glucose utilisation increases, production decreases and steady-state glucose is achieved after some time. The levels of glucose and insulin during this new steady-state and the glucose infusion rate reflect the ability of insulin to stimulate glucose uptake i.e. insulin sensitivity. Assessment of insulin sensitivity in steady-state conditions is based on this paradigm. The most common tests are the glucose clamp (described in Chapter 4) and the insulin suppression test. Surrogate measurements of insulin sensitivity can also be obtained in fasting conditions, without any external intervention.

Insulin sensitivity from fasting measurements

Rationale

Individual fasting plasma glucose level depends upon a controlled balance between hepatic glucose production (HGP) and glucose utilisation. The liver is responsible for providing 90 % of glucose in the fasting state (Eckberg et al. 1999), which is principally utilised (almost two-thirds) by non-insulin-dependent tissues, primarily the central nervous system (Baron et al. 1985). The insulin-dependent tissues utilising the remaining one-third are mostly skeletal muscles and the liver itself. Insulin therefore regulates HGP and glucose uptake to prevent hyper- or hypo-glycaemia. Elevated fasting levels of glucose or insulin are indicative of insulin resistance.

Protocol

Glucose and insulin concentrations are measured from one to three blood samples, usually collected every 10–15 min in the morning after 8–12-hour fasting.

Data analysis

The most common index of insulin resistance in the fasting state is that arising from the homeostasis model assessment formula (HOMA-R). This index is calculated as:

$$\text{HOMA-R} = \frac{G_b \times I_b}{k}$$

where G_b and I_b are basal glucose and insulin concentrations and k is a constant to scale HOMA-R so that it has the value of 1 (or 100 %) with mean normal basal glucose and insulin. For glucose in mmol/l and insulin in μU/ml, $k = 22.5$ (Matthews et al. 1985). k is sometimes omitted.

   HOMA derives from a mathematical model of the glucose-insulin homeostatic system (Levy et al. 1998) and the authors themselves advise using the modeling approach (HOMA2, http://www.dtu.ox.ac.uk./homa/) instead of the raw formula (Wallace et al. 2004), although no evidence has been provided of any clear advantages to using HOMA2 (Mari 2006).

   Another index of fasting insulin sensitivity is the quantitative insulin sensitivity check index, QUICKI (Katz et al. 2000), which is calculated as:

$$\text{QUICKI} = \frac{1}{\log G_b + \log I_b}$$

It is the reciprocal of the logarithm of HOMA calculated with $k = 1$. Therefore, the information obtained with the two indices is virtually the same.

Outcome

Since the liver is the primary organ responsible for maintaining basal glucose homeostasis, the sensitivity measured with basal glucose and insulin values is reputed to be a figure of *hepatic insulin resistance*.

Features and limitations

The agreement between HOMA-R and clamp-measured insulin sensitivity is controversial, ranging from very good to non-existing (Pacini & Mari 2003). HOMA-R and QUICKI are simplified predictors of insulin resistance and sensitivity; they are the only possible option when only fasting measurements are available.

HOMA-R represents insulin resistance, rather than sensitivity; the correlation with the clamp is inverse and curvilinear, thus it is usually linearised by logarithmic transformation of HOMA-R: i.e. 1/log(HOMA-R). QUICKI accomplishes this transformation.

Both indices may be markedly affected by errors in measurements, particularly if a single blood sample is used. Thus, they should preferably be used in studies involving a high number of subjects (e.g. epidemiological studies) where errors associated with a limited group should not pose particular problems.

Insulin sensitivity indices are often used in relation with other variables of interest, for example with insulin secretion, to determine the disposition index (see Chapter 2). Because HOMA is just the product of fasting glucose and insulin, it does not make any sense to use it to explore the relationship between fasting insulin, as a marker of insulin secretion, and insulin sensitivity, as is sometimes done (see comments in Mari et al. 2005c). Similarly HOMA may not be adequate to study the relationship between insulin sensitivity and other variables and in particular the role of insulin sensitivity in a disease in which hyperinsulinaemia itself is a factor in the pathology. Other extensive comments on the limits of fasting indices can be found in several reviews (Ferrannini & Mari 1998; Pacini & Mari 2003; Mari et al. 2005a, 2005c; Mari 2006).

Insulin Suppression Test (IST)

Rationale

This test exploits the effects of insulin on glucose disappearance when endogenous insulin is suppressed and standardised infusions of exogenous glucose and insulin are intravenously administered. Insulin levels are approximately the same in all subjects, while those of glucose vary: higher steady-state plasma glucose levels (SSPG, mg/dl or mmol/l) mean that the subject is more insulin resistant (Greenfield et al. 1981).

Protocol

The original IST protocol requires an injection of 5 mg propranolol, followed by concomitant infusions of epinephrine (6 μg/min), propranolol (80 μg/min), glucose (6 mg/min/kg) and insulin (80 mU/min). After 90 min, blood is sampled every 10 min for 1 h. More recently the use of somatostatin (5 μg/min) instead of epinephrine and propranolol, and different doses of glucose ($240 \, \text{mg/min/m}^2$) and insulin ($25 \, \text{mU/min/m}^2$) have been proposed (Jones et al. 1997).

Outcome

The inverse of SSPG is considered a measure of insulin sensitivity. If different glucose infusion rates are used, insulin sensitivity can be described by the glucose clearance, as infusion rate divided by SSPG.

Features and limitations

Giving glucose and insulin exogenously without beta-cell activity allows a good control of the system and the possibility of reaching desired levels. However, there are several problems with IST. One is the fact that it is unknown whether the given insulin dose completely suppresses HGP in intolerant and diabetic subjects. If HGP is not totally suppressed, SSPG is proportional to the remaining HGP and insulin resistance will be overestimated.

Elevated levels of SSPG for a long time may exceed the renal threshold (insulin independent) and so it is necessary to measure glucose in the urine to correct the sensitivity index. In some situations, for example highly sensitive subjects, SSPG is quite low. In this case the fasting level is sometimes subtracted by SSPG, since its contribution is not negligible and, being primarily determined by insulin independent glucose clearance, is a confounding factor for the sensitivity index. Other aspects of IST have been analysed in detail by Bergman et al. (1985) and Ferrannini & Mari (1998). Despite its limitations, this method is still used (Jones et al. 2000).

Insulin sensitivity from dynamic tests

After a glucose load and the consequent hyperglycaemia and hyperinsulinaemia, insulin-mediated glucose uptake plays a fundamental role in glucose disappearance. Sustained hyperglycaemia, lasting longer than in normal conditions, may be due to the lack of proper amount of insulin secretion or to an impaired action of the hormone (insulin resistance). To evaluate insulin sensitivity in dynamic conditions it is therefore necessary to perturb the glucose/insulin system by exogenously administering glucose or insulin and to relate glucose disappearance to insulin levels. The most common experimental procedures are the intravenous and oral glucose tolerance tests and the insulin tolerance test.

Intravenous Glucose Tolerance Test (IVGTT)

Rationale

With this test the equilibrium is perturbed with an exogenous bolus of glucose. The format of this test has evolved during the last 50 years; the original intravenous test was carried out for 30 to 60 min with sampling every 10–15 min (Amatuzio et al. 1953). Since the late seventies, the glucose dose has been standardised (0.3 g/kg body weight), the experiment extended to 3–4 hours and a more frequent sampling adopted (Bergman et al. 1981). These new tests are called FSIGT, frequently sampled intravenous glucose test. Further, to increase the dynamics of the experiment, additional infusions of tolbutamide (Beard et al. 1986) or insulin (Bergman 1989) can be given after 20 min following the glucose injection. These last types of test have been called modified-FSIGT, to distinguish them from the regular-FSIGT: i.e. that without additional infusions.

After the bolus injection, glucose concentration reaches elevated peak values (around 300 mg/dl for the standard dose of 0.3 g/kg) and then begins declining. Insulin, released in response to the glucose increase, accelerates the glucose decline to a rate depending upon the insulin level and its action. Therefore, the extent to which a given peripheral insulin concentration accelerates glucose disappearance is reflective of insulin sensitivity.

Protocol

Regular-FSIGT   After an overnight (8–12 hr) fast, a catheter is inserted into an antecubital vein for blood sampling and into a controlateral antecubital vein for glucose injection. Usually two basal samples are drawn, e.g. at ten and one minutes before glucose injection. At time 0, glucose (300 mg/kg) is injected over one minute, and then additional samples are collected according to specific protocols that vary among labs. A common sampling schedule is 3, 4, 5, 6, 8, 10, 14, 19, 22, 25, 27, 30, 40, 50, 60, 80, 100, 140, 180 min (Pacini et al. 1998), but other timetables have been carried out, as extensively reviewed by D.T. Finegood (1997). Samples after three hours, e.g. at 210 and 240 min, are advisable when there is the suspicion that subjects are severely resistant or glucose intolerant, as their glucose may not be back to pre-injection basal values by three hours.

Insulin-modified-FSIGT   Until the sample at 19 min, the protocol is the same as for the regular test. At 20 min, a non-primed infusion of insulin begins and lasts for 5 min, in the same vein as the glucose was injected into. Total amount of insulin given varies from 0.03 (in normotolerant subjects) to 0.05 U/kg (in impaired tolerance and type 2 diabetes; see below). The sampling schedule is similar to that of the regular test, though studies exist for a reduced number of samples (Steil et al. 1993). The insulin-modified-FSIGT is nowadays the reference test in any condition.

Data analysis

An index of intravenous glucose tolerance (K_G) was made popular by Lerner & Porte (1971) to quantify the rate of glucose disappearance after the mixing phase: i.e. when the injected glucose is assumed to be distributed homogeneously in its own distribution space. K_G is calculated from the linear regression over time as the slope of the log-transformed glucose concentration values from 10 until 40 min in the regular-FSIGT and until 19 min in the modified-FSIGT.

K_G quantifies glucose disappearance without accounting for insulin. In addition, it is calculated only during the early phase of the test, while the IVGTT comprises other parts where insulin still plays a very important role. For a more comprehensive figure of insulin action, it is necessary therefore to analyse the time course of glucose and insulin concentration during the whole test. This was achieved by describing the glucose-insulin dynamic relationship with a mathematical model, known as the minimal model (Bergman et al. 1979; Bergman et al. 1985; Pacini & Bergman 1986). This renowned model has two equations: one represents glucose disappearance after the glucose bolus, depending upon insulin in a compartment remote from plasma; the other equation describes the kinetics of insulin in the remote compartment. The analysis with the minimal model is used with both the regular and the insulin-modified FSIGT and yields the insulin sensitivity index, S_I. If glucose is measured in mg/dl and insulin in μU/ml, units of S_I are $\min^{-1}/(\mu U/ml)$, that is, a fractional glucose clearance per unit insulin concentration.

Outcome

Since muscle and adipose tissues are the primary organs responsible for returning glucose to pre-test values, S_I can be assumed to mainly represent a figure of the *peripheral insulin resistance* (Mari 1997).

Features and limitations

S_I obtained from both regular and insulin-modified tests has been thoroughly validated against the glucose clamp (Finegood 1997). The performance of the method is generally considered quite good, although some structural model defects have been demonstrated (Caumo et al. 1996; Mari 1997).

The first modified test used tolbutamide to boost endogenous insulin secretion (Yang et al. 1987). Given the difficulties of tolbutamide availability, the insulin-modified FSIGT was introduced, on the basis that endogenous and exogenous insulin elicit the same effects on glucose disappearance. The increment of the test dynamics allows a more precise estimation of S_I and use in subjects with insufficient insulin response, in whom the regular-FSIGT would not yield reliable parameter estimates: for example, negative S_I. In this regard, the correct choice of the insulin dose is important: 0.03 U/kg should be used when subjects are known already not to be very insulin resistant and there is the possibility of their reaching hypoglycaemic levels if a higher dose is used. In fact, if glucose falls below fasting levels following exogenous insulin administration, depending upon the hypoglycaemic level reached, counterregulatory response is stimulated (Vicini et al. 1999) and in this condition the estimation of S_I may not be completely reliable (Brehm et al. 2006). On the other hand, 0.05 U/kg is the advisable dose in subjects expected to be insulin resistant, such as obese, type 2, hypertensive and so forth. It is however wise to use the same dose in those groups that are to be compared (e.g., pathological *vs.* control subjects).

It is prudent to give exogenous insulin as a 5-min infusion instead of a bolus. The main reason is that with the bolus, very high levels of the hormone are reached with a likely saturation of all insulin receptors. Modeling analysis in this case may underestimate the insulin effect. In addition, the slower infusion allows a better distribution of the hormone. If a bolus injection is used, insulin measurements at 22 and 25 min should be taken with caution in the minimal model analysis, since mixing effects could still occur.

Steil et al. (1993) proposed a reduced sampling schedule comprising only 12 (instead of 20) samples at specific times, motivated mainly by the reduction of assay costs. This reduced schedule was developed for the tolbutamide-modified FSIGT, but it has been successfully applied to the insulin-modified test (Saad et al. 1994), although with a loss of precision of the S_I estimate of about 20 %. The reduced sampling is a cost-effective alternative when a large number of subjects is studied or when large differences in S_I are anticipated; however, the full schedule is still preferable when only a few subjects are investigated (Steil et al. 1994).

Even with simplified protocols, the FSIGT remains a far from simple test to perform: meticulous skill is required on the part of the operator(s) performing the necessary coordinated actions (glucose injection, insulin infusion, frequent sampling, patency of catheters), and the expert use of specific equipment (pumps) and computers is indispensable. For these reasons, it can only be used in medium size population samples.

A particular expertise is also essential for data analysis (Godsland & Walton 2001). In fact, the calculation of S_I is not immediate and requires the use of specific software, which can be implemented by describing the model and adding the proper routines for parameter estimation and differential equation integration (Pacini & Bergman 1986). Pre-compiled and easy-to-run versions are available either from R. Bergman (Physiology, Univ. Southern California, Los Angeles, USA), Boston et al. (2003) or at the website http://www.winsaam. com/products.htm.

The minimal model analysis of FSIGT data not only yields S_I, but also other parameters, which can be important for a wide characterisation of the glucose kinetics of a subject. In particular, parameter S_G, the glucose effectiveness (min^{-1}), describes the fractional clearance rate of glucose per se, without any change of dynamic insulin (Best et al. 1996; Pacini et al. 1998). Another parameter derived from the model is the glucose initial distribution volume (V_d, ml), calculated as the glucose dose divided by the estimated glucose intercept at zero-time (Bergman et al. 1987).

Because in the modified-FSIGT the insulin dose is known and the following insulin time course measured, it is possible to obtain a figure of insulin clearance (Gibaldi & Perrier 1982), often co-responsible for hyperinsulinaemia in particular categories of patients (Jones et al. 1997). During IVGTT a direct and immediate stimulation of pancreatic secretion of insulin occurs and can easily be quantified (see Chapter 2); therefore, from just one test, it is possible to obtain information on several of the major processes involved in glucose homeostasis.

Oral Glucose Tolerance Test (OGTT)

Rationale

With this test the equilibrium is perturbed with an oral glucose load. Glucose in blood rises during the first 60 min and, in normal conditions, is back to pre-load values after 2–3 hours. The rationale is similar to that of the IVGTT though in the case of oral load the rate of appearance of glucose in blood is unknown.

Protocol

After an overnight (8–12 hours) fast, a cannula is inserted in an antecubital vein for blood sampling. Basal samples are drawn (for instance at 5 and 2 min) before the oral load is administered, consisting of 75 g glucose (usually dextrose 50 %) diluted in water for a total volume of 300 ml drunk in 5 min. Venous samples are drawn, and again at specific time points for the following 2–3 hours. The sampling schedule depends upon the specific purpose. The OGTT is considered a diagnostic test and so only glucose measured at basal and 2 h sample is necessary (ADA Clinical Practice Recommendations). Of course, no other information is drawn with this limited protocol. In order to assess insulin sensitivity, it is necessary to sample more frequently. A common schedule is 0, 30, 60, 90, 120 min (Matsuda & DeFronzo 1999; Stumvoll et al. 2000).

Data analysis

Insulin sensitivity is calculated from glucose-insulin data using simple formulas programmable on a spreadsheet. Different approaches to developing the formulas (empirical or model-derived assumptions) characterise the various methods.

Here, we have only considered methods that have been validated against the clamp in a relatively large number of subjects. Other existing methods have been described and tested by Matsuda & DeFronzo (1999) and reviewed elsewhere by Pacini & Mari (2003) and Mari et al. (2005c).

Matsuda's Formula   This insulin sensitivity index, originally denoted as ISI_{comp} (Matsuda & DeFronzo 1999), is calculated as:

$$ISI_{comp} = \frac{10000}{\sqrt{G_b \cdot I_b \cdot Gm \cdot Im}}$$

where G_b and I_b are basal pre-load glucose and insulin, respectively, and Gm and Im the mean concentrations during the OGTT (used sampling protocol: 0, 30, 60, 90, 120 min). ISI_{comp} is a sort of 'super-QUICKI' that gives the glucose-insulin relationship in dynamic conditions.

Stumvoll's Method   This insulin sensitivity index, originally denoted as MCR_{est} (Stumvoll et al. 2000), is calculated as:

$$MCR_{est} = 18.8 - 0.27 \cdot BMI - 0.0052 \cdot I_{120} - 0.27 \cdot G_{90}$$

where BMI (kg/m^2) is body mass index, I_{120} insulin at 120 min (pmol/l) and G_{90} glucose at 90 min (mmol/l). This equation compares results with the last 60 min clamp-derived glucose clearance; MCR_{est} units are thus ml $min^{-1}kg^{-1}$. Alternative formulas without BMI or for different sampling times have been also provided (Stumvoll et al. 2000, 2001). The specific functional dependence of MCR_{est} on those particular concentrations and the numerical coefficients are purely empirical.

OGIS Model   This insulin sensitivity index, called OGIS (Mari et al. 2001), is obtained from a model-derived equation:

$$OGIS = f(G_b, G_{90}, G_{120}, I_b, I_{90}, D)$$

where G and I are glucose and insulin concentrations at the time indicated by the subscript and D is the oral glucose dose $(g/m^2$ body surface area). The function f is more complex than those above, but can easily be programmed on a spreadsheet or downloaded from http://www.isib.cnr.it/bioing/ogis/home.html. OGIS is a predictor of the clamp-derived glucose clearance normalised to body surface area; thus units are ml $min^{-1}m^{-2}$. Formulas for a 3 h OGTT are also available (Mari et al. 2001) at the same web address.

Outcome

OGTT is a relatively simple test (much simpler than FSIGT or glucose clamp). It activates the insulin-glucose homeostatic process and in principle provides information on dynamic insulin sensitivity.

Features and limitations

The above three OGTT methods are the most commonly used and have been validated against the glucose clamp in large cohorts of subjects characterised by different metabolic conditions. A recent comparative study (Mari et al. 2005c) with an independent data-base confirmed their good performance, although the methods differed when more severe tests were carried out. This study suggests that the model-based formula OGIS and MCR_{est} better represent genuine sensitivity. OGIS has also been used with a standard 475-kcal meal test after validation against the clamp (Mari et al. 2005b).

The formulas for ISI_{comp} and MCR_{est} are completely empirical, but OGIS also incorporates some empirical assumptions. In fact, OGIS exploits the known quantitative relationship between the observed data and the clamp insulin sensitivity to attempt a genuine prediction of the index. However, empirical assumptions are necessary because the rate of glucose appearance cannot be directly measured. This is the main problem with the OGTT indices and it cannot be easily overcome.

Another limitation of the OGTT is that the interpretation of the data is more uncertain than in the other tests. In fact, in addition to the unknown absorption, glucose production plays a more important role than in the IVGTT. The heterogeneous nature of the OGTT pattern, even within groups similar from a metabolic point of view, has been emphasised since shortly after the advent of insulin radioimmunoassay (Reaven & Miller 1968) and consequently particular attention must be placed on the interpretation of results arising from comparing subjects on the basis of parameters derived by the OGTT, when small differences are expected.

Nonetheless, all three methods are very simple, require a limited number of samples, do not need a specific mathematical expertise and can be implemented on a spreadsheet or with a pocket calculator. Since the 2 h sample is commonly analysed for diagnostic purposes, the OGTT is already widely used and the important metabolic information potentially obtainable should be worth the additional effort of collecting and measuring a few more samples. Finally, as reported in Chapter 2, the OGTT, when properly analysed, provides important information on insulin secretion.

Insulin Tolerance Test (ITT)

Rationale

With this test the equilibrium is perturbed with an exogenous insulin injection that provokes a fall in plasma glucose. The intravenous ITT allows the assessment of insulin sensitivity by determining the rate of glucose decay.

Protocol

In overnight fasted subjects, after collection of basal samples, regular insulin (0.1 U/kg) is rapidly injected and blood is sampled. Since glucose quickly decreases to hypoglycaemic levels, counterregulatory response may be induced; this slows glucose disappearance rate from plasma, creating a confounding factor. In fact, in such a case, the fall of glucose concentration depends both on insulin and stimulated counterregulatory hormones. The users of this test claim that the counterregulation occurs only after 15–20 min and therefore the protocol –5, 0, 3, 5, 7, 10 and 15 min has been proposed.

Data analysis and outcome

An insulin sensitivity index can be calculated either by the ratio $\Delta G/G_b$ (where G_b is fasting glycemia and ΔG the difference between G_b and glucose measured after 15 min), or by the glucose disposal rate (*Kitt*), calculated from the slope of the linear regression of the logarithm of blood glucose against time during the 15 min interval.

Features and limitations

Kitt has been validated against the glucose clamp (Bonora et al. 1989), and ITT is proposed as a simple method of quantifying insulin sensitivity, although the risk of hypoglycemia remains a potential difficulty. In fact, while ITT can be safely applied to both types of diabetes and in general to any insulin resistant subject, caution must be used with healthy insulin sensitive subjects, since the conventional insulin dose of 0.1 U/kg may result in symptomatic hypoglycemia. It has been suggested this problem can be overcome by adopting a lower (0.05 U/kg) dose of insulin (Gelding et al. 1994).

Conclusion

This chapter has described the most common, easily available methods of assessing insulin sensitivity both from steady-state and dynamic tests. The presented approaches are simpler than the gold standard glucose clamp and do not require complicated calculations, except for the minimal model which has nonetheless come to be routinely used. We tried to provide a quick reference manual for the performance of the tests and data analysis, highlighting both the advantages and the possible limitations. Table 3.1 summarises the characteristics of the tests illustrated in this chapter, while Table 3.2 gives some general suggestions for

Table 3.1 Summary of Tests' Characteristics

test	characteristics of the insulin sensitivity index	specific equipment/ pharmacological agents	β-cell function[1]	complexity[2]
HOMA	empirical index of fasting (liver) insulin resistance		yes	+
QUICKI	empirical index of fasting (liver) insulin sensitivity			+
Euglycemic clamp[3]	estimate of glucose uptake at fixed insulin levels	infusion pumps, glucose analyser for quick bedside measurement	no	++++
Hyperglycaemic clamp[3]	estimate of ratio of glucose uptake to prevailing insulin levels	infusion pumps, glucose analyser for quick bedside measurement	yes	++++
IST	estimate of glucose uptake at fixed insulin levels	infusion pumps/somatostatin	no	++++

Table 3.1   Continued

test	characteristics of the insulin sensitivity index	specific equipment/ pharmacological agents	β-cell function[1]	complexity[2]
IVGTT	estimate of fractional glucose clearance (mostly skeletal muscles and adipose tissues) normalised to insulin	infusion pump[4]; modeling software	yes	+++
OGTT	surrogate estimates of clamp insulin sensitivity	spreadsheet	yes	++
ITT	rate of glucose disappearance		no	+++

1. See Chapter 2 for a discussion of the indices.
2. Complexity ranking is somewhat subjective ($+$ = simplest; $++++$ = most complex).
3. See Chapter 4 for use, outcomes and limitations of these tests.
4. The infusion pump is used for insulin infusion in insulin-modified FSIGT.

Table 3.2   Practical Considerations

- Select test considering:

  o The reliability of the insulin sensitivity indices in the specific context of the study;

  o Test complexity;

  o Availability of laboratory equipment and software for data analysis;

  o Possibility of also assessing beta-cell function

- If the assessment of insulin sensitivity is critical for the study, the direct tests (1st choice: glucose clamp; 2nd choice: IVGTT) must be used.

- Keep in mind that very simplified tests have limited reliability.

- Verify on the original references the protocol details: check especially the doses of given substances and the sampling schedules before planning experiments. Strict observance of the protocol is important for test quality and reliability of results.

- Use the appropriate insulin dose with the insulin-modified-FSIGT.

- If the test is used to compare groups, be sure that tests yield results that are comparable. For instance, OGTT and FSIGT are not comparable.

their practical realisation. The final aim was to make the investigator consider the most appropriate test for his/her study, depending on the kind of research, the type of subjects, the available resources and the expected interpretation of the results.

References

Amatuzio DS, Stutzman FL, Vanderbilt MJ, Nesbitt S (1953) Interpretation of the rapid intravenous glucose tolerance test in normal individuals and in mild diabetes mellitus *J Clin Invest* **32**, 428–435

Baron AD, Kolterman OG, Bell J, Mandarino LJ, Olefsky JM (1985) Rates of noninsulin-mediated glucose uptake are elevated in type II diabetic subjects *J Clin Invest* **76**, 1782–1788

Beard JC, Bergman RN, Ward WK, Porte D Jr (1986) The insulin sensitivity index in nondiabetic man: Correlation between clamp-derived and IVGTT-derived values *Diabetes* **35**, 362–369

Bergman RN (1989) Toward physiological understanding of glucose tolerance: Minimal-model approach *Diabetes* **38**, 1512–1527

Bergman RN, Finegood DT, Ader M (1985) Assessment of insulin sensitivity in vivo *Endocrine Reviews* **6**, 45–86

Bergman RN, Ider YZ, Bowden CR, Cobelli C (1979) Quantitative estimation of insulin sensitivity *Am J Physiol Endocrinol Metab* **236**, E667–E677

Bergman RN, Phillips LS, Cobelli C (1981) Physiologic evaluation of factors controlling glucose tolerance in man *J Clin Invest* **68**, 1456–1467

Bergman RN, Prager R, Volund A, Olefsky JM (1987) Equivalence of the insulin sensitivity index in man derived by the minimal model method and the euglycemic glucose clamp *J Clin Invest* **79**, 790–800

Berson SA, Yalow RS (1970) Insulin 'antagonists' and insulin resistance In: M Ellenberg, H Rifkin (Eds) *Diabetes Mellitus: Theory and Practice*, McGraw-Hill, New York, pp 388–423

Best JD, Kahn SE, Ader M et al. (1996) Role of glucose effectiveness in the determination of glucose tolerance *Diabetes Care* **19**, 1018–1030

Bonora E, Moghetti P, Zancanaro C et al. (1989) Estimates of in vivo insulin action in man: comparison of insulin tolerance tests with euglycemic and hyperglycemic glucose clamp studies *J Clin Endocrinol Metab* **68**, 374–378

Boston RC, Stefanovski D, Moate PJ et al. (2003) MINMOD millennium: a computer program to calculate glucose effectiveness and insulin sensitivity from the frequently sampled intravenous glucose tolerance test *Diabetes Technol Ther* **5**, 1003–1015

Brehm A, Thomaseth K, Bernroider E et al. (2006) The role of endocrine counterregulation for estimating insulin sensitivity from intravenous glucose tolerance tests *J Clin Endrocrinol Metab* **91**, 2272–2278

Caumo A, Vicini P, Cobelli C (1996) Is the minimal model too minimal? *Diabetologia* **39**, 997–1000

DeFronzo RA, Ferrannini E, Keen H, Zimmet P (Eds) (2004) *International Textbook of Diabetes Mellitus*, Wiley, Chichester

Ekberg K, Landau BR, Wajngot A et al. (1999) Contributions by kidney and liver to glucose production in the postabsorptive state and after 60 h of fasting *Diabetes* **48**, 292–298

Ferrannini E, Mari A (1998) How to measure insulin sensitivity *J Hypertens* **16**, 895–906

Finegood DT (1997) Application of the minimal model of glucose kinetics In: RN Bergman, JC Lovejoy (Eds) *The Minimal Model Approach and Determinants of Glucose Tolerance*, Louisiana State Univ Press, Baton Rouge, LA, pp. 51–122

Gelding SV, Robinson S, Lowe S, Niththyananthan R, Johnston DG (1994) Validation of the low dose short insulin tolerance test for evaluation of insulin sensitivity *Clin Endocrinol (Oxf)* **40**, 611–615

Gibaldi M, Perrier D (1982) *Pharmacokinetics* (2 ed) Dekker, New York

Godsland IF, Walton C (2001) Maximizing the success rate of minimal model insulin sensitivity measurement in humans: the importance of basal glucose levels *Clin Sci (Lond)* **101**, 1–9

Greenfield MS, Doberne L, Kraemer F, Tobey T, Reaven G (1981) Assessment of insulin resistance with the insulin suppression test and the euglycemic clamp *Diabetes* **30**, 387–392

Jones CN, Abbasi F, Carantoni M, Polonsky KS, Reaven G (2000) Roles of insulin resistance and obesity in regulation of plasma insulin concentration *Am J Physiol Endocrinol Metab* **278**, E501–E508

Jones CN, Pei D, Staris P et al. (1997) Alterations in the glucose-stimulated insulin secretory dose-response curve and in insulin clearance in nondiabetic insulin-resistant individuals *J Clin Endocrinol Metab* **82**, 1834–1838

Katz A, Nambi SS, Mather K et al. (2000) Quantitative insulin sensitivity check index: a simple, accurate method for assessing insulin sensitivity in humans *J Clin Endocrinol Metab* **85**, 2402–2410

Krentz A (2002) *Insulin Resistance* Blackwell, Oxford

Lerner RL, Porte D Jr (1971) Relationship between intravenous glucose loads, insulin responses and glucose disappearance rate *J Clin Endocrinol Metab* **33**, 409–417

Levy JC, Matthews DR, Hermans MP (1998) Correct homeostasis model assessment (HOMA) evaluation uses the computer program *Diabetes Care* **21**, 2191–2192

Mari A (1997) Assessment of insulin sensitivity with minimal model: role of model assumptions *Am J Physiol Endocrinol Metab* **272**, E925–E934

Mari A (2006) Methods of assessment of insulin sensitivity and beta-cell function *Immun Endoc & Metab Agents-Med Chem* **6**, 91–104

Mari A, Ahrén B, Pacini G (2005a) Assessment of insulin secretion in relation to insulin resistance *Curr Opin Clin Nutr Metab Care* **8**, 529–533

Mari A, Gastaldelli A, Foley JE, Pratley RE, Ferrannini E (2005b) Beta-cell function in mild type 2 diabetic patients: effects of 6-month glucose lowering with nateglinide *Diabetes Care* **28**, 1132–1138

Mari A, Pacini G, Brazzale AR, Ahrén B (2005c) Comparative evaluation of simple insulin sensitivity methods based on the oral glucose tolerance test *Diabetologia* **48**, 748–751

Mari A, Pacini G, Murphy E, Ludvik B, Nolan JJ (2001) A model-based method for assessing insulin sensitivity from the oral glucose tolerance test *Diabetes Care* **24**, 539–548

Matsuda M, DeFronzo RA (1999) Insulin sensitivity indices obtained from oral glucose tolerance testing Comparison with the euglycemic insulin clamp *Diabetes Care* **22**, 1462–1470

Matthews DR, Hosker JP, Rudenski AS et al. (1985) Homeostasis model assessment: Insulin resistance and beta-cell function from fasting plasma glucose and insulin concentrations in man *Diabetologia* **28**, 412–419

Moller DE (Ed) (1993) *Insulin Resistance*, Wiley, Chichester

Pacini G, Bergman RN (1986) MINMOD: A computer program to calculate insulin sensitivity and pancreatic responsivity from frequently sampled IVGTT *Comp Methods Programs Biomed* **23**, 113–122

Pacini G, Mari A (2003) Methods for clinical assessment of insulin sensitivity and beta-cell function *Best Pract Res Clin Endocrinol Metab* **17**, 305–322

Pacini G, Tonolo G, Sambataro M et al. (1998) Insulin sensitivity and glucose effectiveness: minimal model analysis of regular and insulin-modified FSIGT *Am J Physiol Endocrinol Metab* **274**, E592–599

Porte D Jr, Sherwin RS, Baron A (Eds) (2003) *Ellenberg and Rifkin's Diabetes Mellitus,* McGraw-Hill, New York

Reaven G, Miller R (1968) Study of the relationship between glucose and insulin responses to an oral glucose load in man *Diabetes* **17**, 560–569

Reaven GM, Laws A (1999) *Insulin Resistance – The Metabolic Syndrome X* Humana Press, Totowa, NJ

Saad MF, Anderson RL, Laws A et al. (1994) A comparison between the minimal model and the glucose clamp in the assessment of insulin sensitivity across the spectrum of glucose tolerance Insulin Resistance Atherosclerosis Study *Diabetes* **43**, 1114–1121

Steil GM, Murray J, Bergman RN, Buchanan TA (1994) Repeatability of insulin sensitivity and glucose effectiveness from the minimal model Implications for study design *Diabetes* **43**, 1365–1371

Steil GM, Vølund A, Kahn SE, Bergman RN (1993) Reduced sample number for calculation of insulin sensitivity and glucose effectiveness from the minimal model Suitability for use in population studies *Diabetes* **42**, 250–256

Stumvoll M, Mitrakou A, Pimenta W et al. (2000) Use of the oral glucose tolerance test to assess insulin release and insulin sensitivity *Diabetes Care* **23**, 295–301

Stumvoll M, Van Haeften T, Fritsche A, Gerich J (2001) Oral glucose tolerance test indexes for insulin sensitivity and secretion based on various availabilities of sampling times *Diabetes Care* **24**, 796–797

Vicini P, Zachwieja JJ, Yarasheski KE et al. (1999) Glucose production during an IVGTT by decon-volution: Validation with the tracer-to-tracee clamp technique *Am J Physiol Endocrinol Metab* **276**, E285–E294

Wallace TM, Levy JC, Matthews DR (2004) Use and abuse of HOMA modeling *Diabetes Care* **27**, 1487–1495

Wolfe RR (1992) *Radioactive and Stable Isotope Tracers in Biomedicine* Wiley, New York

Yang YJ, Youn JH, Bergman RN (1987) Modified protocols improve insulin sensitivity estimation using the minimal model *Am J Physiol Endocrinol Metab* **253**, E595–E602

4

Glucose Clamp Techniques

Attila Brehm and Michael Roden

Introduction

Insulin sensitivity of glucose metabolism is crucial for the understanding of diseases such as diabetes mellitus and related metabolic disorders. In the last few decades, much of the understanding of diabetes mellitus in humans, particularly type 2 diabetes mellitus, has been derived from *in vivo* assessment of insulin sensitivity of glucose metabolism. And much of the insight into the hormonal regulation and pathophysiology of carbohydrate metabolism was generated by studies applying the glucose clamp technique (Andres et al. 1966; Sherwin et al. 1974; Insel et al. 1975; DeFronzo 1988; Cherrington 1999).

History of the *in vivo* assessment of insulin sensitivity

Early attempts to assess the *in vivo* effects of insulin on glucose metabolism analysed the glycaemic response to intravenous injection of insulin (Horgaard & Thayssen 1929). An attempt to standardise protocols for *in vivo* determination of insulin sensitivity was developed in the 1930s by Himsworth & Kerr (Himsworth 1936). These investigators recognised that lean patients with diabetes prone to ketoacidosis were more sensitive to exogenous insulin than obese nonketotic patients with diabetes (Himsworth 1936; Himsworth & Kerr 1939). However, due to the impossibility of quantifying plasma insulin concentrations in those days, the relevance of these findings was questioned. In 1960, the need for a specific tool for the quantification of plasma insulin concentrations was met by the development of a radio immunoassay for insulin by Yalow & Berson (1960a).

In the following years a number of studies applied oral or intravenous glucose tolerance tests with the simultaneous determination of plasma concentrations of glucose and insulin. Indices of tissue sensitivity to insulin and indices of insulin secretion were proposed and derived from the relationship between the plasma glycaemic and insulinaemic responses to glucose (Seltzer et al. 1967). These studies reported insensitivity to insulin in obese, glucose intolerant and overt diabetic patients (Yalow & Berson 1960b; Karam et al. 1963; Reaven & Miller 1968) and several other metabolic conditions such as aging (Soerjodibroto et al. 1979), pregnancy and gestational diabetes (Lind 1979), liver disease (Creutzfeldt et al. 1974; Riggio

Clinical Diabetes Research: Methods and Techniques   Edited by Michael Roden
© 2007 John Wiley & Sons, Ltd   ISBN 978-0-470-01728-9

et al. 1982), uraemia (Horton et al. 1968), primary hyperparathyroidism (Prager et al. 1983) and hypercortisolism (Yasuda et al. 1982). The conclusion of insulin insensitivity in these studies was primarily based on the observation of elevated plasma concentrations of insulin in the presence of normal or elevated plasma concentrations of glucose. Though the conclusion of insulin insensitivity in those metabolic states was correct, the glycaemic response during an oral or intravenous glucose tolerance test in fact results from a complex interaction between numerous hormonal and metabolic processes induced by the application of these techniques. Because a technically simple protocol such as the oral glucose tolerance test does not provide sufficient information to analyse the impact of the various simultaneously active processes, it is not trivial to obtain information of insulin sensitivity of whole body glucose utilisation per se.

Methods for the *in vivo* assessment of insulin sensitivity of glucose metabolism

Several methods for the *in vivo* assessment of insulin sensitivity of glucose metabolism have been developed (for reviews see Bergman et al. 1985; Waldhäusl 1993; Ferrannini & Mari 1998; Del Prato 1999). They can be divided into two categories; those interrupting the physiologically-operating feedback loop between the ambient plasma glucose concentration and insulin secretion (glucose clamp technique, insulin suppression test) and those analysing the physiologically-operating feedback loop (frequently sampled intravenous glucose tolerance with minimal model analysis, insulin tolerance test, homeostasis model of glucose tolerance, indices of insulin sensitivity derived from oral glucose tolerance tests).

Basically, fasting plasma concentrations of glucose and insulin can be related to each other and indices of fasting insulin sensitivity can be derived by the use of mathematical models (Matthews et al. 1985; Katz et al. 2000) (for review see Wallace et al. 2004). These methods require minimal time and personal effort and therefore have been applied in epidemiological studies (Haffner et al. 1997; Matsumoto et al. 1997). Empirical or mathematical models also make it possible to calculate indices of insulin sensitivity from oral glucose tolerance test protocols (Matsuda & DeFronzo 1999; Mari et al. 2001). Most of theses techniques are based on the analysis of the physiologically-operating feedback loop between glucose and insulin and thereby require intact endogenous insulin secretion. In addition, most of these indices exhibit a considerable intraindividual day-to-day variability (coefficient of variation ~20–30 %) (Matthews et al. 1985; Steil et al. 1994).

More complex techniques for the *in vivo* assessment of insulin sensitivity include the insulin tolerance test (Horgaard & Thayssen 1929; Bonora et al. 1989), the quadruple infusion insulin suppression test (Shen et al. 1970), the intravenous glucose tolerance test with minimal model based analysis of the dynamics of the glucose and insulin concentration time curves (Bergman et al. 1979; Bergman 1989) and the hyperinsulinaemic euglycaemic clamp test (Sherwin et al. 1974; Insel et al. 1975; Andres et al. 1966; DeFronzo et al. 1979).

Because of the high reproducibility of the measurements of insulin sensitivity and a considerable flexibility of the protocol, the hyperinsulinaemic glucose clamp test has emerged as the most frequently applied technique and is generally accepted as the 'gold standard' for the *in vivo* assessment of insulin sensitivity of whole body glucose metabolism under insulin stimulated conditions (Waldhäusl 1993; Ferrannini & Mari 1998; Del Prato 1999). The term 'gold standard' should neither imply that only glucose clamp derived measures of insulin action represent 'true' measures of insulin sensitivity nor that the glucose clamp derived measures of insulin sensitivity are generally superior to those obtained by other techniques. Each of the techniques mentioned above provides its own specific advantages and disadvantages (Bergman et al. 1985; Ferrannini & Mari 1998; Wallace et al. 2004).

A literature search performed in August 2006 for the term 'glucose clamp technique', with the results limited to studies performed in humans, yielded 2,559 original articles and 74 review articles. For comparison, the terms 'intravenous glucose tolerance test' and 'insulin suppression test' yielded 984 and 196 original articles, respectively.

Definitions of insulin sensitivity, insulin responsiveness and insulin resistance

Insulin exerts a variety of effects on many types of cell. Its main metabolic action can be summarised as anabolic effecting not only glucose but also lipid and protein metabolism. Despite different biological effects, insulin secretion is tightly coupled to the availability of glucose, allowing the fine tuning of blood glucose concentration within a narrow range. In insulin responsive tissues, insulin stimulates glucose uptake, oxidative and nonoxidative metabolic pathways – which include glucose transport and glycogen synthesis – and the inhibition of lipid oxidation. By regulating these metabolic processes, insulin is responsible for the maintenance of glucose homeostasis throughout the fed and the fasted states.

Sensitivity to insulin can be determined by some of its known biological effects. For example, insulin action on skeletal muscle glucose uptake, hepatic glucose output, adipose tissue lipolysis or the compound action of insulin on whole body glucose metabolism can be determined. The tissue specificity of insulin action also implies that not all biological responses are equally sensitive or responsive to insulin. Even though imprecise, the terms 'insulin sensitivity', 'insulin responsiveness' and 'insulin resistance' are most frequently used to refer to insulin action on glucose metabolism. Insulin resistance can be defined as existing wherever normal concentrations of insulin produce a less than normal biological response (Kahn 1978). This definition requires that insulin concentrations are related to some quantifiable insulin dependent process (insulin action) and that a normal biological response is defined (normal insulin action is defined).

In his *in vitro* experiments on isolated cells, Kahn systematically assessed the activation level of a biological effector system in response to various insulin concentrations in the medium, and summarised the results in terms of a dose-response function of insulin action. This dose-response curve of insulin action was approximately sigmoidal and could be described by Michaelis-Menten kinetics in analogy to saturable enzyme kinetics. In terms of this function, insulin action is characterised by two parameters; insulin sensitivity (EC_{50}) and insulin responsiveness (V_{max}). Insulin sensitivity is defined as the insulin concentration in the medium resulting in a half maximal biological response, while insulin responsiveness is defined as concentration resulting in the maximal biological response (V_{max}) (Kahn 1978) (Figure 4.1A).

Decreased insulin sensitivity is then characterised by a right shift of the dose-response curve, which apparently increases the EC_{50}, whereas decreased insulin responsiveness diminishes the upper asymptotic value (V_{max}), leading to a height reduction of the curve (Figure 4.1B). When two dose-response curves exhibit the same height (comparable maximal response), their EC_{50} exactly expresses their respective sensitivities to insulin. When two curves differ in height (i.e. the maximal response differs), insulin sensitivity should be corrected for

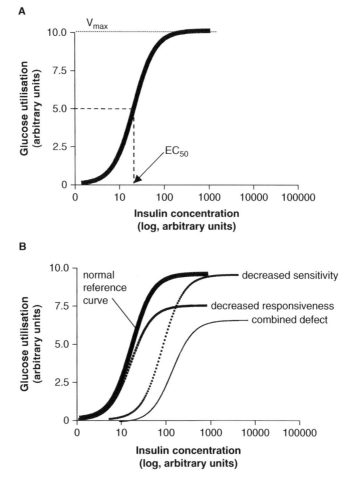

Figure 4.1   A) Characterisation of insulin action on glucose utilisation by means of a dose-response curve with the parameters of insulin sensitivity (EC_{50}) and insulin responsiveness (V_{max}); B) Insulin resistance can result from a decrease in insulin sensitivity, a decrease in insulin responsiveness, or a combination of both. Decreased insulin sensitivity is defined as a right shift of the dose-response curve and a decrease of insulin responsiveness is defined by a reduction of the maximal height of the dose-response curve. Modified from Kahn (1978).

the difference in the maximal responses and needs therefore to be expressed as the ratio V_{max}/EC_{50}.

The characterisation of insulin action in terms of a dose-response curve demonstrates that insulin resistant states can be divided into those caused by decreased sensitivity to insulin, those caused by a decrease in the maximal response to the hormone, and those that are combinations of the two (Kahn 1978; Rizza et al. 1981c). Kahn proposed from his *in vitro* results that disorders associated with alterations at the prereceptor and/or at the receptor level of insulin are more likely to produce decreased insulin sensitivity, whereas disorders associated with alterations at the postreceptor steps in insulin action are more likely to produce decreased responsiveness. This interpretation, however, was recognised to be complicated *in vivo* because of the interrelated nature of the metabolic pathways of insulin action.

Unlike to the *in vitro* conditions, the *in vivo* assessment of insulin action typically determines an integrated whole body response to insulin. Since the hyperinsulinaemic glucose clamp technique provides the possibility of assessing whole body glucose utilisation under conditions of constant glycaemia (substrate) and insulinemia (hormone), it was this technique that enabled the investigators to provide full dose-response relationships for insulin action on glucose metabolism under various metabolic conditions. Numerous laboratories performed serial insulin glucose clamp experiments in humans at various plasma concentrations of insulin and glucose, which characterised insulin action in terms of dose-response curves in states of health and disease (Kolterman et al. 1980; Olefsky & Kolterman 1981; Rizza et al. 1981c; Del Prato et al. 1983; Rowe et al. 1983; Revers et al. 1984b; Laakso et al. 1990). These studies confirmed the sigmoidal shape of the dose-response curve of insulin action on whole body glucose utilisation under various metabolic conditions.

Insulin resistance resulting from a decrease in insulin sensitivity without any decrease of insulin responsiveness was reported in patients with impaired glucose tolerance (Kolterman et al. 1981), in patients with type 2 diabetes mellitus (Rizza et al. 1981b), in the elderly (Rowe et al. 1983), in those with liver cirrhosis (Proietto et al. 1984; Barzilai et al. 1991), under conditions of elevated plasma cortisol concentrations (Rizza et al. 1982), in obesity (Kolterman et al. 1980) and in healthy subjects after one week of bed rest (Stuart et al. 1988). Insulin resistance resulting from a combined decrease in insulin sensitivity and insulin responsiveness has been documented in patients with Cushing syndrome (Nosadini et al. 1983), following musculoskeletal trauma, post-surgery (Brandi et al. 1993), acanthosis nigricans (Cohen et al. 1990), lipodystrophic syndromes (Robert et al. 1990, 1993), liver cirrhosis (Miyamoto et al. 1992), uraemia (Schmitz 1988), pancreas-kidney transplants (Christiansen et al. 1996), obesity (Kolterman et al. 1980; Laakso et al. 1990), poorly controlled type 1 diabetes mellitus (Del Prato et al. 1983; Revers et al. 1984b), type 2 diabetes mellitus (Kolterman et al. 1981; Olefsky & Kolterman 1981; Mandarino et al. 1984; Revers et al. 1984a; Miyamoto et al. 1992), pregnancy and gestational diabetes (Ryan et al. 1985).

These insulin glucose clamp studies also conclusively demonstrated that the rate of glucose utilisation is roughly proportional to the plasma insulin level within the physiological range of plasma insulin concentrations (5-125 μU/ml) (Bergman et al. 1985; Ferrannini & Mari 1998). This holds true for both insulin sensitive and insulin resistant individuals (Figure 4.2). This observation provides the rationale for a valid comparison of rates of whole body glucose metabolism as a measure of insulin sensitivity at a single level of matched hyperinsulinaemia within the physiological range of insulin concentrations.

It must be stated that most published studies involving the insulin glucose clamp technique do not provide complete dose-response relationships for insulin action on whole body glucose metabolism. The most prevalent measure of insulin sensitivity is the M value, which is the rate of whole body glucose metabolism at a single level of hyperinsulinemia during a glucose clamp test. Because insulin stimulated rates of whole body glucose metabolism exhibit considerable inter-individual variability even in glucose tolerant and otherwise healthy subjects, no generally accepted cut-off values exist for the definition of insulin resistance. Bergman et al. (1985) reviewed 18 independent studies in normal, nonelderly and nonobese individuals in whom hyperinsulinaemic ($1\ \mathrm{mU \cdot m^{-2} \cdot min^{-1}}$ or $1\ \mathrm{mU \cdot kg^{-1} \cdot min^{-1}}$) euglycaemic clamp tests were performed, and found the 95 % confidence limits for the mean M values

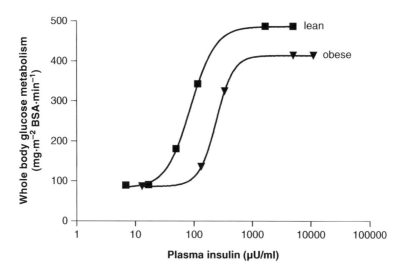

Figure 4.2 Dose-response curve of whole body glucose metabolism as a function of the serum insulin concentration during euglycaemic hyperinsulinaemic clamp tests in lean (squares) and obese (triangles) subjects. Insulin action in the obese is characterised by decreased insulin sensitivity (right shift of the curve) and decreased insulin responsiveness (reduction in the maximal height of the curve), both indicative of insulin resistance. The two curves were originally reported by Laakso et al. (1990) and were reconstructed here by fitting data points from this study with a four-parameter-logistic equation.

in these studies to be 4.7 and 8.7 mg·kg^{-1}·min^{-1}. From these confidence intervals a conservative definition of insulin resistance would be an M value of less than 4.7 mg·kg^{-1}·min^{-1} at the insulin infusion rates applied in these studies.

Despite these efforts to simplify the definition of insulin resistance by introducing cut-off values for insulin stimulated rates of whole body glucose metabolism from standardised clamp protocols, to date the inclusion of age and weight matched individuals serving as a control group remains necessary.

Attempts to find an improved measure of insulin sensitivity from the hyperinsulinaemic euglycaemic clamp test have been made, but they are not widely applied. The initial slope index of insulin sensitivity (ISI) and its rationale should be mentioned (Finegood et al. 1984; Bergman et al. 1985).

As stated above, insulin sensitivity should be defined as the dose-response relationship between plasma insulin concentrations and some measure of insulin action. In addition, the rate of whole body glucose metabolism is roughly proportional to the plasma insulin level within the physiological range of plasma insulin concentrations. Thus, when the maximal response, which is necessary for a complete dose-response relationship, is not determined, but rates of whole body glucose metabolism are measured at three different levels within the range of approximate linear insulin action on glucose metabolism, the initial slope of this incomplete dose-response curve of insulin action can be used as an index of insulin sensitivity (Finegood et al. 1984; Bergman et al. 1985). More recently, another experimental approach was developed by Natali et al. (2000) which enables investigators to obtain both the initial slope index of insulin sensitivity and a complete dose-response relationship for insulin action on glucose metabolism from a single two-step hyperinsulinaemic (20 and

$200 \text{ mU·m}^{-2}\text{·min}^{-1}$) euglycaemic clamp experiment. This technique combines the clamp technique with glucose tracer dilution technology and mathematical modeling of the effects of insulin on whole body glucose disposal.

Basic principles of the euglycaemic hyperinsulinaemic clamp technique

The hyperinsulinaemic euglycaemic clamp technique was developed by Andres et al. (1966) and further developed and widely studied by DeFronzo et al. (1979) (see also Sherwin et al. 1974; Insel et al. 1975). From a mechanistic point of view, this technique breaks the physiologically-operating feedback loop between blood glucose concentration and pancreatic insulin secretion and applies a negative feedback principle to the system regulating the blood glucose concentration (Bergman et al. 1985).

In the postabsorptive state of nondiabetic individuals, the rate of endogenous glucose output originating from hepatic ($\sim$95 %) and renal ($\sim$5 %) glucose release exactly matches the rate of whole body glucose utilisation, resulting in constant glycaemia (Figure 4.3). The administration of exogenous insulin under these conditions reduces endogenous glucose output and increases whole body glucose utilisation, which both result in a decline of blood glucose concentration. This decline can be prevented when an exogenous infusion of glucose exactly matches the insulin induced glucose flux out of the glucose space into glucose utilising cells (i.e. the increase in glucose utilisation) as well as the reduction of endogenous glucose output (Figure 4.4).

With the hyperinsulinaemic euglycaemic clamp technique, exogenous insulin is infused to create a hyperinsulinaemic plateau of plasma insulin concentrations, while the plasma glucose concentration is kept constant at the euglycaemic level by means of a variable exogenous glucose infusion. Thus, the rate of glucose infusion required to maintain constant glycaemia during the period of constant hyperinsulinaemia provides a measure for the net effect of insulin on whole body glucose metabolism (Figure 4.4). In particular, the effects on whole body glucose metabolism comprise stimulation of glucose utilisation and inhibition of endogenous glucose output. Provided that endogenous glucose output is completely suppressed or negligible during the clamp, the amount of glucose infused must equal the amount of glucose being translocated out of the glucose space (i.e. glucose metabolised, M value) (DeFronzo et al. 1979).

The exogenous source of insulin makes it possible to match plasma insulin concentrations under different metabolic conditions and allows the assessment of insulin action independent of intact pancreatic insulin secretion. In addition, by clamping the concentration of plasma glucose at euglycaemic levels, the stimulation of endogenous insulin secretion is prevented and therefore does not disrupt the assessment of insulin action at the desired level of hyperinsulinaemia.

Calculation of whole body glucose metabolism (M value)

Provided that endogenous glucose output is zero or at least negligible, the glucose infused equals the glucose being translocated out of the glucose space (i.e. glucose metabolised, M value) during steady state conditions of hyperinsulinaemic euglycaemia (DeFronzo

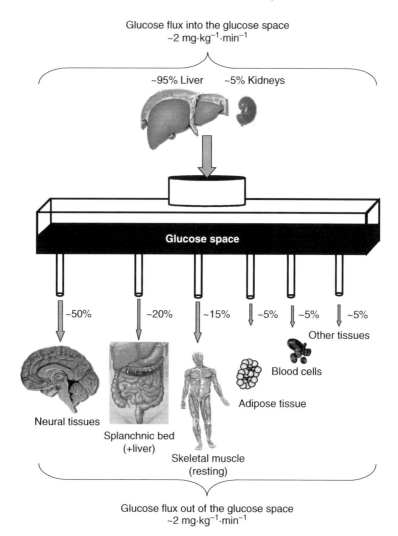

Figure 4.3 Schematic diagram of postabsorptive glucose metabolism in healthy humans. Under postabsorptive conditions the glucose flux into the glucose space (extracellular fluid) equals the glucose flux out of the glucose space, resulting in constant glycaemia. The only source of glucose input is of hepatic and renal origin (endogenous glucose output). The approximate percentage contributions of various tissues to postabsorptive glucose utilisation is summarised and approximated from the following: Björntorp & Sjostrom (1978); Consoli (1992); Dinneen et al. (1992); Boyle et al. (1994); Ekberg et al. (1999); Zierler (1999); Gerich (2000).

et al. 1979). Because the plasma glucose concentration is almost never perfectly maintained (i.e. clamped) at constant, corrections must be done (Figure 4.5). DeFronzo et al. (1979) introduced a correction factor for this under the term 'space correction'. This space correction adjusts the glucose infusion rates from changes in glycaemia and not from real changes in glucose utilisation. For example, when the plasma glucose concentration during a clamp test is raised from 95 mg/dl at 80 minutes to 100 mg/dl at 100 minutes, the glucose

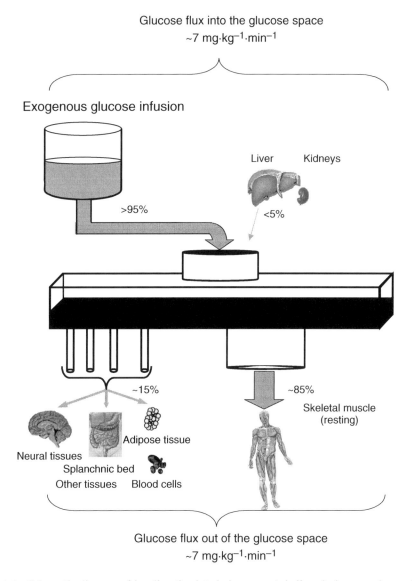

Glucose flux into the glucose space
$\sim$7 mg·kg^{-1}·min^{-1}

Exogenous glucose infusion

Liver   Kidneys

>95%   <5%

$\sim$15% $\sim$85%

Skeletal muscle
(resting)

Neural tissues
Splanchnic bed   Adipose tissue
Other tissues   Blood cells

Glucose flux out of the glucose space
$\sim$7 mg·kg^{-1}·min^{-1}

Figure 4.4 Schematic diagram of insulin stimulated glucose metabolism during a euglycaemic (100 mg/dl) hyperinsulinaemic (40 mU·m^{-2}·min^{-1}) clamp test in healthy humans. Because endogenous glucose output is almost completely suppressed by hyperinsulinaemia, the exogenous glucose infusion accounts for whole body glucose requirements under these conditions. The diagram provides raw approximate percentage contributions of various tissues to insulin stimulated whole body glucose metabolism in healthy humans. The contribution of skeletal muscle may vary with individual insulin sensitivity.

infusion rate in the period between 80 and 100 minutes has actually exceeded the rate of glucose utilisation, otherwise plasma glucose concentration would not have increased. The reverse is true when the plasma glucose concentration declines, indicating that the glucose infusion rate could not completely account for the rate of glucose utilisation in this period.

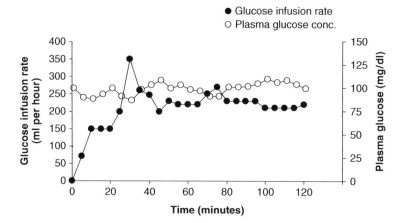

Figure 4.5 Time course of the glucose infusion (filled symbols, scaled on the left ordinate) and plasma glucose concentration (open symbols, scaled on the right ordinate) from a 120-minute eugly-caemic (100 mg/dl) hyperinsulinaemic (40 mU·m^{-2}·min^{-1}) clamp test in a healthy volunteer. The glucose content of the infusion was 20 % weight per volume and the plasma concentration of insulin during the final hour of the clamp test was ∼70 μU/ml. (Unpublished data).

In the original work of DeFronzo et al. (1979) the computation of rates of whole body glucose metabolism (M) during the clamp was calculated from the means of 20-min periods by the following equation:

$$M = GIR - SC - UC$$

where *GIR* is the glucose infusion rate, *SC* the space correction and *UC* the correction for urinary glucose loss. If M is calculated for 20-min periods as recommended, the plasma glucose concentrations at the beginning and the end are computed, for the calculation of the space correction, according to the equations:

$$SC(\text{mg} \cdot \text{kg}^{-1} \cdot \text{min}^{-1}) = \frac{(G_2 - G_1) \cdot 10 \cdot (0.19 \cdot body\ weight)}{20 \cdot body\ weight}$$
$$SC(\text{mg} \cdot \text{kg}^{-1} \cdot \text{min}^{-1}) = (G_2 - G_1) \cdot 0.095$$

where G_2 and G_1 are the plasma glucose concentrations (mg/dl) at the end and the beginning of the 20-min time period, respectively. The multiplication of $(G_2 - G_1)$ with the factor 10 in the numerator converts the units of plasma glucose concentration from mg/dl to mg/l. In the next step, the difference of the glucose concentrations (now mg/l) is multiplied with the whole body distribution volume of glucose expressed in litres [0.19 (litre/kg body-weight) times bodyweight (kg)]. This distribution volume participates in rapid changes of plasma glucose concentrations (i.e. within 20 minutes). Cancelling the litres in the numer-ator results in the difference of whole body glucose mass (milligrams) between the end and the beginning of the 20-min period, which is due to changes in glycaemia. The divi-sion of this difference in glucose mass (mg) by the denominator term (20·bodyweight) accounts for time (20 minutes) and bodyweight (kg) and finally converts the dimension to mg·kg^{-1}·min^{-1}. This is the rate at which glucose was added to or removed from the glucose space independently of changes in glucose utilisation. The space correction represents an approximation derived from a monocompartmental model of glucose metabolism and only performs accurately when plasma glucose concentrations are kept within a narrow range of the target level (± 10 mg/dl). In addition, the time interval between the two measurements of plasma glucose concentrations used for the calculation of the space correction should not exceed 20 minutes. For any other time interval the equation must be adjusted.

Urinary glucose loss does not generally occur during glucose clamp studies performed at euglycaemia. However, when glucose is clamped at hyperglycaemic levels or clamp tests are performed in patients with diabetes at the prevailing fasting plasma glucose concentration (i.e. isoglycaemic clamp studies), the urinary loss of glucose must be accounted for. Urinary glucose loss can be determined by having the participant void just before the start and immediately after the end of the clamp test. The urine from the entire period should be collected and the urinary glucose mass determined. Provided that glycaemia is relatively constant during the clamp experiment, urinary glucose loss can be assumed to be equally distributed over the duration of the clamp test and must be subtracted from the rate of whole body glucose utilisation.

Of all the time periods during a two- or three-hour euglycaemic hyperinsulinaemic clamp test, that between 60 and 120 min after the start of the insulin infusion is the best in which to calculate M values, because that time period exhibits the lowest coefficient of intraindividual variation (Bokemark et al. 2000). In prolonged clamp protocols, later periods are also adequate for the calculation of the M values.

During prolonged hyperinsulinaemic glucose clamp experiments, gradual increases of the glucose infusion rates above those required between 60 and 120 minutes are frequently observed (Roden et al. 1996b). Because rates of nonoxidative glucose metabolism representing glycogen synthesis are constant between one and six hours during hyperinsulinaemic glucose clamps, increases of glucose oxidation account for increasing glucose infusion rates (Roden et al. 1996b). Thus, for the comparison of M values between groups of individuals, the time period used for the calculation of the M values must be matched.

Although glucose infusion rates only approximate but seldom fulfil the mathematical criteria of steady state conditions, the mean value of M during the final 40 or 60 minutes of a two-hour clamp (i.e. 60–120 or 80–120 min) is a satisfactory index of insulin sensitivity for ordinary purposes (Ferrannini & Mari 1998). Representative M values for several metabolic conditions are presented in Table 4.1.

Standardised indices of insulin sensitivity derived from the M value

For purposes of comparison, M values should be standardised (Ferrannini & Mari 1998). The steady state rate of whole body glucose metabolism is frequently normalised for bodyweight (M_{bw}), fat free mass (M_{ffm}), rate of resting energy expenditure (M_{ree}) and steady state plasma insulin concentration during the clamp (M/I) (Bergman et al. 1985; Ferrannini & Mari 1998). Normalisation of the M value for the mean steady state concentration of plasma glucose yields the metabolic clearance rate of glucose (MCR) (Ferrannini & Mari 1998), which is able to account for small differences in glycaemia during a clamp. Any of these normalisations may be advantageous is some cases but bear pitfalls in others. Although several studies could demonstrate adipose tissue glucose uptake under insulin stimulated conditions *in vivo* (Bjorntorp et al. 1971; Virtanen et al. 2002), it is recommended that

Table 4.1 Representative M values (mg glucose per kg bodyweight per minute) from hyperinsulin-aemic (40 mU·m^{-2}·min^{-1} or 1 mU·kg^{-1}·min^{-1}) euglycaemic clamp tests under various metabolic conditions. Some of the listed studies applied glucose tracers during the clamps and reported tracer-determined rates of whole body glucose disposal instead of the M values. To simplify matters, tracer-determined rates of whole body glucose disposal are also indicated as M in this table

Metabolic characteristics	M (mg·kg^{-1}·min^{-1})	Reference
Healthy subjects with normal weight	7.1 ± 2.1	(Ferrannini et al. 1997)
	8.6 ± 1.5	(Ravussin et al. 1983)
Long distance runners	10.0 ± 0.8	(Yki-Jarvinen & Koivisto 1983)
Weight lifters	10.1 ± 1.0	(Yki-Jarvinen & Koivisto 1983)
Glucose tolerant first degree	4.8 ± 1.6	(Perseghin et al. 1997)
relatives of patients with type 2 diabetes	6.6 ± 0.5	(Pratipanawatr et al. 2001)
Obese, otherwise healthy subjects	5.5 ± 2.0	(Ferrannini et al. 1997)
Overweight subjects with impaired glucose tolerance	5.4 ± 0.9	(Bavenholm et al. 2001)
Elderly (age 69 years)	3.8 ± 0.5	(Fink et al. 1983)
Patients with type 2 diabetes mellitus		
poor glycaemic control	2.7 ± 0.4	(Doberne et al. 1982)
poor glycaemic control	2.9 ± 0.2	(Anderwald et al. 2002)
moderate glycaemic control	4.7 ± 1.4	(Bavenholm et al. 2001)
Patients with type 1 diabetes mellitus	4.3 ± 0.6	(Staten et al. 1984)

M-values should be normalised for fat free mass (M_{ffm}) (Ferrannini & Mari 1998). This correction accounts for gender related differences in fat mass (Ferrannini et al. 1997). The normalisation of the M value for bodyweight (per kg bodyweight) instead of fat free mass (per kg of fat free mass) results in an underestimation of insulin sensitivity in obesity (Bokemark et al. 2000). Because M/I is more variable than the M value itself, the correction of the M value for the steady state plasma insulin concentration during a clamp (M/I) is not beneficial (Bergman et al. 1985).

Insulin stimulated whole body glucose metabolism

During euglycaemic hyperinsulinaemia, skeletal muscle is primarily responsible for the insulin dependent increase of whole body glucose metabolism (Figure 4.4 and 4.6A) DeFronzo et al. 1985). The contribution of the liver to whole body glucose metabolism is small under these conditions. However, splanchnic glucose uptake and thus the contribution of the liver to whole body glucose metabolism increases under hyperglycaemic hyperinsulinaemic conditions (Basu et al. 2004; Krssak et al. 2004). Insulin stimulated whole body glucose metabolism depends on two major metabolic pathways: glucose oxidation and nonoxidative glucose metabolism. Nonoxidative glucose metabolism is primarily represented by glycogen synthesis, and skeletal muscle is the tissue accounting for the majority of insulin stimulated glycogen synthesis (Shulman et al. 1990). In insulin resistant states, lower rates of skeletal muscle glycogen synthesis are responsible for the reduction of insulin stimulated whole body glucose metabolism (Figure 4.6B) (Shulman et al. 1990; Roden et al. 1996b; DeFronzo 1988).

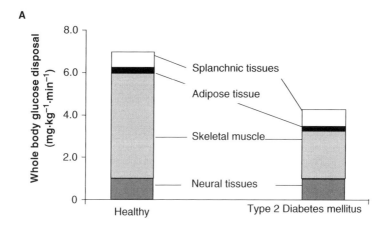

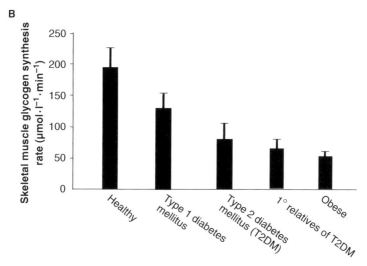

Figure 4.6 A) Summary of whole body glucose metabolism during euglycaemic hyperinsulinaemic clamp tests in healthy individuals and in insulin resistant patients with type 2 diabetes mellitus. Note the difference in skeletal muscle glucose uptake under insulin stimulated conditions between the groups. Modified from DeFronzo (1988); B) Skeletal muscle glycogen synthetic rates during hyperinsulinaemic glucose clamp tests as measured by ^{13}C magnetic resonance spectroscopy in groups of healthy and insulin resistant individuals including patients with type 1 diabetes mellitus, obese, glucose tolerant first degree relatives of patients with type 2 diabetes mellitus and patients with type 2 diabetes mellitus. Modified from Roden & Shulman (1999).

Regulation of endogenous glucose output during euglycaemic hyperinsulinaemia

Hyperinsulinaemia dose dependently inhibits endogenous glucose output (Kolterman et al. 1981; DeFronzo 1988), which is mainly of hepatic origin (Ekberg et al. 1999). An important regulator of hepatic glucose release is the relationship of hepatic sinusoidal concentrations of insulin and glucagon (Cherrington 1999). Although irrelevant during a hyperinsulinaemic clamp test performed at euglycaemia, hyperglycaemia per se also exerts a powerful inhibitory effect on endogenous glucose output (Bell et al. 1986). Because glucoregulatory hormones other than insulin, such as glucagon, are only gradually suppressed during hyperinsulinaemic euglycaemic clamp tests (Prager et al. 1987; Lewis et al. 1998), two other factors essentially impact on endogenous glucose output. These factors are the degree of hyperinsulinaemia per se and the insulin sensitivity of hepatic glucose output. Since insulin is physiologically secreted into the splanchnic circulation, portal vein plasma concentrations of insulin exceed those in peripheral and arterial plasma. The physiological range of the ratio between portal venous and peripheral venous insulin concentrations is approximately 2–2.5:1 (Waldhäusl et al. 1982). During a clamp experiment, endogenous insulin secretion can be monitored by the measurement of plasma C-peptide concentrations because only endogenous insulin secretion and not insulin infusion is accompanied by C-peptide release. Plasma concentrations of C-peptide decline during exogenous insulin infusion, indicating inhibition of endogenous insulin secretion. It is important to note that this inhibition of endogenous insulin secretion abolishes the physiological gradient of insulin concentrations between portal vein and peripheral venous plasma. Thus, peripheral plasma insulin concentrations roughly correspond to portal vein insulin concentrations during a hyperinsulinaemic clamp test, allowing one to assess endogenous glucose output under conditions of known hepatic sinusoidal insulin concentrations.

In nondiabetic subjects the infusion of insulin at rates of 0.2, 0.25, 0.5 and 1 mU per kilogram bodyweight per minute ($mU \cdot kg^{-1} \cdot min^{-1}$) during euglycaemic clamp tests reduce hepatic glucose output by ∼50, ∼68, ∼87 and ∼98 % (Rizza et al. 1981a; DeFronzo et al. 1983). Although the hepatic sinusoidal insulin concentrations remain almost unchanged during low dose insulin infusion, endogenous glucose output is substantially reduced (Prager et al. 1987). This phenomenon is explainable by additional indirect (extrahepatic) effects of insulin on endogenous glucose output, which involve the insulin induced alteration of gluconeogenic substrate flux from the periphery as well as the suppression of adipose tissue lipolysis during peripheral hyperinsulinaemia (Prager et al. 1987; Lewis et al. 1996; McCall et al. 1998; Giacca et al. 1999).

Several metabolic conditions known to be associated with resistance of insulin induced suppression of endogenous glucose output should be considered when a clamp protocol is planned. For example, impaired glucose tolerance (Bavenholm et al. 2001), type 2 diabetes mellitus and obesity (Kolterman et al. 1981; DeFronzo et al. 1985; Butler et al. 1990; Staehr et al. 2001; Krssak et al. 2004), steroid therapy (Rizza et al. 1982), increased availability of free fatty acids and/or triglycerides (Bajaj et al. 2002; Boden et al. 2002) and fat accumulation in the liver (Seppala-Lindroos et al. 2002; Krssak et al. 2004) are associated with defective insulin induced suppression of endogenous glucose output. In terms of a dose-response curve of insulin action on endogenous glucose output, the curve is shifted to the right under these metabolic conditions, indicative of hepatic insulin resistance (Kolterman et al. 1981). In line with these studies, the half maximal effective plasma insulin concentration to suppress endogenous glucose output is increased more than twofold in patients with type 2 diabetes (∼65 µU/ml), compared to nondiabetic controls (∼25 µU/ml) (Campbell et al. 1988).

In summary, in nonobese, glucose tolerant and otherwise healthy individuals, endogenous glucose output can be assumed zero during euglycaemic clamp tests when the insulin infusion rate is in the range of $1\ mU \cdot kg^{-1} \cdot min^{-1}$ or $40\ mU \cdot m^{-2} \cdot min^{-1}$. In any other case, complete inhibition of endogenous glucose output cannot be assumed and has to be measured.

Endogenous glucose output and rates of whole body glucose utilisation

Under several metabolic conditions endogenous glucose output is not zero during eugly-caemic clamp tests with plasma insulin concentrations within the physiological range (Rizza et al. 1982; DeFronzo et al. 1985; Campbell et al. 1988; Staehr et al. 2001; Bajaj et al. 2002; Seppala-Lindroos et al. 2002; Butler et al. 1990). In these cases the glucose infusion rates do not reflect whole body glucose metabolism because the residual endogenous output remains unaccounted for. This implies that as long as complete inhibition of endogenous glucose output is not guaranteed, the M value from a clamp experiment should not be taken as a measure of whole body glucose metabolism. If endogenous glucose output is erroneously assumed null, insulin stimulated rates of whole body glucose metabolism are underesti-mated. Thus, determination of endogenous glucose output is a necessity when plasma insulin concentrations are within the physiological range during a euglycaemic clamp test. In partic-ular, the assessment of endogenous glucose output is required when rates of whole body glucose metabolism are compared between groups of metabolic heterogeneous individuals.

Because of its applicability without the need of additional venous catheterisation during a clamp test, the glucose isotope dilution technique represents the method of choice for the assessment of endogenous glucose output during glucose clamp tests (Steele et al. 1956; Steele 1959; Insel et al. 1975; Bergman 1977; Finegood et al. 1987; Cobelli & Toffolo 1990; Hother-Nielsen et al. 1996). As an alternative, the hepatic vein catheterisation tech-nique provides the possibility of measuring a net balance of splanchnic glucose metabolism (DeFronzo et al. 1978; DeFronzo et al. 1983; Basu et al. 2000).

Methodology

Technical requirements

In order to perform a glucose clamp test, several technical requirements must be met. Two intravenous lines must be kept patent for the duration of the clamp test, one for the infusion of glucose and insulin and the other for frequent blood sampling of arterialised blood. In

Table 4.2 Techniques used in combination with the glucose clamp technique. MRS: magnetic reso-nance spectroscopy; PET: positron emission tomography. Modified from Ferrannini & Mari (1998)

Method	Measure	Reference
Isotope dilution (glucose tracer)	Endogenous glucose output, Rate of disappearance of glucose	(Insel et al. 1975) (DeFronzo et al. 1983)
Forearm/leg catheterisation	Foreram/leg glucose uptake	(Yki-Jarvinen et al. 1987) (DeFronzo et al. 1981)
Hepatic vein catheterisation	Splanchnic glucose balance	(DeFronzo et al. 1983) (Basu et al. 2004)
Indirect calorimetry	Substrate oxidation	(Thiebaud et al. 1983) (Felber et al. 1987)
Glycerol tracer	Lipolysis	(Nurjhan et al. 1986)
Amino acid tracer	Protein synthesis	(Gelfand & Barrett 1987)
Deuterated water	Gluconeogenesis	(Gastaldelli et al. 2001)

Table 4.2   Continued

Method	Measure	Reference
Thermo dilution technique	Insulin induced vasodilatation	(Laakso et al. 1990)
Dye dilution		(DeFronzo et al. 1985)
Plethysmography		(Creager et al. 1985)
Microneurography	Sympathetic nerve activity	(Anderson et al. 1991)
^{31}P MRS	Glucose transport/phosphorylation	(Rothman et al. 1992)
		(Roden et al. 1996b)
	Insulin stimulated ATP-synthesis	(Petersen et al. 2005)
		(Brehm et al. 2006)
^{13}C MRS	Muscle glycogen synthesis	(Shulman et al. 1990)
	Hepatic glycogen synthesis	(Roden et al. 1996a)
		(Krssak et al. 2004)
^{1}H MRS	Intramyocellular lipid content	(Krebs et al. 2001)
		(Boden et al. 2001)
PET	Regional glucose uptake	(Shapiro et al. 1990)
		(Knuuti et al. 1992)
Microdialysis	Refined adipose tissue	(Bernroider et al. 2005)
	and skeletal muscle	(Maggs et al. 1995)
	metabolism	(Hagstrom-Toft et al. 1992)

order to avoid possible interference of ipsilateral infusion and blood sampling, a contralateral placement of the venous catheters is recommended. Two exactly calibrated infusion pumps, one for insulin and the other for glucose, must provide sufficient fine gears for the adjustment of the infusion rates (0.02–0.15 ml/min). The glucose concentration in the blood samples must be determined rapidly (i.e. < 60 seconds) online to facilitate an accurate adjustment of the rate of glucose infusion.

Insulin infusion

The goal of the insulin infusion is to acutely raise and maintain the plasma insulin concentration at a new hyperinsulinaemic plateau for the duration of the clamp experiment. The insulin infusion rate applied depends on the desired steady state plasma insulin concentration during the clamp. In the original experiments reported by Sherwin et al. (1974) and De Fronzo et al. (1979), plasma insulin concentrations were raised to approximately 100 μU/ml above fasting levels by applying a continuous insulin infusion rate of 1 mU per kg bodyweight per minute or 40 mU per square metre body surface area per minute, respectively. Since then, various insulin infusion rates have been applied during glucose clamp tests. However, one should be aware that when plasma insulin concentrations are raised above $\sim$500 μU/ml (corresponding to an insulin infusion rate of $\sim$200 mU$\cdot$m$^{-2}\cdot$min^{-1}), the physiological clearance mechanism of plasma insulin is saturated and plasma insulin concentrations will continuously increase dependent on the duration of the insulin infusion (Bergman et al. 1985).

   The most frequently applied insulin infusion rate has remained 40 mU insulin per square metre body surface area per minute (40 mU$\cdot$m$^{-2}\cdot$min^{-1}), which approximately corresponds to 1 mU insulin per kilogram bodyweight per minute (1 mU$\cdot$kg$^{-1}\cdot$min^{-1}). Importantly, in obese subjects the insulin dose should be normalised for body surface area (mU$\cdot$m$^{-2}\cdot$min^{-1}) instead

Table 4.3 Simple infusion protocol for the administration of a primed (740 mU·m^{-2} body surface area per 10 min) continuous (40 mU·m^{-2}BSA·min^{-1}) insulin infusion for a hyperinsulinaemic euglycaemic clamp test. Modified from DeFronzo et al. (1979).

Time (minutes)	mU Insulin per m^2 BSA per min	Infusion rate (ml/hour)
0–2	100	50
2–4	90	45
4–6	80	40
6–8	60	30
8–end of clamp	40	20

of bodyweight (mU·kg^{-1}·min^{-1}). This may help to avoid relative overinsulinisation in obese individuals. With this insulin infusion rate an insulin dose of ~4.2 I.U. is hourly infused in an individual with 70 kilograms bodyweight and 1.73 square metre body surface area, resulting in constant plasma insulin concentrations between 50 and 130 μU/ml (Bergman et al. 1985). These concentrations are within the range of physiological peripheral hyperinsulinaemia and are comparable to peripheral plasma insulin concentrations after meal ingestion (Singhal et al. 2002; Krssak et al. 2004). Despite the application of almost identical insulin doses during euglycaemic clamp tests in numerous studies performed in nondiabetic subjects, steady state plasma insulin concentrations vary considerably in the literature (~70–132 μU/ml during 1 mU·kg^{-1}·min^{-1}insulin infusion) (Deibert & DeFronzo 1980; Simonson & DeFronzo 1983). This variability is most likely due to differences in the insulin assays, the variability of insulin clearance under different metabolic conditions, differences in the fasting plasma insulin concentrations and differences in the ability of the insulin infusion to suppress endogenous insulin secretion (Bergman et al. 1985).

In order to accelerate the achievement of a desired plateau of plasma insulin concentrations, many investigators apply a priming dose of insulin, administered within the first 10 minutes after the start of the clamp experiment, which is then followed by a lower but continuous rate of insulin infusion. During the 10-minute priming period, the total infused insulin is typically twice that infused in the subsequent 10 minutes of the clamp and the dose is frequently administered in an exponentially declining pattern (Sherwin et al. 1974). Thus, the priming dose for a hyperinsulinaemic clamp performed with an insulin infusion rate of 40 mU·m^{-2}·min^{-1} is ~800 mU insulin per square metre body surface area, administered within the first 10 minutes of the clamp test (Table 4.3) (DeFronzo et al. 1979). It is well documented that this priming dose results in a short term initial overshoot of plasma insulin concentrations above the steady state level achieved later in the test (Sherwin et al. 1974; DeFronzo et al. 1979). On the other hand, unprimed insulin infusion protocols generally need more time to achieve an acceptable plateau of plasma insulin concentration and the experiment should therefore generally last longer than the most frequently applied duration of 120 minutes. The application of an insulin priming dose can therefore be recommended to shorten the time required to approximate steady state conditions.

Preparation of the insulin infusion

The insulin infusate is prepared with human insulin, which is added to isotonic saline. The insulin infusion pump must be calibrated and must provide sufficient fine gears to allow the administration of the calculated insulin dose. In order to prevent the absorption of the hormone in plastic surfaces, 2 ml of the individual's blood per 48 ml of the infusate is added to the infusate (Sherwin et al. 1974; DeFronzo et al. 1979). The effectiveness of this method can be proven by measuring the insulin recovery in the infusate after it is pumped through the infusion lines (Sherwin et al. 1974; Insel et al. 1975; DeFronzo et al. 1979). This may be of special interest when clamp experiments are performed with investigative apparatus such as nuclear magnetic resonance spectrometers or positron emission tomography, which complicate the use of infusion pumps with short infusion lines.

Example of a protocol for insulin infusion

The following paragraph describes the preparation of an insulin infusate for a hyperinsulinaemic ($40 \ mU \cdot m^{-2} \cdot min^{-1}$) euglycaemic clamp test. Table 4.3 provides an infusion scheme for the priming of the insulin space. The continuous infusion rate of the insulin infusion pump is chosen to be 20 ml per hour. 2 ml of blood are drawn from the participant and are promptly added to 48 ml of isotonic saline in a sterile syringe (50 ml). Then the required dose of human insulin is added, calculated as follows:

$$\text{INSULIN (I.U.)} = \frac{Ins(40 \ mU \cdot m^{-2} \cdot \min^{-1}) \cdot BSA(m^2) \cdot 60(\min) \cdot Syringe \ Vol. \ (50 \text{ ml})}{Pump \ factor \ (20 \ ml/h) \cdot 1000}$$

$$\text{INSULIN} \ (I.U.) = 6 \cdot BSA(m^2)$$

where *Ins* represents the rate of insulin infusion normalised to body surface area, *BSA* the body surface area (expressed in square metres), and the *pump factor* is the continuous infusion rate of the insulin infusion pump (ml/h, here chosen to be 20 ml per hour). The number 1,000 in the denominator converts the insulin units from mU to I.U. If more than 50 ml of the insulin infusate is required for a clamp experiment of longer duration, a stem solution of greater volume should be prepared. This reduces the impreciseness in the dosing of insulin and guarantees identical insulin concentrations in sequential infusates.

Instead of adjusting the insulin dose for a predefined infusion rate, it is also feasible to adjust the infusion rate of the insulin pump for a fixed dose of insulin added to the infusate.

Blood sampling site: arterial, venous or arterialised venous blood sampling

Matched hyperinsulinaemia rates of whole body glucose metabolism can only be directly compared among individuals if the concentration of glucose perfusing their glucose utilising tissues is the same (Bergman et al. 1985).

The concentration of plasma glucose physiologically declines during the perfusion of glucose utilising tissues. In addition, pancreatic insulin secretion is regulated by the arterial blood glucose concentration. Early studies applying the glucose clamp technique measured the glucose concentration in arterial plasma drawn from a catheter in the brachial artery (Sherwin et al. 1974; Insel et al. 1975; DeFronzo et al. 1979). In subsequent insulin and glucose clamp studies, several investigators measured glucose concentration in venous plasma, which rendered arterial catheterisation unnecessary and simplified the protocol (Kraegen et al. 1983; Howard et al. 1984; Yki-Jarvinen & Koivisto 1984).

However, the comparison of individuals at equivalent venous plasma glucose concentrations and matched insulinemia results in a systematic error when their sensitivity to insulin is not the same (Bergman et al. 1985). The arteriovenous balance technique demonstrates that the glucose concentration in venous plasma is equivalent to that in arterial plasma minus the decline due to tissue glucose uptake during the perfusion. Because tissue glucose uptake is by definition higher in the insulin sensitive than the insulin resistant individual, the arterial-venous difference of glucose concentration also must be greater in the insulin sensitive individual. Clamping venous glucose concentration at equivalent levels in both individuals results in higher arterial glucose concentration in the sensitive individual – otherwise venous glucose concentration could not be equivalent in both individuals. The difference in arterial glucose concentrations is proportional to the difference in insulin sensitivity and thus systematically impacts on the determination of insulin sensitivity. Interestingly, the M values did not differ within a group of healthy subjects when the glucose concentration was clamped in venous, arterialised venous and capillary blood during repeated clamp experiments (Nauck et al.1996). However, this study only performed intra- and not inter-individual comparisons of insulin sensitivity. Taken together, whole body glucose metabolism should only be compared if the concentration of glucose perfusing glucose utilising tissues is the same, i.e. the arterial glucose concentrations are matched (Bergman et al. 1985). Hence, clamping venous glucose concentration cannot be recommended.

Other investigators avoided arterial catheterisation by sampling arterialised venous blood from veins in the hand heated to ~60 °C; the so-called 'heated hand technique'. For this purpose, heating boxes for the hand were developed, commonly representing thermoregulated Plexiglas boxes. Heat induced vasodilatation and shorter blood transit time result in arterialised venous blood in which the concentration of glucose and other metabolites is similar to that in arterial blood (McGuire et al. 1976). Nowadays, the heated hand technique is widely used and generally accepted for use in metabolic studies (Ferrannini et al. 1983; Maggs et al. 1998; Toft-Nielsen et al. 2001; Bajaj et al. 2005). Because it can prevent differences in the arterial glucose concentration between insulin sensitive and resistant individuals, this technique should be applied during glucose clamp tests.

Measurement of glucose concentration and adjustment of glucose infusion rate

In order to successfully maintain plasma glucose concentration at the desired level, it is necessary to rapidly and repeatedly determine plasma glucose concentrations. Via the negative feedback principle these online measurements of plasma glucose concentration provide the rationale for adjusting the glucose infusion rate and allow maintenance of the plasma glucose concentration at the target value. An exemplary sheet for the documentation of the time course of glucose infusion rates over a three-hour clamp experiment is provided in Table 4.4.

Although several computerised feedback algorithms have been published for the adjustment of the glucose infusion during glucose clamp experiments, many laboratories still prefer empirical adjustment of the glucose infusion rate. The first feedback algorithm for glucose control during a clamp was a simple linear function of the difference between the actual glucose concentration and the target glucose level (Andres et al. 1966). This first algorithm was imperfect and further algorithms were developed: for example, the DeFronzo algorithm,

Table 4.4   Example of a clamp sheet used to document plasma glucose concentration and time course of glucose infusion rates (GIR) during a three-hour clamp (Brehm et al. 2006)

Time	Plasma glucose concentration	Time of GIR change	GIR (ml/h)	Blood drawings	Insulin infusion rate
−15					
−10					
−5					
0					
5					
10					
15					
20					
25					
30					
35					
40					
45					
50					
55					
60					
65					
70					
75					
80					
85					
90					
95					
100					
105					
110					
115					

Time	Plasma glucose concentration	Time of GIR change	GIR (ml/h)	Blood drawings	Insulin infusion rate
120					
125					
130					
135					
140					
145					
150					
155					
160					
165					
170					
175					
180					

which provides glucose infusion rates accounting for the difference between the actual glucose concentration and the target value, and for changes in glucose utilisation (DeFronzo et al. 1979). Other and more complex algorithms based on mathematical models of glucose metabolism followed (for review see Bergman et al. 1985). However, for some of these algorithms reports indicated that manual overriding was necessary to achieve acceptable stability of glycaemia (Greenfield et al. 1981; Del Prato et al. 1983).

Most investigators use a glucose infusion with a glucose content of 20 % (weight per volume). Compared to a 10 % glucose infusion, the 20 % infusion is advantageous because of its lower volume, which can prevent unphysiological overhydration during the clamp experiment.

Plasma glucose concentration is typically determined at five minute intervals (DeFronzo et al. 1978, 1979; Ravussin et al. 1983; Bergman et al. 1985; Maggs et al. 1998), but ten minute intervals have also been successfully applied during glucose clamp experiments (Pacini et al. 1982; Finegood et al. 1984). However, there exists no systematic work on whether greater stability of plasma glucose concentration can be achieved with five or ten minute intervals of blood sampling.

From the five-minute interval between two measurements of plasma glucose concentration it is obvious that only rapid (~60 samples per hour) and precise devices for the measurement of glucose concentration enable the investigator to maintain near constant glycaemia. In addition, frequent calibration measurements with standardised solutions are required to guarantee valid and exact measurement of the glucose concentrations in plasma. Any delay between blood sampling, the measurement of plasma glucose concentration and the ensuing adjustment of the glucose infusion rate shortens the available time and glycaemic effect of the newly adapted glucose infusion rate. Insufficient time between the adjustment of the glucose infusion pump and the subsequent measurement of plasma glucose concentration leads to an underestimation of the effect of the infusion rate and complicates the achievement of steady state conditions during the clamp test. The success of clamping plasma glucose at the desired level can be judged in terms of accuracy (actual mean plasma glucose concentration divided by the desired level times 100) and stability (the coefficient of variation of plasma glucose concentration during the clamp test).

The glucose infusion rates required to maintain euglycaemia typically increase at least within ∼40 minutes from start of the insulin infusion. Much earlier and even sudden increases of the glucose requirements can be observed with primed continuous insulin infusion protocols or after changes in the insulin infusion rate during stepped hyperinsulinaemic clamp test protocols. In these cases, more experience with the performance of clamp experiments is needed to counteract rapid changes with adequate adjustment of the glucose infusion rate. The intensity and onset of insulin action also depend on the insulin dose administered and the individual's insulin sensitivity. When a primed continuous insulin infusion of 40 $mU \cdot m^2 \cdot min^{-1}$ is applied in healthy individuals, many investigators empirically start the glucose infusion four minutes after the start of the insulin infusion, with a rate of 2.0 $mg \cdot kg^{-1} \cdot min^{-1}$ (DeFronzo et al. 1979).

Blood sampling schedule

Blood samples for the determination of glucoregulatory hormones should be drawn before the start of the clamp test and frequently during the final period of the clamp experiment. Many investigators perform blood drawings for the determination of plasma insulin concentration at 10 minute intervals during the final hour of the clamp experiment. This allows one to prove the assumption of steady state hyperinsulinaemia during the period when glucose infusions rates are used to compute the M value.

Reproducibility of insulin sensitivity obtained from clamp tests

Studies on the reproducibility have been performed under several metabolic conditions including lean and obese as well as glucose tolerant and intolerant individuals (DeFronzo et al. 1979; Del Prato et al. 1986; Morris et al. 1997; Bokemark et al. 2000; Soop et al. 2000). The conclusive finding of these studies is that the M value obtained from the hyperinsulinaemic euglycaemic clamp test is a repeatable measure of insulin sensitivity. In these studies the time interval for the repetitive assessment of insulin sensitivity varied from two days to four weeks. The hyperinsulinaemic euglycaemic clamp technique was found to have a coefficient of repeatability of ∼0.85–1.0, which corresponds to an intraindividual coefficient of variation of ∼10 % (Del Prato et al. 1986; Morris et al. 1997; Bokemark et al. 2000; Soop et al. 2000).

Safety considerations for hyperinsulinaemiac euglycaemic clamp test

Hypoglycaemia

Hypoglycaemia and rapid falls of plasma glucose concentration must be avoided during hyperinsulinaemic euglycaemic clamp tests. Hypoglycaemia counterregulatory hormonal response induces posthypoglycaemic insulin resistance (Bolli et al. 1984; Attvall et al. 1987; Bischof et al. 2000) and jeopardises meaningful interpretation of the results. It is almost always necessary to continue glucose infusion after the end of the insulin infusion. The necessary duration and the glucose amount largely depend on the level of hyperinsulinaemia during the clamp and the insulin sensitivity of the individual. In any case, plasma glucose concentrations should be stable without exogenous glucose infusion before the venous catheters are removed and the participant is released.

Hypokalaemia

Hyperinsulinaemia stimulates the cellular uptake of potassium and may therefore result in hypokalemia through a compartmental shift of potassium. This is important since hypokalemia is proarrhythmic and may cause severe complications. Since hyperinsulinaemia decreases plasma potassium concentration dose dependently during the initial two hours, hypokalemia must always be expected when the insulin infusion results in supraphysiological hyperinsulinaemia (Minaker & Rowe 1982).

Interestingly, serum potassium concentration can spontaneously reincrease in the third hour after the start of the insulin infusion (Minaker & Rowe 1982). In order to avoid hypokalemia during hyperinsulinaemic clamp tests, serum potassium concentrations should be repeatedly checked during the first clamp experiments of a new protocol. In the case of supraphysiological hyperinsulinaemia, potassium should a priori be substituted intravenously during the clamp test. To avoid insulin induced hypokalemia, potassium was infused at a rate of 6 milli-equivalent per hour in several studies (Maggs et al. 1998; Hundal et al. 2002).

Modifications of the euglycaemic hyperinsulinaemic clamp test protocol

Nomenclature of glycaemic targets of clamp tests

In healthy subjects an insulin clamp performed at fasting plasma glucose concentration is termed an euglycaemic insulin clamp test. In general, when the target of plasma glucose concentration is above the fasting level, this is termed a hyperglycaemic insulin clamp test. The latter should not be mixed up with the hyperglycaemic glucose clamp test, which is performed without concomitant infusion of insulin and which can be used to assess endogenous insulin secretion in response to glucose (DeFronzo et al. 1979). In diabetic subjects exhibiting fasting hyperglycaemia, insulin clamps may also be performed at the individual fasting plasma glucose concentration, which is termed an isoglycaemic insulin clamp test. However, clamping plasma glucose at 90 or 100 mg/dl in patients with diabetes mellitus is termed an euglycaemic insulin clamp test.

Glucose clamp tests with the target of glucose concentration at or below 60 mg/dl are termed hypoglycaemic insulin clamp tests (DeFronzo & Ferrannini 1982; Fourest-Fontecave et al. 1987; Bischof et al. 2006). The hypoglycaemic insulin clamp test is typically used to assess hypoglycaemic counter regulation.

Pancreatic clamp tests

In order to achieve a maximal possible suppression of endogenous insulin, glucagon and growth hormone release during hyperinsulinaemic clamp tests, a concomitant infusion of somatostatin can be applied (Gottesman et al. 1982; Best et al. 1983; Basu et al. 2000). Glucose clamp tests applying an infusion of somatostatin are commonly referred to as pancreatic clamp tests. Most investigators start the somatostatin infusion a few minutes before or simultaneously with the start of the insulin infusion. The infusion rates of somatostatin vary largely throughout the literature, ranging from 250 µg per hour (Gottesman et al. 1982; Hawkins et al. 2002) to 360 µg per hour (Henriksen et al. 2000) to $0.1 \mu g \cdot kg^{-1} \cdot min^{-1}$ (Krssak et al. 2004). One frequently reported side effect of high dose somatostatin infusions is abdominal discomfort. The use of somatostatin can be advantageous when stimulation of endogenous insulin secretion by substrates or pharmacological agents is to be minimised. One should be aware that somatostatin may affect the rate of glucose utilisation by suppression of the secretion of glucagon and growth hormone or even by other mechanisms (Bergman et al. 1984).

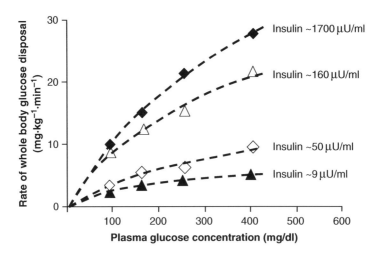

Figure 4.7 Whole body glucose disposal versus glucose concentration at different levels of plasma insulin during pancreatic insulin glucose clamp tests in young healthy subjects. Rates of whole body glucose disposal were measured by isotope dilution technique (glucose tracer) and are corrected for urinary glucose loss. Dashed lines represent best fit. Modified from Yki-Jarvinen et al. (1987).

Stepped hyperinsulinaemic glucose clamp tests

In order to assess whole body glucose metabolism under conditions where more than one insulin dose is given during a single clamp experiment, a stepped hyperinsulinaemic glucose clamp test protocol can be applied (Basu et al. 2000; Bavenholm et al. 2001; Miyazaki et al. 2001; Anderwald et al. 2002). Because each step of hyperinsulinaemia needs at least ~100 minutes to approximate steady state conditions, the total duration of the clamp experiment becomes a limiting factor. Two- or three-step hyperinsulinaemic glucose clamp tests are most commonly applied. In order to avoid carry over effects from the previous insulin infusion step, the experiments should be started with the lowest and end up with the highest insulin infusion rate. For example, the insulin infusion rates of a two-step hyperinsulinaemic glucose clamp test could be 40 mU·m^{-2}·min^{-1} during the first and 160 mU·m^{-2}·min^{-1} during the second step, whereby each step of the insulin infusion rate is maintained for at least 100 minutes. If the duration of each step of the insulin infusion rate is relatively short (i.e. ~100 min), one should apply a primed continuous insulin infusion for each step The advantage of these stepped hyperinsulinaemic clamp test protocols is that the investigator is able to obtain information on insulin action at the lower and upper end of the physiological range of insulin concentrations.

The oral glucose clamp technique

The oral glucose clamp technique (OG-clamp) can be used to non invasively estimate splanchnic glucose uptake after ingestion of an oral glucose load during an euglycemic hyperinsulinemic clamp (Ludvik et al. 1995). The ingestion of a glucose load during steady state conditions of a hyperinsulinaemic glucose clamp leads to a temporarily (~4 hr) reduction of the glucose infusion rates required to maintain constant glycaemia. After completion of the intestinal glucose resorption, glucose infusion rates return to values present before the ingestion of the glucose load. The temporary reduction of the glucose infusion rates during intestinal glucose resorption enables the investigator to estimate splanchnic glucose uptake during this period (Ludvik et al. 1995; Bajaj et al. 2003).

Conclusion

The M value obtained from the hyperinsulinaemic euglycaemic clamp test is a repeatable measure of insulin sensitivity with an intraindividual coefficient of variation of ~10%.

- Because the M value exhibits considerable inter-individual variability, no generally accepted cut-off values exist for the definition of insulin resistance. The inclusion of age and weight matched individuals serving as a control group is a necessity.
- The M value is frequently normalised for bodyweight (M_{bw}), fat free mass (M_{ffm}), rate of resting energy expenditure (M_{ree}) and steady state plasma insulin concentration during the clamp (M/I). The correction M_{ffm} is able to account for gender related differences in fat mass. Normalisation of the M value for bodyweight results in an underestimation of insulin sensitivity in obesity. M/I is more variable than the M value and therefore not beneficial.
- If endogenous glucose output is not zero during an insulin glucose clamp test, the glucose infusion rates do not reflect whole body glucose metabolism because the residual

endogenous output remains unaccounted for. Combining the insulin glucose clamp technique with glucose tracer dilution techniques provides the possibility of quantifying endogenous glucose output and resolves this problem.

- The standard insulin infusion rate during a hyperinsulinaemic euglycaemic clamp test is 40 mU·m^{-2}·min^{-1}, which corresponds to approximately 1 mU·kg^{-1}·min^{-1}. In obese individuals the insulin dose should be normalised for body surface area (i.e. 40 mU·m^{-2}·min^{-1}).
- In order to accelerate the achievement of a plateau of plasma insulin concentrations, primed continuous insulin infusion protocols should be applied.
- The heated hand technique for sampling arterialised blood should be applied during insulin glucose clamp experiments.
- Due to the lack of a perfect feedback algorithm for the adjustment of glucose infusion rates during an insulin glucose clamp test, many laboratories prefer the empirical adjustment of glucose infusion rates.
- Plasma glucose concentrations are typically determined at five-minute intervals during insulin glucose clamp tests, but ten-minute intervals have also been successfully applied.
- Blood for the determination of glucoregulatory hormones should be drawn before and frequently (at 10 minute intervals) during the final period of an insulin glucose clamp experiment.
- Hypoglycaemia and hypokalaemia must be avoided. During high dose insulin infusion, serum levels of potassium should be monitored and potassium should be substituted if necessary.

References

Anderson E A, Hoffman, R P, Balon, T W, Sinkey, C A and Mark, A L (1991) Hyperinsulinemia produces both sympathetic neural activation and vasodilation in normal humans, *J Clin Invest*, **87**, 6, 2246–2252

Anderwald, C, Bernroider, E, Krssak, M, Stingl, H, Brehm, A, Bischof, M G, Nowotny, P, Roden, M and Waldhäusl, W (2002) Effects of insulin treatment in type 2 diabetic patients on intracellular lipid content in liver and skeletal muscle, *Diabetes*, **51**, 10, 3025–3032

Andres, R, Swerdloff, R, Pozefsky, T and Coleman, D (1966) In: Skeggs, L T J (Ed) *Automation in Analytical Chemistry*, New York, Mediad, pp. 486–491

Attvall, S, Eriksson, B M, Fowelin, J, von Schenck, H, Lager, I and Smith, U (1987) Early posthypoglycemic insulin resistance in man is mainly an effect of beta-adrenergic stimulation, *J Clin Invest*, **80**, 2, 437–442

Bajaj, M, Berria, R, Pratipanawatr, T, Kashyap, S, Pratipanawatr, W, Belfort, R, Cusi, K, Mandarino, L and DeFronzo, R A (2002) Free fatty acid-induced peripheral insulin resistance augments splanchnic glucose uptake in healthy humans, *Am J Physiol Endocrinol Metab*, **283**, 2, E346–E352

Bajaj, M, Suraamornkul, S, Pratipanawatr, T, Hardies, L J, Pratipanawatr, W, Glass, L, Cersosimo, E, Miyazaki, Y and DeFronzo, R A (2003) Pioglitazone reduces hepatic fat content and augments splanchnic glucose uptake in patients with type 2 diabetes, *Diabetes*, **52**, 6, 1364–1370

Bajaj, M, Suraamornkul, S, Romanelli, A, Cline, G W, Mandarino, L J, Shulman, G I and DeFronzo, R A (2005) Effect of a sustained reduction in plasma free fatty acid concentration on intramuscular long-chain fatty Acyl-CoAs and insulin action in type 2 diabetic patients, *Diabetes*, **54**, 11, 3148–3153

Barzilai, N, Cohen, P, Karnieli, E, Enat, R, Epstein, O, Owen, J and McIntyre, N (1991) In: vivo insulin action in hepatocellular and cholestatic liver cirrhosis, *J Endocrinol Invest*, **14**, 9, 727–735

Basu, A, Basu, R, Shah, P, Vella, A, Johnson, C M, Nair, K S, Jensen, M D, Schwenk, W F and Rizza, R A (2000) Effects of type 2 diabetes on the ability of insulin and glucose to regulate splanchnic and muscle glucose metabolism: evidence for a defect in hepatic glucokinase activity, *Diabetes*, **49**, 2, 272–283

Basu, R, Basu, A, Johnson, C M, Schwenk, W F and Rizza, R A (2004) Insulin dose-response curves for stimulation of splanchnic glucose uptake and suppression of endogenous glucose production differ in nondiabetic humans and are abnormal in people with type 2 diabetes, *Diabetes*, **53**, 8, 2042–2050

Bavenholm, P N, Pigon, J, Ostenson, C G and Efendic, S (2001) Insulin sensitivity of suppression of endogenous glucose production is the single most important determinant of glucose tolerance, *Diabetes*, **50**, 6, 1449–1454

Bell, P M, Firth, R G and Rizza, R A (1986) Effects of hyperglycemia on glucose production and utilization in humans Measurement with [2^3H]-, [3^3H]-, and [6^{14}C]glucose, *Diabetes*, **35**, 6, 642–648

Bergman, R N (1977) Integrated control of hepatic glucose metabolism, *Fed Proc*, **36**, 2, 265–270

Bergman, R N (1989) Lilly lecture 1989 Toward physiological understanding of glucose tolerance Minimal-model approach, *Diabetes*, **38**, 12, 1512–1527

Bergman, R N, Ader, M, Finegood, D T and Pacini, G (1984) Extrapancreatic effect of somatostatin infusion to increase glucose clearance, *Am J Physiol*, **247**, 3 Pt 1, E370–379

Bergman, R N, Finegood, D T and Ader, M (1985) Assessment of insulin sensitivity in vivo, *Endocr Rev*, **6**, 1, 45–86

Bergman, R N, Ider, Y Z, Bowden, C R and Cobelli, C (1979) Quantitative estimation of insulin sensitivity, *Am J Physiol*, **236**, 6, E667–677

Bernroider, E, Brehm, A, Krssak, M, Anderwald, C, Trajanoski, Z, Cline, G, Shulman, G I and Roden, M (2005) The role of intramyocellular lipids during hypoglycemia in patients with intensively treated type 1 diabetes, *J Clin Endocrinol Metab*, **90**, 10, 5559–5565.

Best, J D, Beard, J C, Taborsky, G J, Jr, Halter, J B and Porte, D, Jr (1983) Effect of hyperglycemia per se on glucose disposal and clearance in noninsulin-dependent diabetics, *J Clin Endocrinol Metab*, **56**, 4, 819–823

Bischof, M G, Brehm, A, Bernroider, E, Krssak, M, Mlynarik, V, Krebs, M and Roden, M (2006) Cerebral glutamate metabolism during hypoglycaemia in healthy and type 1 diabetic humans, *Eur J Clin Invest*, **36**, 3, 164–169

Bischof, M G, Ludwig, C, Hofer, A, Kletter, K, Krebs, M, Stingl, H, Nowotny, P, Waldhausl, W and Roden, M (2000) Hormonal and metabolic counterregulation during and after high-dose insulin-induced hypoglycemia in diabetes mellitus type 2, *HormMetab Res*, **32**, 10, 417–423

Bjorntorp, P, Berchtold, P, Holm, J and Larsson, B (1971) The glucose uptake of human adipose tissue in obesity, *Eur J Clin Invest*, **1**, 6, 480–485

Björntorp, P and Sjostrom, L (1978) Carbohydrate storage in man: speculations and some quantitative considerations, *Metabolism*, **27**, 12 Suppl. 2, 1853–1865

Boden, G, Cheung, P, Stein, T P, Kresge, K and Mozzoli, M (2002) FFA cause hepatic insulin resistance by inhibiting insulin suppression of glycogenolysis, *Am J Physiol Endocrinol Metab*, **283**, 1, E12–E19

Boden, G, Lebed, B, Schatz, M, Homko, C and Lemieux, S (2001) Effects of acute changes of plasma free fatty acids on intramyocellular fat content and insulin resistance in healthy subjects, *Diabetes*, **50**, 7, 1612–1617

Bokemark, L, Froden, A, Attvall, S, Wikstrand, J and Fagerberg, B (2000) The euglycemic hyperinsulinemic clamp examination: variability and reproducibility, *Scand J Clin Lab Invest*, **60**, 1, 27–36

Bolli, G B, Gottesman, I S, Campbell, P J, Haymond, M W, Cryer, P E and Gerich, J E (1984) Glucose counterregulation and waning of insulin in the Somogyi phenomenon (posthypoglycemic hyperglycemia), *N Engl J Med*, **311**, 19, 1214–1219

Bonora, E, Moghetti, P, Zancanaro, C, Cigolini, M, Querena, M, Cacciatori, V, Corgnati, A and Muggeo, M (1989) Estimates of in vivo insulin action in man: comparison of insulin tolerance tests with euglycemic and hyperglycemic glucose clamp studies, *J Clin Endocrinol Metab*, **68**, 2, 374–378

Boyle, P J, Nagy, R J, O'Connor, A M, Kempers, S F, Yeo, R A and Qualls, C (1994) Adaptation in brain glucose uptake following recurrent hypoglycemia, *Proc Natl Acad Sci USA*, **91**, 20, 9352–9356

Brandi, L S, Santoro, D, Natali, A, Altomonte, F, Baldi, S, Frascerra, S and Ferrannini, E (1993) Insulin resistance of stress: sites and mechanisms, *Clin Sci (Lond)*, **85**, 5, 525–35

Brehm, A, Krssak, M, Schmid, A I, Nowotny, P, Waldhausl, W and Roden, M (2006) Increased lipid availability impairs insulin-stimulated ATP synthesis in human skeletal muscle, *Diabetes*, **55**, 1, 136–140

Butler, P C, Kryshak, E J, Schwenk, W F, Haymond, M W and Rizza, R A (1990) Hepatic and extrahepatic responses to insulin in NIDDM and nondiabetic humans Assessment in absence of artifact introduced by tritiated nonglucose contaminants, *Diabetes*, **39**, 2, 217–225

Campbell, P J, Mandarino, L J and Gerich, J E (1988) Quantification of the relative impairment in actions of insulin on hepatic glucose production and peripheral glucose uptake in non-insulin-dependent diabetes mellitus, *Metabolism*, **37**, 1, 15–21

Cherrington, A D (1999) Banting Lecture 1997 Control of glucose uptake and release by the liver in vivo, *Diabetes*, **48**, 5, 1198–1214

Christiansen, E, Vestergaard, H, Tibell, A, Hother-Nielsen, O, Holst, J J, Pedersen, O and Madsbad, S (1996) Impaired insulin-stimulated nonoxidative glucose metabolism in pancreas-kidney transplant recipients Dose-response effects of insulin on glucose turnover, *Diabetes*, **45**,9, 1267–1275

Cobelli, C and Toffolo, G (1990) Constant specific activity input allows reconstruction of endogenous glucose concentration in non-steady state, *Am J Physiol*, **258**, 6 Pt 1, E1037–E1040

Cohen, P, Harel, C, Bergman, R, Daoud, D, Pam, Z, Barzilai, N, Armoni, M and Karnieli, E (1990) Insulin resistance and acanthosis nigricans: evidence for a postbinding defect in vivo, *Metabolism*, **39**, 10, 1006–1011

Consoli, A (1992) Role of liver in pathophysiology of NIDDM, *Diabetes Care*, **15**, 3, 430–441

Creager, M A, Liang, C S and Coffman, J D (1985) Beta adrenergic-mediated vasodilator response to insulin in the human forearm, *J Pharmacol Exp Ther*, **235**, 3, 709–714

Creutzfeldt, W, Frerichs, H and Kneer, P (1974) Liver disease, insulin antagonism and diabetes mellitus, *Horm Metab Res*, Suppl. 4, 135–142

DeFronzo, R A 1988, Lilly lecture (1987) The triumvirate: beta-cell, muscle, liver A collusion responsible for NIDDM, *Diabetes*, **37**, 6, 667–687

DeFronzo, R A, Alvestrand, A, Smith, D, Hendler, R, Hendler, E and Wahren, J (1981) Insulin resistance in uremia, *J Clin Invest*, **67**, 2, 563–568

DeFronzo, R A and Ferrannini, E (1982) Influence of plasma glucose and insulin concentration on plasma glucose clearance in man, *Diabetes*, **31**, 8, 683–688

DeFronzo, R A, Ferrannini, E, Hendler, R, Felig, P and Wahren, J (1983) Regulation of splanchnic and peripheral glucose uptake by insulin and hyperglycemia in man, *Diabetes*, **32**, 1, 35–45

DeFronzo, R A, Ferrannini, E, Hendler, R, Wahren, J and Felig, P (1978) Influence of hyperinsulinemia, hyperglycemia, and the route of glucose administration on splanchnic glucose exchange, *Proc Natl Acad Sci USA*, **75**, 10, 5173–5177

DeFronzo, R A, Gunnarsson, R, Bjorkman, O, Olsson, M and Wahren, J (1985) Effects of insulin on peripheral and splanchnic glucose metabolism in noninsulin-dependent (type II) diabetes mellitus, *J Clin Invest*, **76**, 1, 149–155

DeFronzo, R A, Tobin, J D and Andres, R (1979) Glucose clamp technique: a method for quantifying insulin secretion and resistance, *Am J Physiol*, **237**, 3, E214–E223

Deibert, D C and DeFronzo, R A (1980) Epinephrine-induced insulin resistance in man, *J Clin Invest*, **65**, 3, 717–721

Del Prato, S (1999) Measurement of insulin resistance in vivo, *Drugs*, **58**, Suppl. 1, 3–6; 75–82

Del Prato, S, Ferrannini, E, and DeFronzo, R A (1986) Evaluation of insulin sensitivity in man In: Clarke, W L, Larner, W, Pohl, S L (Eds) *Methods in Diabetes Research Clinical Methods*, John Wiley & Sons, New York, pp. 35–76

Del Prato, S, Nosadini, R, Tiengo, A, Tessari, P, Avogaro, A, Trevisan, R, Valerio, A, Muggeo, M, Cobelli, C and Toffolo, G (1983) Insulin-mediated glucose disposal in type I diabetes: evidence for insulin resistance, *J Clin Endocrinol Metab*, **57**, 5, 904–910

Dinneen, S, Gerich, J and Rizza, R (1992) Carbohydrate metabolism in non-insulin-dependent diabetes mellitus, *N Engl J Med*, **327**, 10, 707–713

Doberne, L, Greenfield, M S, Rosenthal, M, Widstrom, A and Reaven, G (1982) Effect of variations in basal plasma glucose concentration on glucose utilization (M) and metabolic clearance (MCR) rates during insulin clamp studies in patients with non-insulin-dependent diabetes mellitus, *Diabetes*, **31**, 5, 396–400

Ekberg, K, Landau, B R, Wajngot, A, Chandramouli, V, Efendic, S, Brunengraber, H and Wahren, J (1999) Contributions by kidney and liver to glucose production in the postabsorptive state and after 60 h of fasting, *Diabetes*, **48**, 2, 292–298

Felber, J P, Ferrannini, E, Golay, A, Meyer, H U, Theibaud, D, Curchod, B, Maeder, E, Jequier, E and DeFronzo, R A (1987) Role of lipid oxidation in pathogenesis of insulin resistance of obesity and type II diabetes, *Diabetes*, **36**, 11, 1341–50

Ferrannini, E, Barrett, E J, Bevilacqua, S and DeFronzo, R A (1983) Effect of fatty acids on glucose production and utilization in man, *J Clin Invest*, **72**, 5, 1737–1747

Ferrannini, E and Mari, A (1998) How to measure insulin sensitivity, *J Hypertens*, **16**, 7, 895–906

Ferrannini, E, Natali, A, Bell, P, Cavallo-Perin, P, Lalic, N and Mingrone, G (1997) Insulin resistance and hypersecretion in obesity European Group for the Study of Insulin Resistance (EGIR), *J Clin Invest*, **100**, 5, 1166–1173

Finegood, D T, Bergman, R N and Vranic, M (1987) Estimation of endogenous glucose production during hyperinsulinemic-euglycemic glucose clamps Comparison of unlabeled and labeled exogenous glucose infusates, *Diabetes*, **36**, 8, 914–924

Finegood, D T, Pacini, G and Bergman, R N (1984) The insulin sensitivity index Correlation in dogs between values determined from the intravenous glucose tolerance test and the euglycemic glucose clamp, *Diabetes*, **33**, 4, 362–8

Fink, R I, Kolterman, O G, Griffin, J and Olefsky, J M (1983) Mechanisms of insulin resistance in aging, *J Clin Invest*, **71**, 6, 1523–1535

Fourest-Fontecave, S, Adamson, U, Lins, P E, Ekblom, B, Sandahl, C and Strand, L (1987) Mental alertness in response to hypoglycaemia in normal man: the effect of 12 hours and 72 hours of fasting, *Diabetes Metab*, **13**, 4, 405–410

Gastaldelli, A, Toschi, E, Pettiti, M, Frascerra, S, Quinones-Galvan, A, Sironi, A M, Natali, A and Ferrannini, E (2001) Effect of physiological hyperinsulinemia on gluconeogenesis in nondiabetic subjects and in type 2 diabetic patients, *Diabetes*, **50**, 8, 1807–1812

Gelfand, R A and Barrett, E J (1987) Effect of physiologic hyperinsulinemia on skeletal muscle protein synthesis and breakdown in man, *J Clin Invest*, **80**, 1, 1–6

Gerich, J E (2000) Physiology of glucose homeostasis 1, *Diabetes Obes Metab*, **2**, 6, 345–350

Giacca, A, McCall, R, Chan, B and Shi, Z Q (1999) Increased dependence of glucose production on peripheral insulin in diabetic depancreatized dogs, *Metabolism*, **48**, 2, 153–160

Gottesman, I, Mandarino, L, Verdonk, C, Rizza, R and Gerich, J (1982) Insulin increases the maximum velocity for glucose uptake without altering the Michaelis constant in man Evidence that insulin increases glucose uptake merely by providing additional transport sites, *J Clin Invest*, **70**, 6, 1310–1314

Greenfield, M S, Doberne, L, Kraemer, F, Tobey, T and Reaven, G (1981) Assessment of insulin resistance with the insulin suppression test and the euglycemic clamp, *Diabetes*, **30**, 5, 387–392

Haffner, S M, Miettinen, H and Stern, M P (1997) The homeostasis model in the San Antonio Heart Study, *Diabetes Care*, **20**, 7, 1087–1092

Hagstrom-Toft, E, Arner, P, Johansson, U, Eriksson, L S, Ungerstedt, U and Bolinder, J (1992) Effect of insulin on human adipose tissue metabolism in situ. Interactions with beta-adrenoceptors, *Diabetologia*, **35**, 7, 664–670.

Hawkins, M, Gabriely, I, Wozniak, R, Reddy, K, Rossetti, L and Shamoon, H (2002) Glycemic control determines hepatic and peripheral glucose effectiveness in type 2 diabetic subjects, *Diabetes*, **51**, 7, 2179–2189

Henriksen, J E, Levin, K, Thye-Ronn, P, Alford, F, Hother-Nielsen, O, Holst, J J and Beck-Nielsen, H (2000) Glucose-mediated glucose disposal in insulin-resistant normoglycemic relatives of type 2 diabetic patients, *Diabetes*, **49**, 7, 1209–1218

Himsworth, H P (1936) Diabetes mellitus: Its differentiation into insulin-sensitive and insulin-insensitive types, *Lancet*, **1**, 1, 127–30

Himsworth, H P and Kerr, R B (1939) Insulin-sensitive and insulin-insensitive types of diabetes mellitus, *Clin Sci*, **4**, 119–152

Horgaard, A and Thayssen, T E H (1929) Clinical investigation into the effect of the intravenous injection of insulin, *Acta Med Scand*, **72**, 92–95

Horton, E S, Johnson, C and Lebovitz, H E (1968) Carbohydrate metabolism in uremia, *Ann Intern Med*, **68**, 1, 63–74

Hother-Nielsen, O, Henriksen, J E, Holst, J J and Beck-Nielsen, H (1996) Effects of insulin on glucose turnover rates in vivo: isotope dilution versus constant specific activity technique, *Metabolism*, **45**, 1, 82–91

Howard, B V, Klimes, I, Vasquez, B, Brady, D, Nagulesparan, M and Unger, R H (1984) The antipolytic action of insulin in obese subjects with resistance to its glucoregulatory action, *J Clin Endocrinol Metab*, **58**, 3, 544–548

Hundal, R S, Petersen, K F, Mayerson, A B, Randhawa, P S, Inzucchi, S, Shoelson, S E and Shulman, G I (2002) Mechanism by which high-dose aspirin improves glucose metabolism in type 2 diabetes, *J Clin Invest*, **109**, 10, 1321–1326

Insel, P A, Liljenquist, J E, Tobin, J D, Sherwin, R S, Watkins, P, Andres, R and Berman, M (1975) Insulin control of glucose metabolism in man: a new kinetic analysis, *J Clin Invest*, **55**, 51057–1066

Kahn, C R (1978) Insulin resistance, insulin insensitivity, and insulin unresponsiveness: a necessary distinction, *Metabolism*, **27**, 12 Suppl. 2, 1893–1902

Karam, J H, Grodsky, G M and Forsham, P H (1963) Excessive insulin response to glucose in obese subjects as measured by immunochemical assay, *Diabetes*, **12**, 197–204

Katz, A, Nambi, S S, Mather, K, Baron, A D, Follmann, D A, Sullivan, G and Quon, M J (2000) Quantitative insulin sensitivity check index: a simple, accurate method for assessing insulin sensitivity in humans, *J Clin Endocrinol Metab*, **85**, 7, 2402–2410

Knuuti, M J, Nuutila, P, Ruotsalainen, U, Saraste, M, Harkonen, R, Ahonen, A, Teras, M, Haaparanta, M, Wegelius, U, Haapanen, A and et al (1992) Euglycemic hyperinsulinemic clamp and oral glucose load in stimulating myocardial glucose utilization during positron emission tomography, *J Nucl Med*, **33**, 7, 1255–1262

Kolterman, O G, Gray, R S, Griffin, J, Burstein, P, Insel, J, Scarlett, J A and Olefsky, J M (1981) Receptor and postreceptor defects contribute to the insulin resistance in noninsulin-dependent diabetes mellitus, *J Clin Invest*, **68**, 4, 957–969

Kolterman, O G, Insel, J, Saekow, M and Olefsky, J M (1980) Mechanisms of insulin resistance in human obesity: evidence for receptor and postreceptor defects, *J Clin Invest*, **65**, 6, 1272–1284

Kraegen, E W, Lazarus, L and Campbell, L V (1983) Failure of insulin infusion during euglycemia to influence endogenous basal insulin secretion, *Metabolism*, **32**, 6, 622–627

Krebs, M, Krssak, M, Nowotny, P, Weghuber, D, Gruber, S, Mlynarik, V, Bischof, M, Stingl, H, Fürnsinn, C, Waldhäusl, W and Roden, M (2001) Free fatty acids inhibit the glucose-stimulated increase of intramuscular glucose-6–phosphate concentration in humans, *J Clin Endocrinol Metab*, **86**, 5, 2153–2160

Krssak, M, Brehm, A, Bernroider, E, Anderwald, C, Nowotny, P, Man, C D, Cobelli, C, Cline, G W, Shulman, G I, Waldhäusl, W and Roden, M (2004) Alterations in postprandial hepatic glycogen metabolism in type 2 diabetes, *Diabetes*, **53**, 12, 3048–3056

Laakso, M, Edelman, S V, Brechtel, G and Baron, A D (1990) Decreased effect of insulin to stimulate skeletal muscle blood flow in obese man A novel mechanism for insulin resistance, *J Clin Invest*, **85**, 6, 1844–1852

Lewis, G F, Vranic, M and Giacca, A (1998) Role of free fatty acids and glucagon in the peripheral effect of insulin on glucose production in humans, *Am J Physiol*, **275**, 1, E177–E186

Lewis, G F, Zinman, B, Groenewoud, Y, Vranic, M and Giacca, A (1996) Hepatic glucose production is regulated both by direct hepatic and extrahepatic effects of insulin in humans, *Diabetes*, **45**, 4, 454–462

Lind, T (1979) Metabolic changes in pregnancy relevant to diabetes mellitus, *Postgrad Med J*, **55**, 643, 353–357

Ludvik, B, Nolan, J J, Roberts, A, Baloga, J, Joyce, M, Bell, J M and Olefsky, J M (1995) A noninvasive method to measure splanchnic glucose uptake after oral glucose administration, *J Clin Invest*, **95**, 5, 2232–2238

Maggs, D G, Jacob, R, Rife, F, Lange, R, Leone, P, During, M J, Tamborlane, W V and Sherwin, R S (1995) Interstitial fluid concentrations of glycerol, glucose, and amino acids in human quadricep muscle and adipose tissue. Evidence for significant lipolysis in skeletal muscle, *J Clin Invest*, **96**, 1,370–377.

Maggs, D G, Buchanan, T A, Burant, C F, Cline, G, Gumbiner, B, Hsueh, W A, Inzucchi, S, Kelley, D, Nolan, J, Olefsky, J M, Polonsky, K S, Silver, D, Valiquett, T R and Shulman, G I (1998) Metabolic effects of troglitazone monotherapy in type 2 diabetes mellitus A randomized, double-blind, placebo-controlled trial, *Ann Intern Med*, **128**, 3, 176–185

Mandarino, L J, Campbell, P J, Gottesman, I S and Gerich, J E (1984) Abnormal coupling of insulin receptor binding in noninsulin-dependent diabetes, *Am J Physiol*, **247**, 5, E688–692

Mari, A, Pacini, G, Murphy, E, Ludvik, B and Nolan, J J (2001) A model-based method for assessing insulin sensitivity from the oral glucose tolerance test, *Diabetes Care*, **24**, 3, 539–548

Matsuda, M and DeFronzo, R A (1999) Insulin sensitivity indices obtained from oral glucose tolerance testing: comparison with the euglycemic insulin clamp, *Diabetes Care*, **22**, 9, 1462–1470

Matsumoto, K, Miyake, S, Yano, M, Ueki, Y, Yamaguchi, Y, Akazawa, S and Tominaga, Y (1997) Glucose tolerance, insulin secretion, and insulin sensitivity in nonobese and obese Japanese subjects, *Diabetes Care*, **20**, 10, 1562–1568

Matthews, D R, Hosker, J P, Rudenski, A S, Naylor, B A, Treacher, D F and Turner, R C (1985) Homeostasis model assessment: insulin resistance and beta-cell function from fasting plasma glucose and insulin concentrations in man, *Diabetologia*, **28**, 7, 412–419

McCall, R H, Wiesenthal, S R, Shi, Z Q, Polonsky, K and Giacca, A (1998) Insulin acutely suppresses glucose production by both peripheral and hepatic effects in normal dogs, *Am J Physiol*, **274**, 2, E346–E356

McGuire, E A, Helderman, J H, Tobin, J D, Andres, R and Berman, M (1976) Effects of arterial versus venous sampling on analysis of glucose kinetics in man, *J Appl Physiol*, **41**, 4, 565–573

Minaker, K L and Rowe, J W (1982) Potassium homeostasis during hyperinsulinemia: effect of insulin level, beta-blockade, and age, *Am J Physiol*, **242**, 6, E373–377

Miyamoto, I, Miyakoshi, H, Nagai, Y, Ohsawa, K, Nishimura, Y, Noto, Y and Kobayashi, K (1992) Characterization of the insulin resistance in liver cirrhosis: a comparison with non-insulin dependent diabetes mellitus, *Endocrinol Jpn*, **39**, 5, 421–429

Miyazaki, Y, Mahankali, A, Matsuda, M, Glass, L, Mahankali, S, Ferrannini, E, Cusi, K, Mandarino, L J and DeFronzo, R A (2001) Improved glycemic control and enhanced insulin sensitivity in type 2 diabetic subjects treated with pioglitazone, *Diabetes Care*, **24**, 4, 710–719

Morris, A D, Ueda, S, Petrie, J R, Connell, J M, Elliott, H L and Donnelly, R (1997) The euglycaemic hyperinsulinaemic clamp: an evaluation of current methodology, *Clin Exp Pharmacol Physiol*, **24**, 7, 513–518

Natali, A, Gastaldelli, A, Camastra, S, Sironi, A M, Toschi, E, Masoni, A, Ferrannini, E and Mari, A (2000) Dose-response characteristics of insulin action on glucose metabolism: a non-steady-state approach, *Am J Physiol Endocrinol Metab*, **278**, 5, E794–801

Nauck, M A, Blietz, R W and Qualmann, C (1996) Comparison of hyperinsulinaemic clamp experiments using venous, 'arterialized' venous or capillary euglycaemia, *Clin Physiol*, **16**, 6, 589–602

Nosadini, R, Del Prato, S, Tiengo, A, Valerio, A, Muggeo, M, Opocher, G, Mantero, F, Duner, E, Marescotti, C, Mollo, F and Belloni, F (1983) Insulin resistance in Cushing's syndrome, *J Clin Endocrinol Metab*, **57**, 3, 529–536

Nurjhan, N, Campbell, P J, Kennedy, F P, Miles, J M and Gerich, J E (1986) Insulin dose-response characteristics for suppression of glycerol release and conversion to glucose in humans, *Diabetes*, **35**, 12, 1326–1331

Olefsky, J M and Kolterman, O G (1981) Mechanisms of insulin resistance in obesity and noninsulin-dependent (type II) diabetes, *Am J Med*, **70**, 1, 151–168

Pacini, G, Finegood, D T and Bergman, R N (1982) A minimal-model-based glucose clamp yielding insulin sensitivity independent of glycemia, *Diabetes*, **31**, 5, 432–441

Perseghin, G, Ghosh, S, Gerow, K and Shulman, G I (1997) Metabolic defects in lean nondiabetic offspring of NIDDM parents: a cross-sectional study, *Diabetes*, **46**, 6, 1001–1009

Petersen, K F, Dufour, S and Shulman, G I (2005) Decreased Insulin-Stimulated ATP Synthesis and Phosphate Transport in Muscle of Insulin-Resistant Offspring of Type 2 Diabetic Parents, *PLoS Med*, **2**, 9, E233

Prager, R, Kovarik, J, Schernthaner, G, Woloszczuk, W and Willvonseder, R (1983) Peripheral insulin resistance in primary hyperparathyroidism, *Metabolism*, **32**, 8, 800–805

Prager, R, Wallace, P and Olefsky, J M (1987) Direct and indirect effects of insulin to inhibit hepatic glucose output in obese subjects, *Diabetes*, **36**, 5, 607–611

Pratipanawatr, W, Pratipanawatr, T, Cusi, K, Berria, R, Adams, J M, Jenkinson, C P, Maezono, K, DeFronzo, R A and Mandarino, L J (2001) Skeletal muscle insulin resistance in normoglycemic subjects with a strong family history of type 2 diabetes is associated with decreased insulin-stimulated insulin receptor substrate-1 tyrosine phosphorylation, *Diabetes*, **50**, 11, 2572–2578

Proietto, J, Nankervis, A, Aitken, P, Dudley, F J, Caruso, G and Alford, F P (1984) Insulin resistance in cirrhosis: evidence for a post-receptor defect, *Clin Endocrinol (Oxf)*, **21**, 6, 677–88

Ravussin, E, Bogardus, C, Schwartz, R S, Robbins, D C, Wolfe, R R, Horton, E S, Danforth, E, Jr and Sims, E A (1983) Thermic effect of infused glucose and insulin in man Decreased response with increased insulin resistance in obesity and noninsulin-dependent diabetes mellitus, *J Clin Invest*, **72**, 3, 893–902

Reaven, G and Miller, R (1968) Study of the relationship between glucose and insulin responses to an oral glucose load in man, *Diabetes*, **17**, 9, 560–569

Revers, R R, Fink, R, Griffin, J, Olefsky, J M and Kolterman, O G (1984a) Influence of hyperglycemia on insulin's in vivo effects in type II diabetes 1, *J Clin Invest*, **73**, 3, 664–672

Revers, R R, Kolterman, O G, Scarlett, J A, Gray, R S and Olefsky, J M (1984b) Lack of in vivo insulin resistance in controlled insulin-dependent, type I, diabetic patients, *J Clin Endocrinol Metab*, **58**, 2, 353–358

Riggio, O, Merli, M, Cangiano, C, Capocaccia, R, Cascino, A, Lala, A, Leonetti, F, Mauceri, M, Pepe, M, Rossi Fanelli, F, Savioli, M, Tamburrano, G and Capocaccia, L (1982) Glucose intolerance in liver cirrhosis, *Metabolism*, **31**, 6, 627–634

Rizza, R A, Mandarino, L J and Gerich, J E (1981a) Dose-response characteristics for effects of insulin on production and utilization of glucose in man, *Am J Physiol*, **240**, 6, E630–E639

Rizza, R A, Mandarino, L J and Gerich, J E (1981b) Mechanism and significance of insulin resistance in non-insulin-dependent diabetes mellitus, *Diabetes*, **30**, 12, 990–995

Rizza, R A, Mandarino, L J and Gerich, J E (1981c) Mechanisms of insulin resistance in man Assessment using the insulin dose-response curve in conjunction with insulin-receptor binding, *Am J Med*, **70**, 1, 169–176

Rizza, R A, Mandarino, L J and Gerich, J E (1982) Cortisol-induced insulin resistance in man: impaired suppression of glucose production and stimulation of glucose utilization due to a postreceptor detect of insulin action, *J Clin Endocrinol Metab*, **54**, 1, 131–138

Robert, J J, Magre, J, Reynet, C, Darmaun, D, Picard, J and Capeau, J (1990) In: vivo and in vitro characterization of insulin resistance in three cases of lipoatrophic diabetes, *Diabete Metab*, **16**, 3, 240–247

Robert, J J, Rakotoambinina, B, Cochet, I, Foussier, V, Magre, J, Darmaun, D, Chevenne, D and Capeau, J (1993) The development of hyperglycaemia in patients with insulin-resistant generalized lipoatrophic syndromes, *Diabetologia*, **36**, 12, 1288–1292

Roden, M, Perseghin, G, Petersen, K F, Hwang, J H, Cline, G W, Gerow, K, Rothman, D L and Shulman, G I (1996a) The roles of insulin and glucagon in the regulation of hepatic glycogen synthesis and turnover in humans, *J Clin Invest*, **97**, 3, 642–648

Roden, M, Price, T B, Perseghin, G, Petersen, K F, Rothman, D L, Cline, G W and Shulman, G I (1996b) Mechanism of free fatty acid-induced insulin resistance in humans, *J Clin Invest*, **97**, 12, 2859–2865

Roden, M and Shulman, G I (1999) Applications of NMR spectroscopy to study muscle glycogen metabolism in man, *Annu Rev Med*, **50**, 277–290

Rothman, D L, Shulman, R G and Shulman, G I (1992) 31P nuclear magnetic resonance measurements of muscle glucose-6-phosphate Evidence for reduced insulin-dependent muscle glucose transport or phosphorylation activity in non-insulin-dependent diabetes mellitus, *J Clin Invest*, **89**, 4, 1069–1075

Rowe, J W, Minaker, K L, Pallotta, J A and Flier, J S (1983) Characterization of the insulin resistance of aging, *J Clin Invest*, **71**, 6, 1581–1587

Ryan, E A, O'Sullivan, M J and Skyler, J S (1985) Insulin action during pregnancy Studies with the euglycemic clamp technique, *Diabetes*, **34**, 4, 380–389

Schmitz, O (1988) Peripheral and hepatic resistance to insulin and hepatic resistance to glucagon in uraemic subjects Studies at physiologic and supraphysiologic hormone levels, *Acta Endocrinol (Copenh)*, **118**, 1, 125–34

Seltzer, H S, Allen, E W, Herron, A L, Jr and Brennan, M T (1967) Insulin secretion in response to glycemic stimulus: relation of delayed initial release to carbohydrate intolerance in mild diabetes mellitus, *J Clin Invest*, **46**, 3, 323–335

Seppala-Lindroos, A, Vehkavaara, S, Hakkinen, A M, Goto, T, Westerbacka, J, Sovijarvi, A, Halavaara, J and Yki-Jarvinen, H (2002) Fat accumulation in the liver is associated with defects in insulin suppression of glucose production and serum free fatty acids independent of obesity in normal men, *J Clin Endocrinol Metab*, **87**, 7, 3023–3028

Shapiro, E T, Cooper, M, Chen, C T, Given, B D and Polonsky, K S (1990) Change in hexose distribution ume and fractional utilization of [18F]-2-deoxy-2-fluoro-D-glucose in brain during acute hypoglycemia in humans, *Diabetes*, **39**, 2, 175–180

Shen, S W, Reaven, G M and Farquhar, J W (1970) Comparison of impedance to insulin-mediated glucose uptake in normal subjects and in subjects with latent diabetes, *J Clin Invest*, **49**, 12, 2151–2160

Sherwin, R S, Kramer, K J, Tobin, J D, Insel, P A, Liljenquist, J E, Berman, M and Andres, R (1974) A model of the kinetics of insulin in man, *J Clin Invest*, **53**, 5, 1481–1492

Shulman, G I, Rothman, D L, Jue, T, Stein, P, DeFronzo, R A and Shulman, R G (1990) Quantitation of muscle glycogen synthesis in normal subjects and subjects with non-insulin-dependent diabetes by 13C nuclear magnetic resonance spectroscopy, *N Engl J Med*, **322**, 4, 223–228

Simonson, D C and DeFronzo, R A (1983) Glucagon physiology and aging: evidence for enhanced hepatic sensitivity, *Diabetologia*, **25**, 1, 1–7

Singhal, P, Caumo, A, Carey, P E, Cobelli, C and Taylor, R (2002) Regulation of endogenous glucose production after a mixed meal in type 2 diabetes, *Am J Physiol Endocrinol Metab*, **283**, 2, E275–E283

Soerjodibroto, W S, Heard, C R and Exton-Smith, A N (1979) Glucose tolerance, plasma insulin levels and insulin sensitivity in elderly patients, *Age Ageing*, **8**, 2, 65–74

Soop, M, Nygren, J, Brismar, K, Thorell, A and Ljungqvist, O (2000) The hyperinsulinaemic-euglycaemic glucose clamp: reproducibility and metabolic effects of prolonged insulin infusion in healthy subjects, *Clin Sci (Lond)*, **98**, 4, 367–374

Staehr, P, Hother-Nielsen, O, Levin, K, Holst, J J and Beck-Nielsen, H (2001) Assessment of hepatic insulin action in obese type 2 diabetic patients, *Diabetes*, **50**, 6, 1363–1370

Staten, M, Worcester, B, Szekeres, A, Waldeck, N, Ascher, M, Walsh, K M, Rizza, R, Gerich, J and Charles, M A (1984) Comparison of porcine and semisynthetic human insulins using euglycemic clamp-derived glucose-insulin dose-response curves in insulin-dependent diabetes, *Metabolism*, **33**, 2, 132–135

Steele, R (1959) Influences of glucose loading and of injected insulin on hepatic glucose output, *Annals New York Academy of Sciences*, **82**, 420–430

Steele, R, Wall, J S, De Bodo, R C and Altsulzer, N (1956) Measurement of size and turnover rate of body glucose pool by the isotope dilution method, *Am J Physiol Endocrinol Metab*, **187**, 15–24

Steil, G M, Murray, J, Bergman, R N and Buchanan, T A (1994) Repeatability of insulin sensitivity and glucose effectiveness from the minimal model Implications for study design, *Diabetes*, **43**, 11, 1365–1371

Stuart, C A, Shangraw, R E, Prince, M J, Peters, E J and Wolfe, R R (1988) Bed-rest-induced insulin resistance occurs primarily in muscle, *Metabolism*, **37**, 8, 802–806

Thiebaud, D, Schutz, Y, Acheson, K, Jacot, E, DeFronzo, R A, Felber, J P and Jequier, E (1983) Energy cost of glucose storage in human subjects during glucose-insulin infusions, *Am J Physiol*, **244**, 3, E216–221

Toft-Nielsen, M B, Damholt, M B, Madsbad, S, Hilsted, L M, Hughes, T E, Michelsen, B K and Holst, J J (2001) Determinants of the impaired secretion of glucagon-like peptide-1 in type 2 diabetic patients, *J Clin Endocrinol Metab*, **86**, 8, 3717–3723

Virtanen, K A, Lonnroth, P, Parkkola, R, Peltoniemi, P, Asola, M, Viljanen, T, Tolvanen, T, Knuuti, J, Ronnemaa, T, Huupponen, R and Nuutila, P (2002) Glucose uptake and perfusion in subcutaneous and visceral adipose tissue during insulin stimulation in nonobese and obese humans, *J Clin Endocrinol Metab*, **87**, 8, 3902–3910

Waldhausl, W, Bratusch-Marrain, P, Gasic, S, Korn, A and Nowotny, P (1982) Insulin production rate, hepatic insulin retention and splanchnic carbohydrate metabolism after oral glucose ingestion in hyperinsulinaemic Type 2 (non-insulin-dependent) diabetes mellitus, *Diabetologia*, **23**, 1, 6–15

Waldhäusl, W K (1993) In: Belfiore, F, Bergman, R, Molinatti, G M (Eds) *Frontiers in Diabetes: Current topics in Diabetes Research: The Glucose Clamp Technique* 12 Edn, Karger, S, Basel, pp. 24–31

Wallace, T M, Levy, J C and Matthews, D R (2004) Use and abuse of HOMA modeling, *Diabetes Care*, **27**, 6, 1487–1495

Yalow, R S and Berson, S A (1960a) Immunoassay of endogenous plasma insulin in man, *J Clin Invest*, **39**, 1157–1175

Yalow, R S and Berson, S A (1960b) Plasma insulin concentrations in nondiabetic and early diabetic subjects Determinations by a new sensitive immuno-assay technic, *Diabetes*, **9**, 254–260

Yasuda, K, Hines, E, 3rd and Kitabchi, A E (1982) Hypercortisolism and insulin resistance: comparative effects of prednisone, hydrocortisone, and dexamethasone on insulin binding of human erythrocytes, *J Clin Endocrinol Metab*, **55**, 5, 910–915

Yki-Jarvinen, H and Koivisto, V A (1983) Effects of body composition on insulin sensitivity, *Diabetes*, **32**, 10, 965–969

Yki-Jarvinen, H and Koivisto, V A (1984) Continuous subcutaneous insulin infusion therapy decreases insulin resistance in type 1 diabetes, *J Clin Endocrinol Metab*, **58**, 4, 659–666

Yki-Jarvinen, H, Young, A A, Lamkin, C and Foley, J E (1987) Kinetics of glucose disposal in whole body and across the forearm in man, *J Clin Invest*, **79**, 6, 1713–1719

Zierler, K (1999) Whole body glucose metabolism, *Am J Physiol*, **276**, 3, E409–E426

5

Methods of Assessment of Counterregulation to Hypoglycaemia

Pratik Choudhary, Ming Ming Teh and Stephanie A Amiel

Introduction

Hypoglycaemia – literally low blood glucose concentration – occurs infrequently in health but becomes a clinical problem in rare conditions of defective glucose storage or insulin secretion; occasional extremes of human behaviour; rather more common defects in secretion of hyperglycaemic hormones; and most commonly as the result of drug treatment, particularly drug treatment for diabetes mellitus. Iatrogenic hypoglycaemia was first observed in de-pancreatised dogs given pancreatic extracts by Banting and Best during the experiments in which they isolated the glucose-lowering ingredient from the pancreas.(Banting et al. 1923). As insulin came to be used clinically, iatrogenic hypoglycaemia became a common event and recent studies using modern methods of continuous interstitial tissue glucose assessment suggest that up to 70 % of children with type 1 diabetes may have asymptomatic biochemical hypoglycaemia on at least one out of three nights (Kaufman et al. 2002). In adults, 60% of those with short duration of disease and over 80% of those with type 1 diabetes for more than 15 years have interstitial glucose of less than 3.0 mmol/l at least once a week. The equivalent numbers for those with type 2 diabetes are between 20 and 22 % (UK Hypoglycaemia Study Group 2006). These startling statistics are independent of current policies to control blood glucose tightly in diabetes, in order to minimise risk of vascular complications (DCCT 2000; Nathan et al. 2005), which at least in some settings have been associated with a further increase in risk of both symptomatic and severe hypoglycaemia (DCCT 1991, 1993), although intensive education programmes can reduce this. (DAFNE group 2002, 2003; Samann et al. 2005.)

Hypoglycaemia is important because it is associated with fuel deprivation of vital organs, including the brain, which begins to show detectable malfunction at a plasma glucose of around 3 mmol/l, progressing to confusion, disinhibition, reduced conscious level, coma and seizure.

Clinical Diabetes Research: Methods and Techniques   Edited by Michael Roden
© 2007 John Wiley & Sons, Ltd   ISBN 978-0-470-01728-9

Spontaneous hypoglycaemia can present clinically in a variety of ways. Diagnosis of hormone deficiencies such as cortisol and growth hormone may be made on other grounds but must be excluded in the diagnosis. Recurrent hypoglycaemia due to insulin or IGF-secreting tumours may present after months or sometimes years of episodic confusion. Iatrogenic hypoglycaemia may present initially as episodic occurrence of symptoms related to the stress response and stimulation of hunger, which are typical physiological responses to a falling blood glucose concentration, but may later progress to episodes of cognitive impairment and confusion, or even coma and seizure. Iatrogenic hypoglycaemia impacts heavily on the well-being, productivity and quality of life of people with diabetes (Davis et al. 2005) and can sometimes affect performance in the workplace, with impact on employment (Leckie et al. 2005). Fear of hypoglycaemia leads people with diabetes to take sometimes deleterious avoidance activities and people without diabetes to impose restrictions on those perceived at highest risk (DVLA; Pramming et al. 1991; The council of the European Communities 1991).

Rarely, hypoglycaemia can be fatal. Up to 6 % of deaths in patients under 40 with type 1 diabetes are attributed to hypoglycaemia (Sovik & Thordarson 1999), with at least some cases thought to be due to cardiac arrhythmias rather than brain dysfunction; the so-called 'dead in bed syndrome' (Heller 2002). Indeed, fear of hypoglycaemia is an important barrier in achieving tight glucose targets (Cryer et al. 1989). Hypoglycaemia is also a costly condition. The cost of treating a single episode of severe hypoglycaemia has been calculated to be about £380 (Leese et al. 2003), and a German study calculated the cumulative cost of treating severe hypoglycaemia to be US$44,3800/100,000 population (Holstein et al. 2002).

It follows that avoidance of severe hypoglycaemia is a very important clinical target. In order to achieve this, particularly in diabetes therapy, we need to be able to define hypogly-caemia; quantify it clinically; understand the normal physiology of glucose counterregulation, which usually maintains blood glucose concentrations within a very narrow physiological range; understand what goes wrong with these systems in diabetes; and investigate what factors may make particular individuals particularly susceptible to severe hypoglycaemia. This chapter describes the techniques available to investigate hypoglycaemia and counter-regulation to it.

Definitions

We have defined hypoglycaemia by translating it as 'low blood glucose concentration'. Clinically, episodes of hypoglycaemia are defined as either mild or severe. In mild hypo-glycaemia the person experiencing the hypoglycaemia is subjectively aware (symptomatic) of the falling blood glucose concentration at a time when cortical function is sufficiently preserved for the person to recognise the situation and take appropriate action to restore their blood glucose by ingesting carbohydrate. Some authorities also describe a moderate form of hypoglycaemia in which such a symptomatic episode causes significant social disruption. Severe hypoglycaemia is defined as that in which the person experiencing it is too disabled to self-treat and has to be rescued by another person. Again, some authorities add a sub-division of severe hypoglycaemia in which either coma/seizure occurs or in which parenteral therapy has to be administered (DCCT 1991).

There is no consensus on the biochemical definition of hypoglycaemia. Spontaneous patho-logical hypoglycaemia is probably best defined rigorously to avoid extensive investigation of healthy people and is usually considered to exist at glucose concentrations of under 2.8 mmol/l (Marks & Teale 1996). In diabetes, such rigour puts patients at risk of excessive hypoglycaemia exposure. As cortical dysfunction occurs at 3 mmol/l, and avoidance of exposure to blood glucose concentrations of 3 mmol/l reverses some of the defects of counterregulation to hypoglycaemia seen in some people with established diabetes, this is the lowest value that should be considered as definitive and most clinicians would agree that 3.5 mmol/l (the glucose concentration thought to be associated with the onset of adrenergic responses to hypoglycaemia as described below) is more useful. A recent definition as any glucose concentration under 4 mmol/l would describe many healthy people as hypoglycaemic much of the time, although it is a useful number to use as the lower end of the target range for glycaemic control (ADA 2005). Clinically, it is very important to distinguish between a target for therapy (which should indicate a need to adjust therapy if exposure to lower levels is recurrent) and an episode of hypoglycaemia, which requires immediate intervention.

Pathophysiology

In health, the human body protects itself from clinically important hypoglycaemia very efficiently through a series of physiological and neuroendocrine responses, collectively described as 'counterregulation' (Amiel & Gale 1993). The major components of the counterregulatory hormone responses are shown in Figure 5.1. Blood glucose concentrations are normally very strictly regulated at 3.5–7 mmol/l despite massive fluctuations in the rates at which tissues utilise glucose (rest vs exercise) and glucose is entering the circulation (fed vs fasted). It is important to remember that the systems we describe as 'counterregulatory' in the sense that they defend against hypoglycaemia, are in fact 'regulatory' and teleologically are present to maintain normality in health, not defend against pathology or iatrogenic disease. The regulatory mechanisms that are activated by any threat to blood glucose supply start with reduction in endogenous insulin secretion and increased release of pancreatic glucagon. This change in pancreatic endocrine signal disinhibits endogenous, primarily hepatic, glucose release by glycolysis and later gluconeogenesis. Insulin secretion is regulated to the glucose available to the pancreatic β cell, as it is driven by the rate of glucose metabolism in the cell. Glucagon secretion, in response to hypoglycaemia, is additionally driven by cell-cell communication between the insulin secreting β cell and the glucagon-secreting α cell, as any disruption of this link specifically inhibits hypoglycaemia-mediated glucagon release. In health, the pancreatic hormone response to a falling blood glucose occurs as the blood glucose falls below 4 mmol/l (Boyle et al. 1988). At slightly more profound hypoglycaemia (<3.6 mmol/l), the sympathetic nervous system is activated and adrenaline is released, with growth hormone and cortisol release occurring at slightly lower glucose concentrations or during more prolonged exposure to the lowered glucose (Mitrakou et al. 1991). Glucagon increases hepatic glycogenolysis and promotes gluconeogenesis, thereby increasing hepatic glucose production and raising blood sugar. Increase in adrenaline also increases lipolysis and hepatic glucose production (Garber et al. 1976; Hoffman 2006). Adrenergic receptors play an important role in plasma glucose recovery, especially in cases of type 1 diabetes with blunted glucagon responses, as glucose recovery post hypoglycaemia is impeded by the action of beta 1 and 2 receptor blockade (De et al. 1983). Other hormones released in response to hypoglycaemia include prolactin, anti-diuretic hormone (ADH), aldosterone and atrial-natriuretic peptide (ANP), though their role in glucose counterregulation is uncertain

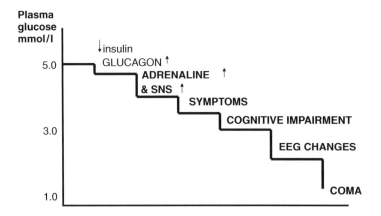

Figure 5.1 Schematic showing hormonal responses to hypoglycaemia, with the approximate glucose concentrations (arterialised venous plasma) for the hierarchy of the response in healthy volunteers. Data from Amiel et al. (1987), Boyle et al. (1988), Mitrakou et al. (1991).

(Woolf et al. 1977; Hayashi et al. 1992). In health, the neurohumoral responses to a falling blood glucose concentration are sufficient to maintain normoglycaemia.

There is a symptomatic response to hypoglycaemia that accompanies the above hormonal responses and is related to them. In disease states, where the normal neurohormonal responses to falling blood glucose may be defective, this subjective awareness is critical to avoidance of severe hypoglycaemia. The symptoms can be roughly divided into those common to any stress response, the so-called adrenergic responses (sweating, shaking, palpitations and hunger) and those related to the beginnings of inadequate fuel supply to the cerebral cortex, such as dizziness, irritability, confusion, lack of energy, drowsiness, poor concentration and difficulty in speaking (Lawrence 1941; Hepburn et al. 1993). Perception of these symptoms, which importantly include the generation of hunger, prompts the individual to eat. However, despite these responses, if blood glucose falls to below 3.0 mmol/l, cognitive dysfunction is detectable and this increases as glucose concentrations continue to fall. At glucose levels of below 2 mmol/l there is usually significant confusion or drowsiness and below 1 mmol/l convulsions and coma can occur.

Even a single episode of hypoglycaemia can blunt the protective, symptomatic and hormonal responses to subsequent hypoglycaemia (Heller & Cryer 1991) and the adrenergic responses can remain blunted for up to five days (George et al. 1995). Probably because of repeated exposure, counterregulatory hormone responses to hypoglycaemia are often impaired in patients with type 1 diabetes and in those patients with type 2 diabetes who are approaching the insulin deficient end of the spectrum (Segel et al. 2002). In particular, the adrenaline response to falling blood glucose is reduced (Dagogo-Jack et al. 1993) and there may be a wider attenuation in autonomic, sympathetic and adrenomedullary activation, giving rise to the clinical syndrome of hypoglycaemia associated autonomic failure (HAAF) (Cryer 1992). An associated loss of symptomatic warning symptoms leads to hypoglycaemia unawareness (Grimaldi et al. 1990). The combination of impaired or absent symptoms and attenuated adrenergic responses sets the scene for repeated hypoglycaemia, putting the individual at high risk of severe hypoglycaemia and significant physical and psychosocial morbidity.

Documentation of hypoglycaemia experience

Glucose meters

Documenting hypoglycaemia in daily life was initially based on description. Unsurprisingly, it is easier to obtain reliable data for severe hypoglycaemia than for mild, because episodes of mild hypoglycaemia are easily forgotten (Frier & Deary 1995). Asymptomatic hypoglycaemia is even more difficult to quantify and cannot by definition be adequately reported by the person experiencing it. Since the advent of home blood glucose monitoring, more quantitative data have been obtainable. Most systems depend on the patient obtaining a small drop of capillary blood by pricking a finger and placing the blood drop on a sensor, which can estimate the glucose concentration from an electro-chemical reaction with the glucose. All sensors incorporate an enzyme system that is highly specific for glucose, such as glucose oxidase, hexokinase or glucose dehydrogenase. The enzyme reacts with the glucose and the product generates either a chromogenic reaction that can be detected photometrically or a change in electron flow that can be measured electrochemically. Quality control of the meters is very important and in research studies, one type of meter should be used for all measurements. Modern glucose meters using very small amounts of blood are less prone to error than earlier versions but considerations of sampling technique and quality control remain particularly important in research, where differences in rates of hypoglycaemia may be subtle. Patients need to be instructed in the proper use of the meter, as errors can easily occur (for example, if the meter is incorrectly calibrated for the strips to be used, the skin is not clean before a blood drop is obtained or a skin region with low blood flow is used at a time when blood glucose concentration is changing rapidly (Ellison et al. 2002)). Traditionally, the fingertip is used for producing a sample due to location and close proximity of the capillary bed to the skin, but recently devices using capillary glucose from alternative sites such as the forearm or thigh have been used. There is however a difference between blood glucose and glucose obtained from alternative sites which is more pronounced in the post prandial state and also when there are large fluctuations of glucose (Bina et al. 2003), which makes these techniques unsuitable for the reliable detection and documentation of hypoglycaemia (Meguro et al. 2005).

Where rates of hypoglycaemia need to be compared objectively between different treatment regimens or patient groups, it is usual to request home blood sampling at specific, pre-defined times. Eight-point glucose profiles, in which the patient measures with specific frequencies before and after meals (usually 90 min to 2 hr), at bedtime and at 3 am, are popular, allowing documentation of pre- and post-prandial glucose concentrations and checking for nocturnal hypoglycaemia. When comparing rates of hypoglycaemia, it is essential to consider the same frequency of test results in each subject – hypoglycaemia is likely to be detected more frequently in someone testing eight times a day every day, than in someone testing once a week.

Glucose diaries

In research, such home glucose monitoring is often recorded in glucose diaries. These diaries may include questionnaires to be completed for each episode of hypoglycaemia experienced, so that the nature of the hypoglycaemia experience can be determined. The questionnaires

Patient Number   Patient Initials   Centre Number   Date

Clinical research fellows to fill in

HYPOGLYCAEMIA RECORDING FORM

Name: _____   Todays date: (dd/mm/yy)   (/   /   )

Date of hypo: (dd/mm/yy)   (/   /   )   Time of hypo: ☐ am
                                                                      _____   ☐ pm

Did you have any warning symptoms?   ☐ YES   ☐ NO

If yes, please indicate which, if any, of the following occurred (tick more than one box if necessary)

Confusion	☐		Double vision	☐
Sweating	☐		Blurred vision	☐
Drowsiness	☐		Hunger	☐
Weakness	☐		Thirst	☐
Dizziness	☐		Nausea	☐
Warmness	☐		Anxiety	☐
Difficulty speaking	☐		Tiredness	☐
Pounding heart	☐		Tingling lips	☐
Inability to concentrate	☐		Trembling	☐
Shivering	☐		Headache	☐
Unsteady on feet	☐		Abdominal pain	☐
Yellow vision	☐		Other (specify)	☐

How did the intensity of these symptoms compare to normal?

The same ☐   Less intense ☐   More intense ☐

What treatment did you require? (please tick all that apply)

Food eaten   ☐   specify
Dextrose tablets   ☐
Glucose drink   ☐   _____
Glucagon injection   ☐
Glucose injected into a vein ☐

Did you measure your blood sugar?   ☐ YES   ☐ NO

If yes, what was it?   _____ mmol/l

Was the blood sugar taken before or after treatment?   ☐ Before   ☐ After

During the hypo, did you need someone else to help you?   ☐ YES   ☐ NO

Did you lose consciousness during the hypo?   ☐ YES   ☐ NO

How long did the hypo last?   _____

Figure 5.2   Hypoglycaemia Questionnaire. An example of a form used for recording details of hypoglycaemia events experienced during daily life in prospective studies detailing hypoglycaemia experience. Reproduced courtesy of the UK Hypoglycaemia Study Group, 2006, with permission.

need to be kept short and simple but may ask the patient to record their blood glucose at the time of the hypoglycaemia, the symptoms experienced and the treatment taken. An example of a hypoglycaemia questionnaire used in a recent UK study is given in Figure 5.2.

There have been several attempts to quantify glycaemic control and lability on the basis of such glucose diaries, and to obtain objective descriptions of glycaemic control and hypoglycaemia experience. Commonly used measurements of glycaemic lability are the mean amplitude of glycaemic excursion (MAGE) (Service et al. 1970), the M value of Schlichtkrull (Schlichtkrull et al. 1965) and the hypoglycaemia burden (see below) and glycaemic labiliy index (Ryan et al. 2004). These estimates are commonly used in studies, although they have not been tested for validity in large numbers of patients. MAGE is calculated by taking the mean of the increment and decrement of blood glucose (from blood glucose troughs to peaks or vice versa) when both the ascending and the descending segments exceed one standard deviation of the blood glucose for the corresponding twenty-four hour period.

M value of Schlichtkrull is calculated by taking the difference between the maximum and minimum blood sugar values (in mg/dl) and dividing that by 20; the resulting product is then added to the average of all blood glucose excursions that have undergone an logarithmic transformation. The M value can also be used as a quantitative index of efficacy of treatment in the individual diabetic patient. The M value formula is as follow:

$$M = M^{BS} + \text{difference between the maximum and minimum blood sugar fluctuations}/20$$
$$M^{BS} = \text{mean of}(10 \times \log \text{blood sugar}/120)^3 \text{over the measured period}$$

Lability index

The lability index for a week is calculated for the month based on the following sum

$$\text{LI mmol/l}^2/\text{h} \cdot \text{week}^{-1} = \sum_{n=1}^{N} \frac{(\text{Gluc}_n - \text{Gluc}_{n+1})^2}{(h_{n+1} - h_n)}$$

where Gluc_n (in millimoles/l) in the *nth* reading taken at time h_n (rounded to the nearest hour). N is the total number of readings in a week.

These methods were developed for use with eight point glucose testing, but are now increasingly being applied to continuous glucose monitoring, where the frequency and number of readings are much larger. There is a need to validate these measurements using continuous glucose monitoring.

Hypoglycaemia questionnaires

In hypoglycaemia research, it may be important to document the quality as well as the quantity of hypoglycaemia. Problematic hypoglycaemia may be described in terms of the frequency of severe hypoglycaemia and there are at least three validated questionnaire-based assessments of subjective awareness of hypoglycaemia. Clarke's questionnaire is a set of questions aiming at self-assessment of hypoglycaemia awareness. A scoring system stratifies the individual as having impaired awareness or being unaware (Clarke et al. 1995). Gold's assessment of hypoglycaemia awareness is based on no subjective change in hypoglycaemia warning symptoms since commencing insulin and the experience of mainly autonomic hypo-glycaemia symptoms, using a visual analogue scale of 1 to 7 for assessment of autonomic, neuroglycopaenic and non-specific hypoglycaemia warning symptoms (Gold et al. 1994). Documenting a patient's ability to detect his or her own awareness of hypoglycaemia is important in many studies looking at the pathogenesis of hypoglycaemia unawareness and severe hypoglycaemia and may be critical in recruiting patients for studies designed to improve glycaemic control and/or protection against hypoglycaemia. Some authorities seek evidence for a minimum frequency of episodes of asymptomatic biochemical hypoglycaemia on home blood glucose monitoring records; others depend on patient report of symptoms during hypoglycaemia; others on a mixture of the two (Maran et al. 1993, 1995). Other assessments have been introduced more specifically to describe hypoglycaemia experience.

More recently, Ryan et al. (2004), working on the islet transplant programme in Canada, set out to quantify the severity of the hypoglycaemia problem experienced by patients and developed the hypoglycaemia burden score.

To calculate the burden of hypoglycaemia, patient are asked to complete a detailed record of blood glucose readings for four weeks, putting particular emphasis on details and number of hypoglycaemic events. Patients are also asked to complete a questionnaire about the frequency of severe hypoglycaemia reactions over the previous year. A score is then generated, based on frequency, severity and degree of unawareness of hypoglycaemia. A higher score indicates a greater problem with hypoglycaemia, with a score of 433 or more indicating problematic hypoglycaemia, while a score of ≥ 1047 is indicative of serious problem with hypoglycaemia. This uniquely provides quantification of the severity of hypoglycaemia, which can be used to compare treatments for their effect on hypoglycaemia experience. It has been mostly used in the islet transplant programme, where it has identified people having much more problematic hypoglycaemia than the norm and has also shown hypoglycaemia to reduce to unmeasurable when the transplant is successful. Its sensitivity for documenting less effective improvements in hypoglycaemia experience remains to be demonstrated (Ryan et al. 2004).

Continuous glucose monitoring (CGMS)

Even with the most intense capillary glucose monitoring, there are vast periods of time when patients are unaware of their glucose values. The emergence of continuous glucose monitoring technologies has introduced new possibilities for measuring exposure to hypoglycaemia in terms of duration and severity. Continuous glucose monitors use a variety of techniques to measure interstitial glucose. The most commonly used method uses a subcutaneous sensor coated with glucose oxidase, which reacts with glucose in the interstitial tissue, producing a current which is measured by the device and converted to a glucose reading (Rebrin et al. 1999). A more direct way of measuring interstitial glucose is microdialysis, in which a dialysate fluid is passed through the interstitial fluid and the glucose equilibrates across the dialysis membrane. The glucose concentration in the dialysate is then measured (Bolinder et al. 1993). Reverse iontophoresis is another technique, in which a small electrical current is used to draw glucose in the interstitium through the skin, which is then measured using an enzymo-electrical reaction (Tamada et al. 1995).

Whichever technique is used, continuous glucose monitoring provides a far greater degree of information about the frequency, duration and severity of hypoglycaemia than was previously possible. It is no surprise that the first reports of clinical use of continuous glucose monitoring commented on the amount of subclinical asymptomatic hypoglycaemia that was detected (Boland et al. 2001). There were however concerns about the accuracy of CGMS devices (Mauras et al. 2004) and in particular there are concerns about over-reporting of nocturnal hypoglycaemia (McGowan et al. 2002). Recent revisions and improvements to the devices have increased reliability and accuracy but it is important to remember that these devices are measuring interstitial glucose and not blood glucose and so the two readings are inherently different, in particular when there are rapid changes in blood glucose concentration.

There has been some recent work to suggest that in patients with type 1 diabetes, interstitial glucose closely parallels blood glucose during hypoglycaemia (Caplin et al. 2003) and there are emerging data suggesting that glucose values obtained from continuous glucose monitoring devices are accurate during symptomatic hypoglycaemia (Choudhary et al. 2006).

Continuous glucose monitoring can provide insight into the frequency and duration of hypoglycaemia and can be used to compare hypoglycaemia burden objectively between groups (UK Hypoglycaemia Study Group 2006). Monitors can be adapted to incorporate hypoglycaemia (and hyperglycaemia) alarms, activated at glucose concentrations selected by the user. Recently, the ability to display the measured glucose recording in real time has been developed. In clinical use, they can reduce the amount of hypoglycaemia experienced (Garg et al. 2006). In research, they are less useful for merely documenting hypoglycaemia rates, as their displays will influence patient behaviour.

Investigating the pathogenesis of problematic hypoglycaemia

In order to investigate counterregulatory mechanisms, it is important to produce hypoglycaemia in a controlled laboratory setting where physiological and cognitive responses can be measured accurately and reproducibly. Two variables can be measured: the ability to counterregulate, in which the subject's ability to arrest a falling glucose is determined; and the elements of the counterregulatory responses themselves, in which the hypoglycaemic challenge is strictly controlled by the investigator, in order to compare the responses to that particular hypoglycaemia in different settings. The former is best assessed by exposure to an unopposed hypoglycaemic agent; in the latter, the hypoglycaemic agent is applied but the rate and magnitude of the response is modified by monitored application of exogenous glucose. In comparing the response to hypoglycaemia between conditions (for example, if it is necessary to compare the effects of different clinical situations or treatments on hypoglycaemia), some attempt must be made to achieve a reproducible stimulus. A hypoglycaemic challenge can vary in timing, magnitude, rate of fall and method of induction.

For a successful study, it is important that all aspects of planning are considered, from logistics and location to selection of appropriate subjects, instructions to the subjects and, of course, decisions regarding the study protocol. It is important to ensure there are enough personnel. Tasks include clinical care of the subject; frequent blood sampling and care of intravenous lines; timely centrifugation and processing of blood samples, with rapid readout of glucose concentrations; frequent appropriate adjustment of glucose infusion rates; collection of physiological data; symptom scores; and cognitive function. The study should be carried out in a spacious, quiet and, ideally, temperature controlled environment, with all equipment in close proximity (Figure 5.3). Safety of the subject and of the researchers

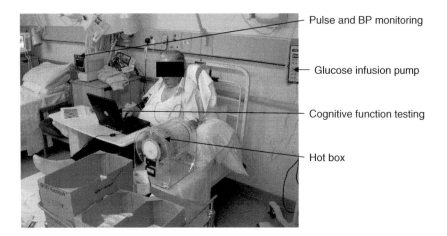

Pulse and BP monitoring

Glucose infusion pump

Cognitive function testing

Hot box

Figure 5.3 Subject in position during experimental induction of hypoglycaemia. In this example, the subject is undergoing a stepped hypoglycaemic clamp.

is of paramount importance. Strict aseptic technique, wearing of disposable gloves and safe disposal of sharps are essential ground rules. Subjects need to be carefully observed both during and after an induced hypoglycaemic challenge. Blood glucose should always be restored to normal and the subject fed after a study, and observation should be continued, including blood glucose monitoring, until the investigator is sure that normoglycaemia is being maintained spontaneously.

It is important to avoid carrying out hypoglycaemia studies on people with ischaemic heart disease, epilepsy, hypertension, untreated hypothyroidism, hypoadrenalism or unstable diabetic retinopathy. It is crucial not to carry out studies on women of childbearing age if radioisotopes or potentially teratogenic or fetotoxic drugs are to be used, because of the potential risk to any future fetus.

For comparative studies, subjects should be age and gender matched, as there are important differences in counterregulatory responses between sexes and age groups (Matyka et al. 1997; Davis et al. 2000). Mixing genders and ages will at the very least increase the variance of the measures made and may obscure differences resulting from other factors. If groups are of mixed gender in a cross sectional study, the gender distribution must be matched. Vigorous exercise and caffeine should be avoided prior to the study as they can also affect counterregulatory responses (Debrah et al. 1996; Sandoval et al. 2006). Subjects should be studied in the same position (lying or standing) as there is a greater perception of hypoglycaemic symptoms in the standing position than in the lying position (Hirsch et al. 1991). It is usual to study subjects in the fasting or post-absorptive state. This allows a steady-state baseline. In the fed state, symptoms of hypoglycaemia are decreased, but counterregulatory hormone responses are increased (Porcellati et al. 2003). Furthermore, there are diurnal rhythms in many counterregulatory hormones – such as cortisol and growth hormone – which may affect both insulin sensitivity and counter-regulatory responses. It is important that comparator studies are done at the same time of day to avoid such confounders. With fasting subjects, this will usually be in the morning.

For subjects with diabetes, it is often necessary to achieve near-normoglycaemia prior to study. Otherwise, the magnitude of the hypoglycaemic challenge may vary enormously, with some subjects falling to hypoglycaemia from significant hyperglycaemia, and others starting with a near-normoglycaemic blood glucose concentration. Based on evidence that exposure to hypoglycaemia during the night will reduce counterregulatory responses to hypoglycaemia next day, it is also very important to avoid such asymptomatic hypoglycaemia the night before study. The gold standard is to admit the patient to an observation bed the evening before the study, omit the usual evening intermediate-acting or long-acting subcutaneous insulin and control blood glucose overnight with a monitored low dose intravenous insulin infusion, given as a sliding scale. Unlike clinical sliding scales, this will be run unopposed (i.e. without a simultaneous glucose infusion) to maintain the fasting state. Blood (or plasma) glucose is measured every 30–60 minutes at the bedside and the rate of the insulin infusion adjusted to maintain near-normoglycaemia. If the blood is sampled from an intravenous cannula by an experienced operator, the subject at least can usually get some sleep!

The nature of the glucose sample

For the purposes of the hypoglycaemic challenge, precision with regard to the measurement of the blood glucose concentration is mandatory. Because of the frequency of sampling, and the need to avoid stress by the action of sampling, an intravenous line is usually placed, using local anaesthetic and aseptic technique, and kept patent by slow infusion of normal saline or heparinised saline (1,000 units heparin in 1 l saline, as used clinically to sustain arterial lines) rather than using a finger prick technique. It is essential that proper techniques are used for blood sampling – the dead space from the cannula must be withdrawn before the sample is taken with a separate syringe. To avoid excess blood loss when sampling is frequent, the dead-space blood is sometimes returned to the patient after the sample has been taken – if this is done, extreme care must be taken to keep the syringes and their connections sterile and to avoid introduction of air or thrombus. Any delay in restoring dead-space blood or any possible contamination should lead to discard of the 'dead space' sample. Careful flushing of the lines after sampling is also essential to avoid clotting.

For prolonged studies, most authorities use plasma rather than venous blood. This necessitates rapid bedside spinning of the sample in a microfuge and sampling of the plasma. Plasma glucose is unaffected by haematocrit and reflects the glucose cells are seeing. For the same reason, the ideal sample would be arterial blood, as this will reflect the glucose that the tissues, particularly the brain, are receiving. Furthermore, muscle is an active tissue that will remove glucose (especially if insulin stimulated and insulin sensitive) and add noradrenaline, for example, to blood. There is thus a significant arterio-venous difference for several substrates, which will vary according to the degree of insulinisation, insulin sensitivity and degree of hypoglycaemia (Liu et al. 1992). Because of the increased risk of arterial cannulation, most authorities use arterialised venous blood where possible. To arterialise venous blood, the cannula is placed in a vein draining a minimally active tissue bed (i.e. as distal as possible), usually using a vein draining just the extremity of the upper limb, in the back of the hand or in the wrist. The hand is kept rested and is warmed in a heating box to increase the flow through the metabolically less active skin (Figure 5.4). The box is designed to accommodate the hand comfortably and heat the air inside to approximately 55 °C. Metal rings should not be worn in the heating box and it must be designed to prevent direct contact

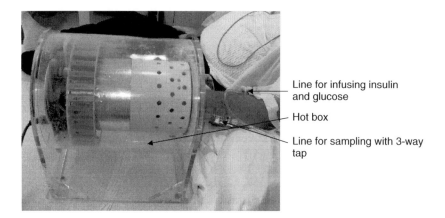

Line for infusing insulin
and glucose

Hot box

Line for sampling with 3-way
tap

Figure 5.4 Close up of arterialised venous sampling during induction of controlled experimental hypoglycaemia.

between the hand and the heating elements. Contact heating of the hand is not recommended as the temperature required may burn the skin. If arterial lines are required, they must be placed by experienced operators in the presence of a documented collateral circulation. They must be kept under direct visual observation and operated by staff trained in using them for sampling.

The nature of the glucose meter is also important. Whatever analyser is chosen, it should be subjected to rigorous quality control both during and between studies. Standards of known glucose concentration should be tested regularly during prolonged studies and the results from them must remain within pre-defined and narrow limits for the study to be considered acceptable. It is important to be able to quote the coefficient of variation for the analyser for the study. The gold standards are usually considered the bench top glucose oxidase analysers, such as those made by Yellow Springs Instrument company or Beckman.

The insulin infusate

Where insulin is to be infused over prolonged periods, it is important to be sure that the concentration of the infusate remains stable. The dose is often estimated in milliunits of insulin per kilogram body weight, although using the body surface area is preferable, especially where subjects of different sizes are to be compared. Body surface area relates more precisely to volume of distribution. The specific requirements for individual studies are discussed below. Insulin sticks to plastic and so an insulin infusate will lose strength over time. To avoid this it is usual to make the insulin up in a 4 % solution of autologous blood, and it is critical that the insulin is mixed by slow rotation (to avoid bubbling). The solution is then run through the entire giving apparatus, to saturate the binding sites in the plastic from the beginning. For infusions lasting more than five hours, fresh solutions should be made. A small amount of all infusions should be kept for later estimation of the exact insulin concentration (in a diluted sample). This is particularly important when the investigator wishes to measure insulin sensitivity. In such studies, accuracy in the making of the insulin solution is critical and use of clinical grade syringes may not be adequate to achieve this reliably.

Sampling for stress hormones

It is important to have an adequate stabilisation period at euglycaemia prior to inducing hypoglycaemia. There may be a marked increase in cortisol and adrenaline due to the stress of cannulation and the stress of being part of a study. This usually settles down within 15–30 minutes.

Hypoglycaemic stimuli for research

Insulin tolerance test

Most experimental hypoglycaemia is induced by insulin. An intravenous insulin challenge, called the insulin tolerance or insulin stress test, was the first test used to determine the effect of hypoglycaemia (Dell'acqua 1951; Hanzlicek & Knobloch 1951). This method was used in early studies that identified the role of the adrenal gland in protective responses to hypoglycaemia (Vogt 1951; De Pergola & Campiello 1953) and has also been used in the past to induce hypoglycaemic seizures as a treatment for severe depression (Mueller et al. 1969) and as a stimulus for gastric acid secretion in the standard Hollander test assessing the completeness of vagotomy (Colin-Jones & Himsworth 1970). It is still used to determine pituitary reserve for growth hormone and cortisol release.

Prior to performing an insulin tolerance test, it is important to rule out complete deficiency of counterrgulatory hormones and establish cardiovascular status. A 9 am cortisol, baseline thyroid function and ECG should be checked as being normal before proceeding. In its simplest form, the insulin tolerance test comprises intravenous injection of soluble insulin

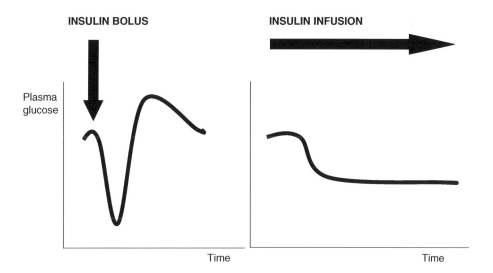

Figure 5.5 The difference between the counterregulatory responses expected between an insulin bolus (left) and insulin infusion (right). In the presence of continued insulin stimulus, counterregulation can arrest but not correct glucose fall. The depth of the fall will depend upon insulin dose. Note the rebound above baseline on recovery in the left panel.

at a dose of 0.1–0.2 mU/kg. Sampling for glucose and insulin is done at regular intervals thereafter for 90–120 minutes (Bloom et al. 1975). The rate of glucose fall, glucose nadir, rate of recovery and counterregulatory hormone responses can be determined. The rate of initial glucose decline has been used as a measure of insulin sensitivity, and where used for this purpose, the test can be terminated at 10 minutes, supposedly before counterregulation has occurred (Lazarus & Volk 1952). The rate of recovery can be taken as a measure of counterregulatory capacity. This model is very effective for inducing hypoglycaemia, but the nadir occurs very quickly and is uncontrolled and the counterregulatory response is correspondingly brisk. In contrast, clinical hypoglycaemia usually develops more gradually and is reversed more slowly. Therefore, a modification of this model was described in 1972 whereby insulin was infused intravenously at the rate of 0.04 units per kg per hour or subcutaneously over 12 hours (Carter et al. 1972). The resulting hypoglycaemia is more gradual and there are small but important differences in counterregulatory findings between the two methods.

Intravenous insulin infusion test

The intravenous insulin infusion test has been used as a tool for identifying type 1 diabetes patients who are at increased risk of hypoglycaemia during intensive therapy. The presence of neurological symptoms of hypoglycaemia or further decline of plasma glucose to below 1.9 mmol/l after intravenous insulin (40 mu/kg/h) were considered a sign of an inadequate counterregulatory response and increased risk of severe hypoglycaemia was predicted on the subsequent application of intensified insulin therapy (White et al. 1983). A similar protocol was used by Ryder et al. to show that severe hypoglycaemia and counterregulatory failure were more common in people with a history of severe hypoglycaemia and that those with classical autonomic neuropathy did not correspond (Abramson et al. 1966).

Bolli and colleagues further modified the insulin tolerance test by suggesting that the subcutaneous route more closely mimicked the clinical situation (Bolli et al. 1985). Overall, the insulin tolerance test provides good insight into the counterregulatory responses to hypoglycaemia. However, the uncontrolled and unpredictable nature of the induced hypoglycaemia makes it very difficult to reproduce and potentially dangerous. It is also difficult to compare specific elements of the hypoglycaemia responses between patients or conditions when the hypoglycaemic challenge is variable. For this, a more controlled hypoglycaemic challenge, which is reproducible in all subjects, is required.

Sulphonylurea induced hypoglycaemia

Sulphonylureas were introduced in the mid 1950s. Some investigators used sulphonylureas such as tolbutamide to study hypoglycaemia. (Visser 1967). The most important differences between insulin and sulphonylurea induced hypoglycaemia are their different effects on the pancreatic β cell and the ratio between peripheral and portal insulin levels, which may have a bearing on counterregulatory hormone release. In insulin induced hypoglycaemia, such as the insulin stress test or the hyperinsulinaemic clamp, endogenous insulin production is suppressed and peripheral and portal insulin levels are similar. However, sulphonylureas stimulate endogenous insulin production, leading to a higher portal to peripheral insulin ratio (Jackson et al. 1973). This may be an important methodological factor in choosing the hypoglycaemic stimulus, particularly when studying effects of the portal glucose sensor. Sulphonylurea induced hypoglycaemia has also been used to examine the influence of the fall in endogenous insulin secretion from pancreatic β cells in determining the glucagon secretory responses from adjacent α cells (Peacey et al. 1997).

In tolbutamide studies, the tolbutamide has been given as a 1.7 g bolus, given intravenously over three minutes, followed by an infusion of 130 mg/h starting 10 minutes after the bolus, to a total dose of 2 g, which is equal to the maximum oral dose (Peacey et al. 1996). With this protocol, the subject must be monitored for a further six hours, to protect against late hypoglycaemia due to the long half-life of tolbutamide. Hypoglycaemia has also been studied using other sulphonylureas (Colin-Jones & Himsworth 1970) infused through the most distal port, so that flow is not interrupted by changes in the glucose infusion rate (Maran & Amiel 1994). The second cannula is inserted for arterialised blood sampling in the dorsum of the hand as described above. There are various protocols for loading the insulin and starting the glucose, which will need to be started before the first plasma glucose measurements are available. In the original descriptions, the insulin is started at 10 times its maintenance rate and adjusted downwards every minute. This requires a pump with a rapidly variable delivery. We use a modified protocol, giving the insulin at three times the desired rate for three minutes, then twice the desired rate for four minutes. In either protocol, the 20 % glucose infusion should be started four minutes after the insulin infusion, at an empirical start rate of 2.0 mg/kg/min; increased to 2.5 mg/kg/min at seven minutes and 3.0 mg/kg/min at nine minutes (DeFronzo et al. 1979). From then on, the investigator adjusts the glucose infusion rate at five-minute intervals, depending on the plasma glucose values, either using a published algorithm or judgement acquired by experience. The adjustment of the glucose infusion rate is carried out based on the principle of negative feedback; if the measured glucose concentration is higher than the desired level the glucose infusion will be reduced and vice versa. Therefore, the investigator has total control of the plasma glucose concentration.

It is important to include a period of normoglycaemia at the start of a study, to allow the insulin to equilibrate and for the glucose infusion rates to stabilise. In euglycaemic clamping, glucose requirements continue to rise for as long as clamping continues, but at the beginning it takes about 20 minutes for the insulin effect to manifest (DeFronzo et al. 1979). Thereafter, the rise in glucose requirements is a slow drift.

The standard dose from clamp studies of insulin sensitivity ($40\,mU/m^2$ per minute) is suboptimal for hypoglycaemia studies, as the degree of insulinisation may be too easily overcome by an intact counterregulatory response and $60\,mU/m^2$ per minute is usual. Very high insulin doses should be avoided as they are not physiological and they may risk unacceptable hypokalaemia. Some authorities replace potassium during clamping but this can cause pain at the infusion site.

One-step hyperinsulinaemic hypoglycaemia clamp

In a one-step study, the infusions of insulin and glucose are initiated as describe above to maintain euglycaemia for a period of stabilisation and then the glucose infusion is reduced or stopped, causing the plasma glucose to drop to the predetermined level within a fixed time (Maran et al. 1991). These can be quick fall or slow fall depending on the relative rates of insulin and glucose. The glucose infusion is then restarted to maintain the hypoglycaemia at a fixed plasma glucose level for a fixed period of time. At the end of the study the glucose infusion is increased and the insulin stopped to restore euglycaemia.

Stepped hypoglycaemic clamp

Stepped clamps are used to create a slow fall in plasma glucose so that the glucose concentration at which any given response begins can be identified (Figure 5.6).

Responses are influenced by the duration of exposure to hypoglycaemia but this is standardised in the stepped clamp procedure. In these clamps, the glucose is held at predetermined plateaus for a fixed duration. The first part of the plateau is used for stabilisation of glucose and the second for measurement of symptoms, cognitive function and counterregulatory hormones, before lowering the glucose to the next plateau. Each plateau must be long enough to allow the plasma glucose to stabilise and the stabilisation of the response, as well as completion of any other measures that the investigator requires. It takes at least 20 minutes for the responses to hypoglycaemia to approach stability (Evans et al. 2000). If a battery of cognitive function tests are being carried out, they will require about 20 minutes to compete, so each plateau will be for about 40 minutes.

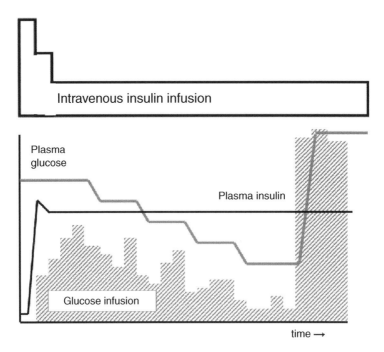

Figure 5.6 Schematic showing the major elements of a stepped hypoglycaemic clamp. A primed continuous intravenous insulin infusion is started (black box) to raise circulating insulin concentrations (black line) rapidly to target. The resultant fall in plasma glucose (grey line) is controlled by a variable rate infusion of glucose solution (hatched bars).

If sophisticated measurements are to be made, these studies usually require at least three team members. Cognitive function tests should be carried out in peaceful surroundings in a reproducible way by an experienced investigator. Blood samples taken for hormone analysis need to be handled with care, often requiring rapid centrifugation, accurate removal of plasma and immediate freezing using dry ice. Teamwork is crucial, with different members completing different parts of the study.

Measurement of physiological responses

Blood pressure, heart rate and ecg

Increments in blood pressure and heart rate are recorded as a safety measure during studies of hypoglycaemia, but increases of 20 % or more in either of the parameters can be used as physiological markers of adrenergic responses to hypoglycaemia (Hepburn et al. 1993). The electrocardiogram can be monitored to obtain accurate continuous measures of heart rate and to monitor for evidence of significant hypokalaemia.

Sweating and tremor

Rate of sweating is measured using a 25 cm^2 ventilated chamber placed on the lower sternum and then corrected for humidity and ambient temperature. Tremor is measured using a ring accelerometer on the index finger of the non-dominant hand, with the hand help outstretched and forearm supported (George et al. 1997).

Measurement of counterregulatory hormones

The hormonal counterregulatory response to hypoglycaemia is a carefully orchestrated release of hormones that has a natural hierarchy in the non-diabetic individual that protects the individual from severe hypoglycaemia (Mitrakou et al. 1991). The first step is a reduction in insulin production, followed by the release of glucagon, adrenaline, cortisol and growth hormone (Cryer et al. 1989).

Studies of counterregulation to hypoglycaemia have looked at either the magnitude of the counterregulatory hormone response to a fixed hypoglycaemic stimulus or the glucose concentration (often referred to as the threshold) at which the response is activated. The former can be done using a single-step design, with hormones collected at a fixed interval after reaching the nadir glucose. These studies are easy to interpret, as simple statistics can be used to compare the hormonal values at the glucose nadir. The latter study requires a slow controlled glucose fall. All studies require adequate baseline sampling. Baseline measurements at euglycaemia must be taken once the insulin and glucose have equilibrated and can then be compared with measurements taken during hypoglycaemia. During a stepped clamp, hormone levels are usually collected at the midpoint and end point of each plateau.

Samples for adrenaline are usually collected in lithium heparin tubes containing EGTA or glutathione preservative. They are then centrifuged at 3,000 rpm for 10 minutes. The plasma is taken off and stored at –80 °C. All samples from a single study should be analysed together, and this is usually done by high performance liquid chromatography (HPLC) with electrochemical detection.

Samples for glucagon are collected in lithium heparin tubes containing 50 μl of trasylol, while cortisol, C-peptide and free insulin are collected in serum tubes. Following immediate centrifugation at 3,000 rpm for 10 minutes, the plasma is decanted of and stored at –80 °C before being analysed by radioimmuno assay.

Calculating glucose thresholds for hormone release

Glucose thresholds for release of counterregulatory hormones or onset of other responses to hypoglycaemia are defined as the plasma glucose concentration at which the response is fisrt significant. They can thus only be reliably identified in slow reductions in plasma glucose, preferably stepped, as described above. The critical issue is to decide before starting what determines a significant change. This can either be to a specific value or by a predefined degree of increase. The gold standard is to perform euglycaemic studies of the same duration in the same patients in the same conditions and compare the hypoglycaemic responses with the euglycaemic absence of response in each subject. For smaller pilot studies, where this is impractical, some investigators have used a statistical definition such as a change in excess of two standard deviations over the mean basal readings – for this, one strictly requires at least five baseline measures for each subject in order to define the standard deviation, which may be very small (Amiel et al. 1987). An alternative method is to predefine a level of response that is of clinical relevance. Based upon studies done in patients with type 1 diabetes, an increase of 410 pmol/l for adrenaline, 0.3 nmol/l for noradrenaline, 190nmol/l for cortisol and 7 microg/l for GH can be used, although it should be appreciated that these definitions are based on cardiovascular responses (Heine 1993; Korzon-Burakowska et al. 1998; Levy et al. 1998).

Measurement of symptoms

Symptoms of hypoglycaemia were first reported in relation to tumours of the pancreas (Wilder 1927). As early as 1927, the symptoms of hypoglycaemia were recognised as forming two groups; the first occurring during mild reactions comprising anxiety, weakness, sweating, hunger, tremor and palpitations and the second more severe group including mood changes, speech and visual disturbances, drowsiness, convulsions and coma (Harrop 1927). It was also noted that some patients did not experience the usual symptoms of hypoglycaemia until their blood glucose had reached much lower concentrations (Lawrence 1941). Symptom profiles provoked by hypoglycaemia are idiosyncratic and vary in character, pattern and intensity between individuals and even within individuals over time (Pennebaker et al. 1981).

Most symptoms experienced during hypoglycaemia are considered to be generated either by the direct effects of low blood glucose on the brain (neuroglycopenia) or through activation of the autonomic nervous system. Both the sympathetic and parasympathetic divisions of the autonomic nervous systems are activated, causing direct neural stimulation of end-organs, and the magnitude of the responses may be augmented by profuse secretion of adrenaline from the adrenal medulla (McAulay et al. 2001).

The modern classification of symptoms depends on symptoms recorded following experimental hypoglycaemia (Hepburn et al. 1991) and also statistical analyses of symptoms

Table 5.1 Symptoms of Hypoglycaemia in Adults with Diabetes

Range of frequencies (%) of individual symptoms of hypoglycaemia reported in eight population studies		Symptoms (and percentage, to nearest 5 %) of people endorsing symptoms as associated with hypoglycaemia	
Sweating	47–84	Sweating	80
Trembling	32–78	Trembling	65
Weakness	28–71	Fatigue/weak	70
Visual disturbance	24–60	Blurred vision	20
Hunger	39–49	Hunger	60
Pounding heart	8–62	Pounding heart	55
Difficulty speaking	7–41	Slurred speech	40
Tingling around mouth	10–39	Numb lips	50
Dizziness	11–41	Light-headed/dizzy	60
Headache	24–36	Headache	30
Anxiety	10–44	Nervous/tense	65
Nausea	5–20	Difficulty concentrating	80
Difficulty concentrating	31–75	Drowsy/sleepy	40
Tiredness	38–46	Uncoordinated	75
Drowsiness	16–33	Cold sweats	40
Confusion	13–53	Slowed thinking	70

Adapted from McAulay et al. 2001.

Table 5.2 Edinburgh Hypoglycaemia Scale: Experimental Hypoglycaemia

Neuroglycopenic symptoms		Autonomic symptoms
Cognitive dysfunction	Neuroglycopenia	
Inability to concentrate	Drowsiness	Sweating
Blurred vision	Tiredness	Trembling
Anxiety	Hunger	Warmness
Confusion	Weakness	
Difficulty speaking		
Double vision		

Adapted from McCrimmon et al. 2001

described by patients in prospective or retrospective studies (Hepburn et al. 1992). The frequency of various symptoms reported in previous population studies is described in Table 5.1 (McAulay et al. 2001). Factor analysis of these symptoms divides them into three groups, 'neuroglycopaenic', 'autonomic' and 'general malaise'. This validated three factor model is commonly used in studies and has been referred to as the Edinburgh hypoglycaemia scale. This has recently been modified for use in experimental hypoglycaemia (Table 5.2) (McCrimmon et al. 2003). Analysis is of total symptoms as well as separately for neuroglycopaenic and adrenergic symptoms.

During experimental studies of hypoglycaemia, it is important to document the symptoms at baseline before the start, and then at regular time points during the study. The subject should be kept blinded to the glucose level at all times. Often studies are carried out to identify thresholds for the development of symptoms and so it is paramount to define the glucose value that will be used as the threshold. Most studies have used the glucose value at which there is an increase of two points or more over the baseline score sustained over at least two time points (Korzon-Burakowska et al. 1998; Spyer et al. 2000). The subject is asked to rate the symptoms in the Edinburgh hypoglycaemic scale on a scale of 1 to 7, where 1 indicates the symptom is absent and 7 indicates the symptom is at its maximum intensity. Other investigators have used a semi-quantitative symptom questionnaire where subjects are scored from 0 to 5 on each of the following symptoms: hunger, dizziness, tingling, blurred vision, difficulty in thinking, faintness (the neuroglycopaenic symptoms) and anxiety, palpitations, sweating, irritability, tremor (the autonomic symptoms) (Fanelli et al. 1998).

Hunger is one of the main symptoms during acute hypoglycaemia but the exact mechanism is unclear. However, it tends to be clustered together with other autonomic symptoms (Deary et al. 1993). Interestingly, craving for particular food rather a general sense of hunger is observed during acute hypoglycaemia, particularly food that is high in carbohydrate content (Strachan et al. 2004).

Measurement of glucose kinetics

A full description of the *in vivo* measurement of glucose kinetics is beyond the scope of this chapter. In human studies, stable isotopes are used in preference to radioisotopes to avoid unnecessary exposure to radiation. The principle is to label the substrate pool with a known amount of labeled substrate, and use the dilution of the labeled substrate as an indicator of the amount of tracee entering the system, from which any exogenous infusion is subtracted. Di-deutrated glucose is commonly used to differentiate endogenous glucose production from glucose uptake by peripheral tissues and the techniques, described in textbooks on measuring insulin sensitivity, can be used in hypoglycaemia research to establish the onset of endogenous glucose counterregulation. In using glucose tracers, it is essential to establish a steady state of tracer labeling in the blood before starting – this is usually achieved by giving a priming dose of tracer (which with stable isotopes does involve a measurable glucose load) and a long infusion ($\sim$2 hours) prior to starting measurements. Baseline measurements can be taken from 90 minutes to 2 hours in a euglycaemic person, but in someone who is hyperglycaemic, a larger bolus and a longer prodromal infusion is required. It is essential to take a sample to assess natural enrichment prior to starting the infusion and to take accurate measurements of tracer concentration in the infusate of the rate of administration. Compartmentalisation of endogenous glucose production can only be achieved by measuring arterio-venous differences and blood flow across the different organs. This has been done for liver, kidney and brain but it requires very invasive selective catheterisation and there are ethical issues to be considered. Such studies have provided very useful information in the past but an investigator should be sure their question is important enough to justify the risks involved and has not been addressed in the literature already.

Animal studies

Various animal models have been used to study hypoglycaemia, including dogs, calves and rats (Dawson 1950; Suzuki & Saito 1951; Bloom et al. 1975). One of the earliest reports of the attenuation of adrenergic responses after repeated hypoglycaemia came from animal studies (Kraicer & Logothetopoulos 1963). Early studies used the insulin tolerance test and focussed on the adrenergic and corticotrophic responses to hypoglycaemia. These early studies were made using the insulin tolerance test, although they tended to use much larger doses of insulin (0.2–1.0 mU/kg) than in human studies as the animals were more insulin resistant than humans.

Many of the techniques described above are used in animal studies, with the advantage that animal studies allow much more invasive monitoring of glucose and allow the possibility of more invasive interventions.

The most commonly used animal model in recent years has been the male Sprague-Dawley rat, with hypoglycaemia being induced using intraperitoneal or intra-cerebro-ventricular insulin (10 units/kg) (McCrimmon et al. 2005). These models have been useful in investigating the role of the cerebral glucose sensor (Evans et al. 2004; Klip & Hawkins 2005), and cannulation of the ventromedial hypothalamus allows brain glucose levels to be measured and modified pharmacologically, independent of peripheral glucose levels (McCrimmon et al. 2005).

A jugular vein catheter and a microdialysis guide catheter are inserted into the male Sprague-Dawley rat. The tip of the microdialysis probe extends to the lateral edge of the anterior portion of the VMH and is fixed in position with dental acrylic cement and anchored to the skull with four stainless steel screws. The animal is given 5–7 days to recover from the stress of the procedure before any experimental procedures are undertaken (Borg et al. 1995).

Investigators have also been using genetically engineered knock-out animals to look at the effects of certain proteins on glucose metabolism and counterregulation (Marty et al. 2005; Jacobson et al. 2006). Animal models also help in establishing molecular pathways for clinical responses, which aid our understanding by providing neurohistological evidence of pathways of activation in response to hypoglycaemia (Han et al. 2005; Paranjape & Briski 2005). Neuroimaging studies such as magnetic resonance spectroscopy allow for quantification of chemicals within the brain and have been developed on animal models before being applied to humans (Oz et al. 2003; Morgenthaler et al. 2006).

Conclusion

Techniques for examining the physiological responses to hypoglycaemia have evolved over the years and have helped us understand a lot about the ways in which humans react to hypoglycaemia and how those processes can be affected in diabetes. There is still a lot to learn, in particular about effects of hypoglycaemia on the brain. New research may also throw up potential pharmacological targets that could support cerebral function or symptom responses in hypoglycaemia. For these studies we need robust and reproducible models for studying hypoglycaemia and over the years, the hyperinsulinaemic hypoglycaemic clamp has been the cornerstone for research in this field. As research moves further towards understanding the role of the brain in subjective awareness of hypoglycaemia, and the interplay between triggers for symptoms and counterregulatory hormone release, neuroimaging techniques will play an increasingly prominent part. Future directions will also include investigating the role of incretins in modulation of hypoglycaemic responses.

Fear of hypoglycaemia remains the main barrier to tighter glycaemic control. Reducing the incidence and severity of hypoglycaemia remains an important goal. A better understanding of the way hypoglycaemia affects individuals will be an important aid to alleviating at least part of the fear.

References

Abramson EA, Arky RA, Woeber KA (1966) Effects of propranolol on the hormonal and metabolic responses to insulin–induced hypoglycaemia *Lancet* **2**(7,478), 1386–8

ADA (2005) Defining and reporting hypoglycemia in diabetes: a report from the American Diabetes Association Workgroup on Hypoglycemia *Diabetes Care* **28**(5), 1245–9

Amiel SA, Gale E (1993) Physiological responses to hypoglycemia: Counterregulation and cognitive function *Diabetes Care* **16**, Suppl. 3, 48–55

Amiel SA, Simonson DC, Tamborlane WV, DeFronzo RA, Sherwin RS (1987) Rate of glucose fall does not affect counterregulatory hormone responses to hypoglycemia in normal and diabetic humans *Diabetes* **36**(4), 518–22

Banting FG, Campbell WR, Fletcher AA (1923) Further clinical experiance with insulin (pancreatic extracts) in the treatment of diabetes mellitus *British Medical Journal* **1**, 8–12

Bina DM, Anderson RL, Johnson ML, Bergenstal RM, Kendall DM (2003) Clinical impact of prandial state exercise and site preparation on the equivalence of alternative-site blood glucose testing *Diabetes Care* **26**(4), 981–5

Bloom SR, Edwards AV, Hardy RN, Malinowska KW, Silver M (1975) Endocrine responses to insulin hypoglycaemia in the young calf *The Journal of Physiology Online* **244**(3), 783–803

Boland E, Monsod T, Delucia M, Brandt CA, Fernando S, Tamborlane WV (2001) Limitations of conventional methods of self–monitoring of blood glucose: lessons learned from 3 days of continuous glucose sensing in pediatric patients with type 1 diabetes *Diabetes Care* **24**(11), 1858–62

Bolinder J, Ungerstedt U, Arner P (1993) Long-term continuous glucose monitoring with microdialysis in ambulatory insulin-dependent diabetic patients *Lancet* **342**(8879), 1080–5

Bolli G, De FP, Perriello G, De CS, Ventura M, Campbell P et al. (1985) Role of hepatic autoregulation in defense against hypoglycemia in humans *J Clin Invest* **75**(5), 1623–31

Borg WP, Sherwin RS, During MJ, Borg MA, Shulman GI (1995) Local ventromedial hypothalamus glucopenia triggers counterregulatory hormone release *Diabetes* **44**(2), 180–4

Boyle PJ, Schwartz NS, Shah SD, Clutter WE, Cryer PE (1988) Plasma glucose concentrations at the onset of hypoglycemic symptoms in patients with poorly controlled diabetes and in nondiabetics *N Engl J Med* **318**(23), 1487–92

Caplin NJ, O'Leary P, Bulsara M, Davis EA, Jones TW (2003) Subcutaneous glucose sensor values closely parallel blood glucose during insulin-induced hypoglycaemia *Diabet Med* **20**(3), 238–41

Carter DC, Dozois RR, Kirkpatrick JR (1972) Insulin infusion test of gastric acid secretion *BrMed J* **2**(807), 202–4

Choudhary P, Davies C, Emery C, Freeman J, Heller SR (2006) Low interstitial glucose detected by CGMS correlates well with clinically significant hypoglycaemia *Diabet Med* **23**(2), 12

Clarke WL, Cox DJ, Gonder-Frederick LA, Julian D, Schlundt D, Polonsky W (1995) Reduced awareness of hypoglycemia in adults with IDDM A prospective study of hypoglycemic frequency and associated symptoms *Diabetes Care* **18**(4), 517–22

Colin-Jones DG, Himsworth RL (1970) The location of the chemoreceptor controlling gastric acid secretion during hypoglycaemia *J Physiol* **206**(2), 397–409

Cryer PE (1992) Iatrogenic hypoglycemia as a cause of hypoglycemia-associated autonomic failure in IDDM: A vicious cycle *Diabetes* **41**(3), 255–60

Cryer PE, Binder C, Bolli GB, Cherrington AD, Gale EA, Gerich JE et al. (1989) Hypoglycemia in IDDM *Diabetes* **38**(9), 1193–9

DAFNE group (2002) Training in flexible intensive insulin management to enable dietary freedom in people with type 1 diabetes: dose adjustment for normal eating (DAFNE) randomised controlled trial *BMJ* **325**(7,367), 746

DAFNE group (2003) Training in flexible intensive insulin management to enable dietary freedom in people with Type 1 diabetes: dose adjustment for normal eating (DAFNE) randomized controlled trial *DiabetMed* **20**, Suppl. 3, 4–5

Dagogo-Jack SE, Craft S, Cryer PE (1993) Hypoglycemia-associated autonomic failure in insulin-dependent diabetes mellitus Recent antecedent hypoglycemia reduces autonomic responses to symptoms of and defense against subsequent hypoglycemia *J Clin Invest* **91**(3), 819–28

Davis RE, Morrissey M, Peters JR, Wittrup-Jensen K, Kennedy-Martin T, Currie CJ (2005) Impact of hypoglycaemia on quality of life and productivity in type 1 and type 2 diabetes *Curr Med Res Opin* **21**(9), 1477–83

Davis SN, Shavers C, Costa F (2000) Gender-related differences in counterregulatory responses to antecedent hypoglycemia in normal humans *J Clin Endocrinol Metab* **85**(6), 2148–57

Dawson R (1950) Studies on the glutamine and glutamic acid content of the rat brain during insulin hypoglycaemia *J Biochem (Tokyo)* **47**(4), 386–91

DCCT (1991) Epidemiology of severe hypoglycemia in the diabetes control and complications trial The DCCT Research Group *Am J Med* **90**(4), 450–9

DCCT (1993) The effect of intensive treatment of diabetes on the development and progression of long-term complications in insulin-dependent diabetes mellitus: The Diabetes Control and Complications Trial Research Group *N Engl J Med* **329**(14), 977–86

DCCT (2000) Retinopathy and nephropathy in patients with type 1 diabetes four years after a trial of intensive therapy: The Diabetes Control and Complications Trial/Epidemiology of Diabetes Interventions and Complications Research Group *N Engl J Med* **342**(6), 381–9

De Pergola E, Campiello G (1953) [Adrenal cortex function during experimental insulin hypoglycemia II: Blood level of cortical hormones] *Minerva Med* **44**(57–58), 214–16

De FP, Bolli G, Perriello G, De CS, Compagnucci P, Angeletti G et al. (1983) The adrenergic contribution to glucose counterregulation in type I diabetes mellitus Dependency on A-cell function and mediation through beta 2-adrenergic receptors *Diabetes* **32**(10), 887–93

Deary IJ, Hepburn DA, MacLeod KM, Frier BM (1993) Partitioning the symptoms of hypoglycaemia using multi-sample confirmatory factor analysis *Diabetologia* **36**(8), 771–7

Debrah K, Sherwin RS, Murphy J, Kerr D (1996) Effect of caffeine on recognition of and physiological responses to hypoglycaemia in insulin-dependent diabetes *Lancet* **347**(8,993), 19–24

DeFronzo RA, Tobin JD, Andres R (1979) Glucose clamp technique: a method for quantifying insulin secretion and resistance *AmJ Physiol* **237**(3), E214–23

Dellacqua G (1951) [Studies on experimental hypoglycemia I Insulin test] *Boll Soc Ital Biol Sper* **27**(3), 451–4

DVLA *At a Glance Guide to the Current Medical Standards of Fitness to Drive – A Guide for Medical Practitioners* Govt of UK

Ellison JM, Stegmann JM, Colner SL, Michael RH, Sharma MK, Ervin KR et al. (2002) Rapid changes in postprandial blood glucose produce concentration differences at finger forearm and thigh sampling sites *Diabetes Care* **25**(6), 961–4

Evans ML, McCrimmon RJ, Flanagan DE, Keshavarz T, Fan X, McNay EC et al. (2004) Hypothalamic ATP-sensitive K + channels play a key role in sensing hypoglycemia and triggering counterregulatory epinephrine and glucagon responses *Diabetes* **53**(10), 2542–51

Evans ML, Pernet A, Lomas J, Jones J, Amiel SA (2000) Delay in onset of awareness of acute hypoglycemia and of restoration of cognitive performance during recovery *Diabetes Care* **23**(7), 893–7

Fanelli CG, Pampanelli S, Porcellati F, Bolli GB (1998) Shift of glycaemic thresholds for cognitive function in hypoglycaemia unawareness in humans *Diabetologia* **41**(6), 720–3

Frier BM, Deary IJ (1995) Unreliability of reports of hypoglycaemia by diabetic patients Hypoglycaemia was validated *BMJ* **310**(6,991), 1407

Garber AJ, Cryer PE, Santiago JV, Haymond MW, Pagliara AS, Kipnis DM (1976) The role of adrenergic mechanisms in the substrate and hormonal response to insulin-induced hypoglycemia in man *JClinInvest* **58**(1), 7–15

Garg S, Zisser H, Schwartz S, Bailey T, Kaplan R, Ellis S et al. (2006) Improvement in glycemic excursions with a transcutaneous real–time continuous glucose sensor: a randomized controlled trial *Diabetes Care* **29**(1), 44–50

George E, Harris N, Bedford C, MacDonald IA, Hardisty CA, Heller SR (1995) Prolonged but partial impairment of the hypoglycaemic physiological response following short-term hypoglycaemia in normal subjects *Diabetologia* **38**(10), 1183–90

George E, Marques JL, Harris ND, MacDonald IA, Hardisty CA, Heller SR (1997) Preservation of physiological responses to hypoglycemia 2 days after antecedent hypoglycemia in patients with IDDM *Diabetes Care* **20**(8), 1293–8

Gold AE, MacLeod KM, Frier BM (1994) Frequency of severe hypoglycemia in patients with type I diabetes with impaired awareness of hypoglycemia *Diabetes Care* **17**(7), 697–703

Grimaldi A, Bosquet F, Davidoff P, Digy JP, Sachon C, Landault C et al. (1990) Unawareness of hypoglycemia by insulin–dependent diabetics *Horm Metab Res* **22**(2), 90–5

Han SM, Namkoong C, Jang PG, Park IS, Hong SW, Katakami H et al. (2005) Hypothalamic AMP-activated protein kinase mediates counter–regulatory responses to hypoglycaemia in rats *Diabetologia* **48**(10), 2170–8

Hanzlicek L, Knobloch V (1951) [Biochemical investigation on insulin hypoglycemia; blood potassium level following insulin shock] *Cas Lek Cesk* **90**(8), 227–9

Harrop GA (1927) Hypoglycaemia and the toxic effects of insulin *Archives of Internal Medicine* **40**, 216–25

Hayashi Y, Murata Y, Seo H, Miyamoto N, Kambe F, Ohmori S et al. (1992) Modification of water and electrolyte metabolism during head–down tilting by hypoglycemia in men *J Appl Physiol* **73**(5), 1785–90

Heine RJ (1993) Methods of investigation of insulin induced hypoglycaemia In: Frier BM, Fisher BM (Eds) *Hypoglycaemia and Diabetes*, Edward Arnold, London, pp. 165–75

Heller SR (2002) Abnormalities of the electrocardiogram during hypoglycaemia: the cause of the dead in bed syndrome? *Int J Clin Pract Suppl* **129**, 27–32

Heller SR, Cryer PE (1991) Reduced neuroendocrine and symptomatic responses to subsequent hypoglycemia after 1 episode of hypoglycemia in nondiabetic humans *Diabetes* **40**(2), 223–6

Hepburn DA, Deary IJ, Frier BM (1992) Classification of symptoms of hypoglycaemia in insulin–treated diabetic patients using factor analysis: relationship to hypoglycaemia unawareness *Diabet Med* **9**(1), 70–5

Hepburn DA, Deary IJ, Frier BM, Patrick AW, Quinn JD, Fisher BM (1991) Symptoms of acute insulin-induced hypoglycemia in humans with and without IDDM Factor-analysis approach *Diabetes Care* **14**(11), 949–57

Hepburn DA, MacLeod KM, Frier BM (1993) Physiological symptomatic and hormonal responses to acute hypoglycaemia in type 1 diabetic patients with autonomic neuropathy *Diabet Med* **10**(10), 940–9

Hirsch IB, Heller SR, Cryer PE (1991) Increased symptoms of hypoglycaemia in the standing position in insulin–dependent diabetes mellitus *Clin Sci (Lond)* **80**(6), 583–6

Hoffman RP (2006) Antecedent hypoglycemia does not alter increased epinephrine-induced lipolysis in type 1 diabetes mellitus *Metabolism* **55**(3), 371–80

Holstein A, Plaschke A, Egberts EH (2002) Incidence and costs of severe hypoglycemia *Diabetes Care* **25**(11), 2109–10

Jackson WP, Van Mieghem W, Keller P (1973) Observations of the mechanism of action of the sulfonylureas under clinical conditions *Metabolism* **22**(9), 1,155–62

Jacobson L, Ansari T, Potts J, McGuinness OP (2006) Glucocorticoid-deficient corticotropin-releasing hormone knockout mice maintain glucose requirements but not autonomic responses during repeated hypoglycemia *Am J Physiol Endocrinol Metab*

Kaufman FR, Austin J, Neinstein A, Jeng L, Halvorson M, Devoe DJ et al. (2002) Nocturnal hypoglycemia detected with the Continuous Glucose Monitoring System in pediatric patients with type 1 diabetes *J Pediatr* **141**(5), 625–30

Klip A, Hawkins M (2005) Desperately seeking sugar: glial cells as hypoglycemia sensors *J Clin Invest* **115**(12), 3403–5

Korzon-Burakowska A, Hopkins D, Matyka K, Lomas J, Pernet A, Macdonald I et al. (1998) Effects of glycemic control on protective responses against hypoglycemia in type 2 diabetes *Diabetes Care* **21**(2), 283–90

Kraicer J, Logothetopoulos J (1963) Adrenal Cortical response to insulin-induced hypoglycemia in the rat 1 Adaptation to repeated daily injections of Protamine Zinc Insulin *Acta Endocrinol (Copenh)* **44**, 259–71

Lawrence RD (1941) Insulin Hypoglycaemia Changes in nervous manifestations *Lancet* **238**(6,168), 602

Lazarus SS, Volk BW (1952) The estimation of insulin sensitivity by the modified glucose insulin tolerance test *J Lab Clin Med* **39**(3), 404–13

Leckie AM, Graham MK, Grant JB, Ritchie PJ, Frier BM (2005) Frequency severity and morbidity of hypoglycemia occurring in the workplace in people with insulin-treated diabetes *Diabetes Care* **28**(6), 1333–8

Leese GP, Wang J, Broomhall J, Kelly P, Marsden A, Morrison W et al. (2003) Frequency of severe hypoglycemia requiring emergency treatment in type 1 and type 2 diabetes: a population-based study of health service resource use *Diabetes Care* **26**(4), 1176–80

Levy CJ, Kinsley BT, Bajaj M, Simonson DC (1998) Effect of glycemic control on glucose counter-regulation during hypoglycemia in NIDDM *Diabetes Care* **21**(8), 1330–8

Liu D, Moberg E, Kollind M, Lins PE, Adamson U, MacDonald IA (1992) Arterial arterialized venous venous and capillary blood glucose measurements in normal man during hyperinsulinaemic euglycaemia and hypoglycaemia *Diabetologia* **35**(3), 287–90

Maran A, Amiel S (1994) Research methodologies in hypoglycaemia: counterregulation phenomena and nerve/brain dysfunction In: *Research methodologies in Human Diabetes – Part 1*

Maran A, Lomas J, Archibald H, MacDonald IA, Gale EA, Amiel SA (1993) Double blind clinical and laboratory study of hypoglycaemia with human and porcine insulin in diabetic patients reporting hypoglycaemia unawareness after transferring to human insulin *BMJ* **306**(6,871), 167–71

Maran A, Lomas J, MacDonald IA, Amiel SA (1995) Lack of preservation of higher brain function during hypoglycaemia in patients with intensively-treated IDDM *Diabetologia* **38**(12), 1412–18

Maran A, Macdonald I, Amiel SA (1991) The euglycaemic-hypoglycaemic clamp – a reliable tool for the investigation of responses to hypoglycaemia? *Diabetes* **40**, Suppl. 1, A543

Marks V, Teale JD (1996) Investigation of hypoglycaemia *Clin Endocrinol (Oxf)* **44**(2), 133–6

Marty N, Dallaporta M, Foretz M, Emery M, Tarussio D, Bady I et al. (2005) Regulation of glucagon secretion by glucose transporter type 2 (glut2) and astrocyte-dependent glucose sensors *Journal of Clinical Investigation* **115**(12), 3545–53

Matyka K, Evans M, Lomas J, Cranston I, Macdonald I, Amiel SA (1997) Altered hierarchy of protective responses against severe hypoglycemia in normal aging in healthy men *Diabetes Care* **20**(2), 135–41

Mauras N, Beck RW, Ruedy KJ, Kollman C, Tamborlane WV, Chase HP et al. (2004) Lack of accuracy of continuous glucose sensors in healthy nondiabetic children: results of the Diabetes Research in Children Network (DirecNet) accuracy study *J Pediatr* **144**(6), 770–5

McAulay V, Deary IJ, Frier BM (2001) Symptoms of hypoglycaemia in people with diabetes *Diabet Med* **18**(9), 690–705

McCrimmon RJ, Deary IJ, Gold AE, Hepburn DA, MacLeod KM, Ewing FM et al. (2003) Symptoms reported during experimental hypoglycaemia: effect of method of induction of hypoglycaemia and of diabetes per se *Diabet Med* **20**(6), 507–9

McCrimmon RJ, Evans ML, Fan X, McNay EC, Chan O, Ding Y et al. (2005) Activation of ATP–sensitive K+ channels in the ventromedial hypothalamus amplifies counterregulatory hormone responses to hypoglycemia in normal and recurrently hypoglycemic rats *Diabetes* **54**(11), 3169–74

McGowan K, Thomas W, Moran A (2002) Spurious reporting of nocturnal hypoglycemia by CGMS in patients with tightly controlled type 1 diabetes *Diabetes Care* **25**(9), 1499–503

Meguro S, Funae O, Hosokawa K, Atsumi Y (2005) Hypoglycemia detection rate differs among blood glucose monitoring sites *Diabetes Care* **28**(3), 708–9

Mitrakou A, Ryan C, Veneman T, Mokan M, Jenssen T, Kiss I et al. (1991) Hierarchy of glycemic thresholds for counterregulatory hormone secretion symptoms and cerebral dysfunction *Am J Physiol* **260**(1), Pt 1, E67–74

Morgenthaler FD, Koski DM, Kraftsik R, Henry PG, Gruetter R (2006) Biochemical quantification of total brain glycogen concentration in rats under different glycemic states *Neurochem Int*

Mueller PS, Heninger GR, McDonald RK (1969) Insulin tolerance test in depression *Arch Gen Psychiatry* **21**(5), 587–94

Nathan DM, Cleary PA, Backlund JY, Genuth SM, Lachin JM, Orchard TJ et al. (2005) Intensive diabetes treatment and cardiovascular disease in patients with type 1 diabetes *N Engl J Med* **353**(25), 2643–53

Oz G, Henry PG, Seaquist ER, Gruetter R (2003) Direct noninvasive measurement of brain glycogen metabolism in humans *NeurochemInt* **43**(4–5), 323–9

Paranjape SA, Briski KP (2005) Recurrent insulin-induced hypoglycemia causes site-specific patterns of habituation or amplification of CNS neuronal genomic activation *Neuroscience* **130**(4), 957–70

Peacey SR, George E, Rostami-Hodjegan A, Bedford C, Harris N, Hardisty CA et al. (1996) Similar physiological and symptomatic responses to sulphonylurea and insulin induced hypoglycaemia in normal subjects *Diabet Med* **13**(7), 634–41

Peacey SR, Rostami-Hodjegan A, George E, Tucker GT, Heller SR (1997) The use of tolbutamide-induced hypoglycemia to examine the intraislet role of insulin in mediating glucagon release in normal humans *J Clin Endocrinol Metab* **82**(5), 1458–61

Pennebaker JW, Cox DJ, Gonder-Frederick L, Wunsch MG, Evans WS, Pohl S (1981) Physical symptoms related to blood glucose in insulin-dependent diabetics *Psychosom Med* **43**(6), 489–500

Porcellati F, Pampanelli S, Rossetti P, Cordoni C, Marzotti S, Scionti L et al. (2003) Counterregulatory hormone and symptom responses to insulin–induced hypoglycaemia in the postprandial state in humans *Diabetes* **52**(11), 2774–83

Pramming S, Thorsteinsson B, Bendtson I, Binder C (1991) Symptomatic hypoglycaemia in 411 type 1 diabetic patients *Diabet Med* **8**(3), 217–22

Rebrin K, Steil GM, van Antwerp WP, Mastrototaro JJ (1999) Subcutaneous glucose predicts plasma glucose independent of insulin: implications for continuous monitoring *Am J Physiol* **277**(3), Pt 1, E561–71

Ryan EA, Shandro T, Green K, Paty BW, Senior PA, Bigam D et al. (2004) Assessment of the severity of hypoglycemia and glycemic lability in type 1 diabetic subjects undergoing islet transplantation *Diabetes* **53**(4), 955–62

Samann A, Muhlhauser I, Bender R, Kloos C, Muller UA (2005) Glycaemic control and severe hypoglycaemia following training in flexible intensive insulin therapy to enable dietary freedom in people with type 1 diabetes: a prospective implementation study *Diabetologia* **48**(10), 1965–70

Sandoval DA, Aftab Guy DL, Richardson MA, Ertl AC, Davis SN (2006) Acute Same Day Effects of Antecedent Exercise on Counterregulatory Responses to Subsequent Hypoglycemia in Type 1 Diabetes Mellitus *Am J Physiol Endocrinol Metab*

Schlichtkrull J, Munck O, Jersild M (1965) The M Value an index of blood sugar control in diabetics *Acta Med Scand* **177**, 95–102

Segel SA, Paramore DS, Cryer PE (2002) Hypoglycemia-associated autonomic failure in advanced type 2 diabetes *Diabetes* **51**(3), 724–33

Service FJ, Molnar GD, Rosevear JW, Ackerman E, Gatewood LC, Taylor WF (1970) Mean amplitude of glycemic excursions a measure of diabetic instability *Diabetes* **19**(9), 644–55

Sovik O, Thordarson H (1999) Dead-in-bed syndrome in young diabetic patients *Diabetes Care* **22**, Suppl. 2, B40–2

Spyer G, Hattersley AT, MacDonald IA, Amiel S, MacLeod KM (2000) Hypoglycaemic counter–regulation at normal blood glucose concentrations in patients with well controlled type–2 diabetes *Lancet* **356**(9,246), 1970–4

Strachan MW, Ewing FM, Frier BM, Harper A, Deary IJ (2004) Food cravings during acute hypogly-caemia in adults with Type 1 diabetes *Physiol Behav* **80**(5), 675–82

Suzuki T, Saito K (1951) On the adrenaline secretion of the suprarenal glands during the insulin hypoglycemia in dogs anesthetized with evipan-sodium *Tohoku J Exp Med* **54**(4), 309–12

Tamada JA, Bohannon NJ, Potts RO (1995) Measurement of glucose in diabetic subjects using noninvasive transdermal extraction *Nat Med* **1**(11), 1198–1201

The European Communities Council directive of 29 July 1991 on driving licenses

UK Hypoglycaemia Study Group (2006) *Stratifying Hypoglycemic Event Risk in Insulin-Treated Diabetes*, Department for Transport, London

Visser SL (1967) Significance of the tolbutamide (hypoglycaemia) test as a method of provoking EEG changes: comparison with the bemegride provocation test *Psychiatr Neurol Neurochir* **70**(6), 467–80

Vogt M (1951) The role of hypoglycaemia and of adrenaline in the response of the adrenal cortex to insulin *J Physiol* **114**(1–2), 222–33

White NH, Skor DA, Cryer PE, Levandoski LA, Bier DM, Santiago JV (1983) Identification of type I diabetic patients at increased risk for hypoglycemia during intensive therapy *N Engl J Med* **308**(9), 485–91

Wilder RM (1927) Carcinoma of the islands of the pancreas: Hyperinsulinism and hypoglycemia *JAMA* **89**, 348–55

Woolf PD, Lee LA, Leebaw W, Thompson D, Lilavivathana U, Brodows R et al. (1977) Intracellular glucopenia causes prolactin release in man *J Clin Endocrinol Metab* **45**(3), 377–83

6

Glucose Kinetics: Measurement of Flux Rates

Jerry Radziuk and Susan Pye

Introduction

The maintenance of the 'internal milieu' (Bernard 1878) is the central issue in physiology – and in clinical medicine. The homeostatic processes responsible for this state do not yield a static situation characterised by the presence of appropriate concentrations of body constituents or metabolites but a 'dynamic steady state' (Schoenheimer 1964) in which these concentrations are preserved by the precisely balanced fluxes of the molecules of which the system is composed. Perturbations from the 'external' milieu are dealt with by the body through adaptive responses in these fluxes, the goal of which is the restoration of the dynamic equilibrium. A chronic alteration in a system component, such as a metabolite concentration, is then the final manifestation of a maladaptive response, resulting from a failure in regulation. It is evident therefore that it is metabolite fluxes that are regulated by endocrine and neural controls (e.g. Cahill et al. 1966) and whose dysregulation could result in disease.

The circulating concentration of glucose is both representative of and central to these homeostatic processes. Under normal, basal conditions, it is maintained within a remarkably tight range by an exquisite balance of the rate at which it is produced (primarily by the liver) and the rate at which it is utilised. Perturbations such as meals, stress or exercise result in altered glucose fluxes, such as the entry of additional glucose from intestinal absorption. Negative feedback effects rapidly restore any altered glucose concentrations to their steady state concentration. The underlying fluxes are generally reinstated more slowly. Type 2 diabetes is characterised by chronic alterations in glucose levels. Probing of the normal homeostatic responses, and of the dysregulation that occurs in diabetes, clearly needs to take place at the level of the fluxes.

Clinical Diabetes Research: Methods and Techniques   Edited by Michael Roden
© 2007 John Wiley & Sons, Ltd   ISBN 978-0-470-01728-9

Measurement of glucose production and uptake by the liver – tissue balance techniques

The major part of glucose production occurs in the liver, although the kidney (Gersosimo et al. 1994; Stumvoll et al. 1995) and the intestinal bed (Croset et al. 2001) have also been shown to contribute. The most direct approach to measuring this flux is simply to measure the efflux of glucose from the liver and subtract the influx, yielding a net output. This can be accomplished in animal models by simultaneously sampling arterial, portal and hepatic venous blood (Madison 1969; Cherrington et al. 1982). Although the portal vein is generally inaccessible in humans, splanchnic metabolism may nevertheless be assessed since hepatic venous blood may be accessed by the fluoroscopically guided retrograde insertion of a catheter from the femoral vein (Felig et al. 1978; Sacca et al. 1982; Basu et al. 2001). Net splanchnic glucose output can then be calculated as:

$$Net\ SGO = HBF \cdot (C_A - C_H) \qquad (6.1)$$

Where C_A = arterial glucose concentration, C_H = hepatic venous concentration and HBF = hepatic blood flow.

The most accurate determinations can be made when glucose concentrations correspond to blood levels. Hepatic blood flow is most commonly determined through the extraction of indocyanine green dye (ICG) by the liver (Felig et al. 1978; Sacca et al. 1982; Basu et al. 2001). Since plasma levels of ICG are measured, plasma flow is obtained by dividing the rate of infusion of ICG by the difference between arterial and hepatic venous concentrations. Correction to blood flow is made, when appropriate, by dividing by 1/(1-haematocrit).

The liver and the gut also take up glucose for storage and/or energy requirements. In order to calculate the total splanchnic production of glucose, this uptake must be accounted for. This can be accomplished using tracers.

A tracer is essentially a glucose molecule or analogue that is labeled (isotopically or chemically) so that it is distinguishable from glucose, but continues to have the equivalent kinetic behaviour to that of glucose. It is introduced in quantities much smaller than the glucose so that it does not perturb glucose dynamics. If labeled glucose is systemically infused to equilibrium then the splanchnic uptake of tracer (SGU^*) can be expressed as:

$$SGU^* = HBF \cdot (C_A^* - C_H^*) \qquad (6.2)$$

Where C_A^*, C_H^* are the measured arterial and hepatic concentrations of the tracer.

We now invoke a central assumption of the tracer method: the kinetic/biochemical equivalence of the tracer and the glucose (tracee) molecule. Mathematically, this means that:

$$\frac{SGU^*}{SGU} = \frac{C_A^*}{C_A} \qquad (6.3)$$

Or that the uptake of glucose and tracer are proportional to their concentrations. We can now estimate the total SGO:

$$Total\ SGO = Net\ SGO + SGU$$

$$= Net\ SGO + (C_A/C_A^*) \cdot SGU^* \qquad (6.4)$$

$$= Net\ SGO + f \cdot HBF \cdot C_A$$

Where $f = (C_A{}^* - C_H{}^*)/C_A{}^*$ and f is the fractional extraction of the glucose tracer (or glucose) by the liver. The fact that f is the same for both molecules is a restatement of the tracer indistinguishability principle.

The above derivations assume equilibrium conditions or a steady state – no change in measured concentrations or fluxes with respect to time. Under non-steady state conditions, the problem is more difficult. Tracer or glucose molecules which enter the liver simultaneously will undergo variable delays as they transit through the inhomogeneous labyrinth of sinusoids, resulting in the dispersion of their arrival times at the outflow (Sheppard 1962). If one now conceptually subdivides the influx of glucose or tracer into a series of boluses, each bolus of molecules will yield a distribution at the outflow. Because under steady state conditions all the inflow 'boluses' are equal, the summation of the distributed outflows will also remain constant, with the applicability of Equations 6.2–4. As influx concentrations change, however, the dispersion-induced delays in transit will alter the efflux concentration profile so that, even with zero input/uptake, the differences will be non-zero. To circumvent this problem, injection of a (unit amount of) kinetic analogue of glucose/tracer that is not produced or taken up by the liver (e.g. labeled sucrose) at the inflow, but which is distributed in the same way, will yield a dispersion or distribution function, $h(t)$, at the outflow. The theoretical efflux profile of glucose, $C'_H(t)$, or tracer, $C_H^{*\prime}(t)$, had there been no output or uptake of glucose by the liver, can then be calculated as the sum of these bolus effects. In the limit, as the boluses become very small and large in number, these profiles become the convolution integrals:

$$C'_H(t) = \int_{-\infty}^{t} h(t-\tau)C_A(\tau)d\tau \qquad C_H^{*\prime}(t) = \int_{-\infty}^{t} h(t-\tau)\cdot C_A^*(\tau)d\tau \qquad (6.5)$$

The difference between $C_H^{*\prime}(t)$ and $C_H^*(t)$, the measured hepatic venous tracer concentration multiplied by HBF, would yield a better estimate of the uptake of the tracer, and the difference between $C_H(t)$ and $C'_H(t)$, a better approximation of net glucose production. Such an approach was used in non-steady experiments in perfused livers (Zhang & Radziuk 1991, 1994), a situation analogous to the measurement of splanchnic fluxes in situ.

The above discussion outlines the measurement of glucose production and uptake by the liver, an approach which is immediately generalisable to other tissues. We have introduced the concept of tracers as quantitatively small, kinetically equivalent but separately measurable molecules that enable the measurement of total fluxes. The following discussion of tracer properties serves to outline the strategy of choosing appropriate tracers for the desired flux measurements and the considerations which enter into their use.

Properties of glucose tracers

Since the liver can exchange glucose with the circulation (via the glucokinase/glucose-6-phosphatase cycle), all labeled glucose tracers are distinguished from each other by their behaviour in the liver.

Property one: measurement distinguishability

This simply means that glucose and tracer must be separately measurable. Usually it means that glucose is isotopically labeled. The most frequently used labels are ^{14}C or [3]H (radioactive) and ^{12}C or [2]H (stable). Labels are not all equivalent and the method of measurement may affect the results. For example, the use of [U-^{13}C]glucose and the measurement of the M+6 isotopomer (all six carbons of each glucose molecule are labeled) yields results equivalent to the use of [3-^{3}H]glucose. Both will lose their (measured) label in the equilibration in the triose phosphate pool. [U-^{14}C]glucose, which appears to be similarly labeled, only has a uniformly distributed label; not all carbons in each molecule are labeled. Any measurement of [U-^{14}C]glucose will therefore include label that has been recycled via glycolysis and gluconeogenesis, which is not the case for [U-^{13}C]glucose. If both these carbon labels undergo combustion to CO_2, however, an analogous measurement of their enrichment will be obtained. Label choices and methods of measurement must therefore always be made with the metabolic application in mind.

Property two: kinetic equivalence

From a kinetic, transport, metabolic standpoint, the tracer must be indistinguishable from glucose. For splanchnic glucose uptake, this is stated in Equation 6.3. More generally:

$$\frac{R^*}{R} = \frac{C^*}{C} \tag{6.6}$$

Where R^* and R are equivalent tracer and glucose fluxes and C^* and C are the concentrations in the pool from which the flux takes place. In practice, one must take into account the process that the tracer actually tracks. The loci in the metabolic pathway at which tracers lose their label, and thus the processes tracked, are summarised below:

[2-^{3}H] or [2-^{2}H]glucose

[2-^{3}H] or [2-^{2}H]glucose is detritiated or de-deuterated in the hydrogen exchanges that take place at phosphoglucose isomerase. This has no quantitative consequence in peripheral tissues but is important in the liver because tracer that has lost its label can be immediately dephosphorylated and re-released as unlabeled glucose. This would not be appropriate in the determination of an irreversible uptake of glucose in the liver or, by extrapolation, systemically – since it would include some part of this 'futile' cycle (glucose $\rightleftharpoons$ glucose-6-phosphate) (Katz & Dunn 1967; Hers & Hue 1983). Because the equilibration with water at the isomerase step might not be complete, a portion of the label may be retained both in the second and the first positions. Approximately 80 % of the cycle is however accounted for by the detritiation/de-deuteration (Wajngot et al. 1989), with the result that estimates of endogenous glucose production (*EGP*) made using this label in normal humans were found to be $\sim$ 17 % higher than those made with (recycling corrected) [6-^{14}C]glucose and 29 % higher than those using [3-^{3}H]glucose (Bell et al. 1986). In type 2 diabetes, this cycle may be increased (Efendic et al. 1988) and thus the overestimate may be greater. On the other hand, the comparison of estimates of *EGP* using e.g. [2-^{3}H]glucose and [6-^{3}H]glucose will yield a reasonable estimate of the flux through the glucose cycle (Bell et al. 1986).

[3-^{3}H]glucose

The tritium from this label ends up on the first position of dihydroxyacetone phosphate (DHAP). Assuming no redistribution of this label to the second position in the isomerase reaction, it will be removed either by exchange with water or in the glyceraldehyde-3-phosphate dehydrogenase equilibration. Any tritium which is transferred to the second position will nevertheless be removed at the enolase step. To the extent that this equilibration is complete, [3-^{3}H]glucose will provide an estimate of *EGP* that includes the 'fructose cycle' (Topper 1957). Approximately 80 % of this cycle would be accounted for using [3-^{3}H]glucose (Landau 1993). A direct comparison showed that *EGP* estimated with this tracer was about 9 % lower than that using (recycling corrected) [6-^{14}C]glucose (Bell et al. 1986). The estimate with [3-^{3}H]glucose was lower, although not significantly. This is consistent with other recent observations and suggests that the 'fructose cycle' is not significant in humans (Wajngot et al. 2001). It does not completely agree, however, with previous work, which indicated that up to 25 % of the *EGP* determined using [3-^{3}H]glucose could be due to triose-phosphate cycling (Shulman et al. 1985). When [3-^{3}H] and [6-^{3}H]glucose were compared directly (Karlander et al. 1986), this type of difference was found to occur in fewer than half the subjects studied.

[6-^{3}H] or [6,6-^{2}H$_2$]glucose

This label is randomised to the first and sixth positions in the aldolase triose-phosphate isomerase reaction. Following this, some of the label will be removed from the first position in the phosphoglucose isomerase reaction. A large part of the remainder is removed in the oxaloacetate $\rightleftharpoons$ malate $\rightleftharpoons$ fumarate equilibration (Dunn et al. 1967) or the 'phospho-enolpyruvate cycle'. About 10 % of the label could remain and be recycled back to glucose (Wajngot et al. 1989). Since the [6,6-^{2}H$_2$]glucose is measured as the M+2 isotopomer and one of the ^{2}H would be lost in the above reactions, the recycling of label that might occur for this tracer would be negligible. Relative to the stable label, the tritiated tracer would therefore sightly underestimate *EGP*.

[^{2}H$_4$-2,3,6,6]glucose

[^{2}H$_4$-2,3,6,6]glucose will lose its labels at the steps in the glycolytic/gluconeogenetic pathways already outlined. When measured as the M + 4 isotopomer, it will behave as [2-^{2}H]glucose, since the label in the second position will be lost most quickly.

[1-^{14}C], [6-^{14}C], [1-^{13}C] and [6-^{13}C]glucose

Carbon label is not 'lost' in the glycolytic or gluconeogenetic processes as ^{3}H or ^{2}H are in exchanges with hydrogen from water. It is, however, redistributed within the glucose molecule as this proceeds through the metabolic pathways and some of it will eventually be removed as ^{14}CO$_2$/^{13}CO$_2$. Label in the first position will appear in the sixth, as a result of the triose phosphate isomerase reaction. The inverse (sixth – first) redistribution will also take place. Further downstream, redistribution will occur in the exchange of carbons with the tricarboxylic acid cycle in the oxaloacetate/malate pool. Assuming symmetry, the infused label in the first and sixth positions can be corrected for recycling by subtracting what has been redistributed to the opposite position. If both measurements are not made, unrecycled label can be estimated by comparing total label to label in one of these positions (Reichard et al. 1963). It is usually assumed that four times the label in the complementary position arises from recycling. More complex calculations can be used (e.g. Hetenyi 1982; Kelleher 1986; Radziuk 1989) if greater knowledge of the exchanges that take place is desired. When the ^{13}C label is used, isotopomer analysis will yield similar information (Katz et al. 1991;

Lee 1989). Simultaneously, the more complex analyses can optimise the estimation of unrecycled glucose label concentrations. When careful corrections for recycling are made, this type of estimate should yield rates of *EGP* that are near the 'actual' rate – i.e. don't include any of the 'futile' cycles. The complementary calculation based on these label redistributions will also yield estimates of the rate of passage of glucose carbons through the Cori cycle. These range from 15% in normal humans to 30% in subjects with type 2 diabetes.

[U-^{13}C]glucose

The measurement of the M+6 isotopomer will preclude any recycled glucose. The reason is that if the amounts of tracer administered are small (<5% of R_a), the probability of recombination of two 3-carbon metabolic products to the M+6 molecule is neglible. Thus, no cycling through any 3-carbon pools will be included in the estimates of *EGP*. This tracer is therefore equivalent to [3-^{3}H]glucose, [6,6-^{2}H$_2$]glucose (measured as the M+2 moiety) or [1-*C] or [6-*C]glucose (when the latter are appropriately corrected for recycled label). If the M+6 and M+3 isotopomers are both considered then the [U-^{13}C]glucose would be nearly equivalent to [6-^{3}H]glucose.

Chemical analogues of glucose

Chemical analogues of glucose, such as 3-O-methylglucose and 2-deoxyglucose (2DG), track different properties of the glucose molecule: the former yields glucose distribution within total body water, the latter is trapped after phosphorylation in tissues that do not possess glucose-6-phosphatase activity. Labeled 2DG is therefore a very useful tracer for the determination of relative uptakes in different tissues and in the fluorine-18 labeled moiety is one of the major tools in positron emission tomography. These molecules do not follow the same kinetics as glucose, however. This is compensated for by the 'lumped constant', which represents the differences in kinetics (Sokoloff et al. 1977; Phelps et al. 1978; Utriainen et al. 2000).

A more detailed description of the different tracers can be found in e.g. Wolfe (1992). From the above, it would be expected that [U-^{13}C], [3-*H] or [6-*H]glucose would provide the most consistent estimates of *EGP*. It should be noted, however, that the kinetic equivalences of tracers will refer to different fluxes depending on the tracer used.

Property three: quantitatively negligible

The quantities of tracer administered are always small relative to the glucose fluxes being measured. This is necessary in a nonlinear system, such as the glucose system, as it is critical that the tracer not perturb parameters/processes that are concentration-dependent.

In many tissues, glucose uptake involves carrier-mediated transport into cells (Baldwin & Lienhard 1981) – primarily by glucose transporters (e.g. Koistinen & Zierath 2002) – so it can be defined by:

$$uptake = \frac{V_{max}C}{(K_m + C)} \tag{6.7}$$

Where V_{max} and K_m are Michaelis-Menten constants representing appropriate approximations in the equations for carrier-mediated transport (Gottesman et al. 1984). Adding tracer to the system, we have:

$$uptake\,(glu\cos e + tracer) = V_{max}(C + C^*)/(K_m + C + C^*)$$

$$\cong V_{max}C/(K_m + C) + V_{max}C^*/(K_m + C) \quad (6.8)$$

With $C + C^* \sim C$ in the denominator, since $C^* << C$. The glucose and tracer components of the uptake are thus separable. It is important to note that while $V_{max}/(K_m + C)$ depends on C, the uptake of tracer is linear in C^*, albeit multiplied by a factor that is (from the perspective of the tracer, C^*) time-dependent. $V_{max}/(K_m + C)$, which defines a 'cellular extraction efficiency', is a time-varying factor that can be calculated when tracer uptake and concentration are measured (Radziuk & Lickley 1985).

This efficiency is not just a function of glucose concentration but will also change in response to altered insulin levels (and many other factors). Glucose concentration stimulates insulin secretion. As we have seen, a tracer cannot stimulate the cellular efficiency of glucose extraction. Neither, due to its low quantity, can it contribute to the stimulation of insulin secretion. In effect, a tracer linearises the nonlinear glucose system, making it much more tractable to analysis.

A linear system is one where the following property holds:

If inputs R_1 and R_2 produce the concentrations C_1 and C_2 , then the input $\alpha R_1 + \beta R_2$ produces the concentration $\alpha C_1 + \beta C_2$

Property four: equivalent entry

We have seen that metabolite concentrations in blood entering the liver may not be representative of concentrations at the outflow, even if no input or uptake of the metabolite takes place, because of tissue heterogeneity. A recirculating system, such as the whole body, will display additional heterogeneities. For example, during absorption of a meal, tracer is infused into a peripheral vein. Newly absorbed glucose enters the portal vein and a fraction is removed on first passage through the liver, prior to entering the peripheral circulation. Clearly meal glucose and tracer are not entering at equivalent points. It is not likely therefore that Equation 6.6 will hold for meal glucose and tracer. By using a second tracer in the meal glucose, however, this situation can be exploited to calculate the fractional extraction of glucose by the liver (Radziuk et al. 1978; Radziuk 1987). Equivalent entry is even more problematic for other metabolites, such as lactate, which enter diffusely throughout the body (Katz et al. 1981), since tracer can realistically only be administered at one (or perhaps a few) points. What well-designed protocols are likely to yield in both cases is a 'first entry' of the metabolite into the sampled pool. Outside of meals, glucose from the liver enters the hepatic vein, or else it is infused at one site, and first entry is generally synonymous with actual entry, minimising these interpretational problems.

Measurement of glucose production and uptake by the liver – systemic techniques

Accounting for organ glucose uptake using tracers can be generalised to the whole body. Direct measurement across organs is replaced by the tracer dilution principle and a mathematical description of the distribution of glucose throughout the body.

The behaviour of glucose within the whole body is characterised by the law of conservation of mass, or:

$$\frac{dM}{dt} = R_a - R_d \tag{6.9}$$

Where M is the mass of glucose in the system and R_a and R_d are its rate of production and removal. The analogous equation holds for tracers:

$$\frac{dM^*}{dt} = R_a^* - R_d^* \tag{6.10}$$

Where M^* is the mass of tracer and R_a^* and R_d^* are the rates of tracer administration (e.g. infusion) and its irreversible removal. How accurately R_a and R_d are determined from the measured concentrations will be determined by the extent that the tracer conforms to the properties discussed above and how well the physical distribution of glucose is described mathematically.

The steady state

The metabolic steady state is characterised by both constant concentrations and fluxes. Under these conditions, $dM/dt = 0$ and $R_a = R_d$. If the tracer is also in steady state, we have: $dM^*/dt = 0$ and $R_a^* = R_d^*$. From Equation 6.6, the removal rates of glucose and tracer are proportional to their concentrations. Hence:

$$R_a = MCR \cdot C \text{ where } MCR = R_a^*/C^* \text{ or } R_a = R_a^*/a \text{ where } a = C^*/C \tag{6.11}$$

a is defined as the specific activity (radioactive tracers) or enrichment (stable labels).

It should be noted that, for stable isotopically labeled glucose, the tracer has a small but finite mass and therefore its rate of administration needs to be subtracted from R_a

$$R_a = R_a^*/a - R_a^* = ((1-a)/a) \cdot R_a^* \tag{6.12}$$

This subtraction is implied in subsequent descriptions. *MCR* in Equation 6.11 defines the metabolic clearance rate and is analogous to the 'cellular extraction efficiency' defined above. The identity of *MCR* for glucose and for tracer is the systemic expression of the equivalence in kinetic behaviour of the two molecules (Radziuk & Lickley 1985).

It should be noted that, under steady state conditions, both tracer infusions and injections are comparable approaches for determining R_a (e.g. Radziuk et al. 1978). Only tracer infusions will be considered here.

The non-steady state

Broadly, the non-steady state is defined by Equations 6.9 and 6.10. Unlike the steady state condition, knowledge of M (and M*) is required for the calculation of R_d^*, R_d and R_a.

Because, in general, glucose concentration is non-uniform and will thus not be identical to that in the sampling compartment, the determination of its total mass, M, requires a structure or model for the system (Cobelli & Caumo 1998). Such models can be highly complex or very simple (Radziuk & Hetenyi 1982). The complexity of the model structure is not only determined by the system it describes but by the purpose for which it is used. With respect to glucose dynamics, metabolism takes place against a background of the mixing of the newly-formed glucose throughout the system (as well as replacement of glucose that is removed by cells). The principle consideration becomes the relative speed of mixing and of changes in metabolic processes or fluxes. If such changes take place over hours, and complete mixing of a glucose tracer throughout the extracellular space takes place in minutes, then the system may be considered well-mixed with respect to that process. This is undoubtedly why the assumption of a uniform distribution (a one-compartment model) has worked so well when assessing the responses of the liver, for example, to moderate exercise, meals, etc. (reviewed in Radziuk & Pye 2002). If, on the other hand, the two processes (mixing and metabolism) approach each other in their time-constants, additional structure is required to properly describe the distribution of the glucose, since this distribution or mixing will be a determinant of the time course of the metabolic process. This becomes evident in the response of the liver to insulin (hyper-insulinaemic, euglycaemic or hyperglyacemic clamps), which is also of the order of minutes. Its calculation against a background of rapid changes in uptake and of glucose distribution becomes a more difficult modeling problem (e.g. Katz et al. 1993; Hother-Nielsen et al. 1996).

A well-mixed sampling compartment (the blood) within an otherwise inhomogeneous system can be modeled (Radziuk 1976; Radziuk & Pye 2002). The lowest orders of approximation for this non-uniform system are the one- and two-compartment models. The equations for these are summarised below:

The one-compartment model

$$\frac{dC}{dt} = -k \cdot C + \frac{R_a}{V} \quad and \quad \frac{dC^*}{dt} = -k \cdot C^* + \frac{R_a^*}{V} \tag{6.13}$$

Where k is the fractional disappearance rate of glucose and V its volume of distribution. These equations can be solved for the metabolic clearance rate, MCR, and R_a:

$$MCR = k \cdot V = R_a^* - V \cdot \frac{dC^*}{dt}; \quad R_d = MCR \cdot C \quad and \quad R_a = \frac{R_a^*}{a} - \frac{V \cdot C}{a} \cdot \frac{da}{dt} \tag{6.14}$$

Where R_d is the rate of disappearance or removal of glucose.

It can be noted that MCR is a function only of tracer quantities, as already discussed for organs and the steady state situation. It should also be pointed out that the volume of distribution V is often estimated as a fraction of the extracellular fluid (pV, where p is a 'pool fraction'). Better precision in the calculation is achieved if it is estimated from the data (Radziuk & Pye 2002).

The two-compartment model

$$\frac{dC_1}{dt} = -(k_{21} + k_{01}) \cdot C_1 + k_{12}C_2 + \frac{R_a}{V_1} \quad and \quad \frac{dC_2}{dt} = k_{21} \cdot C_1 - (k_{12} + k_{02}) \cdot C_2$$

$$\tag{6.15}$$

Where C_1 and C_2 are the glucose concentrations in the sampling compartment (#1) and a more distal compartment (#2, which would, for example, include part of the interstitial space); k_{12} and k_{21} are exchange coefficients and k_{01} and k_{02} are fractional disappearance rates; V_1 is the volume of distribution of the first (sampled) pool.

An exactly analogous set of equations holds for the tracer with C_1, C_2 replaced by C_1^*, C_2^* and R_a by R_a^*. For the special case of the two-compartment model where $k_{02} = 0$, there is a closed form solution:

$$R_a(t) = \frac{R_a^*}{a_1} - \frac{V_1 \cdot C_1}{a_1} \cdot \frac{da_1}{dt} + V_1 \cdot k_{12} \cdot k_{21} \cdot \int_0^t e^{-k_{12}(t-\tau)} \left[\frac{C_1^*(\tau)}{a_1(t)} - C_1(\tau) \right] d\tau$$

$$+ \; terms \; defining \; initial \; conditions \tag{6.16}$$

$$R_d = MCR \cdot C_1 = V_1 \cdot k_{01} \cdot C_1 \tag{6.17}$$

Where $a_1 = C_1^*(t) \big/ C_1(t)$ is the specific activity in the sampled compartment (Radziuk et al. 1978).

k_{12}, k_{21} and V_1 are estimated from initial tracer data (when no variation in k_{01} takes place). Interestingly, each level of relative complexity, from steady state through one- and two-compartment models, provides an additional correction term in the formula for glucose production, R_a.

Basal conditions

Basal conditions prevail at rest when no exogenous perturbations, such as meals, are taking place. They are characterised by a state which is stable and thus predictable in time. Most commonly these conditions occur in the fasting or postprandial state. There is a widespread association of basal and steady state conditions, and indeed in non-diabetic individuals this is the case, and all of glucose production, removal and concentration are constant. Under these circumstances, the usual method of assessing glucose turnover (production = removal) is tracer infusion and Equation 6.11. Fasting glucose production – and its contribution to fasting hyperglycaemia in type 2 diabetes – has been a topic of some discussion (reviewed in Radziuk & Pye 2002). Some studies showed an increase, whereas others showed a glucose production (*EGP*) identical to normal, and occasionally lower. The reasons for this appeared to be the patient populations studied, the time of day at which measurements were made and the techniques, both experimental and analytical, that were used (Radziuk & Pye 2002).

Studies were therefore made without the assumption of a steady state, using Equation 6.14, to re-evaluate the nature of the fasting *EGP* in type 2 diabetes (Radziuk & Pye 2001, 2002). The results (Figure 6.1) showed that glycaemia was high in the morning and fell throughout the day. This was caused by a corresponding decrease in *EGP*, against the background of a nearly constant *MCR*. This contrasted with the near constant fluxes seen in control subjects and demonstrated the lack of steady state under basal conditions in diabetes.

These data appear to reveal an instability in *EGP* in diabetic patients. To determine how glycaemia and *EGP* rose to morning levels, patients fasted from 8 am on day 1 of a study until 2 pm on day 2. Glucose levels and fluxes were monitored using Equation 6.14 for the last 24 h of the study (Radziuk & Pye 2006). In contrast to controls, whose glucose levels remained near constant, it was observed that glycaemia rose spontaneously throughout the

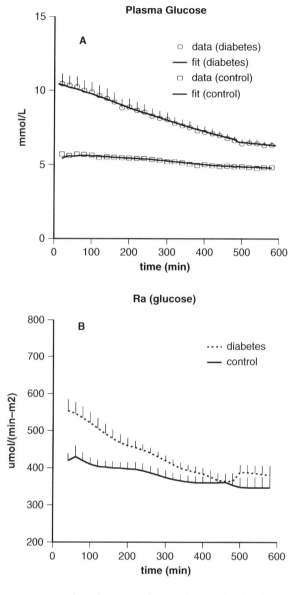

Figure 6.1   A) glucose concentrations (means and mean fitted values) collected from 8 am to 6 pm in patients with type 2 diabetes and in control subjects, who were previously fasted for 12–14 h; B) rates of endogenous glucose production (R_a) calculated using non-steady state methods and a simultaneously infused tracer. Reproduced with permission from Radziuk J, Pye A. (2001) Production and metabolic clearance of glucose under basal conditions in type II (non-insulin dependent) diabetes. *Diabetologia* **44** 983–991, Springer.

night in these fasting patients, peaking in the early morning and declining through the day to reach levels near those of the previous afternoon (Figure 6.2).

This was reflected in the underlying glucose production, which followed the same pattern, anticipating that in glycaemia. Again, the *MCR* did not change appreciably throughout this period. *EGP* in type 2 diabetes is seen to never be in steady state, displaying rather

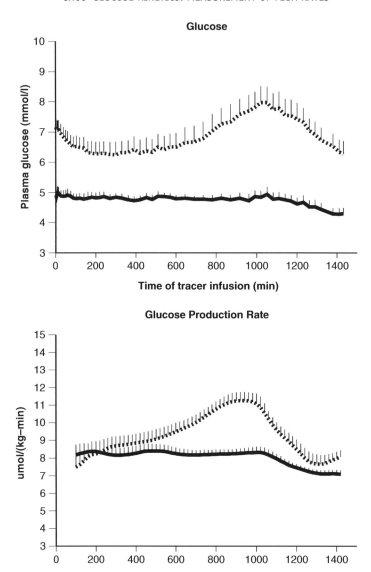

Figure 6.2   Top Panel: glucose concentrations in type 2 diabetic (dashed line) and control (solid line) subjects, collected from 2 pm on day 1 until 2 pm on day 2 of a 24 h study. All subjects were fasted from 8 am on day 1. Lower Panel: rate of endogenous glucose production calculated using a simultaneous constant infusion of [U-^{13}C]glucose. Reproduced with permission from Radziuk J, Pye S (2006) *Diabetologia* **49**, 1614–28.

a cyclical (diurnal) temporal pattern. This phasic behaviour is restricted to diabetes and is not seen in normal controls. It drives the glucose concentrations throughout the day and is likely extended; diabetic patients with isoglycaemic clamps who were fasted for 72 h also demonstrated a cyclical glucose requirement, most likely attributable to *EGP* (Boden et al. 1996).

The pattern of changes in *EGP* may be related to suprachiasmatic nucleus activity and circadian rhythms (Boden et al. 1996; Kalsbeek et al. 2004). Alternatively, it could reflect the intrinsic nonlinear behaviour of (primarily hepatic) metabolism that determines glucose levels but might also subsume central regulatory pathways. The transition from the normal to the diabetic state would then be characterised by the switch in *EGP* from steady state behaviour to the stable limit cycle behaviour (Mackey & Glass 1977; Boden et al. 1996). Interestingly, a group of diseases termed 'dynamical diseases' is typified by such relatively abrupt transitions, based on complex behaviour of the system in question, acting as a whole (Guyton et al. 1956; Mackey & Glass 1977).

Basal conditions, therefore, can be characterised by a steady state, but other states, such as a limit cycle, are possible and may distinguish the normal from the diabetic state (Radziuk & Pye 2006).

Perturbed conditions

Activities of daily living, such as meals or exercise, constitute perturbations of the basal state. Regulatory mechanisms involved in the maintenance of homeostasis restore basal conditions. Type 2 diabetes is not only characterised by altered basal conditions but also by intolerance to glucose, indicating dysregulation at this level. The determination of, for example, postprandial glucose fluxes is therefore critical to understanding these deviations. A large part of glucose intolerance is due to insulin insensitivity, which is manifested both at the level of peripheral tissues and of the liver. It is generally measured using euglycaemic hyperinsulinaemic or hyperglycaemic clamps (DeFronzo et al. 1979). In order to differentiate between changes in glucose production and removal, tracer is infused prior to and during the clamp procedure. System parameters can be calculated from the basal tracer infusion (Radziuk & Pye 2002). Total glucose appearance is calculated using either Equation 6.14 or 6.16. Endogenous glucose production is then determined by subtracting the variable glucose infusion rate from the total R_a. Peripheral insulin sensitivity is calculated by dividing *MCR* by the insulin concentrations, and hepatic sensitivity by estimating the suppression of endogenous glucose production relative to basal.

The situation becomes more complex when the more physiological handling of meal glucose is addressed.

Measurement of postprandial glucose fluxes: the double tracer method

Following absorption during a meal, glucose enters the portal vein, where it mixes with circulating glucose. It then enters the liver, where a portion will be removed for storage as glycogen or metabolism. The remainder enters the general circulation and is further sequestered in peripheral tissues, mainly muscle. The fluxes which then determine the 'tolerance' to this meal glucose are: 1) the absorption rate of ingested glucose; 2) its first-pass uptake by the liver; 3) its uptake by peripheral tissues; and 4) the concurrent suppression of endogenous glucose production. These fluxes can all be estimated by using a dual tracer approach (Radziuk et al. 1978). The first tracer is infused intravenously and the second is used to label the glucose part of the meal (which has to be known and exist as glucose to mix with the tracer). Both tracers must display kinetics equivalent to glucose, losing their labels only with irreversible uptake of glucose (e.g. [U-^{13}C] and [3-^{3}H]glucose). The concentration of ingested tracer can be converted to the concentration of the glucose that has its origin in the meal (C^+) simply by dividing it by the ratio of label to glucose in the meal. The concentration of endogenously produced glucose, C_{endog}, can then be calculated as: $C_{endog} = C - C^+$. If a one-compartment model for glucose kinetics is used, we calculate the appearance of both ingested and endogenous glucose using Equation 6.14:

$$R_a^+ = \frac{R_a^*}{a^+} - \frac{V \cdot C^+}{a^+} \cdot \frac{da^+}{dt} \text{ and } R_{a,endog} = \frac{R_a^*}{a_{endog}} - \frac{V \cdot C_{endog}}{a_{endog}} \cdot \frac{da_{endog}}{dt} \tag{6.18}$$

Where R_a^+ and $R_{a,endog}$ are the appearance of the ingested and endogenous glucose respectively; C^+ and C_{endog} are their concentrations; $a^+ = C^*/C^+$ and $a_{endog} = C^*/C_{endog}$. Suppression of endogenous production is obtained by comparing $R_{a,endog}$ (EGP) to the basal (pre-meal) R_a.

Postprandial suppression of EGP has been calculated in a number of laboratories. It is generally considered to be impaired in type 2 diabetes. Although postprandial EGP is frequently found to be higher in diabetic than in control subjects, fractional suppression has often been found not to differ in the two groups except in severe disease (reviewed in Radziuk 1989). We have recently therefore 1) used individual parameter estimates to calculate EGP; and 2) examined the postprandial changes in this rate relative to the decreasing basal EGP that precedes the perturbation induced by a meal (Figure 6.3) (Radziuk & Pye 2004).

When compared to an average basal EGP, suppression was similar in normal and diabetic subjects ($\sim 60\,\%$). When basal EGP was extrapolated in a linear fashion into the postprandial period, the deviation of the measured EGP from the extrapolated rate became very small ($\sim 10\,\%$). Such data suggest that, in the diabetic state, EGP falls during the day more or less independently of postprandial hormonal influences, but rather in response to those factors that determine its diurnal rhythm. This could be an expression of a more severe resistance to insulin in the liver than might be anticipated. Such data also underline the importance of the perspective when evaluating the behaviour of EGP before and after meals in diabetes.

MCR and R_d are calculated from Equation 6.14.

Finally, a mean estimate of the first-pass splanchnic uptake (Radziuk et al. 1978; Radziuk 1987) of the ingested glucose during the period of glucose absorption can be obtained by subtracting $\int_{\substack{absorption \\ period}} R_a^+ dt$ (the area under the curve of glucose appearance) from the amount of glucose ingested. Dividing this by the amount of glucose ingested yields a fractional extraction of glucose by the liver, which then also applies to the recirculating glucose (and is about 80\,% of the portal glucose). A rough estimate of total splanchnic glucose uptake can be obtained by multiplying the fractional extraction by the splanchnic plasma flow and an estimated portal glucose concentration. This calculation has proven to be approximately equivalent to the total liver glycogen formed during the absorption time (Radziuk 1989).

Splanchnic glucose extraction has also been calculated by arterio-hepatic venous differences directly in humans (Basu et al. 2001) using Equations 6.2–4. Fractional extractions very similar to those seen using the indirect method ($\sim 8\,\%$ in normals and 5\,% in type 2 diabetes) were found (Basu et al. 2001).

Sources of errors

The determination of glucose fluxes takes place in the context of biological systems that are complex and inhomogeneous. This necessitates their modeling. Models do not need to

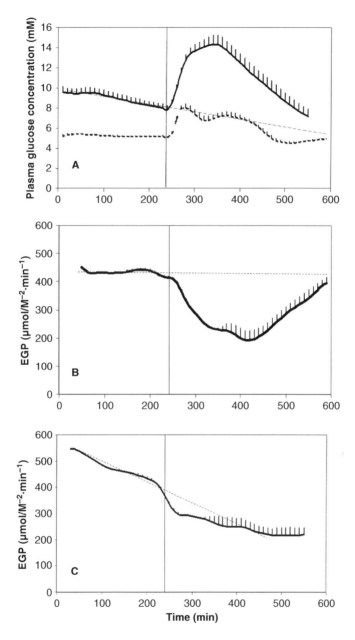

Figure 6.3 A) plasma glucose concentrations in diabetic (solid line) and control (dashed line) subjects who were fasted overnight for 12–14 h and ingested a mixed meal at t = 240 min of the study. [U-^{13}C]glucose was infused intravenously at a constant rate, and the ingested glucose was labeled with [6-^{3}H]glucose. Endogenous glucose production (*EGP*) was calculated from the two tracer concentrations and glucose levels as described in the text; B) *EGP* in control subjects before and after the meal; C) *EGP* in subjects with type 2 diabetes before and after the meal. The dotted lines are basal rates of *EGP* extrapolated to the postprandial period. Reproduced with permission from Radziuk J, Pye S (2004) Glucose production in health and type 2 diabetes: measurement, regulation, and molecular basis. An overview. *J Invest Med* **52** (6), 379–388, Courtesy of the American Federation for Medical Research.

be isomorphic with the system but do need to provide enough structure that distribution dynamics occuring on the same timescale as the changes in the fluxes of interest can be accounted for.

Errors arise when there is a mismatch between the timescale on which the dynamics of interest (glucose production, metabolic clearance, etc.) are changing and the timescale on which mixing occurs. Since fluxes often change slowly, this accounts for the adequacy of the one-compartment (completely mixed) model in their measurement.

Structural errors can arise from an inappropriate model order – e.g. using a one-compartment model when a two-compartment model would be more appropriate to describe the timecourse of glucose distribution when it is similar to the flux changes (Radziuk & Hetenyi 1982; Cobelli et al. 1987; Mari 1993). They could also arise when parameters are used that do not conform to those actually operative in the study subject. Errors due to sampling occur when sampling frequency is inadequate to describe the changes being examined (Livesey et al. 1998). For example, sampling every 15 min is insufficient when studying a flux that oscillates with a period of 30 min.

Primers and specific activity clamping: avoiding difficulties due to system structure

Primers under basal conditions

When the tracer is in steady state (i.e. *MCR* is constant), the concentration response to its infusion is a sum of integrated exponentials:

$$C_{\text{inf}}^*(t) = \sum_{i=1}^{n} (A_i/b_i) \cdot (1 - e^{-b_i t}) \tag{6.19}$$

If an injection of the tracer is administered at

$$t = 0, C_{inj}^*(t) = \sum_{i=1}^{n} D_i \cdot e^{-b_i t} \tag{6.20}$$

a primed infusion would show the response:

$$C_{primed}^*(t) = \sum_{i=1}^{n} [(A_i/b_i) + (D_i - (A_i/b_i)) \cdot e^{-b_i t}] \tag{6.21}$$

If $b_1 > b_2 > \dots$, so that b_n is the smallest time constant, then an injection of mass, $D_n = A_n/b_n$, would eliminate the last term in Equation 6.21 and thus significantly accelerate the convergence of the tracer concentrations to a steady state, $(\sum_{i=1}^{n} (A_i/b_i))$.

This can be illustrated by the solution to Equation 6.13 for the tracer infusion, R_a^*, and injection, $I \cdot \delta(t)$, where $\delta(t)$ is the mathematical delta function:

$$C^*(t) = \frac{R_a^*}{V \cdot k} + \frac{1}{V}\left(I^* - \frac{R_a^*}{k}\right) \cdot e^{-kt} \tag{6.22}$$

In a one-compartment system, then, an injection $I^* = R_a^*/k$ will yield an instant tracer steady state. In normals, $k \approx 0.01$, so an I^* of 100 times the tracer infusion rate is generally used. In type 2 diabetes, *MCR* is impaired and $k < 0.01$. The strategy adopted in diabetes is therefore to estimate k as $k \cdot$(fasting glucose in normals)/(fasting glucose in the diabetic subject) (Hother-Nielsen & Beck-Nielsen 1990).

A rapid convergence of tracer concentrations to a constant value also allows the simplification of the formula for R_a to:

$$R_a = MCR \cdot C + V \cdot \frac{dC}{dt} \qquad (6.23)$$

Where $MCR = V \cdot k$ and is constant (Radziuk & Pye 2002).

It has been demonstrated that theoretical strategies that use an appropriate system structure are completely equivalent to experimental strategies that obviate the need for these structures (Radziuk & Pye 2002).

Specific activity clamping

Under steady state conditions, when the tracer concentration is constant, so is the specific activity. Priming the tracer infusion is therefore a rapid way of achieving these clamp conditions for the special case of the steady state.

Under quite general non-steady state circumstances (Norwich 1973) it can also be shown that: 1) if the tracer infusion is kept at a constant ratio to the rate of glucose appearance then the specific activity will be constant everywhere and equal to this ratio; and, conversely, 2) if the specific activity, a, at the sampling site remains constant throughout the course of the experiment then tracer and glucose appearance will also be related by the same (constant) ratio so that:

$$R_a(t) = \frac{R_a^*(t)}{a} \qquad (6.24)$$

This can easily be seen in the special cases described by Equations 6.14 and 6.16.

Changing the tracer infusion rate to match the unknown glucose production presupposes knowledge of this rate, seemingly obviating the need for its measurement. In an experimental situation, this will not be feasible. However, good approximations can be obtained, for example by frequent and rapid sampling of both glucose and tracer concentrations, and it has been shown experimentally that small deviations from a constant specific activity introduce minimal error (Hother-Nielsen et al. 1995). This can be illustrated using Equation 6.14; if an incorrect volume of distribution, V', is used then:

$$R_a' = \frac{R_a^*}{a} - \frac{V'C}{a} \cdot \frac{da}{dt} \text{ and } error = R_a' - R_a = \frac{(V - V') \cdot C}{a} \cdot \frac{da}{dt} \qquad (6.25)$$

It is evident that the error in volume, $(V - V')$, is amplified by the slope of the specific activity, da/dt. As long as this slope remains small, the error in the R_a calculation will remain small. If rapid changes in a occur, the slope will increase greatly, as will the error.

A near-constant specific activity will therefore minimise the error in R_a or EGP, due to a lack of structural knowledge of the system.

Insulin clamps

The infused tracer is varied so as to ensure a constant plasma specific activity (Butler et al. 1993). Alternatively, a reasonable approximation can be obtained if it is added to the glucose infusion used to maintain euglycaemia, in the same ratio that is found in the basal (pre-clamp) plasma concentrations.

Glucose meals

Intravenous glucose infusions were used as a surrogate for meal. These infusions were labeled with tracer so as to maintain a near-basal specific activity (Levy et al. 1989). Alternatively, the intravenous tracer is infused in a pattern which simulates the estimated rate of absorption and maintains the specific activity found in the basal (pre-clamp) plasma concentrations (Krššák et al. 2004). This allows accurate calculation of the appearance of ingested and total glucose.

Endogenous glucose production

During either clamps or meals, tracer is infused in a pattern which anticipates the decline in *EGP* during these protocols (Singhal et al. 2001; Basu et al. 2003; Krššák et al. 2004). This selects for the precise measurement of this critical rate during its suppression. It helps to avoid the problem of negative R_a, which can occur if the error in e.g. Equation 6.25 is sufficiently negative.

Triple-tracer technique

This has been recently developed (Basu et al. 2003) for the simultaneous optimal estimation of the postprandial appearance of total and ingested glucose, and the suppression of its endogenous production. The first tracer is infused at a constant rate during the basal period and in a pattern which simulates an average absorption of glucose (as previously estimated) postprandially; the second tracer is infused during the basal period and postprandially its infusion rate is altered to simulate the declining postprandial *EGP*; the third tracer is added to the meal to allow the exact calculation of the peripheral appearance of ingested glucose.

Conclusion

Both simpler experimental techniques and more complex models of the system, and experimental protocols that match the tracer infusion to anticipated rates of glucose appearance but require only the simplest models for analysis, are equivalent in the determination of glucose flux rates during physiological procedures in both health and the diabetic state.

Acknowledgements

This work has been made possible by grants from the Canadian Diabetes Association and the Canadian Institutes for Health Research.

References

Baldwin S, Lienhard G (1981) *Trends Biochem Sci* **6**, 208–11

Basu A, Basu R, Shah P, Vella A, Johnson M, Jensen M et al. (2001) *Diabetes* **50**, 1351–62

Basu R, Di Camillo B, Toffolo G, Basu A, Shah P, Vella A et al. (2003) *Am J Physiol* **284**, E55–69

Bell PM, Firth RG, Rizza RA (1986a) *Diabetes* **35**, 642–8 s

Bell PM, Firth RG, Rizza RA (1986b) *J Clin Invest* **78**, 1479–86

Bernard C (1878) *Lecons sur les Phenomenes de la Vie Communs aux Animaux et aux Vegetaux*, J. Baillere, Paris

Boden G, Chen X, Urbain JL (1996) *Diabetes* **45**, 1044–50

Butler PC, Caumo A, Zerman A, O'Brien PC, Cobelli C, Rizza RA (1993) *Am J Physiol* **264**, E548–60

Cahill GF Jr, Herrera MG, Morgan AP (1966) *J Clin Invest* **45**, 1751–69

Cersosimo E, Judd RL, Miles JM (1994) *J Clin Invest* **93**, 2584–9

Cherrington AD, Williams PE, Shulman GI, Lacy WW, Liljenquist JE (1982) *Am J Physiol* **5**, 98–101

Cobelli C, Mari A, Ferrannini E (1987) *Am J Physiol* **252**, E679–89

Croset M, Rajas F, Zitoun C, Hurot J-M, Montano S, Mithieux G (2001) *Diabetes* **50**, 740–6

DeFronzo RA, Tobin JD, Andres R (1979) *Am J Physiol* **237**, E214–23

Dunn A, Chenoweth M, Schaeffer LD (1967) *Biochemistry* **6**, 6–11

Efendic S, Karlander S, Vranic ML (1988) *J Clin Invest* **81**, 1953–61

Felig P, Wahren J, Hendler R (1978) *Diabetes* **27**, 121–6

Gottesman I, Mandarino L, Gerich J (1984) *Diabetes* **33**, 184–91

Guyton AC, Crowell JW, Moore JW (1956) *Am J Physiol* **187**, 395–8

Hers HG, Hue L (1983) *Annual Review of Biochemistry* **52**, 617–53

Hetenyi G Jr (1982) *Fed Proc* **41**, 104–9

Hother-Nielsen O, Beck-Nielsen H (1990) *Diabetologia* **33**, 603–10

Hother-Nielsen O, Henriksen JE, Holst JJ, Beck-Nielsen H (1996) *Metabolism* **45**, 82–91

Hother-Nielsen O, Henriksen JE, Staehr P, Beck-Nielsen H (1995) *Endocrinol Metab* **2**, 275–87

Kalsbeek A, laFleur S, Van Heijningen C, Buijs RM (2004) *J Neurosci* **24**, 7604–13

Mackey MC, Glass L (1977) *Science* **197**, 287–9

Karlander S, Roovete A, Vranic M, Efendic S (1986) *Am J Physiol* **251**, E530–6

Katz H, Butler P, Homan M, Zerman A, Caumo A, Cobelli C et al. (1993) *Am J Physiol* **264**, E561–6

Katz J, Dunn A (1967) *Biochemistry* **6**, 1–5

Katz J, Okajima F, Chenoweth M, Dunn A (1981) *Biochem J* **194**, 513–24

Cobelli C, Caumo A (1998) *Metabolism* **47**, 1009–35

Katz J, Wals PA, Lee W-NP (1991) *Proc Natl Acad Sci USA* **88**, 2103–7

Kelleher JK (1986) *Am J Physiol* **250**, E296–305

Krššák M, Brehm A, Bernroider E, Anderwald C, Nowotny P, Dalla Man C et al. (2004) *Diabetes* **53**, 3048–56

Koistinen HA, Zierath JR (2002) *Ann Med* **34**, 410–18

Landau BR (1993) **42**, 457–62

Lee W-NP (1989) *J Biol Chem* **264**, 13002–4

Levy JC, Brown G, Matthews DR, Turner RC (1989) *Am J Physiol* **257**, E531–40

Livesey G, Wilson PDG, Dainty JR, Brown JC, Faulks RM, Roe MA et al. (1998) *Am J Physiol* **275**, E717 28

Madison LL (1969) *Arch Intern Med* **123**, 284–92

Mari A (1993) *J Theor Biol* **160**, 509–31

Norwich KH (1973) *Can J Physiol Pharmacol* **51**, 91–101

Phelps ME, Huang SC, Hoffman EJ, Selin CJ, Kuhl DE (1978) *J Nucl Med* **19**, 1311–19

Radziuk J (1976) *Bull Math Biol* **38**, 679–93

Radziuk J (1987) *Diabetes/Metabolism Reviews* **3**, 231–67

Radziuk J (1989) *Am J Physiol* **257**, E158–69

Radziuk J, Hetenyi G Jr (1982) In: Cramp D (Ed) *Quantitative Approaches to Metabolism: The Role of Tracers and Models in Clinical Medicine* John Wiley and Sons, London, pp. 73–142

Radziuk J, Lickley HLA (1985) *Diabetologia* **28**, 315–22

Radziuk J, McDonald TJ, Rubenstein D, Dupre J (1978) *Metabolism* **27**, 657–69

Radziuk J, Norwich KH, Vranic M (1978) *Am J Physiol* **234**, E84–93

Radziuk J, Pye S (2001) *Diabetologia* **44**, 983–91

Radziuk J, Pye S (2002) *Diabetologia* **45**, 1053–84

Radziuk J, Pye S (2004) *J Invest Med* **52**, 379–88

Radziuk J, Pye S (2006) *Diabetologia* **49**, 1614–28

Reichard GA Jr, Moury NF Jr, Hochella NJ et al. (1963) *J Biol Chem* **238**, 495–501

Sacca L, Cicala M, Trimarco B, Ungaro B, Vigorito C (1982) *J Clin Invest* **70**, 117–26

Schoenheimer R (1964) *The Dyamic State of Body Constituents*, reprinted by Haffner Publishing Co., New York and London

Shulman GI, Ladenson PW, Wolfe MH et al. (1985) *J Clin Invest* **76**, 757–64

Sheppard CW (1962) *Basic Principles of the Tracer Method*, John Wiley and Sons, New York

Singhal P, Caumo A, Carey PE, Cobelli C, Taylor R (2001) *Am J Physiol* **283**, E275–83

Sokoloff L, Reivich M, Kennedy C, Des Rosiers MH, Patlak KD, Sakurada O et al. (1977) *J Neurochem* **28**, 897–916

Stumvoll M, Chintalapudi U, Perriello G, Welle S, Gutierrez O, Gerich J (1995) *J Clin Invest* **96**, 2528–33

Topper YJ (1957) *Journal of Biological Chemistry* **225**, 419–25

Utriainen T, Lovisatti S, Makimattila S, Bertoldo A, Weintraub S, DeFronzo R et al. (2000) *Am J Physiol* **279**, E228–33

Wajngot A, Chandramouli V, Schumann WC et al. (1989) *Am J Physiol* **256**, E668–75

Wajngot A, Chandramouli V, Schumann WC et al. (2001) *Metabolism* **50**, 47–52

Wolfe RR (1992) *Radioactive and Stable Isotope Tracers in Biomedicine: Principles and Practice of Kinetic Analysis*, Wiley-Liss, New York

Zhang Z, Radziuk J (1991) *Biochem J* **280**, 415–19

Zhang Z, Radziuk J (1994) *Am J Physiol* **266**, E583–91

7

Xenobiotics as Probes of Carbohydrate Metabolism

Bernard Landau

Introduction

Substances foreign to the body, i.e. xenobiotics (Mason et al. 1965), are conjugated in the liver by glucuronidation, glutamination, ribosylation, acetylation and glycination (Figure 7.1). Monitoring the excretion of these conjugates provides a means of noninvasively quantitating the pathways of carbohydrate metabolism in the liver, by which the glucuronic acid, glutamic acid, ribose, acetate and glycine used in the conjugations are formed (Landau 1991). A substrate that is a precursor in the formation of the conjugate, labeled with a radioactive or stable isotope, is administered along with the xenobiotic, and the fate of the label in the excreted conjugate is determined. Interpretation of the incorporation of the label depends upon a knowledge of the site(s) of formation of the conjugate. This approach is analogous to the use of a needle to biopsy the liver for analysis (Landau 1991). The xenobiotic is the needle – a probe – and the biopsy sample the conjugate. The size of the biopsy sample depends on the amount of xenobiotic that can safely be given.

Glucuronidation

Glucuronidation is the most widespread process for the conjugation of drugs in the body (Dutton 1980). It functions mainly in the liver. The conjugation to glucuronic acid increases the drug's water solubility, resulting in more rapid urinary excretion. Acetaminophen is excreted both as its glucuronide and sulfate conjugates, the former in larger percentage the higher the dose of the acetaminophen. The enzyme catalyzing its coupling is UDPglucuronyl transferase, acetaminophen + UDPglucuronic acid → acetaminophen glucuronide (Figure 7.1). The precursor of the UDPglucuronic acid is UDPglucose, which is also the immediate precursor of glycosyl units of glycogen. The UDPglucose can be formed from glucose via glucose-6-P and from galactose via galactose-1-P (Figure 7.2). There is no rearrangement of the carbons and hydrogens of the glucose and galactose during these conversions, but the

Clinical Diabetes Research: Methods and Techniques   Edited by Michael Roden
© 2007 John Wiley & Sons, Ltd   ISBN 978-0-470-01728-9

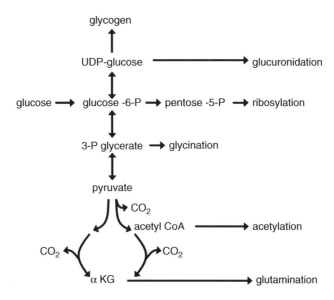

Figure 7.1 Conjugation of xenobiotics.

two hydrogens bound to their carbon 6 are removed in the formation of the carboxyl group of the glucuronic acid, $-CH_2OH + 2NAD \rightarrow -COOH + 2NADH$, Thus, when acetaminophen and a radioactive or stable labeled substrate are administrated and the label is incorporated into the glucuronic acid moiety of the excreted glucuronide, its labeling reflects this in the UDPglucose from which it was formed, and in any glycogen made. Hepatic glycogen in an early study was concluded to be formed from a different pool of UDPglucose than the glucuronide, but that conclusion was in error (Hellerstein et al. 1986, 1995; Magnusson et al. 1987).

0.5–2.0 g of acetaminophen can be safely given to subjects, the larger quantities often in divided dose, orally or infused over several hours. Hypersensitivity to acetaminophen is rare. Commercial preparations for intravenous administration are available in Europe, but not the United States. Enrichments of ^2H and ^{13}C in the glucuronic acid moiety of glucuronate in blood collections have been measured using chromatography/mass spectrometry (Hellerstein et al. 1997; Bischof et al. 2002). Assays of label have usually been in glucuronide from urine collected over 1–2 h. Subjects have usually been encouraged to drink water to enhance urine output. Glucuronidation of acetaminophen in rat liver is estimated to occur 30 to 60 minutes before the conjugate is excreted in the urine (Taylor et al. 1996). The half-life of the glucuronide in the circulation, before its excretion, has been estimated to be 21 minutes.

Glucuronide in urine has been concentrated, precipitated and then reduced to its glucoside. The glucoside has been enzymatically hydrolyzed and the glucose released purified, usually by HPLC (Magnusson et al. 1987, 1988; Ekberg et al. 1995). Specific activities of the glucose when labeled with ^3H and ^{14}C can be measured in a liquid scintillation counter. The ^{14}C specific activity of each of the carbons of the glucose labeled were determined by bacterial, followed by chemical, degradation, isolating each carbon of the glucose in $BaCO_3$ for assay of radioactivity (Magnusson et al. 1988; Shulman et al. 1990; Ekberg et al. 1995). When labeled with ^{2}H and ^{13}C the enrichments in the hydrogens and carbons of the glucose have been determined using its 1,2-isopropylidene derivative and NMR spectroscopy (Burgess et al. 2003a). Alternatively, the hydrogens have been isolated in formaldehyde, which is then reacted with ammonia to form hexamethylenetetramine for assay of enrichment by mass spectrometry (Burgess et al. 2003b; Stingl et al. 2005). When labeled with ^{13}C the enrichment in the carbons can also be determined by mass spectrometry (Shulman et al. 1990; Landau 2000; Petersen et al. 2001).

While glucuronidation occurs in sites other than the liver (Dutton 1980), glucuronidation of acetaminophen is so much greater in the liver that acetaminophen glucuronide in blood and urine can be assumed to originate in the liver. However, that glucuronidation occurs more in the perivenous and periportal zones of the liver lobule (Jungermann & Katz 1989), which could affect interpretation of results. Thus, when normal subjects were infused with labeled glycerol and lactate and given acetaminophen, labeling of the glucose by glycerol was more than by lactate, compared to their relative labeling of the glucuronide. Therefore, the glucose and glucuronide were not formed completely from the same glucose-6-P pool (Ekberg et al. 1995). Presumably, that is because gluconeogenesis occurs to a greater extent in periportal than perivenous zones. Because of glycerol's avid uptake by the liver, glycerol's concentration – compared to lactate's concentration – was much less in perivenous than periportal zones.

In equating UDPglucose flux to the rate of glycogen synthesis using labeled galactose, all the galactose infused is assumed to be converted to UDPglucose and hence to glycogen. To the extent the UDPglucose phosphorylase reaction proceeds in the direction UDPglucose + 2P → glucose-1-P + UTP, the rate of glycogen formation will be overestimated, i.e. UDPglucose will not convert completely to glycogen (Landau 2000). That may contribute to the 50 % higher rate of UDPglucose flux than glycogen synthesis reported in Hellerstein et al. (1997). Furthermore, by the Leloir pathway galactose can be converted to glucose in the liver without glycogen being a required intermediate (Landau 2000).

The nature of the pentose cycle and its contribution to glucose utilisation in the liver of normal subjects have been determined from the distribution of ^{14}C in glucuronide on infusing [2-^{14}C]glucose and acetaminophen (Magnusson et al. 1988). The contribution of the direct pathway to hepatic glycogen formation was determined from the ^{13}C enrichment in the glucuronide and its carbons 1 and 6 compared to that in blood glucose on giving [1-^{13}C]glucose and acetaminophen to normal subjects after an overnight fast and with feeding (Magnusson et al. 1987; Taylor et al. 1996; Petersen et al. 2001b), in type 1 diabetes after insulin therapy (Bischof et al. 2002) and on stimulation by insulin of glycogen synthesis on giving a low dose of fructose (Petersen et al. 2001a). The contribution of the direct pathway was also estimated from the specific activities of the glucuronide and blood glucose on administering [6-^{14}C]glucose to fed and fasted normal subjects (Shulman et al. 1990), on giving a glucose load labeled with [5-^{3}H]glucose (Magnusson et al. 1987) and in type 1 and 2 diabetics infused with [3-^{3}H]glucose (Basu et al. 2000; Vella et al. 2001). It was also estimated in normal subjects in fed and fasted states from the ratio of ^{2}H enrichment in the excreted glucuronide to that in plasma glucose on giving [1-^{2}H]glucose and acetaminophen (Hellerstein et al. 1995).

The contribution of glycogen cycling, UDPglucose→ glycogen→ glucose-1-P→ UDPglucose, was estimated on giving a glucose load, again by estimating the contribution of the direct pathway of glycogen formation using [5-^{3}H]glucose, but at the same time giving ^{2}H$_2$O and estimating the contribution of the indirect pathway from the ratio of the enrichments

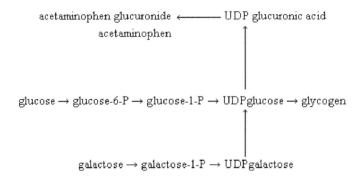

Figure 7.2   Acetaminophen Glucuronide.

```
acetaminophen glucuronide ←———————— UDP glucuronic acid
        acetaminophen                      ↑
                                           |
                                           |
                                           |
glucose → glucose-6-P → glucose-1-P → UDPglucose → glycogen
                                           ↑
                                           |
                                           |
        galactose → galactose-1-P → UDPgalactose
```

Figure 7.3   Pathway of Formation of Acetaminophen Glucuronide.

in the hydrogens bound to carbon 5 to two of the glucuronic acid moiety, thus % cycling = 100 % – (% direct + % indirect) (Stingl et al. 2005). Cycling was also estimated in normal and type 2 diabetic subjects given a glucose load, acetaminophen and [2-^{3}H, 6-^{14}C]galactose from the ^{3}H/^{14}C ratio in the glucuronide excreted in urine and in the galactose (Wajngot et al. 1991).

Rates of glycogen synthesis, equated to the flux of UDPglucose, have been estimated on administering ^{2}H, ^{13}C, or ^{14}C galactose and acetaminophen from the rate of infusion of the galactose and its specific activity or enrichment, and that of the excreted glucuronide (Rother & Schwenk 1995). Estimates have been made of the rate of glycogen synthesis on giving insulin and glucose to type 2 diabetic subjects (Basu et al. 2000), patients with liver cirrhosis (Schneiter et al. 1999) and obese patients (Allick et al. 2004).

Glutamination

Phenylacetate is conjugated to glutamine in primates and the conjugate is excreted in urine (Thierfelder & Sherwin 1915; James et al. 1972). The enzyme activating the phenylacetate to its coenzyme A derivative and catalyzing the conjugation, acyl CoA: L-glutamine N-acyltransferase, is present in the liver and kidney (Moldave & Meister 1957). Glutamine via glutamate is formed from α-ketoglutarate, an intermediate in the Krebs cycle.

Phenylacetate is normally found in small quantity in human urine, a minor end product in phenylalanine's metabolism. It is rapidly absorbed following oral ingestion and mostly excreted as its glutamine conjugate. Many grams can be ingested safely (Ambrose et al. 1933). It has been given to children with urea enzyme deficiencies to increase their excretion

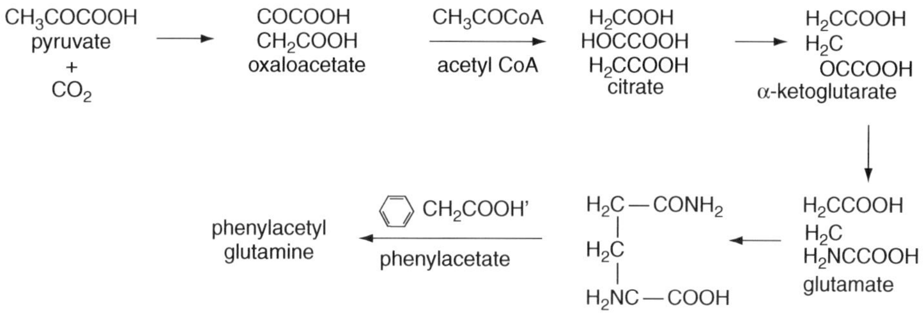

CH$_3$COCOOH   COCOOH   CH$_3$COCoA   H$_2$COOH   H$_2$CCOOH
pyruvate   CH$_2$COOH   acetyl CoA   HOCCOOH   H$_2$C
  +   oxaloacetate   H$_2$CCOOH   OCCOOH
CO$_2$ citrate   α-ketoglutarate

                                                                     H$_2$CCOOH
                                                                     H$_2$C
              CH$_2$COOH'   H$_2$C—CONH$_2$ H$_2$NCCOOH
phenylacetyl   H$_2$C   glutamate
glutamine   phenylacetate   H$_2$NC—COOH

Figure 7.4 Pathway of formation of Phenylacetyl Glutamine (Magnusson et al. 1994).

of nitrogenous waste (Simell et al. 1986; Brusilow & Maestri 1996; Praphanphoj et al. 2000). Sodium phenylacetate in solution has a 'soapy' taste and an unpleasant odour that persists in urine. Phenylbutyrate is also excreted, conjugated to glutamine, and does not have the odour. While phenylbutyrate has not as yet been used in tracer studies, it has been given to children with urea enzyme deficiencies (Brusilow & Maestri 1996).

Phenylacetate has been administered to normal and diabetic subjects along with ^{13}C- and ^{14}C-labeled gluconeogenic substrates. From the distribution of label in the carbons of glutamine from the excreted conjugate, assuming that distribution to be the same as in hepatic α-ketoglutarate, rates of reaction in the Krebs cycle and contributions of gluconeogenesis to glucose production have been estimated (Yang & Brunengraber 2000). Phenylacetate administration has been shown not to affect rates of gluconeogenesis (Wajngot et al. 2000).

Five grams of sodium phenylacetate, its taste masked by solution in a beverage, was given to normal subjects, fasted overnight or fasted for 60 h, given a glucose load and infused with [3-^{14}C]lactate. Glutamine was isolated from the conjugate in urine, collected at 1½ h intervals over a 6 h period, and chemically degraded to yield each of its carbons as CO_2 for assay for ^{14}C specific activity. Comparison of the ^{14}C distribution in blood glucose samples collected at the same time supported the assumption that the distributions found in glutamate were the same as in α-ketoglutarate. Corrections to the distributions for the fixation of $^{14}CO_2$ formed from the lactate were made from measurements of ^{14}C incorporation into the carbons of the glutamine and glucose when ^{14}C-labeled bicarbonate, rather than lactate, was administered. The specific activity of the $^{14}CO_2$ fixed when the [3-^{14}C]lactate was infused was estimated from the specific activity of carbon in urea from the urine. In the fasted state pyruvate carboxylation was twice the rate of Krebs cycle flux and one-twenty-fifth the rate of decarboxylation. In the fed state the rate of pyruvate carboxylation was one-half to one-sixth the rate of carboxylation. The conversion of oxaloacetate to fumarate was many fold the rate of Krebs cycle flux.

The phenylacetate probe has also been used to estimate hepatic rates of gluconeogenesis on administering ^{14}C-bicarbonate (Ensemo et al. 1992), [U-^{14}C]propionate (Landau et al. 1993) and [U-^{13}C]propionate (Jones et al. 1998), the latter using NMR spectrometry to measure the distribution of ^{13}C in the glutamine. Support for the validity of using carbon labeled lactate to estimate rates of Krebs cycle activity and gluconeogenesis was obtained by comparing distributions in glutamine and glutamate, obtained on perfusions with labeled isolated substrates of rat livers, with distributions found on their *in vivo* administrations (Beylot et al. 1995). Also, rates in rats under various conditions *in vivo*, estimated from labeled glutamate distributions, were as expected (Large et al. 1997).

When ^{14}C-labeled acetate, rather than lactate, was infused into normal subjects, distributions in glutamine indicated much of the labeling occurred in peripheral tissues, presumably muscle, rather than liver (Schumann et al. 1991). When carbon-labeled lactate and acetate were infused into rats, the distributions of label in the carbons of plasma glucose and liver glutamate supported the patterns obtained, with the labeled lactate measuring liver metabolism, while the labeled acetate reflected metabolism mainly in non-gluconeogenic tissues (Beylot et al. 1995).

In type 1 diabetes, withdrawn from insulin and infused with [3-^{14}C]lactate, rates estimated from the distribution in glutamine, chemically determined, were similar to those in 60 h fasted normal subjects (Landau et al. 1995). The effect of type 1 diabetes on rates of hepatic glycogen synthesis and flux through hepatic pyruvate dehydrogenase was determined during a hyperglycemic hyperinsulinemic clamp by infusing [1-^{13}C]glucose and using ^{13}C nuclear magnetic resonance spectroscopy to monitor glycogen, acetaminophen to sample hepatic UDPglucose (see 'Glucuronidation' above), and phenylacetate to sample hepatic glutamine (Cline et al. 1994). An increased rate of gluconeogenesis and a decreased contribution of pyruvate oxidation to Krebs cycle flux were reported.

Type 2 diabetic and normal subjects were infused with [3-^{13}C]lactate and given aspartame as a source of phenylacetate. The labeling pattern in the glutamine isolated from the urinary conjugate was determined by mass spectrometry, correcting for $^{13}CO_2$ incorporation by a separate $NaH^{13}CO_3$ infusion. There was no evidence of increased hepatic fatty acid oxidation or gluconeogenesis in the diabetics, despite increased lactate turnover (Diraison et al. 1998). [13]C distributions in the glutamine from the conjugate in the urine and in glutamine from apolipoprotein B-100 of plasma very-low-density lipoprotein were similar, providing further support for idea that the distribution in the glutamine from the conjugate reflected intrahepatic metabolism (Diraison et al. 1999).

Ribosylation

Imidazole acetic acid (IMA) has been used in a few studies to 'chemically biopsy' hepatic ribose. IMA is a naturally occurring metabolite of histamine, readily synthesised (Bauer & Tabor 1957) and commercially available. In animals and humans it is excreted in urine conjugated to ribose (Imamura et al. 1984; Khandelwal et al. 1989), i.e. as ribosylimidazole acetic acid (IMAR) (Figure 7.5). An enzyme, IMAR synthetase, catalyzes the condensation of the IMA with 5-phosphoribosyl-1-pyrophosphate (PRPP), utilising ATP, to yield IMA ribosylphosphate (IMARP), i.e. IMA + ATP + PRPP → IMARP + ADP + PP + P (Crowley 1964). That enzyme is found mainly in the liver and kidney. Relative activity values in rat tissues are liver 100, kidney 160, brain, lung, small intestine, heart muscle, and spleen <10. A phosphatase catalyzes the hydrolysis of the IMARP to the excreted IMAR.

Pyrophosphatase kinase catalyzes the formation of PRPP from ribose-5-P (R5P), R5P + ATP → PRPP + AMT. R5P is formed from glucose-6-P in the oxidative portion of the pentose cycle with the loss of carbon 1 as CO_2, i.e. glucose-6-P → CO_2 + R5P. Pentose-5-P is also formed in the reversal of the non-oxidative portion of the cycle, i.e. 2 fructose-6-P + glyceraldehyde-3-P → 3 pentose-5-P, and in the glucuronic acid pathway. Hence, when a labeled precursor of ribose-5-P is given along with IMA, the label in ribose in the excreted IMAR can be used to trace the pathways of its formation. IMA has been given to subjects

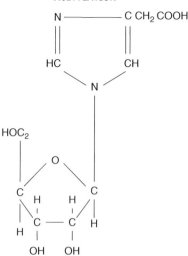

Figure 7.5 Ribosylimidazole Acetic Acid (Gowley, GM 1964).

in a dose of ~15–30 umoles/kg bodyweight (Hiatt 1958a, 1958b). About one-third the dose has been excreted in urine as the riboside.

IMA is a γ-aminobutyric acid (GABA) agonist. It is reported to have an analgesic effect in rodents at a dose of 0.3 mmol/kg (Tunnicliff 1998). However, no toxic effect was reported in mice, rats, or guinea pigs at a dose of 3 mmoles/kg or in dogs at a much higher dose (Hiatt 1958b). No toxicity effects were reported in a trial in which patients with Huntington's disease were treated with IMA (Shoulson et al. 1975). Oral dosages began at 0.8 mmoles/day and reached 80 mmoles/day, and up to 8 mmoles were administered intravenously over a 2 h period.

The excreted IMAR is hydrolyzed and the ribose released is isolated and purified using chromatographic procedures. The hydrolysis is accomplished using acid in sealed tubes at 145 °C with recovery of 80 % (Karjala 1955) or by incubation with a nucleosidase from lactobacillus delbruckii (Tabor & Hayaishi 1955).

Hiatt (1958b) found the ^{14}C distribution in the carbons of ribose isolated from IMAR excreted by subjects given [2-^{14}C]glucose was in accord with its synthesis by the reactions of the pentose cycle. Ribose biosynthesis via the glucuronic pathway was evidenced by giving ^{14}C-labeled gluconolactone to subjects along with IMA (Hiatt 1958a), providing support for a defect in that pathway being responsible for the excretion of L-xylulose in individuals with chronic essential pentosuria.

Acetylation

A number of drugs are acetylated in the liver, including sulfamethazole (SMX), SMX + acetyl CoA → acetylsulfamethazole (SMX Ac) (Figure 7.6). SMX has been administered to humans along with ^{13}C-labeled acetate (Hellerstein et al. 1991a). The ^{13}C enrichment in the SMXAc excreted in the urine has been measured by HPLC-mass spectrometry and the ^{13}C enrichment of acetyl CoA used in the synthesis of the very-low-density lipoproteins in the

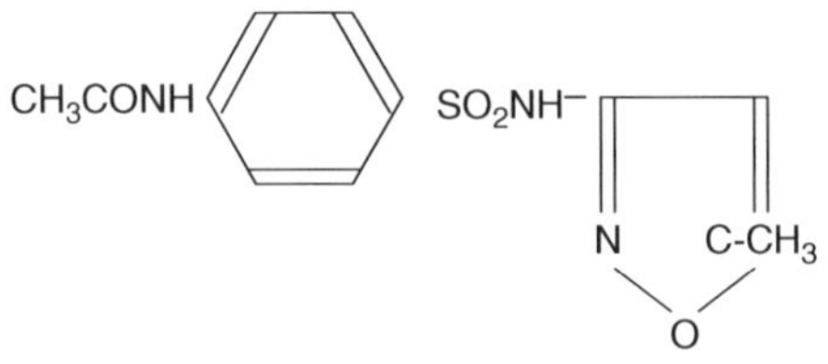

Figure 7.6 Acetylsulfamethazole (Human Biochemistry ninth edition (1975) pp. 738–739, the CV Mosby Company).

circulation estimated by mass isotopomer distribution analysis (MIDA). There was no difference in the enrichments, confirming an SMX study in the rat (Hellerstein et al. 1991b) and supporting the use of MIDA to estimate the hepatic cytosolic acetyl CoA in humans. De novo hepatic lipogenesis was then estimated from the isotopomer calculated precursor acetyl CoA enrichment and the ^{13}C incorporations into isotopomers of VLDL fatty acids (Hellerstein et al. 1991c). Rats were also infused with [U-^{13}C]glucose and hepatic acetyl CoA sampled using SMX, and hepatic UDP-glucose using acetaminophen (see 'Glucuronidation' above), to estimate the fraction of hepatic acetyl CoA derived from glucose (Kaempfer et al. 1991).

For these estimates, a constant enrichment of lipogenic acetyl CoA in hepatocytes was assumed. Evidence exists for a zonation of labeling of acetyl CoA across the liver, a resulting gradient in enrichment along the liver lobule then leading to underestimation of lipogenesis (Bederman et al. 2004a). Isotopomer spectral analysis has been used to calculate the degree of underestimation (Bederman et al. 2004b). Other evidence for the heterogeneity in the hepatic acetyl CoA pool is found in previous uses of other acetylated xenobiotics to study metabolism in rat liver. Bloch & Rittenberg (1945) gave rats phenylaminobutyric acid and two aromatic amines, p-aminobenzoic acid and sulfanilamide, along with deuterated alanine. The acetylated phenylaminobutyric acid had a much higher deuterium content than the acetylated aromatic amines. Anker (1948) confirmed these findings. The possibility of aromatic and aliphatic amines being acetylated in different cellular environments was raised (Crandall et al. 1949). When Hemmelgarn et al. (1977, 1982) gave specific ^{14}C-labeled fatty acids along with phenylaminobutyric acid and p-aminobenzoic acid to rats, the distribution of ^{14}C in acetate from the two acetylated amino acids differed, the distribution from the phenylaminobutyric being that expected if its acetylation occurred in the environment of hepatic peroxisomes, where ω-oxidation of fatty acids occurs. Randomisation of ^{14}C from [2-^{14}C]acetate was found in the carbons of acetate from the acetylated phenylaminobutyric acid, but none in the carbons of hydroxybutyrate, presumably formed from the mitochondrial acetyl CoA. In accord with those observations, Cerdan (1988), on administering ^{13}C-labeled dicarboxylic acids to rats, detected products of β-oxidation by NMR in liver, but no signal characteristic of intramitochondrial oxidation of ^{13}C-labeled acetyl CoA and no labeling of Krebs cycle metabolites or ketone bodies.

Glycination

For completeness, benzoic acid is presented as a probe for the sampling of carbons 1 and 2 of hepatic 3-phosphoglyceric acid. Benzoic acid on ingestion is conjugated almost

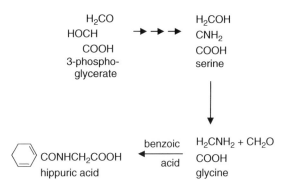

Figure 7.7   Pathway of Formation of Hippuric Acid (Fieser, LF 1941)

quantitatively to glycine, forming hippuric acid, which is excreted in urine (Figure 7.7). Glycine is formed from 3-phosphoglyceric acid via serine.

Safety in giving a dose of five grams of benzoic acid is well established. Benzoic acid is one of the most frequently used food preservatives (Lueck 1980). Children with urea enzyme deficiencies are given benzoic acid to increase their excretion of nitrogen wastes, in one study in a dose of 0.24 g/kg bodyweight intravenously as its sodium salt over a 90 minute period (Simell et al. 1986). A standard laboratory demonstration in the past (Fieser 1941) was having undergraduate chemistry students ingest five grams of sodium benzoate in 200–300 ml of water and then having them isolate hippuric acid from their urine (3 g average yield in 12 hours). There is good evidence for the synthesis of hippuric acid occurring in the liver, the severity of liver disease having been assessed by the ability of patients to form hippuric acid on being infused with benzoate in an intravenous tolerance test (Akira et al. 1997).

Hippuric acid readily precipitates from urine following concentration, acidification and salting with ammonium sulfate. It can then be hydrolyzed in acid and the released benzoic acid can be removed by ether extraction. The glycine remaining can be degraded using ninhydrin, yielding carbon 1 in CO_2 and carbon 2 as in formaldehyde (Siekevitz & Greenberg 1950; Freidemann et al. 1956). Evidence, by giving ^{13}C or ^{14}C-labeled substrates along with benzoic acid, that label in glycine from the hippuric acid excreted can serve as the measure of the label in carbon 1 and 2 of phosphoglyceric is yet to be reported. The label in glycine from VLDL has also not yet been compared with that in the glycine from the hippuric acid to provide evidence that the glycine that is conjugated has a hepatic origin. Furthermore, metabolic heterogeneity of glycine in the liver may be a confounding factor in interpreting results (Schwab et al. 2003).

References

Akira, K, Negishi, E, Yamamoto, C, Baba, S (1997) Evaluation of liver function by co-administration methodology using 13C-labelled benzoic acid and hippuric acid coupled with nuclear magnetic resonance spectroscopy *J Pharm Pharmacol* **49**, 1242–1247

Allick, G, Sprangers, F, Weverling, GJ, Ackermans, MT, Meijer, AJ, Romijn, JA, Endert, E, Bisschop, PH, Sauerwein, HP (2004) Free fatty acids increase hepatic glycogen content in obese males *Metabolism* **53**, 886–893

Ambrose, AM, Power, FW, Sherwin, CP (1933) Further studies on the detoxification of phenylacetic acid *J Biol Chem* **110**, 669–678

Anker, HS (1948) Some aspects of the metabolism of pyruvic acid in the intact animal *J Biol Chem* **176**, 1337–1352

Basu, A, Basu, R, Shah, P, Vella, A, Johnson, CM, Nair, KS, Jensen, MD, Schwenk, WF, Rizza, RA (2000) Effects of type 2 diabetes on the ability of insulin and glucose to regulate splanchnic and muscle glucose metabolism, evidence for a defect in hepatic glucokinase activity *Diabetes* **49**, 272–283

Bauer, H, Tabor, H (1957) The synthesis of imidazoleacetic acid *Biochem Prep* **5**, 97–99

Bederman, IR, Kasumov, J, Reszko, AE, David, F, Brunengraber, H, Kelleher, JK (2004) In vitro modeling of fatty acid synthesis under conditions simulating the zonation of lipogenic [^{13}C]acetyl-CoA enrichment in the liver *J Biol Chem* **279**, 43,217–43,226

Bederman, IR, Reszko, AE, Kasumov, J, David, F, Wasserman, DH, Kelleher, JK, Brunengraber, H (2004) Zonation of labeling of lipogenic acetyl-CoA across the liver, implications for studies of lipogenesis by mass isotopomer analysis *J Biol Chem* **279**, 43,207–43,216

Beylot, M, Soloviev, MV, David, F, Landau, BR, Brunengraber, H (1995) Tracing hepatic gluconeogenesis relative to citric acid cycle activity in vitro and in vivo *J Biol Chem* **270**, 1509–1514

Bischof, MG, Bernroider, E, Krssak, M, Krebs, M, Stingl, H, Nowotny, P, Yu, C, Shulman, GI, Waldhäusl, W, Roden, M (2002) Hepatic glycogen metabolism in type 1 diabetes after long-term near normoglycemia *Diabetes* **51**, 49–54

Bloch, K, Rittenberg, D (1945) An estimation of acetic acid formation in the rat *J Biol Chem* **159**, 45–58

Brusilow, SW, Maestri, NE (1996) Urea cycle disorders, diagnosis, pathophysiology and treatment In: Barness LA (Ed) *Advances in Pediatrics* Vol 43 Mosby-Year Book, Chicago, pp. 127–170

Burgess, SC, Nuss, M, Chandramouli, V, Hardin, DS, Rice, M, Landau, BR, Malloy, CR, Sherry, AD (2003) Analysis of gluconeogenic pathways in vivo by distribution of 2H in plasma glucose, comparison of nuclear magnetic resonance and mass spectrometry *Anal Biochem* **318**, 321–324

Burgess, SC, Weis, B, Jones, JG, Smith, E, Merritt, ME, Margolis, D, Sherry, AD, Malloy, CR (2003) Non-invasive evaluation of liver metabolism by ^{2}H and ^{13}C NMR isotopomer analysis of human urine *Anal Biochem* **312**, 228–234

Cerdan, S, Kunnecke, B, Dolle, A, Seelig, J (1988) In situ metabolism of 1,ω- medium-chain dicarboxylic acids in the liver of intact rats as detected by ^{13}C and ^{1}H NMR *J Biol Chem* **263**, 11664–11674

Cline, GW, Rothman, RL, Magnusson, I, Katz, LD, Shulman, GI (1994) ^{13}C-Nuclear magnetic resonance spectroscopy studies of hepatic glucose metabolism in normal subjects and subjects with insulin-dependent diabetes mellitus *J Clin Invest* **94**, 2369–2376

Crandall, DI, Brady, RO, Gurin, S (1949) Studies of acetoacetate formation from labeled carbon II The conversion of ^{14}C-labeled octanoate to acetoacetate *J Biol Chem* **181**, 845–852

Crowley, GM (1964) The enzymatic synthesis of 5'- phosphoribosylimidazoleacetic acid *J Biol Chem* **239**, 2593–2601

Diraison, F, Large, V, Brunengraber, H, Beylot, M (1998) Non-invasive tracing of liver intermediary metabolism in normal subjects and in moderately hyperglycaemic NIDDM subjects Evidence against increased gluconeogenesis and hepatic fatty acid oxidation in NIDDM *Diabetologia* **41**, 212–220

Diraison, F, Large, V, Maugeais, C, Krempf, M, Beylot, M (1999) Noninvasive tracing of human liver metabolism, comparison of phenylacetate and apoβ-100 to sample glutamate *Am J Physiol* **277**, E529–E536

Dutton, GT (1980) *Glucuronidation of Drugs and Other Compounds*, CRC Press Inc, Boca Raton, FL, USA

Ekberg, K, Chandramouli, V, Kumaran, K, Schumann, WC, Wahren, J, Landau, BR (1995) Gluconeogenesis and glucuronidation in liver in vivo and heterogeneity of hepatocyte function *J Biol Chem* **270**, 21,715–21,717

Ensemo, E, Chandramouli, V, Schumann, WC, Kumaran, K, Wahren, J, Landau, BR (1992) Use of $^{14}CO_2$ in estimating rates of hepatic gluconeogenesis *Am J Physiol* **263**, E36–E41

Fieser, LF (1941) *Experiments in Organic Chemistry* 2 edn, DC Health and Co., Boston, pp. 113–116

Freidemann, B, Levin, HW, Weinhouse, S (1956) Metabolism of glycolaldehyde in the rat *J Biol Chem* **221**, 665–77

Hellerstein, MK, Christiansen, M, Kaempfer, S, Kletke, C, Wu, K, Reid, JS, Mulligan, K, Hellerstein, NS, Shackelton, CHL (1991) Measurement of de novo hepatic lipogenesis in humans using stable isotopes *J Clin Invest* **87**, 1841–1852

Hellerstein, MK, Greenblatt, DJ, Munro, HM (1986) Glycoconjugates as non-invasive probes of intrahepatic metabolism Pathways of glucose entry into compartmentalised hepatic UDP-glucose pools driving glycogen accumulation *Proc Natl Acad Sci USA* **81**, 7044–7048

Hellerstein, MK, Greenblatt, DJ, Munro, HN (1987) Conjugates as non-invasive probes of intrahepatic metabolism I Kinetics of label incorporation with evidence of a common precursor UDP-glucose pool for secreted glycoconjugates *Metabolism* **36**, 988–994

Hellerstein, MK, Kaempfer, S, Reid, JS, Wu, K, Shackleton, CHL (1995) Rate of glucose entry into hepatic uridine diphosphoglucose by the direct pathway in fasted and fed states in normal humans *Metabolism* **44**, 172–182

Hellerstein, MK, Kletke, C, Kaempfer, S, Wu, K, Shackleton, CHL (1991) Use of mass isotopomer distributions in secreted lipids to sample lipogenic acetyl-CoA pool in vivo in humans *Am J Physiol* **261**, E479–E486

Hellerstein, MK, Letscher, A, Schwarz, JM, Cesar, D, Shakleton, CHL, Turner, S, Neese, R, Wu, K, Bock, S, Kaempfer, S (1997) Measurement of hepatic Ra UDP-glucose in vivo in rats, relation to glycogen deposition and labeling patterns *Am J Physiol* **272**, E155–E162

Hellerstein, MK, Neese, RA, Linfoot, P, Christiansen, M, Turner, S, Letscher, A (1997) Hepatic gluconeogenic fluxes and glycogen turnover during fasting in humans A stable isotope study *J Clin Invest* **100**, 1305–1319

Hellerstein, MK, Wu, K, Kaempfer, S, Kletke, C, Shackleton, CHL (1991) Sampling the lipogenic hepatic acetyl-CoA pool in vivo in the rat *J Biol Chem* **266**, 10,912–10,919

Hemmelgarn, E, Kumaran, K, Landau, BR (1977) Role of ω-oxidation of fatty acids in the formation of the acetyl unit for acetylation *J Biol Chem* **252**, 4379–4383

Hemmelgarn, E, Schumann, WC, Margolis, J, Kumaran, K, Landau, BR (1982) ω-oxidation of fatty acids and the acetylation of p-aminobenzoic acid *Biochim Biophys Acta* **572**, 298–306

Hiatt, H (1958a) Studies of ribose metabolism, IV The metabolism of D-glucuronolactone in normal and pentosuric subjects *Biochim Biophys Acta* **28**, 645–647

Hiatt, H (1958b) Studies of ribose metabolism, VI Pathways of ribose synthesis in man *J Clin Invest* **37**, 1461–1464

Imamura, I, Kazutaka, M, Wada, H, Watanabe, T (1984) Determination of imidazoleacetic acid and its conjugate(s) levels in urine, serum and tissues of rats, Studies on changes in their levels under various conditions *Br J Pharmacol* **82**, 701–707

James, MO, Smith, RL, Williams, RT, Reidenberg, M (1972) The conjugation of phenylacetic acid in man, subhuman primates, some nonprimate species *Proc R Soc Lond Biol* **182**, 25–35

Jones, JG, Solomon, MA, Sherry, AD, Jeffrey, FM, Malloy, CR (1998) ^{13}C NMR measurements of human gluconeogenic fluxes after ingestion of [U-$^{13}C_3$]propionate, phenylacetate, acetaminophen *Am J Physiol* **225**, E843–E852

Jungermann, K, Katz, N (1989) Functional specialisation of different hepatocyte populations *Physiol Rev* **69**, 708–764

Kaempfer, S, Blackham, M, Christiansen, M, Wu, K, Cesar, D, Vary, T, Hellerstein, MK (1991) Fraction of hepatic cytosolic acetyl-CoA derived from glucose in vivo, relation to PDH phosphorylation state *Am J Physiol* **260**, E865–E875

Karjala, SA (1955) The partial characterisation of a histamine metabolite from rat and mouse urine *J Am Chem Soc* **77**, 504–505

Khandelwal, JK, Prell, GD, Morrishow, AM, Green, JP (1989) Presence and measurement of imida-zoleacetic acid, a γ-aminobutyric acid agonist, in rat brain and human cerebrospinal fluid *J Neurochem* **52**, 1107–1113

Landau, BR (1991) Noninvasive approaches to tracing pathways in carbohydrate metabolism *J Parenteral Enteral Nutr* **15**, 74S–77S

Landau, BR (2000) Problems with the assumed biochemical basis for estimating hepatic glycogen turnover using glucuronide formation and labeled galactose *Metabolism* **49**, 1374–1378

Landau, BR, Chandramouli, V, Schumann, WC, Ekberg, K, Kumaran, K, Kalhan, SC, Wahren, J (1995) Estimates of Krebs cycle activity and contributions of gluconeogenesis to hepatic glucose production in fasting healthy subjects and IDDM patients *Diabetologia* **38**, 831–838

Landau, BR, Schumann, WC, Chandramouli, V, Magnusson, I, Kumaran, K, Wahren, J (1993) ^{14}C-labeled propionate metabolism in vivo and estimates of hepatic gluconeogenesis relative to Krebs cycle flux *Am J Physiol* **265**, E636–E647

Large, V, Brunengraber, H, Odeon, M, Beylot, M (1997) Use of labeling pattern of liver glutamate to calculate rates of citric acid cycle and gluconeogenesis *Am J Physiol* **272**, E51–E58

Lueck, E (1980) *Antimicrobial Food Additives* Chapter 27, Springer-Verlag, pp. 210

Simell, O, Sipila, I, Rajantie, J, Valle, DL, Brusilow, SW (1986) Waste nitrogen excretion via amino acid acylation, benzoate and phenylacetate in lysinuric protein intolerance *Pediatr Res* **20**, 1117–1121

Magnusson, I, Chandramouli, V, Schumann, WC, Kumaran, K, Wahren, J, Landau, BR (1987) Quantation of the pathways of hepatic glycogen formation on ingesting a glucose load *J Clin Invest* **80**, 1748–1754

Magnusson, I, Chandramouli, V, Schumann, WC, Kumaran, K, Wahren, J, Landau, BR (1988) Pentose pathway in liver *Proc Natl Acad Sci USA* **85**, 4682–4685

Magnusson, I, Schumann, WC, Bartsch, GE, Chandramouli, V, Kumaran, K, Wahren, J, Landau, BR (1991) Noninvasive tracing of Krebs cycle metabolism in liver *J Biol Chem* **266**, 6975–6984

Mason, HS, North, JC, Vanneste, M (1965) Microsomal mixed-function oxidations, the metabolism of xenobiotics *Fed Proc* **24**, 1172–80

Moldave, K, Meister, A (1957) Synthesis of phenylacetylglutamine by human tissue *J Biol Chem* **229**, 463–476

Peterson, KF, Cline, GW, Gerard, DP, Magnusson, I Rothman, DL, Shulman, GI (2001) Contribution of net hepatic glycogen synthesis to disposal of an oral glucose load in humans *Metabolism* **50**, 598–601

Petersen, KF, Laurent, D, Yu, C, Cline, GW, Shulman, GI (2001) Stimulating effects of low-dose fructose on insulin-stimulated hepatic glycogen synthesis in humans *Diabetes* **50**, 1263–1268

Rother, KI, Schwenk, WF (1995) Hepatic glycogen accurately reflected by acetaminophen glucuronide in dogs refed after fasting *Am J Physiol* **269**, E766–E773

Praphanphoj, V, Boyadjiev, SA, Waber, LJ, Brusilow, SW, Geraghty, MT (2000) Three cases of intravenous sodium benzoate and sodium phenylacetate toxicity occurring in the treatment of acute hyperammonaemia *J Inherit Metab Dis* **23**, 129–136

Schneiter, P, Gillet, M, Chiolero, R, Jequier, E, Tappy, L (1999) Hepatic nonoxidative disposal of an oral glucose meal in patients with liver cirrhosis *Metabolism* **48**, 1260–1266

Schwab, AJ, Tao, L, Kang, M, Meng, L, Pang, KS (2003) Moment analysis of metabolic heterogeneity, conjugation of benzoate with glycine in rat liver studied by multiple indicator dilution technique *J Pharmacol Exp Ther* **305**, 279–89

Schumann, WC, Magnusson, I, Chandramouli, V, Kumaran, K, Wahren, J, Landau, BR (1991) Metabolism of [2-14C]acetate and its use in assessing hepatic Krebs cycle activity and gluconeogenesis *J Biol Chem* **266**, 6985–6990

Shoulson, I, Chase, TN, Roberts, E, Van Balgooy, JNA (1975) Huntington's disease, treatment with imidazole-4-acetic acid *New Eng J Med* **293**, 504–505

Shulman, GI, Cline, G, Schumann, WC, Chandramouli, V, Kumaran, K, Landau, BR (1990) Quantitative comparison of pathways of hepatic glycogen repletion in fed and fasted humans *Am J Physiol* **215**, E335–E341

Siekevitz, P, Greenberg, DM (1950) The biological formation of formate from methyl compounds in liver slices *JBiolChem* **186**, 275–86

Simell, O, Sipila, I, Rajantie, J, Valle, DL, Brusilow, SW (1986) Waste-nitrogen excretion via amino acid acylation, Benzoate and phenylacetate in lysinuric protein intolerance *Pediatr Res* **20**, 1117–1121

Stingl, H, Chandramouli, V, Schumann, WC, Brehm, H, Nowotny, P, Waldhäusl, W et al. (2005) Changes in hepatic glycogen cycling during a glucose load in healthy humans *Diabetologia* (abstract)

Tabor, H, Hayaishi, O (1955) The excretion of imidazoleacetic acid riboside following the administration of imidazoleacetic acid or histamine to rats *J Am Chem Soc* **77**, 505–506

Taylor, R, Magnusson, I, Rothman, DL, Cline, GW, Caumo, A, Cobelli, C, Shulman, GI (1996) Direct assessment of liver glycogen storage by ^{13}C nuclear magnetic resonance spectroscopy and regulation of glucose homeostasis after a mixed meal in normal subjects *J Clin Invest* **97**, 126–132

Thierfelder, H, Sherwin, CP (1915) Phenylacetylglutamin und seine bildung im menschlichen korper nach lingabe von phenylessigsaure Hoppe Seylers *Z Physiol Chem* **94**, 1–9

Tunnicliff, G (1998) Pharmacology and function of imidazole-4-acetic acid in brain *Gen Pharmacol* **31**, 503–509

Vella, A, Shah, P, Basu, R, Basu, A, Camilleri, M, Schwenk, WF, Rizza, RA (2001) Type I diabetes mellitus does not alter initial splanchnic glucose extraction or hepatic UDP-glucose flux during enteral glucose administration *Diabetologia* **44**, 729–737

Wajngot, A, Chandramouli, V, Schumann, WC, Brunengraber, H, Efendic, S, Landau, BR (2000) A probing dose of phenylacetate does not affect glucose production and gluconeogenesis in humans *Metabolism* **49**, 1211–1214

Wajngot, A, Chandramouli, V, Schumann, WC, Efendic, S, Landau, BR (1991) Quantitation of glycogen/glucose-1-P cycling in liver Metabolism 40, 877–881

Yang, D, Brunengraber, H (2000) Glutamate, a window on liver intermediary metabolism *J Nutr* **130**, 9915–9945

8

Tracing Hepatic Glucose and Glycogen Fluxes with ^2H_2O

John G Jones

Introduction

Labeled water has long been used as a tracer of mammalian biosynthetic pathways, including gluconeogenesis and lipogenesis. The study of lipid metabolism with deuterated water was among the first biological isotope tracer studies to be performed (Schoenheimer & Rittenberg 1936). From the 1950s to the 1970s, mechanistic studies of gluconeogenic and glycolytic enzymes established that the incorporation of labeled water hydrogen into gluconeogenic precursors was highly specific with respect to a given enzyme and metabolite labeling site. This led to the realisation that 1) hepatic glucose-6-phosphate (G6P) synthesised in the presence of tritiated water (^3H_2O) has a non-uniform distribution of tritium amongst its backbone hydrogens; and 2) the amount of tritium in one position relative to another is related to the contribution of gluconeogenic versus non-gluconeogenic sources of G6P synthesis (Rognstad et al. 1974; Postle & Bloxham 1980). For determining the contribution of gluconeogenic substrates to hepatic G6P production, labeled water has some important advantages over carbon tracers. The equilibration of labeled water with total body water means that the precursor enrichment can be determined precisely from plasma or urine water, whereas the true precursor enrichment of many gluconeogenic carbon tracers may require a direct analysis of liver tissue. Also, exchanges of gluconeogenic carbons with those of other metabolic pathways via the hepatic Krebs cycle and transamination pathways have no effect on the labeling of G6P from water, whereas they contribute significantly to the dilution of carbon tracers.

To study hepatic glucose metabolism in humans, the amount of ^3H_2O that would be required to achieve sufficient specific activity in plasma glucose is unacceptably high, therefore deuterated water (^2H_2O) is used instead. Within the experimental errors of ^3H-specific activity and ^2H-enrichment measurements, the distributions of label among the hydrogens of hepatic G6P from either ^2H_2O or ^3H_2O are assumed to be equivalent.

Clinical Diabetes Research: Methods and Techniques   Edited by Michael Roden
© 2007 John Wiley & Sons, Ltd   ISBN 978-0-470-01728-9

Methodology

Administration of ^2H_2O and metabolite sampling

For both safety and practical purposes, body-water ^{2}H-enrichment levels in humans is limited to 0.3–0.5 mol %. For attainment of 0.5 mol % body-water enrichment in a 75 kg male, a loading dose of 253 grams of pure ^2H_2O is required (assuming body water content is 60 % of bodyweight. For females, body water content is assumed to be 50 % of bodyweight). The development of transient vertigo – sometimes accompanied by mild nausea – is a well-documented effect of drinking a bolus of highly enriched deuterated water. To avoid this, the loading dose is divided into two or three portions, which are taken over a 1–2 h period. The deuterated water can be made more palatable by dilution with around two volumes of bottled spring water to give a ~33 %-enriched solution. The additional water does not significantly dilute the body water enrichment. Body water enrichment is maintained over the duration of the study by providing drinking water with the same ^{2}H-enrichment as the target enrichment level. Steady state enrichment of body water is obtained within four hours of ingesting the last of the loading dose portions. For studies of fasting glucose production from glycogenolysis and gluconeogenesis, which rely on the assumption that endogenous glycogen stores are not enriched with ^{2}H, the ^2H_2O must be given after meal absorption is complete, typically no earlier than 5–6 hr after the meal. In healthy fasted subjects, steady state enrichment of plasma glucose requires an additional 2–3 hr for the plasma glucose pool to be completely turned over. In diabetic patients, this may take more time if the plasma glucose pool is bigger and clearance is impaired. These factors impose a minimum fasting interval to accommodate absorption and attainment of isotopic steady state, as shown in Figure 8.1. Urinary glucuronide can be sampled slightly earlier because of the relatively small hepatic metabolite pool sizes and the fact that 'old' glucuronide can be disposed of by simply voiding the bladder. As a result, after allowing for 30–60 minutes of transit time from liver to bladder, urinary glucuronide can be harvested around one hour after

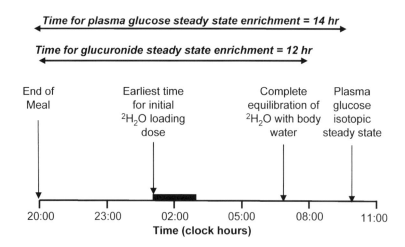

Figure 8.1 Timeline for isotopic equilibration of body water, urinary glucuronide and plasma glucose in humans following ingestion of ^2H_2O after the meal absorption period.

body water has reached steady state enrichment. Non-steady state measurements (such as determining the fractional rate of gluconeogenesis from the glucose 5:2 ^{2}H-enrichment ratio) can be performed as soon as there is sufficient ^{2}H-enrichment in these positions for accurate quantification. Studies of postprandial fluxes with ^{2}H$_2$O utilise a similar overnight dosing procedure to establish steady-state body water enrichment ahead of the feeding protocol (Jones et al. 2006b).

Metabolite analyses

Positional analysis of plasma glucose obtained from human ^{2}H$_2$O ingestion studies by gas chromatography-mass spectrometry (GC-MS) is challenging because of low ^{2}H-enrichment in multiple sites. The analysis of glucose positional hydrogens by GC-MS involves the periodate oxidation of a sugar –CH$_2$OH functionality to give formaldehyde (Landau et al. 1995, 1996). As a result, plasma glycerol has to be removed from the sample since it is also oxidised to the same formaldehyde intermediate, and may therefore interfere with the enrichment measurement (Chandramouli et al. 1997; Saadatian et al. 2000). The incorporation of 6 moles of formaldehyde into a hexamethylenetetramine (HMT) adduct results in a six-fold amplification of the heavy isotope (m + 1) signal in the MS spectrum (Landau et al. 1995, 1996). Additional sensitivity can be obtained by analysis of the isotope fractionation that occurs during the gas-chromatographic separation (Katanik et al. 2003). Enrichment of the position 6 hydrogens can be obtained by direct periodate oxidation of glucose and conversion of the formaldehyde to the hexamethylenetetramine (HMT) adduct (Landau et al. 1995, 1996). The synthesis of HMT from other sites of glucose, including positions 2 and 5, requires more elaborate dehomologation steps (Landau et al. 1996; Chandramouli et al. 1997, 1999). The diisopropylidene-3-O-acetyl derivative of glucose (DIPA) is relatively simple to prepare and provides enrichment information on hydrogen 5 plus 6, hence enrichment in both sites can be resolved when this measurement is combined with the HMT assay of position 6 (Saadatian et al. 2000). At this time, there are no published methods for obtaining positional enrichments of either hydrogen 3 or 4 of glucose by GC-MS. A GC-MS analysis of ^{2}H-enrichment in positions 2, 5 and 6 of glucose via the HMT derivative can be performed on 1 ml of plasma or less, allowing studies to be performed in infants (Kalhan & Parimi 2000). In principle, the HMT method can be applied to the analysis of urinary glucuronide ^{2}H-enrichments following the conversion of glucuronide to glucose as described by Magnusson et al. (1987, 1988). This approach has not been widely adopted because the conversion of glucuronide to glucose substantially adds to an already laborious derivatisation procedure. In addition, the position 6 hydrogens are lost during the metabolism of G6P to glucuronide. Since the HMT derivative incorporates both the positional hydrogen and carbon of glucose, enrichment of the same position by a ^{13}C-tracer will also contribute to the m + 1 signal and will therefore inflate estimates of ^{2}H-enrichment. Since there is currently no simple procedure for resolving or subtracting the ^{13}C enrichment contribution, the HMT assay of positional ^{2}H-enrichment cannot easily accommodate simultaneous ^{13}C-enrichment from complementary ^{13}C-tracers of glucose metabolism.

The ^{2}H-enrichment distribution of glucose can also be quantified by ^{2}H NMR following relatively simple derivatisation protocols (Schleucher 1999; Jones et al. 2000; Kunert et al. 2003). The preparation and analysis of the 1,2-O-isopropylidene derivative, also known as monoacetone glucose (MAG), developed by Schleucher (1999), is currently the most effective of these, since positional ^{2}H-enrichment information for all seven aliphatic hydrogens of glucose is obtained. The derivatisation procedure can be performed on a deproteinised extract of plasma glucose with yields of 50–70%. Compared to GC-MS, the NMR analysis has much less sensitivity but given a sufficient sample mass, glucose ^2H-enrichment distributions down to natural abundance levels can be reliably quantified (Schleucher 1999). ^2H NMR analysis of ^2H-enrichment is also unaffected by low levels of glucose ^{13}C-enrichment thus allowing ^{13}C-tracers and ^2H_2O to be administered at the same time (Jones et al. 2001; Burgess et al. 2003; Perdigoto et al. 2003). For a modern NMR system with standard probe-heads (500/600 MHz spectrometer, 5 mm probe), deuterium enrichments in the 0.1–0.5 % range can be quantified from 40 μmol of MAG using a collection time of 12 hours. The quantity of plasma required for this, assuming a fasting plasma glucose level of 80 mg/dl and a 50 % derivatisation yield, is about 20 ml (i.e. ~40 ml of whole blood). With microprobes, the sensitivity is improved ~1.5-fold, hence the sample mass can be halved for the same collection time, or alternatively, the collection time can be halved for the same sample mass (for a given signal to noise ratio, a 1.5-fold improvement in sensitivity means a reduction of $(1.5)^2$ or 2.25 in the number of scans or the sample mass). Cryoprobes provide a 3–4-fold increase in sensitivity, translating to a 9–16-fold reduction in collection time or sample size. In comparison to plasma glucose, urinary glucuronide samples yield more sample mass, ranging from 100–1,000 μmol. Paracetamol glucuronide needs to be derivatised to MAG for ^2H NMR analysis of positional enrichments (Burgess et al. 2003; Jones et al. 2006a). Urinary menthol glucuronide, generated by ingestion of peppermint oil, has fully resolved glucuronide ^2H NMR signals and can therefore be analysed directly by ^2H NMR following a simple purification procedure (Ribeiro et al. 2005).

Theoretical considerations

^2H Incorporation into hepatic glucose-6-phosphate

Hepatic G6P represents the metabolic crossroads for hepatic glucose and glycogen metabolism. Under fasting conditions, when the liver is a net producer of glucose, virtually all hepatic glucose production is derived from G6P via glucose-6-phosphatase. In turn, G6P is derived from the hydrolysis of glycogen or from gluconeogenesis. Under fed conditions when there is net hepatic glycogen synthesis, most of the glucosyl units of glycogen are derived via G6P. The synthesis of glycogen from galactose is an important exception to this.

   The exchange reactions that result in the incorporation of ^2H into the metabolic precursors of G6P involve extensive equilibration between reactants and products. This minimises the influence of kinetic isotope effects on the incorporation of ^2H into one position of G6P relative to another. As a result, the ^2H-enrichment of a given G6P site is assumed to depend entirely on the completeness of exchange between the hydrogen of the metabolic precursor and that of body water and the fractional contribution of that precursor to G6P synthesis. For determining the sources of hepatic G6P synthesis during either fed or fasted conditions, the ^2H-enrichment distribution in positions 2, 3, 5 and 6 of plasma glucose or positions 2, 3 and 5 of urinary glucuronide have to be considered. The exchange reactions that are relevant to enrichment in these sites are shown in Figure 8.2. Exchange of G6P with F6P via glucose-6-phosphate isomerase is rapid and extensive under both fed and fasted conditions. As a result, position 2 of G6P is quantitatively enriched from body water regardless of the source

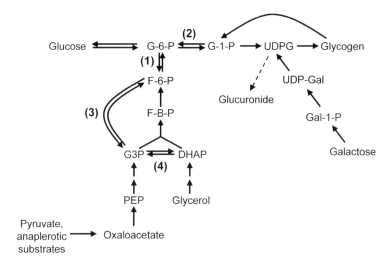

Figure 8.2 Metabolic model showing the principal exchange reactions that result in enrichment of glucose-6-phosphate and gluconeogenic precursors from ^2H_2O. 1) glucose-6-phosphate isomerase; 2) phosphoglucomutase; 3) transaldolase; 4) triose phosphate isomerase.

(glucose, glycogen or gluconeogenesis). Under fasting conditions, when the liver is a net exporter of glucose, enrichment of plasma glucose position 2 represents all glucose derived from G6P. Under isotopic steady state conditions, enrichment of plasma glucose position 2 approaches that of body water, indicating that G6P hydrolysis is the only significant source of plasma glucose (Glycogen debranching enzyme generates glucose directly from glycogen without exchange at position 2 but this process is not a significant source of glucose production). Under fed conditions, plasma glucose hydrogen 2 will not be enriched to the same level as body water because of the presence of unlabeled glucose derived from digestive absorption.

During the fed condition, where there is net hepatic glycogen synthesis, enrichment of UDP-glucose position 2 represents all flux contributions from G6P. However, galactose is metabolised to UDP-glucose by a pathway that does not involve exchange of hexose and body water hydrogens. As a result, enrichment of UDP-glucose position 2 may be significantly less than that of body water to the extent that galactose contributes to UDP-glucose flux. The effects of galactose metabolism on position 2 enrichment of UDP-glucose may be quite significant depending on the composition of the meal. For example, a 250 ml cup of milk taken as part of a high-carbohydrate breakfast meal contains enough galactose to contribute up to ~35 % of the postabsorptive UDP-glucose flux (Jones et al. 2006b).

Incorporation of ^2H into position 5 involves the obligatory addition of water hydrogen to precursor metabolites via the reactions catalyzed by enolase and triose phosphate isomerase. This applies to all gluconeogenic precursors including glycerol, therefore enrichment of position 5 is considered to be a quantitative marker for the total gluconeogenic contribution to G6P synthesis (Landau et al. 1996). This is supported by the observation that position 5 enrichment approaches that of position 2 and of body water under prolonged fasting conditions, where essentially all G6P is derived from gluconeogenesis (Landau et al. 1996).

Enrichment of the prochiral hydrogen 6 positions of G6P is mediated by several exchange steps and one addition reaction. Enrichment of the individual 6R and 6S positions reflects ^{2}H-incorporation into the respective 3S and 3R hydrogens of oxaloacetate. Addition of water via fumarase contributes to enrichment of the 3R hydrogen while enrichment of the 3S hydrogen is completely dependent on exchange reactions. These two sites are extensively randomised and subjected to additional exchange with body water due to extensive hepatic oxaloacetate-pyruvate recycling. As a result, the 6R and 6S sites of G6P are enriched to equivalent levels (Jones 2001; Burgess et al. 2003; Weis et al. 2004) and the extent to which the oxaloacetate 3R and 3S precursor sites are enriched relative to body water is believed to be extensive (at least 80 % complete). Since metabolism of glycerol to glucose via triose phosphates does not result in enrichment of either 6R or 6S positions of G6P, their enrichment specifically reflects the contribution of gluconeogenesis via PEP and the Krebs cycle. Consequently, enrichment of both position 6 sites is less than that of position 5 and the difference between position 5 and 6 enrichments reflects the fractional contributions of glycerol to total gluconeogenic flux (Landau et al. 1996).

Position 3 of G6P is enriched following the isomerisation of glyceraldehyde-3-phosphate (GA3P) to dihydroxyacetone phosphate (DHAP) and subsequent incorporation of DHAP into hexose phosphate via aldolase. When the gluconeogenic substrate is glycerol, incorporation of body water into this position is dependent on exchange of dihydroxyacetone phosphate and GA3P via triose phosphate isomerase. Given that triose phosphate isomerase exchange is very extensive and that the gluconeogenic contribution from glycerol in postabsorptive humans is typically small (20 % or less of the total gluconeogenic flux), position 3 enrichment is anticipated to reflect the total gluconeogenic fraction. However, at the time of writing, it has not been verified that position 3 attains the same enrichment levels as position 2 and body water after prolonged fasting.

Effect of transaldolase exchange

It has long been known that transaldolase will reversibly exchange the glyceraldehyde-3-phosphate moiety of F6P (i.e. carbons 4, 5 and 6) with free GA3P in many tissues including liver (Ljungdahl et al. 1961; Landau & Bartsch 1966). For F6P derived via gluconeogenesis, this process has no significant effect on the ^{2}H-enrichment distributions. However, for F6P molecules derived from glucose or glycogen where the 4,5,6-triose moiety is unlabeled, transaldolase can exchange this moiety with that of a gluconeogenic GA3P molecule enriched from body water. Consequently, position 5 enrichment of G6P reflects the sum of the gluconeogenic contribution plus the fraction of G6P derived from glycogen or glucose that experienced transaldolase exchange. Therefore, measurement of gluconeogenesis based on position 5 enrichment may be an overestimate to the extent that transaldolase exchange is occurring. Unlike position 5, position 3 enrichment of G6P is not modified by transaldolase exchange. Pending verification that it is a quantitative marker of gluconeogenesis, position 3 enrichment may more accurately reflect the gluconeogenic contribution than position 5 enrichment. The observation that position 3 enrichment is significantly less than position 5 in both fasted and postprandial states is consistent with the presence of transaldolase activity under these conditions (Perdigoto et al. 2003; Jones et al. 2006b).

Effects of glycogen cycling

The term 'glycogen cycling' refers to a futile cycle between glycogen and glucose-1-phosphate (G1P). Since G1P is also in rapid exchange with G6P, glycogen cycling influences the ^{2}H-enrichment of G6P by trapping labeled G6P molecules in glycogen and replacing them with unlabeled equivalents. Under fasting conditions, glycogen cycling will therefore diminish G6P enrichment from gluconeogenic precursors, hence the gluconeogenesis contribution will appear to be reduced while the glycogenolysis contribution will be correspondingly increased. The same process operating under fed conditions will result in underestimates of gluconeogenic and overestimates of direct pathway contributions to hepatic glycogen synthesis.

Equivalence of plasma glucose and urinary glucuronide ^{2}H-enrichment patterns during fasting

Given the assumption that all fasting plasma glucose is directly derived from G6P via glucose-6-phosphatase, the enrichment patterns of plasma glucose and hepatic G6P are equivalent at isotopic steady state. Hepatic G6P is also in rapid exchange with G1P, which in turn supplies a basal flux of hexose units for UDP-glucose synthesis and glucuronidation activities. As a result, the enrichment distribution of G6P is also preserved in glucuronide, with the important exception of the position 6 hydrogens, which are removed from the hexose skeleton following the oxidation of UDP-glucose to UDP-glucuronic acid and are therefore absent from the glucuronide. Urinary glucuronide and plasma glucose enrichments appear to be equivalent in overnight-fasted healthy subjects, although only a small number of subjects have been studied to date.

Quantifying hepatic glucose and glycogen metabolism

The analysis of glucose or glucuronide positional enrichment following ingestion of ^{2}H$_2$O can provide information on the sources of hepatic glucose production during fasting and hepatic glycogen synthesis during feeding. The metabolic models for fasted and fed states are shown in Figures 8.3 and 8.4, respectively. The mechanisms of ^{2}H incorporation and the rates of metabolite/body water hydrogen exchange are assumed to be the same for both nutritional states.

Fasted state (net glucose synthesis from hepatic G6P)

Under these conditions, hepatic G6P is assumed to be entirely derived from gluconeogenesis and glycogenolysis activities and to be the sole source of plasma glucose synthesis, as shown in Figure 8.3. Because of extensive G6P-F6P exchange, position 2 is assumed to be enriched to the same level as body water and therefore it represents all G6P sources. Meanwhile, position 5 enrichment reflects the total gluconeogenic contribution. On this basis, the ratio of position 5 to position 2 enrichment (H5/H2) of plasma glucose provides an estimate of the percent contribution of gluconeogenesis to hepatic glucose production (equation 1), with the glycogenolysis contribution obtained by difference (equation 2). The difference between

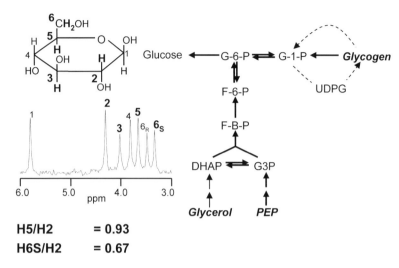

H5/H2   = 0.93

H6S/H2   = 0.67

Figure 8.3 Metabolic Model for the Sources of Hepatic Glucose Output During Fasting Also shown is a ^2H NMR spectrum of a MAG derivative prepared from plasma glucose of a heart failure patient with new-onset diabetes. The number above each signal represents the glucose position where the signal originated. The ratio of position 5 to position 2 (H5/H2) and position 6S to position 2 (H6S/H2) enrichments as determined from the relative areas of the NMR signals are also shown. Applying these data to equations 1–4 gives the following estimates of flux contributions to fasting glucose production: 7 % from glycogenolysis, 67 % from PEP and 26 % from glycerol.

position 5 and position 6 enrichments (H5 and H6) reflects the contributions of glycerol to the gluconeogenic fraction. The contribution of glycerol and PEP gluconeogenesis to fasting glucose production can thus be calculated according to equations 3 and 4.

1) Percentage of glucose derived by glycogenolysis = [1–(H5/H2)] × 100
2) Percentage of glucose derived by total gluconeogenesis = (H5/H2) × 100
3) Fraction of glucose derived by glycerol gluconeogenesis = [(H5 – H6)/H2] × 100
4) Fraction of glucose derived by PEP gluconeogenesis = (H6/H2) × 100

Since all flux parameters are based on relative rather than absolute glucose ^2H-enrichment values, they can be obtained before plasma glucose and body water have reached isotopic steady state. These equations do not account for the effects of transaldolase exchange and will therefore give overestimates of gluconeogenic flux in the presence of transaldolase activity. (For example, after overnight fasting H5/H2 is typically 0.50, hence the estimated contribution of gluconeogenesis to glucose production is 50 % and that of glycogenolysis is 50 %. Assume that 20 % of G6P molecules also underwent transaldolase exchange and let x be the real percentage of glucose molecules formed by glycogenolysis with 100 – x being the percentage formed by gluconeogenesis. Then, 100 – x % would be enriched at position 5 by gluconeogenesis and 0.2x % would be enriched at position 5 by transaldolase exchange. Thus, H5/H2 = 0.5 = (100 – x + 0.2x)/100. Solving for x gives 62.5 % – the real contribution of glycogenolysis. The real contribution of gluconeogenesis is therefore 37.5%. From the NMR spectrum shown in Figure 8.3, the lower intensity of the position 3 signal relative to

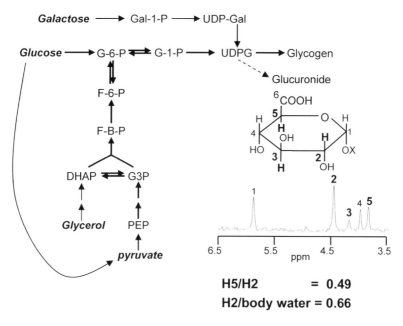

H5/H2 = 0.49
H2/body water = 0.66

Figure 8.4 Metabolic Scheme Representing Hepatic Glycogen Synthesis During Feeding Also shown is a ^{2}H NMR spectrum of a MAG derivative prepared from Paracetamol glucuronide of a healthy subject that had ingested ^{2}H$_2$O and Paracetamol some hours before a morning breakfast meal. The number above each signal represents the glucuronide position where the signal originated. The ratio of position 5 to position 2 (H5/H2) enrichments as determined from the relative areas of the NMR signals and the enrichment of position 2 relative to body water (H2/body water) are also shown. Applying these data to equations 5–7 gives the following estimates of UDP-glucose flux contributions: 33 % from galactose, 33 % from gluconeogenesis and 34 % from direct pathway metabolism of glucose.

those of positions 4 and 5 reflects a reduced enrichment in position 3 relative to positions 4 and 5, which is consistent with transaldolase activity.

Fed state (net glycogen synthesis from hepatic G6P)

As shown in Figure 8.4, both galactose and G6P can supply glucosyl units for glycogen synthesis via UDP-glucose. G6P in turn is derived directly from glucose or is synthesised from gluconeogenic precursors. The gluconeogenic fraction includes the indirect pathway of glucose conversion to glycogen plus contributions from non-glucose precursors such as glycerol and amino acids. The fraction of UDP-glucose derived from galactose, direct pathway glucose and gluconeogenesis can be estimated from the enrichments of positions 2 and 5 of glucuronide (glucuronide H2, H5) and that of body water as shown in equations 5–7.

5) Percentage of glycogen from galactose = (glucuronide H2/body water) × 100
6) Percentage of glycogen from gluconeogenesis = (glucuronide H5/body water) × 100
7) Percentage of glycogen from direct pathway = 100 – percentage from gluconeogenesis– percentage from galactose

These measurements are based on absolute enrichments of glucuronide and body water and therefore require isotopic steady state of body water and glucuronide to be attained beforehand. Transaldolase activity will result in overestimates of the gluconeogenic contribution to glycogen synthesis in an analogous manner to the fasted condition (Stingl et al. 2006). From the NMR spectrum shown in Figure 8.4, position 3 enrichment is notably less than either position 4 or 5, which is consistent with transaldolase activity.

Conclusion

Sources of hepatic glucose production during fasting and glycogen synthesis during feeding can be derived by analysis of glucose and glucuronide enrichment following ^2H_2O ingestion. The measurement is simple to implement and can be performed in a standard clinical setting. For obtaining realistic estimates of the gluconeogenic contribution to hepatic glucose production or glycogen synthesis, the effect of transaldolase exchange on the glucose/glucuronide ^2H-enrichment distributions may have to be considered. This requires the quantification of ^2H-enrichment in position 3 as well as in positions 2, 5 and 6. Provided that sufficient sample mass is available, ^2H NMR analysis of glucose or glucuronide derivatives is the most effective method for quantifying ^2H-enrichment in these sites.

References

Burgess SC, Weis B, Jones JG, Smith E, Merritt ME, Margolis D et al. (2003) *Analy Biochem* **312**, 228–34

Chandramouli V, Ekberg K, Schumann WC, Kalhan SC, Wahren J, Landau BR (1997) *Am J Physiol* **273**, E1,209–15

Chandramouli V, Ekberg K, Schumann WC, Wahren J, Landau BR (1999) *Am J Physiol* **277**, E717–23

Jones JG, Barosa C, Gomes F, Mendes AC, Delgado TC, Diogo L et al. (2006a) *J Carbohydr Chem* **25**, 203–17

Jones JG, Carvalho RA, Sherry AD, Malloy CR (2000) *Anal Biochem* **277**, 121–6

Jones JG, Fagulha A, Barosa C, Bastos M, Barros L, Baptista C et al. (2006b) *Diabetes* **55**, 2294–2300

Jones JG, Solomon MA, Cole SM, Sherry AD, Malloy CR (2001) *Am J Physiol* **281**, E848–51

Kalhan S, Parimi P (2000) *Seminars in Perinatology* **24**, 94–106

Katanik J, McCabe BJ, Brunengraber DZ, Chandramouli V, Nishiyama FJ, Anderson VE et al. (2003) *Am J Physiol* **284**, E1043–8

Kunert O, Stingl H, Rosian E, Krššák M, Bernroider E, Seebacher W et al. (2003) *Diabetes* **52**, 2475–82

Landau BR, Bartsch GE (1966) *J Biol Chem* **241**, 741–9

Landau BR, Wahren J, Chandramouli V, Schumann WC, Ekberg K, Kalhan, SC (1995) *J Clin Invest* **95**, 172–8

Landau BR, Wahren J, Chandramouli V, Schumann WC, Ekberg K, Kalhan SC (1996) *J Clin Invest* **98**, 378–85

Ljungdahl L, Wood HG, Couri D, Racker E (1961) *J Biol Chem* **236**, 1622–5

Magnusson I, Chandramouli V, Schumann WC, Kumaran K, Wahren J, Landau BR (1987) *J Clin Invest* **80**, 1748–54

Magnusson I, Chandramouli V, Schumann WC, Kumaran K, Wahren J, Landau BR (1988) *Proc Nat Acad Sci USA* **85**, 4682–5

Perdigoto R, Rodrigues TB, Furtado AL, Porto A, Geraldes C, Jones JG (2003) *NMR in Biomedicine* **16**, 189–98

Postle AD, Bloxham DP (1980) *Biochem J* **192**, 65–73

Ribeiro A, Caldeira MM, Carvalheiro M, Bastos M, Baptista C, Fagulha A et al. (2005) *Magn Reson Med* **54**, 429–34

Rognstad R, Clark G, Katz J (1974) *Eur J Biochem* **47**, 383–8

Saadatian M, Peroni O, Diraison F, Beylot M (2000) *Diabetes and Metab* **26**, 202–9

Schleucher J, Vanderveer P, Markley JL, Sharkey TD (1999) *Plant Cell and Environ* **22**, 525–33

Schoenheimer R, Rittenberg D (1936) *J Biol Chem* **114**, 373–9

Stingl H, Chandramouli V, Schumann WC, Brehm A, Nowotny P, Waldhausl W et al. (2006) *Diabetologia* **49**, 360–8

Weis BC, Margolis D, Burgess SC, Merritt ME, Wise H, Sherry AD et al. (2004) *Mag Res Med* **51**, 649–54

9
Lipid Kinetics

John M Miles and Robert H Nelson

Introduction

There has been increasing interest in lipid fuel metabolism over the past 15 years, in part due to recognition of the key role of lipids as mediators of insulin resistance in individuals with obesity, dyslipidemia and type 2 diabetes (McGarry 1992; Boden 1997). In particular, the production and delivery of circulating triglycerides to tissues for fat storage or oxidation is not well understood. The development of methods to probe lipid fuel metabolism has been challenging, but considerable progress has been made in recent years. This chapter will focus on new methodologies for studying adipose tissue lipolysis and triglyceride-rich lipoprotein metabolism. The study of lipoprotein particle metabolism with protein tracers (i.e. the administration of amino acid precursors to label a lipoprotein product) is an important area that will not be reviewed in detail here.

Tracers for the study of adipose tissue lipolysis

Free fatty acids

Free fatty acids (FFAs) are the major lipid fuel in the circulation, with a relatively high flux rate that can be estimated at approximately 100 g/day in healthy adults (Miles et al. 2004). The use of tracers for the study of FFA kinetics is nearly 50 years old (Frederickson & Gordon 1958), but there has been a renewed interest in FFA metabolism in recent years because of evidence that elevated FFA levels are likely mediators of insulin resistance (Boden et al. 1991), endothelial dysfunction (Steinberg et al. 1997) and hypertension (Stojiljkovic et al. 2001). Although there is in general an excellent correlation between plasma FFA concentration and FFA turnover (Armstrong et al. 1961), there are dramatic examples of how measurement of FFA concentration fails to detect changes in flux. For example, in normal and diabetic subjects, submaximal exercise results in a near-doubling of oleate turnover rate without a significant increase in the arterial concentration of this fatty acid (Wahren et al. 1975). Another example of the value of kinetic measurements is the difference that has

Clinical Diabetes Research: Methods and Techniques   Edited by Michael Roden
© 2007 John Wiley & Sons, Ltd   ISBN 978-0-470-01728-9

been reported in FFA turnover between men and women, with no difference in plasma FFA concentration (Nielsen et al. 2003). This lack of difference in concentration is due to an offsetting increase in FFA clearance in women compared to men, again requiring the use of a tracer for its detection. Measurement of FFA flux can be an extremely sensitive indicator of changes in plasma insulin concentration. When insulin was infused in dogs at a rate that was so low that it did not produce a measurable increase in plasma insulin concentrations, a significant decrease in palmitate appearance was observed (Cersosimo & Miles, unpublished results).

FFAs are quite insoluble in aqueous media, and are avidly bound to circulating albumin (Spector 1975), a characteristic that makes their measurement more difficult. For many years, plasma FFA concentrations were determined colourimetrically (Dole 1956). Enzymatic assays for FFAs (Miles et al. 1983) represented an improvement on the older methods, but have their own limitations (see below). An early report describing the *in vivo* use of FFA tracers involved separate bolus injections of ^{14}C palmitate, ^{14}C oleate and ^{14}C linoleate in mostly healthy volunteers, and found that the flux and half life of total FFAs in plasma were 600–700 μmol/min and 2–3 min respectively after an overnight fast (Frederickson & Gordon 1958). These results differ slightly from more recent estimates but are surprisingly accurate considering that 1) the injected tracer was frozen prior to use and 2) relatively crude methods, the only ones available at the time, were employed for the isolation of FFA radioactivity and measurement of FFA concentration (Frederickson & Gordon 1958). Some investigators have used simple extraction into an organic solvent to isolate FFA radioactivity (Hagenfeldt & Wahren 1968); this procedure lacks specificity for FFAs because of the *in vivo* incorporation of labeled FFAs into neutral lipids (Frederickson & Gordon 1958). Thin layer chromatography (Most et al. 1969; Dagenais et al. 1976) or back extraction into dilute base (Armstrong et al. 1961; Gold et al. 1964) is more specific, but tedious and somewhat imprecise. Furthermore, it lacks accuracy because the extraction of FFAs from plasma with organic solvents is often not quantitative (Duncombe & Rising 1973).

The advantage of the bolus injection technique is that it requires a relatively small tracer dose and a short sampling interval (10–30 min) after the injection. Its disadvantage is that its accuracy depends substantially on frequent early sampling (every 0.5–2 minutes) and it is not valid under non-steady state conditions. Because of these limitations, constant tracer infusion (Barter & Nestel 1972) has become more popular. The constant infusion allows measurement of FFA kinetics under non-steady state conditions using a modification of the equations of Steele; an effective volume of distribution of 90 mL/kg provides the most accurate estimates of FFA inflow (Jensen et al. 1990). Fortunately, the methodologic problems that plague measurements of glucose kinetics under non-steady state conditions (Finegood et al. 1987) do not occur with plasma FFA, owing to the very short (2–3 min) half life of the latter.

Subsequently, a stable isotope method was introduced for the measurement of palmitate kinetics (Wolfe et al. 1980). This method utilises an FFA tracer labeled with ^{13}C or ^{2}H and represents a major advance in precision, sensitivity and specificity of tracer analysis. The avoidance of radioactivity allows studies in children and pregnant women. The sample is extracted from plasma (often after addition of a stable isotopic internal standard to allow quantification of concentration), purified by thin layer chromatography and derivatised. The procedure is based on the use of gas chromatography/mass spectrometry using selected ion monitoring. It allows accurate and precise measurement of low individual and total FFA concentrations, such as are observed during insulin infusion (Mittendorfer et al. 2003).

Moreover, it is more specific and precise in the determination of tracer enrichment than older methods for FFA specific activity (Frederickson & Gordon 1958). Because of its specificity, it can be used for the simultaneous measurement of the kinetics of several fatty acids (Mittendorfer et al. 2003). However, considerable amounts of tracer, along with significant amounts of albumin, must be infused in order to achieve tracer enrichment sufficient for detection. Several hundred milliliters of 4 % albumin can be required for studies of 4–8 hours in duration, a perturbation that is not desirable.

The development of a method using ultra-low infusion rates of uniformly labeled ^{13}C palmitate, based on combustion isotope ratio mass spectrometry (IRMS) in which $^{13}CO_2$ enrichment is actually measured (Guo et al. 1997), was a major advance in FFA tracer methodology. The sensitivity of IRMS allows tracer (and thus albumin) infusion rates to be reduced by more than an order of magnitude. Uniformly labeled tracer of oleate (and potentially other fatty acids; see below) can be utilised in place of palmitate.

Significant improvements have also been made in the use of radiolabeled FFA tracers. We reported a method for determining FFA kinetics in which modest amounts of tracer (0.2–0.3 μCi/min of e.g. ^3H palmitate or ^3H oleate) are infused and the specific radioactivity of the individual fatty acid is determined with high performance liquid chromatography (HPLC). Plasma is extracted into an organic solvent and the extract is taken to dryness without need for isolation by thin layer chromatography. A phenacyl derivative is then prepared (Miles et al. 1987). The addition of $[^2H_{31}]$ palmitate as an internal standard (Jensen et al. 1988) allowed the precise and accurate measurement of plasma palmitate, oleate and linoleate concentrations. Subsequent modification of column and mobile phase conditions expanded the measurement to a total of nine long chain FFAs (Miles et al. 1995). Recent improvements in the procedure allow determination of total FFAs (i.e. the sum of the concentrations of the nine FFAs) in a 30 minute run. This is accomplished by using a 4 μm, 15 cm ODS column in a 50 °C water bath eluted with 78 % acetonitrile in water at 2.0 mL/min. A chromatogram of plasma FFAs is shown in Figure 9.1. For human studies, a relatively large aliquot (usually 1.0 mL) of plasma is analysed to allow lower tracer infusion rates. To accommodate this larger amount of FFA, it is necessary to set the UV detector at a less sensitive wavelength (254 or 260 nm; maximum absorbance is at ~242 nm). Using this modified method, plasma total FFA concentrations were 26 ± 2 (range, 13–38) μ mol/L in 20 subjects during a euglycemic, hyperinsulinemic clamp (unpublished data), illustrating the method's sensitivity. A chief limitation of enzymatic methods (Miles et al. 1983) is the inability to accurately detect such low concentrations.

Unfortunately, it is usually necessary to choose a tracer from one of the circulating fatty acids as representative of the aggregate of FFAs. There are significant differences in the regional metabolism of the different classes of fatty acids (Harris et al. 1962; Miller et al. 1962; Hagenfeldt 1975), indicating a potential for misleading conclusions when a single tracer is used. Mittendorfer et al. (2003) infused five FFA tracers (myristate, palmitate, oleate, linoleate and stearate) simultaneously in healthy subjects under basal conditions, during epinephrine infusion and during insulin infusion. Palmitate, oleate and linoleate each provided estimates of total FFA flux that were within 15 % of actual values, whereas myristate and stearate consistently overestimated and underestimated, respectively, total FFA flux. This indicates that the latter two tracers should not be used to estimate total FFA kinetics except under special circumstances.

Another advantage of continuous tracer infusion is that it allows determination of regional kinetics in tissues such as the extremity (Martin & Jensen 1991; Miles et al. 2004),

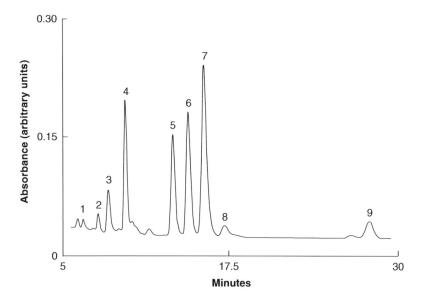

Figure 9.1   A Chromatogram of Plasma FFAs using High Performance Liquid Chromatography $1 = \alpha$-linolenic acid; 2 = myristic acid; 3 = palmitoleic acid + arachidonic acid; 4 = linoleic acid; $5 = [^2H_{31}]$ palmitate (internal standard); 6 = palmitic acid; 7 = oleic acid; 8 = elaidic acid; 9 = stearic acid.

myocardium (Wisneski et al. 1987) and splanchnic bed (Nielsen et al. 2004). The combination of net balance (based on arteriovenous concentration differences) and tracer balance allows partitioning of uptake and release and provides an extremely powerful probe of tissue bed kinetics. However, it is invasive and requires steady state conditions with respect to both tracer and tracee. The relationship between plasma FFA concentration and FFA transport in tissues can be markedly non-linear, as shown in Figure 9.2. Six subjects received an infusion of ^{14}C oleate during a diagnostic cardiac catheterisation in which simultaneous arterial and coronary sinus blood samples were taken (Nelson et al. 2007a). The data show a striking negative correlation between arterial plasma oleate concentration and the fractional extraction of ^{14}C oleate (the latter a reflection of tissue clearance) by the myocardium.

FFA oxidation

FFA carbon tracers (^{13}C or ^{14}C) can be used to estimate plasma FFA oxidation. However, in order to obtain accurate data, a correction for CO_2 fixation must be made (Sidossis et al. 1995). When indirect calorimetry is used to estimate total fat oxidation, it is clear that unlabeled fat is being oxidised, especially during exercise (Goodpaster et al. 2002). The observation that total body fat oxidation often exceeds plasma FFA oxidation, even when a correction is made for CO_2 fixation, is an indication that intracellular pools of unlabeled fatty acids are being directly oxidised. These unlabeled fatty acids likely reside in cytosolic triglyceride droplets in the liver, skeletal muscle and elsewhere, and are in isotopic disequilibrium with plasma FFA. Another technique that appears to be satisfactory for the measurement of fatty acid oxidation is ^3H water generation. There is a good correlation between measurement of meal fat oxidation with ^{14}C and ^3H-labeled fat (Romanski et al. 2000).

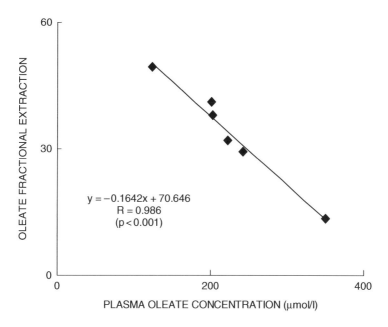

Figure 9.2 Relationship Between Myocardial Fractional Extraction of Radiolabeled Oleate and Arterial Plasma Oleate Concentrations in Six Subjects (unpublished data).

Glycerol

Glycerol kinetics have been extensively studied as a measure of adipose tissue lipolysis. Some investigators have suggested that glycerol provides a more accurate indicate of lipolysis because it is not re-esterified in adipose tissues. In contrast, FFAs produced by hormone sensitive lipase can be reincorporated into triglyceride without exiting the adipocyte (Vaughan 1962). In post-absorptive subjects, local adipose tissue fatty acid re-esterification is minimal, but it increases when hormone sensitive lipase is suppressed by insulin (Coppack et al. 1999). Glycerol flux may be a less specific indicator of hormone sensitive lipase activity, considering that unlike FFA, glycerol produced by the action of adipose tissue lipoprotein lipase (LPL) on lipoproteins is quantitatively released into the circulation because of the absence of glycerol kinase in that tissue (Lin 1977).

Most studies of glycerol kinetics employ a primed, continuous infusion (Klein et al. 1986; Coppack et al. 1999). It is not clear why a priming dose is needed, considering that the half life of glycerol is if anything shorter than that of FFA (Beylot et al. 1987), with a clearance rate much higher than that of FFA (Coppack et al. 1999).

Unlike FFA, glycerol is water soluble and is not bound to plasma proteins. Analysis of plasma glycerol can be challenging because of its relatively low concentrations, hydrophilic properties, poor UV absorbance and surprising volatility when isolated and subjected to a vacuum during a drying procedure. This may account for the divergent and sometimes implausible results when radiolabeled glycerol is used to determine glycerol kinetics. FFA:glycerol turnover ratios have been reported to range from 1.4:1 to 5.2:1 (Bjorntorp et al. 1969; Winkler et al. 1969). Glycerol radioactivity can be isolated with borate columns (Nurjhan et al. 1986), but the procedure is tedious. Moreover, the need for a separate measurement of glycerol concentration reduces precision. This problem was overcome by the use of gas chromatography/mass spectrometry (Klein et al. 1986) and HPLC (Judd et al. 1998), both of which provide excellent accuracy and precision because of their specificity and because of the linkage between the measurement of tracer and tracee.

Practical considerations

The use of FFA or glycerol tracers is relatively free of difficulties compared with measuring the kinetics of longer-lived substances such as glucose (Finegood et al. 1987) because there is less need for priming doses and non-steady state errors are minimal (Miles et al. 1987). For the same reason, minimal time (30–60 minutes) is required for tracer equilibration during a continuous infusion. Radiolabeled FFA tracers are inexpensive, and relatively low infusion rates (0.2–0.3 μCi/min) with favourable whole-body radiation dosimetry considerations make their use attractive. Experiments of 6–8 hr duration or longer can be undertaken, allowing the investigator to obtain data during a baseline (often post-absorptive) period and again during a perturbation such as a meal or infusion of a hormone or drug. Infusion in a peripheral vein and sampling of arterialised venous blood (Jensen & Heiling 1991) is satisfactory for measurement of whole-body kinetics. However, for studies of regional metabolism in a tissue bed such as the forearm or myocardium, the need for additional precision requires arterial sampling.

Tracers for the study of triglyceride-rich lipoprotein kinetics

Chylomicrons

Chylomicrons are large lipoprotein particles that are formed by the small intestine during fat absorption. The amount of lipid fuel that traverses the circulation in the form of chylomicrons obviously varies with dietary fat consumption. In individuals on high-fat diets, however, it can equal or exceed FFA flux (Miles et al. 2004). The triglyceride transported in chylomicrons is metabolised by LPL, which is widely distributed in tissues but is most abundant in adipose tissue and skeletal muscle (Eckel 1989). Nascent chylomicrons have a short residence time in the circulation, with a half life of approximately five minutes (Park et al. 2001). Chylomicron half life is prolonged at higher chylomicron triglyceride concentrations (Park et al. 2001).

Triglyceride uptake from the circulation can under some circumstances occur independent of enzymes such as LPL and hepatic lipase. Saturation of transport appears to occur at plasma triglyceride concentrations of $\sim$400 mg/dL^{-1} (Brunzell et al. 1973, 1979) or lower (Nikkila & Kekki 1973). It is important to note that chylomicron-sized lipid particles can be removed via nonenzymatic pathways, particularly the reticuloendothelial system (Seidner et al. 1989). When large amounts of a lipid emulsion were administered to rats by bolus injection, there was evidence of non-enzymatic lipid clearance (Lutz et al. 1989). Karpe et al. (1997) concluded that, during mild chylomicronaemia after a high fat meal in normal subjects, the removal of triglycerides by non-lipolytic tissues was negligible. Quantitatively significant reticuloendothelial uptake may occur only at plasma triglyceride concentrations above those at which maximal rates of LPL-mediated triglyceride hydrolysis are observed, i.e. $\sim$300–400 mg/dL^{-1} or 3.4–4.5 mmol/L^{-1} (Miles et al. 2001).

Mere measurement of triglyceride concentrations (and triglyceride-rich lipoprotein concentrations) in plasma cannot distinguish defects in production from abnormalities in removal and provide no insight into kinetic events. Many investigators have therefore utilised experimental procedures for this purpose. A variety of techniques, using native chylomicrons, lipid emulsions as a surrogate for chylomicrons, and both labeled and unlabeled materials, have been employed.

The choice of method for tracking the metabolism of chylomicrons depends substantially on the intended focus of the investigation: the triglyceride fatty acids in the nascent particle or the particle itself, together with its remnants. There is substantial evidence to suggest that chylomicron remnants are atherogenic (Redgrave 2004). An older method for studying chylomicron particle metabolism involved labeling of a fat meal with retinol palmitate (Hazzard & Bierman 1976). However, the fact that retinol palmitate appears in very low density lipoprotein (VLDL) particles (Lemieux et al. 1998) and that it is hydrolysed and taken up by adipose tissue LPL (Blaner et al. 1994) indicates that it is not an ideal tracer for this purpose. An alternative approach suitable for tracing the metabolism of chylomicron remnants is the labeling of apolipoprotein B-48 with a stable isotope (Lichtenstein et al. 1992). Finally, labeled cholesterol esters can be added to a synthetic lipid emulsion and administered intravenously (Redgrave & Maranhao 1985). The cholesterol ester disappears much more slowly from plasma than does labeled triglyceride (Redgrave & Maranhao 1985), as would be expected with a tracer that is retained in the particle after its interaction with LPL.

The fate of dietary fatty acids can be traced by adding a radiolabeled triglyceride to a mixed meal and tracking the appearance of the labeled fatty acid in the plasma space and its subsequent uptake in regional fat depots (Roust & Jensen 1993; Romanski et al. 2000; Jensen et al. 2003). Triglycerides or fatty acids labeled with stable isotopes can be administered as part of a meal in order to generate labeled chylomicrons (Evans et al. 2002; Barrows et al. 2005). The technique can be extremely useful in assessing patterns of dietary fat storage. It has the advantage that the secreted chylomicrons contain physiological mixed triglycerides. A limitation is that tracer input (i.e. the rate of absorption of labeled chylomicrons) is unknown.

Nestel et al. (1962) administered chylomicrons harvested surgically from thoracic duct lymph to normal volunteers to study triglyceride-rich lipoprotein metabolism. Whereas this represents a physiological approach, the invasiveness of the method limits its usefulness. Because of such limitations, investigators have since then employed a lipid emulsion as a surrogate for native chylomicrons. Although some investigators have used a bolus injection of unlabeled lipid (Rossner 1974), this also has limitations because it perturbs the same intrinsic parameters (clearance; half life; residence time) that the technique is attempting to measure, increasing plasma triglyceride concentrations to >1000 mg/dL^{-1} (11.3 mmol/L^{-1}). In fact, triglyceride clearance estimated from intravenous fat tolerance tests is 100–200 % slower (Rossner 1974; Cohen 1989) than the clearance of a tracer dose of radioactive lipid (Nakandakare et al. 1994). Moreover, the intravenous fat tolerance test may result in significant, if brief, reticuloendothelial uptake of lipid because of the temporary high triglyceride concentrations achieved, as described above. A bolus injection of a radiolabeled lipid emulsion of relatively high specific activity (Nakandakare et al. 1994), on the other hand, allows the investigator to give what is in essence a massless amount of lipid as a tracer.

One of the key questions with this experimental approach is whether the artificial lipid emulsion is metabolised in a fashion that approximates that of chylomicrons. Infused lipid particles rapidly acquire apolipoprotein C2 (Iriyama et al. 1988). However, this does not ensure that the emulsion particles are metabolised similarly to chylomicrons. It is clear that the absence of cholesterol and cholesterol esters in artificial lipid emulsions results in the *in vivo* production of remnants that are cleared much more slowly than chylomicron remnants. To make it possible to trace chylomicron remnant metabolism with a radiolabeled artificial lipid emulsion, Redgrave developed (Redgrave & Maranhao 1985) and validated (Redgrave et al. 1993) a technique in which cholesterol and cholesterol esters are incorporated in chylomicron-like particles, and radiolabeled phospholipid-rich vesicles are removed by ultracentrifugation. This method allows the investigator to trace chylomicron triglyceride and remnant particle metabolism by adding radiolabeled triglyceride and cholesterol ester, respectively, during emulsion preparation, and produces clearance data that are very similar to results with chylomicrons (Redgrave & Maranhao 1985; Redgrave et al. 1993). From available data, it appears that a chylomicron-like particle requires cholesterol and cholesterol esters in order to undergo normal remnant metabolism, but these components have little effect on particle interaction with LPL, based on the observations of Redgrave & Maranhao (1985).

For *in vivo* investigations, a tracer-containing lipid emulsion can be prepared from oil, water, an emulsifying agent and other ingredients using sonication and density grandient ultracentrifugation. This approach has been used for studies in rodents (Redgrave & Maranhao 1985; Redgrave et al. 1993) and in humans (Redgrave et al. 1993; Nakandakare et al. 1994). Alternatively, a radiolabeled triglyceride can be incorporated into a commercial lipid emulsion (Park et al. 2000). Although triolein is not an entirely physiological triglyceride, most investigators (Redgrave & Maranhao 1985; Redgrave et al. 1993; Nakandakare et al. 1994; Hultin et al. 1995; Martins et al. 1996; Park et al. 2000) have found that emulsions labeled with this material provide good estimates of chylomicron triglyceride metabolism, with no evidence of exchange of labeled triolein with other lipoproteins when administered to humans (Nakandakare et al. 1994).

When labeled triolein is added to a commercial lipid emulsion, it is distributed roughly equally between large triglyceride-rich, chylomicron-sized (mean diameter $\sim$340 nm) particles and much smaller phospholipid-rich vesicles (Park et al. 2000). A size exclusion HPLC purification step is therefore required to isolate the large particles in pure form; a radiochromatogram showing the separation of the two species of particles is shown in Figure 9.3. The material is immediately collected in a vial containing unlabeled lipid emulsion, which maintains its stability by restoring the phospholipid excess present in the commercial preparation, and is then autoclaved. The particle size spectrum of this preparation is almost identical to that of native chylomicrons (Park et al. 2000), as shown in Figure 9.4.

The labeled lipid emulsion prepared in this fashion appears to be stable for at least a month (unpublished results). Infused at a rate of 0.6–1.2 μCi/min, it has a sufficiently high specific activity ($\sim$400,000 dpm/μmol fatty acid) that the infusion does not result in an increase in plasma triglyceride concentrations. Limitations on the amount of material that can be incorporated into the emulsion preclude using this technique to prepare an emulsion labeled with a stable isotopic tracer. Isolation of chylomicrons from plasma, separate from particles containing apolipoprotein B-100, is a challenge. A reasonably pure chylomicron isolate can be obtained with triple ultracentrifugation, although it still contains a small ($\sim$4 % of total triglyceride) contribution from VLDL (Park et al. 2000). This indicates that roughly half of the particles in the specimen are VLDL, and half are chylomicrons. Immunoaffinity

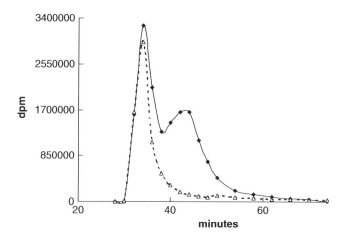

Figure 9.3 A size exclusion HPLC radiochromatogram of unpurified lipid emulsion (solid line) and a rechromatographed, purified 30–40 min fraction containing chylomicron sized particles (dashed line). Reproduced courtesy of Park Y, Grellner WJ, Harris WS, Miles JM, (2000) A new method for the study of chylomicron kinetics in vivo. *Am J Physiol 279*, E1258–E1263.

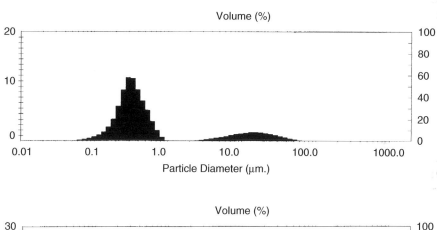

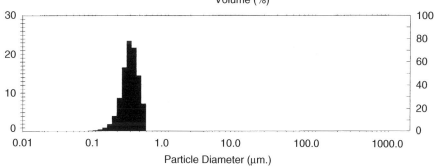

Figure 9.4 Size distribution of human chylomicrons isolated by triple-spin ultracentrifugation (A) and the purified lipid emulsion (B), both measured by laser light scattering spectroscopy. Reproduced courtesy of Park Y, Grellner WJ, Harris WS, Miles JM (2000) A new method for the study of chylomicron kinetics in vivo. *Am J Physiol 279*, E1258–E1263.

chromatography could potentially produce a more pure chylomicron specimen, but a method for this purpose is not yet available.

This tracer appears to be metabolised by LPL in a way similar to native chylomicrons (Park et al. 2000). Preliminary results from splanchnic balance studies using this technique in dogs are consistent with previous data on dietary triglyceride uptake in both animals and humans (Nelson et al. 2007b). The labeled lipid emulsion can be used to estimate the spillover of LPL-generated fatty acids into the circulation. In order to accomplish this, the emulsion (usually labeled with ^{3}H triolein) is administered along with a separate FFA tracer, either ^{14}C oleate or ^{13}C oleate. The rate of appearance of ^{3}H oleate is estimated in a calculation in which the carbon-labeled oleate is the tracer and the ^{3}H oleate is the tracee. Utilising this principle, both systemic and regional spillover can be determined. In an initial study in healthy volunteers, systemic and forearm fractional spillover were ~36 % and ~14 % respectively (Miles et al. 2004). The degree of spillover that occurs during meal absorption is not known since these studies were conducted after an overnight fast. However, considering the amount of dietary fat that traverses the circulation, it is possible that dietary fat makes a major contribution to plasma FFA. Others have estimated postprandial spillover in adipose tissue to be as high as 80 % in healthy subjects (Evans et al. 2002).

VLDL

Very low density lipoproteins (VLDL) are of interest for two reasons. First, they are the obligate precursor of low density lipoproteins (LDL) (Dietschy et al. 1993). Second, together with chylomicrons, VLDLs represent the major vehicle for transport of triglycerides in the circulation. VLDL triglyceride secretion by the liver is controlled to some extent by the supply of FFA to that tissue (Lewis et al. 1995), with additional acute regulation by insulin (Sparks & Sparks 1994).

Hepatic VLDL production can be determined using several different techniques. One of the first methods utilised by investigators was the hepatic balance technique (Basso & Havel 1970). This approach requires arterial, portal vein and hepatic vein sampling, together with a measurement of hepatic blood flow, and thus can only be used in animal studies. Splanchnic triglyceride balance (sampling arterial and hepatic venous blood, without portal venous sampling) has been measured in humans (Havel et al. 1970). The procedure is reasonably safe in experienced hands. However, it likely produces underestimates of actual hepatic VLDL triglyceride secretion rates because of uptake of VLDL triglyceride from arterial blood by nonhepatic splanchnic tissues, primarily visceral adipose tissue. Tracer techniques are far preferable to splanchnic balance measurements because they avoid this pitfall and in addition are noninvasive.

One of the first attempts to apply such a tracer technique was a study by Reaven et al. (1965). The investigators determined plasma triglyceride kinetics in normotriglyceridemic and hypertriglyceridemic subjects after an overnight fast using a bolus injection of radiolabeled glycerol, and measured tracer disappearance for eight hours after the injection. VLDL was isolated by ultracentrifugation and triglycerides were subsequently isolated using thin layer chromatography. Using a two-compartmental model for data analysis, the hypertriglyceridemic subjects had markedly higher triglyceride production rates and markedly lower fractional catabolic rates compared with the normotriglyceridemic subjects. Subsequently, numerous investigators published studies using a similar technique, in some instances using a fatty acid tracer instead of a glycerol tracer to label VLDL (Quarfordt et al. 1970).

Perhaps the most detailed investigation of tracer methodology for VLDL kinetics was conducted by Patterson et al. (2002), who administered a bolus of $[^2H_5]$ glycerol (16 subjects) or $[^{13}C]$ palmitate (7 subjects) to normotriglyceridemic subjects and applied both monoexponential and compartmental analysis to the data. An additional five subjects received a constant infusion of $[^{13}C]$ palmitate to determine turnover from the rise-to-plateau of VLDL triglyceride enrichment, as described by Parks et al. (1999). Laboratory analyses were performed using gas chromatography/mass spectrometry (GC/MS). Fractional turnover was slower with the fatty acid tracer than with glycerol. When kinetics of an endogenous substance are determined by administering a labeled precursor, calculations are based on the disappearance of the labeled product. If there is ongoing production of that product during the time that disappearance is being measured, the slope of disappearance will be less steep and an error will be introduced. In the case of VLDL, the precursor (glycerol or a fatty acid) enters the intrahepatic VLDL triglyceride pool and resides there for a finite period of time before secretion into the circulation. Previous studies have shown that the systemic clearance of glycerol from plasma is 3 to 4-fold higher than that of FFA (Coppack et al. 1999). If the intrahepatic clearance of glycerol is similarly greater than that of fatty acids, then intrahepatic labeled glycerol disappears more rapidly than intrahepatic labeled palmitate, making it unavailable for further VLDL triglyceride synthesis. This may explain why a fatty acid tracer provides lower estimates of VLDL turnover than a glycerol tracer.

Patterson et al. (2002) also found that compartmental modeling produced an estimate of fractional VLDL turnover that was nearly double the value obtained with monoexponential analysis. The discrepancy was even greater when compared with previous reports using $[^3H]$ glycerol, whether or not compartmental analysis was used. This could indicate greater tracer recycling with $[^3H]$ glycerol compared to $[^2H_5]$ glycerol, or could simply be related to the fact that different subjects were studied and fractional turnover varies among subjects. Another possibility, however, relates to isotope effects, which are generally more of a problem with hydrogen labeled tracers than with carbon labeled tracers. The potential for isotope effects can be greater for tritium than for deuterium (Northrop 1981). In general, an isotope effect results in a slowing of enzyme-mediated reactions, and thus would produce slower flux rates, lower clearance and lower fractional turnover.

Whether glycerol or a fatty acid tracer is used, high quality laboratory analyses are important. Older methods for VLDL kinetics analysed tracer and tracee in separate procedures (Reaven et al. 1965; Quarfordt et al. 1970). This adds to analytical imprecision and can be a limiting factor. When HPLC (Miles et al. 1987; Judd et al. 1998) or GC/MS (Guo et al. 1997; Gilker et al. 1992) are used, the measurement of tracer and tracee are linked, minimising imprecision. This is particularly important when conducting extended sampling, as is needed for compartmental analysis. An example of VLDL disappearance curves (in this case using $[^2H_5]$ glycerol as a precursor) is shown in Figure 9.5. As can be seen, $[^2H_5]$ enrichment in VLDL triglyceride peaked later in individuals with type 2 diabetes than in control subjects (Isley et al. 2006). The explanation for this is not clear, but it could represent slower fractional turnover of either intrahepatic VLDL triglyceride or its precursor fatty acid pool.

A limitation in many studies of lipoprotein kinetics has been the use of a precursor to label a product of interest, as discussed above. There have been attempts to develop techniques

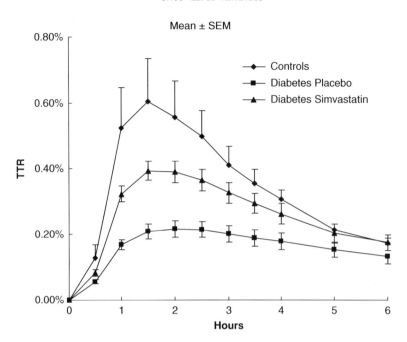

Figure 9.5 Isotopic enrichment curves in normal subjects (diamonds) and in type 2 diabetic subjects before (triangles) and after (squares) 12 weeks of therapy with high dose (80 mg) simvastatin. TTR = tracer:tracee ratio. Reproduced from Isley WL, Miles JM, Patterson BW, Harris WS (2006) The effect of high-dose simvastatin on triglyceride-rich lipoprotein metabolism in patients with type 2 diabetes mellitus. *J Lipid Res* **47**: 193–200. Courtesy of The American Society for Biochemistry and Molecular Biology.

for labeling VLDL for subsequent intravenous administration. Two potential approaches have been used. A radiolabeled glycerol or fatty acid can be administered, and VLDL can be harvested from the plasma 1–2 hours later for subsequent use. Wolfe et al. (1985) used this technique to obtain labeled VLDL from donor dogs for subsequent infusion into other animals in a study of VLDL kinetics in sepsis. Sidossis et al. (2004) gave oral doses of [U-^{13}C] glycerol to normal volunteers and harvested labeled VLDL by plasmapheresis. The labeled VLDL was administered using a two-hour constant infusion 2–3 days later. The infusion was 'primed' with a bolus dose equal to three times the hourly infusion rate. Fractional turnover rates were 1.9–2.2 pools/h after an overnight fast on normal and high fat diets, and somewhat lower (1.3–1.7 pools/h) on a high fat diet and during a glucose infusion. Considering the relatively long half-life of VLDL triglyceride in plasma, the adequacy of the isotopic steady state achieved in this study is not entirely clear, since samples were limited to a 20 minute interval 100–120 minutes after the start of the infusion. However, this report represents a major advance in the development of a novel technique for the measurement of VLDL kinetics in humans.

Early investigators harvested VLDL from study subjects and prepared a radioiodinated VLDL ex vivo, followed by filter sterilisation prior to autologous use (Sigurdsson et al. 1975). Studies such as this suggest that ex vivo labeling of lipoproteins might be feasible, with the same caveats about sterility. However, use of radioiodinated tracers has fallen from favour because of the radiation exposure involved, in addition to concerns that iodination alters the metabolism of the lipoprotein particle. Recently, Gormsen et al. (2006a) reported a technique for ex vivo preparation of a VLDL tracer using a radiolabeled triglyceride (triolein) for subsequent autologous use. It was necessary to sonicate the material at 37 °C for six hours in order to fully incorporate the radiolabeled triglyceride into VLDL. When tracer thus prepared was infused into the subject, very little spillover of LPL-generated fatty acids was observed. This is consistent with the work of Wolfe et al. (1985), who found <5 % fractional spillover of endogenously labeled VLDL in dogs. The use of an ex vivo labeled VLDL tracer avoids the difficulties presented when a labeled precursor is given and the VLDL disappearance curve is altered by ongoing secretion of labeled VLDL. In addition, the low rates of spillover observed indicate minimal potential for tracer recycling.

Gormsen et al. (2006b) have reported additional VLDL kinetic data in 25 normotriglyceridemic subjects using a modification of this technique. Sampling for five hours and using monoexponential analysis, they found VLDL fractional turnover of ~0.25 pools/h. This is strikingly different than the results of Patterson et al. (2002), who reported fractional turnover rates of 0.64 and 1.06 pools/h using monoexponential and compartmental analysis, respectively, with the $[^2H_5]$ glycerol method. The implications of this are not entirely clear. Individuals with higher fractional turnover would be expected to have lower plasma triglyceride concentrations (Reaven et al. 1965). Comparison of the two studies is difficult, especially considering that Patterson found essentially identical results with monoexponential and compartmental analysis when fractional turnover was <0.4 pools/h. It is possible that tracer recycling, in relative terms, creates a larger error in the measurement when fractional VLDL turnover is high and half life is short, at least when a precursor labeling method is used. Significant enrichment in plasma glycerol one and two hours after the injection of labeled glycerol, as shown by Patterson et al. (2002), would contribute a greater error to apparent monoexponential disappearance of VLDL when VLDL fractional turnover is higher, because of a greater contribution on ongoing synthesis and secretion of labeled VLDL during the first several hours after the injection to VLDL triglyceride enrichment/specific activity. Recycling of ^2H or ^3H through the body-water pool would be an unlikely factor because of the enormous dilution that would be expected to occur with recycling via this pathway. Ex vivo labeling has theoretical advantages over *in vivo* labeling, as discussed above. However, additional studies of the ex vivo method, in which it is directly compared with the $[^2H_5]$ glycerol method, and perhaps (if feasible) extended sampling and compartmental analysis, are warranted. A comparison of the two methods using only monoexponential analysis in individuals with low (say <0.8 mmol/L) plasma total triglyceride concentrations would be particularly informative, since these subjects would be expected to have higher fractional turnover rates. In addition to a need for further validation experiments, any method that involves tracer preparation in the laboratory, including isolation of biosynthetic tracer (Sidossis et al. 2004), obviously requires scrupulous sterile technique and safeguards against contamination.

A limitation of the methods that involve benchtop processing of an autologous VLDL tracer is that the material is reinfused within a relatively short period of time – 2–7 days (Sidossis et al. 2004; Gormsen et al. 2006a, 2006b). If a method that would allow long term storage of a biosynthesised or ex vivo prepared tracer were available, the tracer could be collected under baseline conditions (e.g. before weight loss or before drug therapy), then administered after the intervention. Plasmapheresis and subsequent cryopreservation of tracer has been applied successfully to low density lipoproteins (Rumsey et al. 1992, 1994) and could potentially be used to administer VLDL tracer several months after harvesting.

Practical considerations

The study of lipoprotein triglyceride fatty acid kinetics has been challenging because of the unavailability, until recently, of primary pool tracers. When chylomicron or VLDL triglycerides are labeled with a precursor (e.g. oral ingestion of a labeled triglyceride or fatty acid in the case of chylomicrons; oral or intravenous administration of labeled glycerol in the case of VLDL), the rate of tracer appearance into the primary pool is not known. Measurement of kinetics under non-steady state conditions is problematic because there is often ongoing tracer appearance at an unknown rate and therefore simultaneous tracer disappearance at an unknown rate. This problem can be circumvented with the direct administration of labeled chylomicrons (or a surrogate thereof, such as a lipid emulsion) or labeled VLDL. The relatively recent availability of such tracers should improve the reliability of measurements made under steady state conditions and should also make it possible to attempt non-steady state measurements. Like FFA, chylomicron tracers do not require a priming dose, and a short tracer equilibration time is sufficient. VLDL triglyceride tracers more closely resemble glucose with respect to their longer half life and, in the case of continuous infusion experiments, need for a priming dose.

Conclusion

Methods for the study of lipid kinetics have been in use for ~50 years. Early techniques, however, were relatively crude and imposed interpretive limitations due to nonphysiological conditions, artifacts and analytical imprecision. The availability of robust new techniques has allowed investigators to overcome these limitations and gain new insights into the *in vivo* transport, storage and oxidation of lipid energy. These new techniques include improved methods for tracer isolation and purification as well as sophisticated analytical tools such as mass spectrometry and high performance liquid chromatography. The future should bring continued validation and refinement of these techniques.

Acknowledgements

Supported in part by grants from the USPHS (HL67933) and the Mayo Foundation.

References

Armstrong DT, Steele R, Altszuler N, Dunn A, Bishop JS, DeBodo RC (1961) Regulation of plasma free fatty acid turnover *Am J Physiol* **201**, 9–15

Barrows BR, Timlin MT, Parks EJ (2005) Spillover of dietary fatty acids and use of serum nonesterified fatty acids for the synthesis of VLDL-triacylglycerol under two different feeding regimens *Diabetes* **54**, 2668–2673

Barter PJ, Nestel PJ (1972) Plasma free fatty acid transport during prolonged glucose consumption and its relationship to plasma triglyceride fatty acids in man *J Lipid Res* **13**, 483–490

Basso LV, Havel RJ (1970) Hepatic metabolism of free fatty acids in normal and diabetic dogs *J Clin Invest* **49**, 537–547

Beylot M, Martin C, Beaufrère B, Riou JP, Mornex R (1987) Determination of steady state and nonsteady-state glycerol kinetics in humans using deuterium-labeled glycerol *J Lipid Res* **28**, 414–422

Bjorntorp P, Bergman H, Varnauskas E, Lindholm B (1969) Lipid mobilization in relation to body composition in man *Metabolism* **18**, 840–851

Blaner WS, Obunike JC, Kurlandsky SB, al-Haideri M, Piantedosi R, Deckelbaum RJ, Goldberg IJ (1994) Lipoprotein lipase hydrolysis of retinyl ester Possible implications for retinoid uptake by cells *J Biol Chem* **269**, 16, 559–16, 565

Boden G (1997) Role of fatty acids in the pathogenesis of insulin resistance and NIDDM *Diabetes* **46**, 3–10

Boden G, Jadali F, White J, Liang Y, Mozzoli M, Chen X, Coleman E, Smith C (1991) Effects of fat on insulin stimulated carbohydrate metabolism in normal men *J Clin Invest*, 960–966

Brunzell JD, Hazzard WR, Porte D, Jr, Bierman EL (1973) Evidence for a common, saturable, triglyceride removal mechanism for Chylomicrons and very low density lipoproteins in man *J Clin Invest* **52**, 1578–1585

Brunzell J, Porte DJ, Bierman E (1979) Abnormal lipoprotein-lipase-mediated plasma triglyceride removal in untreated diabetes mellitus associated with hypertriglyceridemia *Metabolism* **28**, 901–907

Cohen J (1989) Chylomicron triglyceride clearance, comparison of three assessment methods *Am J Clin Nutr* **49**, 306–313

Coppack SW, Persson M, Judd RL, Miles JM (1999) Glycerol and nonesterified fatty acid metabolism in human muscle and adipose tissue in vivo *Am J Physiol* **276**, E233–E240

Dagenais GR, Tancredi RG, Zierler KL (1976) Free fatty acid oxidation by forearm muscle at rest, and evidence for an intramuscular lipid pool in the human forearm *J Clin Invest* **58**, 421–431

Dietschy JM, Turley SD, Spady DK (1993) Role of liver in the maintenance of cholesterol and low density lipoprotein homeostasis in different animal species, including humans *J Lipid Res* **34**, 1637–1659

Dole VP (1956) A relation between non-esterified fatty acids in plasma and the metabolism of glucose *J Clin Invest* **35**, 150–154

Duncombe WG, Rising TJ (1973) Quantitative extraction and determination of nonesterified fatty acids in plasma *J Lipid Res* **14**, 258–261

Eckel RH (1989) Lipoprotein lipase, a multifunctional enzyme relevant to common metabolic diseases *N Engl J Med* **320**, 1060–1068

Evans K, Burdge GC, Wootton SA, Clark ML, Frayn KN (2002) Regulation of dietary fatty acid entrapment in subcutaneous adipose tissue and skeletal muscle *Diabetes* **51**, 2684–2690

Finegood DT, Bergman RN, Vranic M (1987) Estimation of endogenous glucose production during hyperinsulinaemic euglycaemic glucose clamps, comparison of unlabelled and labelled exogenous glucose infusates *Diabetes* **36**, 914–924

Fredrickson DS, Gordon RS (1958) The metabolism of albumin-bound C^{14-} labelled unesterified fatty acids in normal human subjects *J Clin Invest* **37**, 1504–1515

Gilker CD, Resola GR, Matthews DE (1992) A mass spectrometric method for measuring glycerol levels and enrichments in plasma using ^{13}C and ^{2}H stable isotopic tracers *Anal Biochem* **205**, 172–178

Gold M, Spitzer JJ (1964) Metabolism of free fatty acids by myocardium and kidney *Am J Physiol* **206**, 153–158

Goodpaster BH, Wolfe RR, Kelley DE (2002) Effects of obesity on substrate utilization during exercise *Obes Res* **10**, 575–584

Gormsen LC, Jensen MD, Nielsen S (2006a) Measuring VLDL-triglyceride turnover in humans using ex vivo-prepared VLDL tracer *J Lipid Res* **47**, 99–106

Gormsen LC, Jensen MD, Schmitz O, Moller N, Christiansen JS, Nielsen S (2006b) Energy expenditure, insulin, and VLDL triglyceride production in humans *J Lipid Res*

Guo Z, Nielsen S, Burguera B, Jensen MD (1997) Free fatty acid turnover measured using ultralow doses of [U-13C]palmitate *J Lipid Res* **38**, 1888–1895

Hagenfeldt L (1975) Turnover of individual free fatty acids in man *Federation Proc* **34**, 2246–2249

Hagenfeldt L, Wahren J (1968) Human forearm muscle metabolism during exercise II Uptake, release and oxidation of individual FFA and glycerol *Scand J Clin Lab Invest* **21**, 263–276

Harris P, Chlouverakis C, Gloster J, Jones JH (1962) Arterio-venous differences in the composition of plasma free fatty acids in various regions of the body *Clin Sci* **22**, 113–118

Havel RJ, Kane JP, Balasse EO, Segel N, Basso LV (1970) Splanchnic metabolism of free fatty acids and production of triglycerides of very low density lipoproteins in normotriglyceridemic and hypertriglyceridemic humans *JClinInvest* **49**, 2017–2035

Hazzard WR, Bierman EL (1976) Delayed clearance of chylomicron remnants following vitamin-A-containing oral fat loads in broad-beta disease (type III hyperlipoproteinemia) *Metabolism* **25**, 777–801

Hultin M, Carneheim C, Rosenqvist K, Olivecrona T (1995) Intravenous lipid emulsions, removal mechanisms as compared to chylomicrons *J Lipid Res* **36**, 2174–2184

Iriyama K, Nishiwaki H, Terashima H, Tonouchi H, Miki C, Suzuki H, Carpentier Y (1988) Apolipoprotein C-II modifications associated with an infusion of artificial lipid particles *JPEN* **12**, 60–62

Isley WL, Miles JM, Patterson BW, Harris WS (2006) The effect of high-dose simvastatin on triglyceride-rich lipoprotein metabolism in patients with type 2 diabetes mellitus *J Lipid Res* **47**, 193–200

Jensen MD, Heiling VJ (1991) Heated hand vein blood is satisfactory for measurements during free fatty acid kinetic studies *Metabolism* **40**, 406–409

Jensen MD, Heiling VJ, Miles JM (1990) Measurement of non-steady-state free fatty acid turnover *Am J Physiol* **258**, E103–E108

Jensen MD, Rogers PJ, Ellman MG, Miles JM (1988) Choice of infusion-sampling mode for tracer studies of free fatty acid metabolism *Am J Physiol* **254**, E562–E565

Jensen MD, Sarr MG, Dumesic DA, Southorn PA, Levine JA (2003) Regional uptake of meal fatty acids in humans *Am J Physiol Endocrinol Metab* **285**, E1282–1288

Judd RL, Nelson R, Klein S, Jensen MD, Miles JM (1998) Measurement of plasma glycerol specific activity by high performance liquid chromatography to determine glycerol flux *J Lipid Res* **39**, 1106–1110

Karpe F, Humphreys S, Samra J, Summers L, Frayn K (1997) Clearance of lipoprotein remnant particles in adipose tissue and muscle in humans *J Lipid Res* **38**, 2335–2343

Klein S, Young VR, Blackburn GL, Bistrian BR, Wolfe RR (1986) Palmitate and glycerol kinetics during brief starvation in normal weight young adult and elderly subjects *J Clin Invest* **78**, 928–933

Lemieux S, Fontani R, Uffelman KD, Lewis GF, Steiner G (1998) Apolipoprotein B-48 and retinyl palmitate are not equivalent markers of postprandial intestinal lipoproteins *J Lipid Res* **39**, 1964–1971

Lewis G, Uffelman K, Szeto L, Weller B, Steiner G (1995) Interaction between free fatty acids and insulin in the acute control of very low density lipoprotein production in humans *J Clin Invest* **95**, 158–166

Lichtenstein AH, Hachey DL, Millar JS, Jenner JL, Booth L, Ordovas J, Schaefer EJ (1992) Measurement of human apolipoprotein B-48 and B-100 kinetics in triglyceride-rich lipoproteins using [5,5,5-2H3]leucine *J Lipid Res* **33**, 907–914

Lin EC (1977) Glycerol utilization and its regulation in mammals *Annu Rev Biochem* **46**, 765–795

Lutz O, Meraihi Z, Mura J-L, Riess GH, Back AC (1989) Fat emulsion particle size, influence on the clearance rate and the tissue lipolytic activity *Am J Clin Nutr* **50**, 1370–1381

Martin ML, Jensen MD (1991) Effects of body fat distribution on regional lipolysis in obesity *J Clin Invest* **88**, 609–613

Martins IJ, Mortimer BC, Miller J, Redgrave TG (1996) Effects of particle size and number on the plasma clearance of chylomicrons and remnants *J Lipid Res* **37**, 2696–2705

McGarry JD (1992) What if Minkowski had been ageusic? An alternative angle on diabetes *Science*, **258**, 766–770

Miles JM, Glasscock R, Aikens J, Gerich JE, Haymond MW (1983) A microfluorometric method for the determination of free fatty acids in plasma *J Lipid Res* **24**, 96–99

Miles JM, Ellman MG, McClean KL, Jensen MD (1987) Validation of a new method for determination of free fatty acid turnover *Am J Physiol* **252**, E431–E438

Miles JM, Judd RL, Persson M, Coppack SW (1995) Methods for estimating the kinetics of lipid fuels in vivo In *Research Methodologies in Human Diabetes* Mogensen CE, Standl W, Eds New York, Walter de Gruyter, 345–359

Miles JM, Park Y, Harris WS (2001) Lipoprotein lipase and triglyceride-rich lipoprotein metabolism *Nutr Clin Pract* **16**, 273–279

Miles J, Park Y, Walewicz D, Russell-Lopez C, Windsor S, Isley W, Coppack S, Harris W (2004) Systemic and forearm triglyceride metabolism, fate of lipoprotein lipase-generated glycerol and free fatty acids *Diabetes* **53**, 521–527

Miller HI, Gold M, Spitzer JJ (1962) Removal and mobilization of individual free fatty acids in dogs *Am J Physiol* **202**, 370–374

Mittendorfer B, Liem O, Patterson BW, Miles JM, Klein S (2003) What does the measurement of whole-body fatty acid rate of appearance in plasma by using a fatty acid tracer really mean? *Diabetes* **52**, 1641–1648

Most AS, Brachfeld N, Gorlin R, Wahren J (1969) Free fatty acid metabolism of the human heart at rest *J Clin Invest* **48**, 1177–1188

Nakandakare E, Lottenberg S, Oliveira H, Bertolami M, Vasconcelos K, Sperotto G, Quintao E (1994) Simultaneous measurements of chylomicron lipolysis and remnant removal using a doubly labeled artificial lipid emulsion, studies in normolipidemic and hyperlipidemic subjects *J Lipid Res* **35**, 143–152

Nelson RH, Prasad A, Lerman A, Miles J (2007) Myocardial uptake of circulating triglycerides in nondiabetic patients with heart disease. *Diabetes* **56**, 527

Nelson RH, Edgerton DS, Basu R, Roesner JC, Cherrington AD, Miles JM (in press) Triglyceride uptake and lipoprotein lipase-generated fatty acid spillover in the splanchnic bed of dogs *Diabetes*

Nestel P, Denborough M, O'Dea J (1962) Disposal of human chylomicrons administered intravenously in ischaemic heart disease and essential hyperlipemia *Circ Res* **10**, 786–791

Nielsen S, Guo Z, Albu JB, Klein S, O'Brien PC, Jensen MD (2003) Energy expenditure, sex, and endogenous fuel availability in humans *J Clin Invest* **111**, 981–988

Nielsen S, Guo Z, Johnson CM, Hensrud DD, Jensen MD (2004) Splanchnic lipolysis in human obesity *J Clin Invest* **113**, 1582–1588

Nikkila E, Kekki M (1973) Plasma triglyceride transport kinetics in diabetes mellitus *Metabolism* **22**, 1–22

Northrop DB (1981) The expression of isotope effects on enzyme-catalyzed reactions *Annu Rev Biochem* **50**, 103–131

Nurjhan N, Campbell PJ, Kennedy FP, Miles JM, Gerich JE (1986) Insulin dose-response characteristics for suppression of glycerol release and conversion to glucose in humans *Diabetes* **35**, 1326–1331

Park Y, Damron BD, Miles JM, Harris WS (2001) Measurement of human chylomicron triglyceride clearance with a labeled commercial lipid emulsion *Lipids* **36**, 115–120

Park Y, Grellner WJ, Harris WS, Miles JM (2000) A new method for the study of chylomicron kinetics in vivo *Am J Physiol* **279**, E1258–E1263

Parks EJ, Krauss RM, Christiansen MP, Neese RA, Hellerstein MK (1999) Effects of a low-fat, high-carbohydrate diet on VLDL-triglyceride assembly, production, and clearance *J Clin Invest* **104**, 1087–1096

Patterson BW, Mittendorfer B, Elias N, Satyanarayana R, Klein S (2002) Use of stable isotopically labeled tracers to measure very low density lipoprotein-triglyceride turnover *J Lipid Res* **43**, 223–233

Quarfordt SH, Frank A, Shames DM, Berman M, Steinberg D (1970) Very low density lipoprotein triglyceride transport in type IV hyperlipoproteinemia and the effects of carbohydrate-rich diets *J Clin Invest* **49**, 2281–2297

Reaven G, Hill D, Gross R, Farquhar J (1965) Kinetics of triglyceride turnover of very-low-density lipoproteins of human plasma *J Clin Invest* **44**, 1826–1833

Redgrave TG (2004) Chylomicron metabolism *Biochem Soc Trans* **32**, 79–82

Redgrave T, Ly H, Quintao E, Ramberg C, Boston R (1993) Clearance from plasma of triacylglycerol and cholesteryl ester after intravenous injection of chylomicron-like lipid emulsions in rats and man *Biochem J* **290**, 843–847

Redgrave TG, Maranhao RC (1985) Metabolism of protein-free lipid emulsion models of chylomicrons in rats *Biochim Biophys Acta* **835**, 104–112

Romanski SA, Nelson RM, Jensen MD (2000) Meal fatty acid uptake in human adipose tissue, technical and experimental design issues *Am J Physiol* **279**, E447–454

Rossner S (1974) Studies on an intravenous fat tolerance test Methodological, experimental and clinical experiences with Intralipid *Acta Med Scand* **564**, 1–24

Roust LR, Jensen MD (1993) Postprandial free fatty acid kinetics are abnormal in upper body obesity *Diabetes* **42**, 1567–1573

Rumsey SC, Galeano NF, Arad Y, Deckelbaum RJ (1992) Cryopreservation with sucrose maintains normal physical and biological properties of human plasma low density lipoproteins *J Lipid Res* **33**, 1551–1561

Rumsey SC, Stucchi AF, Nicolosi RJ, Ginsberg HN, Ramakrishnan R, Deckelbaum RJ (1994) Human plasma LDL cryopreserved with sucrose maintains in vivo kinetics indistinguishable from freshly isolated human LDL in cynomolgus monkeys *J Lipid Res* **35**, 1592–1598

Seidner DL, Mascioli EA, Istfan NW, Porter KA, Selleck K, Blackburn GL, Bistrian BR (1989) Effects of long-chain triglyceride emulsions on reticuloendothelial system function in humans *JPEN* **13**, 614–619

Sidossis LS, Coggan AR, Gastaldelli A, Wolfe RR (1995) A new correction factor for use in tracer estimations of plasma fatty acid oxidation *Am J Physiol* **269**, E649–656

Sidossis LS, Magkos F, Mittendorfer B, Wolfe RR (2004) Stable isotope tracer dilution for quantifying very low-density lipoprotein-triacylglycerol kinetics in man *Clin Nutr* **23**, 457–466

Sigurdsson G, Nicoll A, Lewis B (1975) Conversion of very low density lipoprotein to low density lipoprotein A metabolic study of apolipoprotein B kinetics in human subjects *J Clin Invest* **56**, 1481–1490

Sparks JD, Sparks CE (1994) Insulin regulation of triacylglycerol-rich lipoprotein synthesis and secretion *Biochim Biophys Acta* **1215**, 9–32

Spector AA (1975) Fatty acid binding to plasma albumin *JLipid Res* **16**, 165–179

Steinberg HO, Tarshoby M, Monestel R, Hook G, Cronin J, Johnson A, Bayazeed B, Baron AD (1997) Elevated circulating free fatty acid levels impair endothelium-dependent vasodilation *J Clin Invest* **100**, 1230–1239

Stojiljkovic MP, Zhang D, Lopes HF, Lee CG, Goodfriend TL, Egan BM (2001) Hemodynamic effects of lipids in humans *Am J Physiol* **280**, R1674–R1679

Vaughan M (1962) The production and release of glycerol by adipose tissue incubated in vitro *J Biol Chem* **237**, 3354–3358

Wahren J, Hagenfeldt L, Felig P (1975) Splanchnic and leg exchange of glucose, amino acids, and free fatty acids during exercise in diabetes mellitus *J Clin Invest* **55**, 1303–1314

Winkler B, Steele R, Altszuler N (1969) Effects of growth hormone administration on free fatty acid and glycerol turnover in the normal dog *Endocrinology* **85**, 25–30

Wisneski JA, Gertz EW, Neese RA, Mayr M (1987) Myocardial metabolism of free fatty acids Studies with ^{14}C- labelled substrates in humans *J Clin Invest* **79**, 359–366

Wolfe RR, Evans JE, Mullany CJ, Burke JF (1980) Measurement of plasma free fatty acid turnover and oxidation using [1–^{13}C]palmitic acid *Biomed Mass Spectrom* **7**, 168–171

Wolfe RR, Shaw JHF, Durkot MJ (1985) Effects of sepsis on VLDL kinetics, responses in basal state and during glucose infusion *Am J Physiol* **248**, E732–E740

10

Protein and Amino Acid Kinetics

Stephen F Previs, Danielle A Gilge and **Nadia Rachdaoui**

Introduction

Proteins serve numerous functions by acting as structural supports, receptors, signaling molecules and enzymes. In addition, proteins facilitate nutrient transport and maintain immunological responses. Although the abundance of certain proteins (e.g. circulating albumin) may not change appreciably over short intervals, proteins are continuously remodeled. For example, in spite of the fact that healthy individuals may consume ~1 g of protein per kg bodyweight per day, ~3–4 times that amount may be degraded and synthesised per day (Figure 10.1) (Waterlow 1995).

In this chapter we discuss the use of isotope tracer methods for quantifying protein dynamics; attention is given to new developments in the field of proteomics. Since the maintenance of protein (nitrogen) homeostasis depends on the balance of amino acid flux rates, e.g. dietary intake and oxidative disposal, we consider methods for measuring amino acid and urea kinetics. A simple scenario may highlight the importance of using isotopes to facilitate research in these areas. For example, clinicians are typically faced with the challenge of affecting the abundance of a protein(s), e.g. circulating albumin provides a measure of protein nutritional status and is a good predictor of a patient's recovery from disease (D'Erasmo et al. 1997; Jones et al. 1997; Gariballa et al. 1998). However, since the fractional turnover of albumin is relatively slow (~3–5 % of the pool is newly made per day), several weeks of therapeutic intervention may be required to affect the concentration of plasma albumin. Jeejeebhoy et al. (1973) recognised that the concentration of albumin is a delayed-onset marker of nutritional status and tested whether the synthesis of albumin is an acute marker of protein intake. They demonstrated that albumin synthesis is decreased within ~24 hours of inadequate nitrogen intake and that diet-induced impairments in albumin synthesis are readily corrected by restoring nitrogen intake. Similar observations were reported by others, who found that albumin synthesis is stimulated during the fasted→fed transition (De Feo et al. 1992). Thus, the ability to measure albumin synthesis may allow a clinician to immediately evaluate the efficacy of an intervention and may suggest whether a patient is likely to benefit from a particular treatment.

Clinical Diabetes Research: Methods and Techniques   Edited by Michael Roden
© 2007 John Wiley & Sons, Ltd   ISBN 978-0-470-01728-9

Overview of protein and amino acid dynamics.

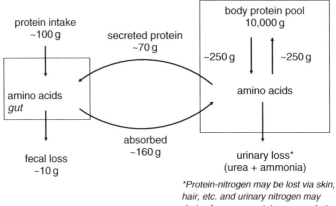

Figure 10.1 Overview of Whole-Body Protein Dynamics A generalised scheme of protein and amino acid metabolism is considered.

A number of innovative methods have been developed to address an array of questions regarding protein and amino acid kinetics *in vivo* (Wolfe & Chinkes 2004). Our goal is to discuss the fundamental underpinnings regarding the use of isotopes to quantify flux rates. In addition, we briefly consider the advances made by investigators who have combined the tools used in molecular biology with tracer methods to examine the mechanisms that control protein dynamics. An apology is extended to those researchers whose work is not cited here; references were selected to explain the development and the application of methods. Finally, it is beyond the scope of our discussion to elaborate on the interpretation(s) of data regarding physiological homeostasis; we consider here general points of knowledge regarding protein and amino acid metabolism in diabetes.

Measuring amino acid turnover

Isotope tracers are typically used to measure the turnover rate of a compound (Patterson 1997), defined here as the quantity of that compound moving through its pool per unit time. Assuming that tracers and tracees are metabolised in an equivalent fashion and that tracer administration does not modify the kinetics under investigation, investigators often consider three factors when designing tracer studies: 1) the use radioactive or stable isotopes; 2) the approach that is used to measure the kinetics; and 3) the positional location of the isotope in the tracer. We review these topics, using examples to facilitate the discussion. Finally, it should be noted that the mode of tracer infusion and sampling can affect the results (Abumrad et al. 1981); however, since studies in humans are generally limited to venous infusion and 'arterial' sampling we do not provide an elaborate discussion of this matter, we refer the reader to several excellent resources (Layman & Wolfe 1987; Katz 1992; Sacca et al. 1992).

Radioactive vs stable isotopes

The study of amino acid kinetics is typically concerned with measuring the flow of carbon and/or nitrogen. The choice of whether to use radioactive or stable isotopes typically depends on an investigator's experience, the research question(s) being asked and the facilities that are available. We consider here three factors that have likely contributed to the increased use of stable isotopes over radioactive isotopes.

First, concerns for safety and improvements in nuclear magnetic resonance spectroscopy and mass spectrometry have led to an increased use of stable isotopes. In particular, since gas chromatography methods allow for rapid high-resolution separations of analytes it is possible to measure the concentration and/or the rates of appearance of numerous amino acids in a single assay. In addition, commonly available quadrupole mass spectrometers provide relatively high precision measurements of isotope labeling. For example, investigators demonstrated the ability to measure the ^{15}N-labeling of 18 amino acids in a single run, with an average coefficient of variation of $\sim 0.35\%$ of the background labeling (Patterson et al. 1993). In another report, investigators analysed a number of amino acids via gas chromatography-mass spectrometry (GC-MS) and were able to detect $\sim 0.08\%$ atom excess labeling; neither the ionisation mode nor the type of derivative affected the measurements (Matthews et al. 1979). It is reasonable to expect that future advances in the design of GC-MS hardware will continue to increase the limits of detection and improve the reproducibility of measurements. We recently developed a new method for integrating GC-MS data (Katanik et al. 2003), suggesting that improvements in data processing software will also facilitate studies. Another important area where advances in instrument development have facilitated investigations centres on the use of gas chromatography-isotope ratio mass spectrometers (Preston & McMillan 1988; Brand 1996; Corso & Brenna 1997; Meier-Augenstein 1999). For example, the measurement of very low levels of isotopic enrichment typically requires that the compound of interest be isolated, degraded to a simple molecule (e.g. [^{13}C]leucine $\rightarrow$ $^{13}CO_2$) and then analysed using an isotope ratio mass spectrometer. New instruments couple gas chromatography on-line with isotope ratio mass spectrometry and thereby permit high-throughput measurements of very low levels of isotope labeling. In addition, modern instruments can readily convert parent analytes (e.g. labeled amino acids) to various simple products (e.g. H_2, CO_2 or N_2 gas), allowing investigators to use amino acid tracers of different isotopic composition (Hofmann et al. 2003; Kulik et al. 2003).

A second factor that likely contributes to the preferential use of stable isotopes over radioactive isotopes is related to practical matters regarding certain radioactive tracers. For example, although investigators have used radiolabeled carbon tracers (e.g. [^{14}C]leucine), radioactive nitrogen (^{13}N) has a half-life of ~ 10 min (Baumgartner et al. 1981). Thus, when studying processes involving nitrogen transfer, one is limited to centres with the requisite equipment for preparation and measurement of ^{13}N.

Third, suppose that an investigator was interested in determining the rate of appearance of an amino acid and determining its concentration in plasma, e.g. glutamate. The application of radioactive isotopes (e.g. [^{14}C]glutamate) requires that samples are split for two different assays, where one portion is used to measure the radioactivity and the other is used to measure the concentration; one then calculates the rate of appearance from the specific activity (i.e. dpm per μmol). When using stable isotopes and GC-MS the two parameters can be determined using one assay (Darmaun et al. 1985). To simplify our discussion, let the molecular weight of endogenous glutamate equal 147 (represented by the notation M0). To measure the rate of appearance, one infuses [2-^{15}N]glutamate (molecular weight 148, M1) and collects samples at the desired times. A known amount of [^{2}H$_3$]glutamate (molecular weight 150, M3) is added to a known volume of plasma and the sample is processed for GC-MS analysis. Although the three isotopes of glutamate elute at the same time during the chromatographic separation, since each species has a unique molecular weight the mass spectrometer measures the abundance of the individual molecules. The rate of appearance of glutamate is determined from the ratio of (M1) / (M0 + M1) and the total concentration of glutamate from the ratio of (M0 + M1) / M3. The ability to simultaneously measure the kinetics and the concentration of an amino acid using one sample minimises the quantity of blood that must be collected and decreases the analysis time.

   The use of stable isotopes offers a very practical advantage, especially when studying glutamate and glutamine metabolism, a major nitrogen transport system. Darmaun et al. (1985) recognised that during sample preparation a substantial portion of glutamine is converted to glutamate. They developed a clever strategy to circumvent this artifact and avoid an erroneous interpretation of the data. Briefly, they demonstrated that when a known amount of [^{2}H$_5$]glutamine (M5) is added to a sample before preparation, one can correct the glutamate concentration and labeling by measuring the amount of M5 glutamate (i.e. if [^{2}H$_5$]glutamine (M5) is degraded it will appear as [^{2}H$_5$]glutamate (M5)). This method was used to study glutamate and glutamine kinetics in patients with type 1 diabetes under conditions similar to those experienced after a night of poor metabolic control (Darmaun et al. 1991). In support of the hypothesis that insulin deficiency leads to increased proteolysis and muscle wasting, Darmaun et al. observed increased rates of leucine appearance and oxidation; however, glutamate and glutamine flux were apparently unaltered.

Approaches for measuring kinetics

The turnover of a compound can be determined by administering stable isotope tracers via a bolus injection, a constant infusion or a primed-infusion (Matthews et al. 1980; Cobelli et al. 1991; Wolfe & Chinkes 2004). An abbreviated discussion of each approach is presented. Unless noted, we assume that the system is in a metabolic steady state, therefore the rate of appearance (Ra) of an amino acid equals its rate of disappearance (Rd); readers are referred to additional resources that discuss modeling other conditions (Shipley & Clark 1972; Cobelli et al. 2000).

   When a tracer is administered via a bolus injection, the Rd is calculated from the elimination of the isotope using the equation:

$$labeling_{time\ z} = labeling_{time\ 0} \times e^{-kt} \tag{10.1}$$

where $labeling_{time\ 0}$ is the labeling of the tracee pool at zero time (the initial dilution), t is the time at which a sample is collected, $labeling_{time z}$ is the labeling of the tracee pool at the time when the sample is collected and k equals the elimination constant (i.e. the fraction of the pool leaving per unit time). The Rd (the mass of the pool leaving per unit time) is determined by solving the equation for k, and then multiplying k by the pool size (which can be determined from the initial dilution of the tracer). This approach (and equation) requires that the tracer rapidly enters and evenly distributes in a well-mixed pool and that tracer and tracee metabolism follow first-order kinetics. Slow mixing of the tracer and/or the presence of more than one pool will result in multi-exponential rates of elimination. Although the mathematical treatment of such scenarios is somewhat straightforward, the ability to obtain sufficient biological samples to confirm the complex models often presents a challenge.

The constant infusion offers an alternative to the bolus for administering isotope tracers. Using this approach, an isotope is continuously infused to establish a steady state labeling. The Ra is calculated using the equation:

$$labeling_{time\ z} = labeling_{plateau} \times (1 - e^{-kt}) \tag{10.2}$$

where t is the time at which a sample is collected, $labeling_{timez}$ is the labeling of the tracee pool at the time when the sample is collected, $labeling_{plateau}$ is the labeling of the tracee pool at plateau (steady state) and k equals the elimination constant (i.e. the fraction of the pool leaving per unit time). Analogous to the bolus method, this equation assumes a single tracee pool.

Finally, the primed-infusion is a hybrid technique that involves administering a bolus of an isotope, followed immediately with a constant infusion. The quantity of the priming dose is estimated from the pool size and the desired steady state isotope labeling, and the constant infusion rate is that rate that is required to maintain the initial labeling. The Ra is calculated from the steady state labeling using the equation:

$$infusion\ rate\ of\ the\ tracer \times [(labeling_{infusate}/labeling_{sample}) - 1] \tag{10.3}$$

where $labeling_{infusate}$ is the isotopic enrichment of the infused tracer and $labeling_{sample}$ is the isotopic enrichment of the tracee pool. The units of Ra are the same as those used to define the infusion rate of the tracer. Although the rationale behind using the primed-infusion is that less time is required to reach an isotopic steady state, one must consider what happens if the priming bolus does not reach the anticipated steady state labeling. For example, if the priming bolus results in an enrichment that is higher than that expected from the constant infusion then, in theory, ~4 half-lives will be required to clear excess tracer and arrive at the approximate enrichment of the constant infusion. Since most amino acids are generally present in low abundance and display a rapid turnover one would expect that errors in the priming bolus would have a modest impact on the data, however, this matter becomes somewhat important when studying urea metabolism (as discussed later).

Influence of tracer labeling

Investigators should consider the positional location of an isotope within a given tracer since isotope exchange and/or recycling will affect determinations of tracee turnover. For example, suppose that an investigator wanted to measure the rate of appearance of leucine in an overnight fasted subject: is there a difference between using [1-^{13}C]leucine or [2-^{15}N]leucine? Assuming that both isotopes are administered under identical conditions, the principle of calculating the rate of appearance is the same regardless of the tracer, i.e. one administers the isotope and then determines its rate of elimination and/or dilution. However, although leucine is an essential amino acid and the net appearance of leucine is only via protein breakdown, leucine labeling is affected by two processes; protein breakdown and transamination (leucine↔ketoisocaproate). Since transamination removes ^{15}N but not ^{13}C, the rate of protein breakdown will be overestimated when [2-^{15}N]leucine is used as compared to when [1-^{13}C]leucine is used. Nair et al. (1983, 1995) capitalised on this aspect of leucine tracer metabolism during studies of leucine kinetics in diabetes. They observed an elevated leucine nitrogen flux (transamination) in poorly controlled diabetics and noted that treatment with insulin reduces leucine nitrogen flux (transamination) in patients with either type 1 or type 2 diabetes.

Using rates of amino acid flux to determine whole-body protein turnover

As noted earlier in this section, investigators are faced with several choices regarding measurements of amino acid flux and protein turnover. One of the more widely applied methods for quantifying amino acid and protein turnover centres on the use of a primed-infusion of $[1\text{-}^{13}\text{C}]$leucine (Figure 10.2). The flux of an amino acid (e.g. leucine) is described using the equation:

$$Q = S + C = B + I \qquad (10.4)$$

where Q is the rate of amino acid turnover in plasma (or the flux), S is the rate of incorporation of the amino acid into protein, C is the rate of amino acid oxidation (or catabolism), B is the rate of amino acid release from protein breakdown and I is the rate of exogenous intake of an amino acid (typically from the diet). In cases where subjects are studied in postabsorptive state, $I = 0$ and $Q = B$. Q and C are experimentally determined from the dilution of the infused tracer (e.g. $[1\text{-}^{13}\text{C}]$leucine) and the rate of production of expired $^{13}\text{CO}_2$ respectively; S is then calculated by solving the equation, i.e. $S = Q - C$.

The approach outlined above provides a measure of amino acid flux and whole-body protein turnover. In their seminal study, Matthews et al. (1980) thoroughly discuss the determination of these parameters during the infusion of $[1\text{-}^{13}\text{C}]$leucine; their report also considers the extent to which analytical error(s) could impact the data. Although subsequent studies suggested that a multicompartmental model yields a more accurate determination

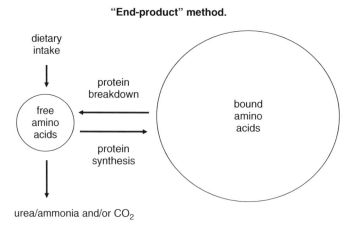

"End-product" method.

dietary intake

protein breakdown

free amino acids

bound amino acids

protein synthesis

urea/ammonia and/or CO_2

Figure 10.2 'Black Box' Model of Protein and Amino Acid Metabolism Studies often consider a two-pool model of protein and amino acid dynamics. Assuming a constant mass of free amino acids, different tracer methods (e.g. $[1\text{-}^{13}\text{C}]$leucine or $[^{15}\text{N}]$glycine) can be used to quantify the various flux rates in fasted or fed subjects.

of leucine kinetics (Cobelli et al. 1991), investigators typically rely on simpler 'primary' (Matthews et al. 1980) or 'reciprocal' (Horber et al. 1989; Matthews et al. 1982) models. It is important to note that determination of $^{13}CO_2$ production is complicated by the fact that $^{13}CO_2$ molecules will exchange with unlabeled CO_2 and be deposited in the body; Matthews and others have addressed this matter (Downey et al. 1986; Toth et al. 2001).

Numerous tracer studies of leucine flux and whole-body protein turnover have been performed in diabetic subjects. The data suggest a tendency for increased protein breakdown in poorly controlled type 1 diabetics, and that intensive insulin therapy normalises leucine flux in most cases (Luzi et al. 1990; Lariviere et al. 1992). It appears that insulin action on whole-body protein turnover plays a greater role in modulating splanchnic vs leg muscle protein turnover *in vivo* (Nair et al. 1995). In contrast to studies done in type 1 diabetics, there appears to be some discrepancy regarding leucine flux and protein turnover in those with type 2 diabetes and related conditions. For example, studies performed in subjects with type 2 diabetes report no alterations in leucine flux during basal or insulin-stimulated conditions in patients with impaired regulation of glucose metabolism (Luzi et al. 1993). However, studies done in the offspring of patients with type 2 diabetes found evidence of impaired insulin-mediated suppression of leucine appearance, comparable to that observed for the defect in insulin-stimulated glucose metabolism (Lattuada et al. 2004). Investigators have also demonstrated impaired insulin-mediated activation of whole-body protein synthesis in obese insulin-resistant women (Chevalier et al. 2005). Clearly, the discrepancies between the data reported in various states of insulin resistance may reflect different patient populations and/or variable degrees of disease.

Measuring protein turnover

We review three general approaches that have been used to study protein turnover *in vivo*. Attention is directed toward a discussion of the strengths and the assumptions of specific methods in each of the sections that are outlined.

Coupling nitrogen balance and isotope tracers

Measurements of total nitrogen intake and output can be used to calculate protein nutritional status (Leverton & Gram 1949; Hegsted 1978). This approach is based on principles of chemical mass-balance, and although practical matters concerning collecting total nitrogen waste make this method difficult to implement, measurements of nitrogen balance generally permit a reliable determination of protein homeostasis. Use of the method requires special consideration since urinary nitrogen may occur in the forms of urea and ammonia (derived from amino acid and protein catabolism) and uric acid and creatinine (derived from non-protein sources), and since nitrogen may be lost in faeces, sweat and other products (Figure 10.1). To facilitate studies, investigators have proposed correction factors that account for the relationship between total urinary nitrogen and urinary urea nitrogen (Mackenzie et al. 1985) and for miscellaneous non-urinary nitrogen losses (Calloway et al. 1971).

While measurements of whole-body nitrogen balance can be used to address questions related to the wasting of lean mass and to determine the efficiency of nitrogen retention, nitrogen balance does not yield a measure of the turnover of specific proteins or the remodeling rate(s) of an individual tissue(s) within the body, i.e. one cannot determine whether changes in nitrogen balance reflect changes in protein synthesis and/or protein breakdown. To quantify endogenous protein turnover, and to examine interactions between dietary intake and stored nitrogen, investigators have proposed the use of 'end-product' methods (Figure 10.2). Briefly, these methods consider two pools of endogenous nitrogen, a pool of bound nitrogen (amino acids in existing proteins) and a pool of free nitrogen (amino acids circulating in plasma). The flux of nitrogen in the free pool is described using Equation 10.4, where we let Q represent nitrogen flux.

Investigators have demonstrated that the metabolism of a ^{15}N-labeled precursor affects the excretion of [15]N (Fern et al. 1985). To quantify nitrogen flux, investigators typically administer [^{15}N]glycine (San Pietro & Rittenberg 1953; Matthews et al. 1981; Stein et al. 1980) and then measure the ^{15}N-labeling of urea and/or ammonia. The rate of nitrogen flux is calculated using the equation:

$$nitrogen\ flux\ in\ the\ free\ pool = dose\ of\ the\ administered\ isotope/labeling\ of\ the$$
$$end\text{-}product \tag{10.5}$$

Rates of protein synthesis (S) and protein breakdown (B) are calculated by measuring the quantity of the excreted end-products (urea and ammonia) and using equations:

$$S = nitrogen\ flux - quantity\ of\ excreted\ end\text{-}products \tag{10.6}$$

and

$$B = nitrogen\ flux - dietary\ nitrogen\ intake \tag{10.7}$$

where the conversion factor of 1 g nitrogen is equal to 6.25 g protein. As noted earlier, if subjects are studied during a post-absorptive state, dietary nitrogen intake is equal to 0 and the rate of protein breakdown is equal to nitrogen flux in the free pool.

Duggleby & Waterlow (2005) present a thorough critique of the studies that have used the [^{15}N]glycine method. They discuss the implications of measuring the ^{15}N-labeling in the end-products of ammonia or urea and the effect of using a single bolus or constant administration of [^{15}N]glycine. We comment on the elaborate experiments done by Gougeon et al. (1994, 1997, 1998, 2000), who used the [^{15}N]glycine method to examine protein metabolism in obese patients with type 2 diabetes. Studies were typically performed over the course of several weeks, during which time subjects lived in a clinical research centre. [^{15}N]glycine was administered over ~60 hour intervals several times during the study. Using this method, the investigators made several important overall observations including that: 1) there is an increased nitrogen flux in poorly controlled patients, i.e. those with glycated hemoglobins of ~12 % and fasting glucose of ~12 mM; and 2) normalisation of glycemia (either via insulin or oral hypoglycemic agents) leads to a reduction in protein breakdown thereby decreasing nitrogen flux and promoting nitrogen retention.

To further dissect the nature of endogenous protein turnover, Gougeon et al. (2000) estimated the contribution of muscle protein breakdown to whole-body nitrogen flux by measuring the excretion of methylhistidine. Briefly, the excretion of a modified amino acid (e.g. methylhistidine, hydroxyproline) can be used to measure protein breakdown, i.e. since post-translational modifications render amino acids unsuitable for use during the synthesis of new proteins, the excretion of modified amino acids reflects protein breakdown (Bilmazes et al. 1978; Elia et al. 1980; Marchesini et al. 1982; Selby et al. 1995).

Arterio-venous balance measurements using isotope tracers

The regulation of protein homeostasis can be studied in specific anatomical locations by measuring the plasma (or blood) flow and the concentration difference of amino acids across limbs and/or tissue beds of interest. A simple equation that describes net protein balance is:

$$flow \times (concentration_{\text{artery}} - concentration_{\text{vein}}) \qquad (10.8)$$

where $concentration_x$ is the concentration of an amino acid in a blood vessel; ideally one should calculate the balance of all amino acids.

This approach is based on principles of chemical mass-balance and requires certain assumptions. First, the intracellular pool of free amino acids must remain constant, therefore changes in amino acid balance reflect changes in protein turnover. Second, oxidative disposal of amino acids must not change, e.g. if an intervention increases the uptake of amino acids across the splanchnic bed, one assumes that more protein is being made and that amino acids are not being oxidised, converted to glucose, etc. Lastly, since blood cells make a substantial contribution to amino acid transport, one must consider whether to calculate the balance of amino acids in plasma or blood (Felig et al. 1973). Although the requirement for catheterisation procedures complicate the application of arterio-venous balance measurements, the classic studies of Wahren et al. (1975, 1976) demonstrated that catheterisation of numerous organs is possible and that studies are not limited to bed-ridden sedentary patients – Wahren often studied subjects during exercise.

As with measurements of whole-body nitrogen balance, arterio-venous balance measurements do not allow conclusions regarding the rates of protein synthesis and protein breakdown. However, just as the use of [^{15}N]glycine enhances the study of whole-body protein turnover, the use of isotope tracers greatly facilitates arterio-venous balance measurements of amino acid and protein dynamics, as seen in arterio-venous balance studies using infusions of isotopically labeled phenylalanine to study muscle protein dynamics (Barrett et al. 1987; Thompson et al. 1989). The rationale behind the use of phenylalanine in studies of muscle protein turnover is that phenylalanine has only one fate in muscle, incorporation into newly-made protein.

The fractional uptake of a labeled amino acid is determined using the equation:

$$[(concentration_{artery} \; x \; labeling_{artery}) - (concentration_{vein} \times labeling_{vein})]/$$
$$(concentration_{artery} \times labeling_{artery}) \qquad (10.9)$$

where $concentration_x$ and $labeling_x$ represent the concentration and isotopic enrichment of an amino acid, e.g. phenylalanine. Assuming that the tracer follows the same metabolic fate as the tracee, the absolute quantity of the amino acid that is removed (protein synthesis) is determined using the equation:

$$flow \times concentration_{artery} \times \text{Equation 10.9} \qquad (10.10)$$

i.e. multiply the quantity of tracee that is delivered to the tissue by the fractional uptake of the tracer. Finally, the number of unlabeled molecules that are released (protein breakdown) can be calculated using the equation:

$$flow \times [(concentration_{artery} \times (1 - labeling_{artery}))$$
$$- (concentration_{vein} \times (1 - labeling_{vein}))] \qquad (10.11)$$

Arterio-venous isotope balance studies have been widely used in the study of insulin action and diabetes on muscle protein turnover. For example, Gelfand & Barrett (1987) demonstrated that the anabolic action of insulin was primarily a consequence of decreased protein breakdown and not increased protein synthesis. Nair et al. (1983, 1995) extended the use of the arterio-venous balance method to include measurements of muscle and splanchnic protein balance in type 1 diabetes, concluding that insulin decreases protein breakdown in both sites but with different apparent sensitivities.

One important assumption that is made when using the arterio-venous balance of isotope tracers to measure protein turnover concerns whether the tracer completely mixes with the organ under investigation; incomplete mixing could result from heterogeneous tissue perfusion and/or limited transport across cell membranes. Compartmental models of muscle amino acid balance have been developed to address this matter (Bonadonna et al. 1993; Biolo et al. 1995). In particular, the addition of mannitol and methylaminoisobutyrate to tracer studies yield measures of tracer distribution in blood and diffusion through capillary walls into interstitial fluid and system A membrane transport without metabolism, respectively. Data suggest two important points regarding muscle amino acid balance and protein turnover. First, physiologic hyperinsulinemia stimulates the activity of system A amino acid transport, which may play an important role in the overall response of muscle amino acid flux and protein turnover (Bonadonna et al. 1993). Second, transmembrane transport of phenylalanine may be limiting under certain conditions (Biolo et al. 1995).

Precursor: product-labeling techniques

Protein synthesis can be determined by administering a labeled amino acid and then measuring its incorporation into a protein(s) (Figure 10.3). This 'direct' approach allows one to study the synthesis of total and/or specific proteins. If one can obtain multiple samples of the protein(s) of interest then Equation 10.2 can be used to determine the fractional turnover (k). However, if one obtains samples of the protein(s) of interest during the period of time when there is a linear change in the labeling of the respective protein(s), the fractional rate of protein synthesis can be calculated using the equation:

$$(protein\ labeling_{time\ 2} - protein\ labeling_{time\ 1})/$$
$$[precursor\ labeling \times (time2 - time1)] \qquad (10.12)$$

The use of precursor:product-labeling ratios has been plagued by two central problems; identification of the true precursor and measurement of its labeling. We consider some of the approaches that have been used to circumvent these problems; briefly, since the presumed precursor is a tRNA-bound amino acid and since measurement of its labeling is not routine, investigators have developed various surrogates.

Precursor-product method.

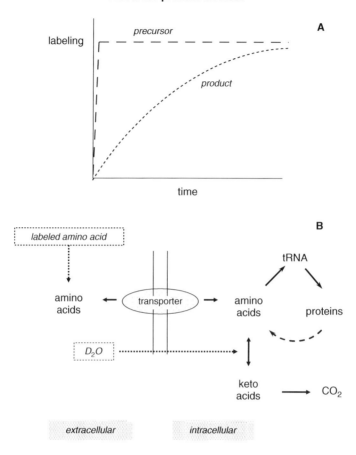

Figure 10.3 Direct Measurements of Protein Synthesis Using Precursor:Product-Labeling Methods
Panel A outlines a general isotope labeling scheme where an isotopic precursor is administered and
maintained at a steady state of labeling, and newly made protein molecules (products) incorporate
the isotope. Panel B demonstrates that in cases when a labeled amino acid is administered, the
isotope must be transported from the extracellular to the intracellular space, whereas when ^2H_2O is
administered, cells may be labeled directly in the intracellular space.

As described earlier, [1-^{13}C]leucine can be used to measure total protein turnover by
measuring the rates of appearance and oxidation of leucine, using samples of plasma
and breath respectively (Matthews et al. 1980). The rate of protein synthesis can also be
determined by administering a primed infusion of [1-^{13}C]leucine and then measuring the
^{13}C-labeling of protein-bound leucine (Rennie et al. 1982, 1994). However, since concentration gradients exist between amino acids in plasma and amino acids in intracellular
fluid and since there is compartmentation of isotope distribution within cells (Airhart et al.
1974; Khairallah & Mortimore 1976), investigators have raised questions regarding the true
precursor labeling (Ahlman et al. 2001). Watt et al. (1991) rigorously examined this matter
by measuring the labeling of arterial, venous and intracellular leucine and α-ketoisocaproate,

as well as that of tRNA-bound leucine from muscle. They demonstrated that the labeling of venous α-ketoisocaproate and the labeling of intracellular leucine provide reasonable surrogates for the labeling of tRNA-bound leucine.

Ballmer et al. (1990) proposed a novel 'flooding dose' method, the principle being that if one administers a large quantity of a labeled amino acid, its labeling in plasma will accurately reflect its labeling within a cell, i.e. increasing the plasma concentration will stimulate (saturate) the uptake of the amino acid by a tissue(s) and thus reduce any labeling gradients between a free amino acid and its respective tRNA-bound form (Caso et al. 2002). Using this method, one can assume that the precursor labeling is that of the amino acid in plasma. The flooding dose method offers a major advantage over the primed-infusion method since the experimental period is substantially reduced; a typical flooding dose experiment takes less than 60 minutes, whereas a primed-infusion experiment may require several hours. While this makes the method attractive, one must consider whether the increase in the pool size of the tracee alters the metabolism under investigation. The elegant studies of Rennie and colleagues examined the effect of 'flooding' with different amino acids on muscle protein synthesis (Smith et al. 1998). The data suggest that flooding with certain essential amino acids stimulates protein synthesis whereas flooding with certain non-essential amino acids has little or no effect on protein synthesis. (Note: although muscle protein synthesis was not stimulated by non-essential amino acids, the administration of certain non-essential amino acids led to a slight increase in circulating insulin.)

In a clever study aimed at measuring the synthesis of prealbumin, Reeds et al. (1992) administered $[^2H_3]$leucine and used the ^{2}H-labeling of leucine in VLDL-apoB-100 as a marker of the intrahepatic precursor labeling. The rationale was that since apoB-100 has a much shorter half life than prealbumin, the ^{2}H-labeling of apoB-100 leucine was expected to rapidly reach its maximum steady state level and thereby reflect the true labeling of intrahepatic leucine. This method is based on the assumptions that apoB-100 and prealbumin are synthesised in the same cells and that there is no zonation of leucine labeling.

The methods discussed above have a common constraint; since experiments must be performed in a controlled environment, the data will likely reflect the fact that a subject's behavior is somewhat artificial. To study protein dynamics in free-living subjects, Gersovitz et al. (1980) developed an innovative $[^{15}N]$glycine method for studying albumin synthesis. The rationale of the method is that if subjects continuously ingest $[^{15}N]$glycine over multiple days, one can assume that the precursor labeling is equivalent to that of urea (which is synthesised in the liver from arginine) and the product labeling is that of albumin-bound arginine. While suitable for use in free-living subjects, they must ingest $[^{15}N]$glycine every few hours over ~2.5 days (Gersovitz et al. 1980).

Perhaps the oldest, and least recognised, precursor:product-labeling approach centres on the use of ^2H_2O (Schoenheimer & Rittenberg 1940; Ussing 1941). The principle is that following the administration of ^2H_2O, ^{2}H atoms will distribute in body water and undergo rapid and stable incorporation into the carbon-bound hydrogens of amino acids (e.g. alanine), before those amino acids are incorporated into newly synthesised proteins. It is of interest to note that in the original studies (Ussing 1941) the observation that some amino acids were less labeled than others suggested that certain amino acids must be derived from the diet (e.g. lysine), since they are not synthesised *in vivo*.

We hypothesised that the use of ^2H_2O should minimise precursor labeling gradients as ^2H_2O labels cells from the 'inside' whereas labeled amino acids label cells from the 'outside' (Figure 10.3) (Previs et al. 2004; Dufner et al. 2005). Our attention has been focused on alanine since it undergoes a very rapid turnover (Yang et al. 1984, 1986; Hoffer et al. 1988), consequently we expected that the ^{2}H-labeling of alanine would reflect that of body water under many conditions. In our initial study, we measured albumin synthesis and breakdown over a prolonged period in patients receiving hemodialysis (Previs et al. 2004). Since we observed nearly 100 % equilibration of ^{2}H-labeling between body water and plasma alanine, we hypothesised that precursor:product-labeling ratios can be determined with confidence, i.e. the precursor is the ^{2}H-labeling of body water and the product is either the ^{2}H-labeling of the α-hydrogen of protein-alanine or the total ^{2}H-labeling of protein-alanine divided by n, the number of incorporated deuteriums. While the ^{2}H$_2$O method appears well-suited for measuring protein synthesis, especially in free-living subjects, our study highlights a concern regarding the use of ^{2}H$_2$O for measuring protein breakdown. To measure protein breakdown, the elimination of ^{2}H from the precursor pool must be substantially greater than the elimination of ^{2}H from the product (Bederman et al. 2005). Using the ^{2}H$_2$O method in patients receiving haemodialysis entails an extreme physiological setting since $\sim$80 % of total body water is turned over during a single dialysis session (Previs et al. 2004).

We initiated a follow-up study to further examine the equilibration of ^{2}H-labeling in alanine following the administration of ^{2}H$_2$O to rats (Dufner et al. 2005). The ability to use the total labeling of protein-bound alanine (as the product) offers an advantage when studying protein synthesis over short intervals (e.g. after feeding) and/or when studying the turnover of proteins with long half lives (e.g. if all four carbon-bound hydrogens are replaced by deuterium before free alanine is incorporated into newly made protein, the sensitivity of the analytical measurements is increased). We determined that even during substantial perturbations, the ^{2}H-labeling of body water rapidly equilibrates with the carbon-bound hydrogens of free alanine (Dufner et al. 2005). Those observations, in the rodent model, are consistent with what one might predict based on the central role of alanine in intermediary metabolism – the carbon-bound hydrogens of plasma alanine are replaced several times per hour (Yang et al. 1984, 1986; Hoffer et al. 1988) – and agree with experimental data regarding the ^{2}H-labeling of alanine during hemodialysis; we observed parallel decreases in the ^{2}H-labeling of body water and circulating alanine (Previs et al. 2004).

Proteome dynamics

Although a number of instruments and methods can be used in proteomic research, we consider certain general concepts in the field and highlight recent advances towards measuring proteome dynamics *in vivo*.

In spite of the fact that measurements in the field of proteomics typically yield information regarding static gene expression profiles, i.e. experiments typically consider measurements of the abundance of a protein(s) at one point in time (Aebersold & Mann 2003; Wu et al. 2004; Julka & Regnier 2005), investigators have used isotope tracer kinetics to explain how expression profiles develop (Papageorgopoulos et al. 1999; van Eijk & Deutz 2003; Andersen et al. 2005; Doherty et al. 2005). Although the *in vitro* application of tracer methods is somewhat straightforward (Andersen et al. 2005), studies of *in vivo* proteome dynamics face certain obstacles, including: 1) how does one administer a dose of isotope (typically a labeled amino acid) over a prolonged period; and 2) how does one determine the true precursor labeling (since a labeled amino acid will be diluted) (Papageorgopoulos et al. 1999; van Eijk & Deutz 2003; Doherty et al. 2005)? As noted earlier, ^2H_2O offers certain advantages regarding the ease of tracer administration and confidence in determining precursor labeling. Therefore, we hypothesised that one could couple the administration of ^2H_2O with proteomic-based assays and measure proteome turnover *in vivo* (Sun et al. 2004). We briefly explain the initial development of this approach and present an example of its application.

^2H_2O was administered to C57BL/6J mice and blood samples were collected over 10 days (Figure 10.4). Plasma albumin was isolated and hydrolyzed and the ^2H-labeling of albumin-alanine was determined using GC-MS methods (Dufner et al. 2005). The fractional rate of albumin synthesis was determined by fitting the ^2H-labeling of albumin-alanine; similar rates were determined regardless of whether we fitted the ^2H-labeling of the α-hydrogen or that of the total hydrogens (Figure 10.4, Panel A) – ~36 % or 33 % of the albumin was newly made per day, respectively. Next, we simulated the mass isotopomer distribution profile of tryptic peptide DVFLGTFLYEYSR (molecular ion 1609) derived from mouse albumin, assuming that albumin was made in the presence of H_2O or 2.5 % ^2H_2O (Figure 10.4, Panel B). To predict the isotope profile of the ^2H-labeled peptide, we considered that hydrogens are either solvent exchangeable or stably incorporated in carbon-hydrogen bonds of amino acids. Since solvent exchangeable hydrogens will re-exchange with buffer during tryptic digestion, the ^2H-labeling of a peptide reflects only those hydrogens (deuteriums) that are incorporated in the carbon-hydrogen bonds of the precursor amino acids. We used data in the literature to estimate the equilibration of ^2H-labeling between carbon-bound hydrogens of individual amino acids and body water (Commerford et al. 1983). We then mixed the 'virtual' peptides together, simulating the mass isotopomer profile assuming that albumin had been synthesised at ~34.5 % per day (the average rate of albumin synthesis determined in Panel A). Samples from the mice shown in Panel A were digested with trypsin and the ^2H-labeling of peptide DVFLGTFLYEYSR was determined using matrix assisted laser desorption ionisation-time of flight mass spectrometry (MALDI-TOF). We observed excellent agreement between the expected isotope profile (solid bars) and the measured isotope profile (open bars) (Figure 10.4, Panel C).

The data shown in Figure 10.4 demonstrate that proteomic-based assays (e.g. MALDI-TOF) reliably detect small changes in peptide labeling (MacCoss et al. 2005) and suggest that it is possible to obtain a functional image of gene action by measuring protein dynamics *in vivo* (Sun et al. 2004); subsequent studies have demonstrated the ability to determine an acute response of albumin synthesis following consumption of a meal. However, before we can propose the widespread use of ^2H_2O-proteomics, we must consider that the current limitation of the method is the need for knowledge regarding the equilibration of ^2H-labeling between body water and all proteogenic amino acids under different conditions. Studies are addressing the latter issue, thus it should soon be possible to reliably determine the synthesis of numerous proteins in a single proteomic assay *in vivo*.

Urea kinetics

Since urea is the major 'sink' for nitrogen that is derived from amino acid degradation, urea output is often used to estimate whole-body protein homeostasis. However, since quantitation of urea production via chemical mass-balance methods is not always practical, investigators

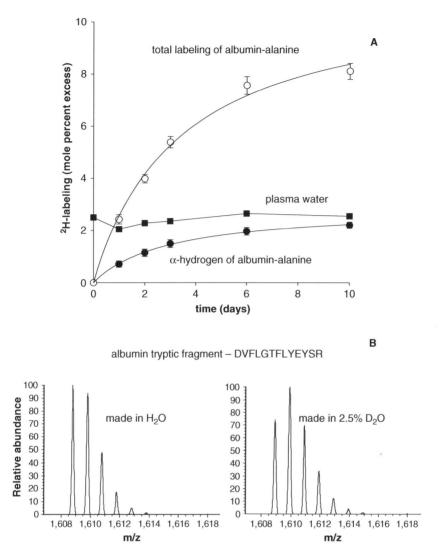

Figure 10.4 ^2H_2O-Proteomics Panel A demonstrates that a steady-state labeling of body water can be achieved using 'primed-infusion' of ^2H_2O; on day 0 mice were given a bolus of ^2H-labeled saline (20 ul per g body weight) and then maintained on 5% ^2H-labeled drinking water (days 0 to 10). Mice had ad libitum access to food and were killed on various days ($n = 3$ per day) and blood was collected. The rate of albumin synthesis was determined by fitting the labeling profiles of the α-hydrogen and the total labeling of albumin-alanine, resulting in rates of 36% and 33% newly made albumin per day, respectively. Panel B displays the theoretical mass isotopomer distribution profiles of tryptic peptide DVFLGTFLYEYSR, derived from mouse albumin made in the presence of H_2O or 2.5% ^2H_2O. Panel C demonstrates that MALDI-TOF analyses detect the expected shift in the mass isotopomer distribution profile of the tryptic peptide DVFLGTFLYEYSR (solid bars = expected labeling assuming 34.5% newly made albumin per day; open bars = measured labeling).

C

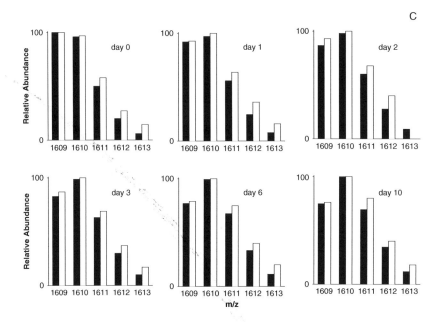

Figure 10.4 Continued

have used stable isotopes to measure urea production *in vivo*. We discuss two central issues that should be considered when using isotope tracers to study urea synthesis.

The first issue that requires consideration is, how should a tracer of urea be administered; does one use a bolus, constant infusion or primed-infusion? Matthews & Downey (1984) carefully examined this question and clearly demonstrated that the mode of isotope administration can have a large impact on the data if certain precautions are not exercised and/or substantial knowledge of the system is not available on which to base isotope dose calculations. Since the fractional turnover of urea is relatively slow (only ~ 8 % of the pool is newly made per hour), the use of a primed-infusion will lead to a substantial error in the calculated rate of urea synthesis (Hamadeh & Hoffer 1998) if the priming dose and the infusion rate are not properly matched.

Matthews & Downey (1984) demonstrated that an accurate rate of urea synthesis can be obtained in humans by measuring the elimination of labeled urea following an intravenous bolus. They developed a compartmental model with two pools of urea; presumably the intravascular pool rapidly mixes with intracellular pools of urea in well-perfused sites and slowly mixes with intracellular pools of urea in sites with reduced blood perfusion. Their report provides an excellent description of the approach and demonstrates that one can clearly identify the elimination constants and fit the model. Hibbert et al. (1992) extended the single bolus approach by considering the use of an oral bolus. However, oral administration of the isotope tracer is complicated by the presence of H pylori infection (since the labeled urea is hydrolysed before it is absorbed).

The second issue that requires consideration is, how does the tracer labeling affect the apparent rate of urea synthesis? This question arises when one considers the sources of nitrogen that are used to synthesise urea. For example, urea nitrogen is derived from amino acid catabolism (amino acids→NH_3 →urea) and from urea that undergoes degradation by bacteria in the gut (urea→NH_3→urea). The recycling of urea nitrogen via urease activity will lead to an overestimation of the rate of amino acid catabolism. To avoid problems related to urea recycling, investigators typically use doubly-labeled tracers, e.g. [$^{15}N_2$]urea (M2 labeled) (Wolfe 1981), the logic being that the appearance of M1 labeled urea ([$^{14}N,^{15}N$]urea) can be used to determine the degree to which urea is (re)synthesised from urea-derived nitrogen. However, when using a bolus injection of [$^{15}N_2$]urea, one will likely underestimate the true contribution of recycling since the [^{15}N]ammonia released during hydrolysis of the doubly-labeled tracer will be diluted by the generation of free ammonia in the gut (glutamine→NH_3+ glutamate). Quantitation of total urea synthesis and the contribution of recycling can be determined by using a constant infusion of urea and fitting the rise to steady state labeling in M2 and M1 urea.

Given the importance of urea as a major end-product of protein degradation/amino acid catabolism, it is surprising that relatively few isotope tracer studies have been done in diabetics. Mass-balance methods have been combined with isotope tracer methods to determine that the conversion of alanine-derived nitrogen to urea is increased in type 1 diabetes and in poorly controlled type 2 diabetes. Those studies did not examine urea turnover using isotopes of urea; rather, the rate of urea excretion was measured over a short interval and compared against the rate of alanine turnover (Almdal et al. 1990, 1994). Kalhan et al. (1982, 1993) examined the impact of gestational diabetes on urea production. They concluded that urea synthesis is not altered in patients with well-controlled gestational diabetes and that maternal diabetes does not have a significant effect on urea synthesis in infants.

Determining the molecular control of protein dynamics

Isotope tracer studies provide information regarding rates of protein turnover, however tracer methods do not identify the mechanisms that could affect protein turnover. Since tissue biopsies are often obtained (and used in determining protein synthesis via precursor:product-labeling ratios), we briefly consider additional parameters that can be measured and thereby used to facilitate the interpretation of isotope labeling data (Figure 10.5) (Prod'homme et al. 2004).

First, one can examine the role of gene transcription in the control of protein levels by using real-time polymerase chain reaction assays to quantify the amount of transcribed mRNA or by performing *in vitro* translation assays to quantify the amount of translatable mRNA. In an interesting study, Peavy et al. (1978) used the flooding dose method to determine that alloxan-induced diabetes leads to a reduction in albumin synthesis *in vivo*. They then used an *in vitro* translation assay and determined that impaired gene transcription plays an important role in limiting albumin synthesis.

Second, to quantify 'translation efficiency', one can measure the polyribosome profile. Peavy et al. (1985) found no differences in the polyribosome profiles of livers from normal vs alloxan-induced diabetic rodents, suggesting that diabetes-related decreases in albumin synthesis are not the result of impaired translation efficiency. These observations support their initial studies, in which the abundance of mRNA appeared to limit albumin synthesis (Peavy et al. 1978).

Third, investigators can examine the signal transduction cascades that control translation, e.g. one can quantify the phosphorylation and the activity of regulatory molecules in signaling pathways (Reiter et al. 2005).

Control of protein turnover.

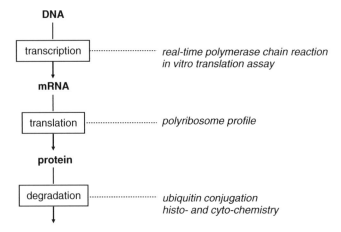

Figure 10.5 Control of Protein Turnover A number of mechanisms control the abundance of a protein. To identify potential molecular mechanisms that may affect protein turnover, one can normalise isotope tracer determinations of biochemical flux against various parameters.

Finally, protein breakdown occurs via lysosomal and non-lysosomal (ubiquitin-proteasome) mediated reactions; markers of some processes can be quantified (van Noorden 1991; Ciechanover 2005) and have been shown to be elevated in diabetes (Lecker et al. 1999).

Conclusion

There are a number of isotope tracer methods for studying protein and amino acid kinetics *in vivo*. Stable isotopes hold advantages over radioactive isotopes that influence the quantity and the quality of the data that can be obtained. The approach that is used to administer the tracer and determine the kinetics deserves attention, and although mathematical modeling techniques are often used to describe the parameters under investigation, the ability to obtain the necessary data may be challenging. The choice of amino acid tracer (both the amino acid species and its positional labeling) deserves attention since labeled tracers may be diluted via 1) protein breakdown, 2) de novo synthesis of an amino acid and 3) reversible metabolism and/or exchange reactions. 'Black box' or stochastic methods (e.g. $[1\text{-}^{13}C]$leucine, $[^{15}N]$glycine) yield estimates of total amino acid flux and whole-body protein turnover. The use of arterio-venous balance methods, with the infusion of isotopes, permits the quantitation of protein turnover in distinct tissues provided that there is sufficient mixing of the isotope between intracellular pools of amino acids and those in circulation. Precursor:product labeling ratios permit the determination of the dynamics of a specific protein; however, this assumes that the protein of interest can be isolated, its labeling measured and that a reliable measure of the precursor labeling can be obtained. Advances in the field of proteomics suggest that it is possible to simultaneously quantify the dynamics of numerous proteins in a 'proteome scan'. Finally, it is possible to determine molecular mechanisms that explain altered rates of protein turnover.

Acknowledgements

We thank Drs. Henri Brunengraber, Faramarz Ismail-Beigi and Bernard Landau for collaboration with the initial development of the ^2H_2O method and Drs. Vernon Anderson, Gang Sun and Benlian Wang for collaboration with the development of the ^2H_2O-proteomic method. This work was supported by the Mt. Sinai Health Care Foundation of Cleveland, OH and the NIH (Roadmap grant 1R33DK070291-01 and training fellowship DK007319 to DAG).

References

Abumrad, NN, Rabin, D, Diamond, MP, Lacy, WW (1981) Use of a heated superficial hand vein as an alternative site for the measurement of amino acid concentrations and for the study of glucose and alanine kinetics in man *Metabolism* **30**, 936–940

Aebersold, R and Mann, M (2003) Mass spectrometry-based proteomics *Nature* **422**, 198–207

Ahlman, B, Charlton, M, Fu, A et al. (2001) Insulin's effect on synthesis rates of liver proteins A swine model comparing various precursors of protein synthesis *Diabetes* **50**, 947–954

Airhart, J, Vidrich, A, Khairallah, EA (1974) Compartmentation of free amino acids for protein synthesis in rat liver *Biochem J* **140**, 539–545

Almdal, TP, Jensen, T, Vilstrup, H (1990) Increased hepatic efficacy of urea synthesis from alanine in insulin-dependent diabetes mellitus *Eur J Clin Invest* **20**, 29–34

Almdal, TP, Jensen, T, Vilstrup, H (1994) Control of non-insulin-dependent diabetes mellitus partially normalizes the increase in hepatic efficacy for urea synthesis *Metabolism* **43**, 328–332

Andersen, JS, Lam, YW, Leung, AK et al. (2005) Nucleolar proteome dynamics *Nature* **433**, 77–83

Ballmer, PE, McNurlan, MA, Milne, E et al. (1990) Measurement of albumin synthesis in humans: a new approach employing stable isotopes *Am J Physiol* **259**, E797–E803

Barrett, EJ, Revkin, JH, Young, LH et al. (1987) An isotopic method for measurement of muscle protein synthesis and degradation in vivo *Biochem J* **245**, 223–228

Baumgartner, FJ, Barrio, JR, Henze, E et al. (1981) 13N-labeled L-amino acids for in vivo assessment of local myocardial metabolism *J Med Chem* **24**, 764–766

Bederman, IR, Dufner, DA, Alexander, JC, Previs, SF (2005) Novel application of the 'doubly-labeled' water method: Measuring CO2 production and the tissue-specific dynamics of lipid and protein in vivo *Am J Physiol Endocrinol Metab*

Bilmazes, C, Uauy, R, Haverberg, LN et al. (1978) Musle protein breakdown rates in humans based on Ntau-methylhistidine (3–methylhistidine) content of mixed proteins in skeletal muscle and urinary output of Ntau-methylhistidine *Metabolism* **27**, 525–530

Biolo, G, Fleming, RY, Maggi, SP, Wolfe, RR (1995) Transmembrane transport and intracellular kinetics of amino acids in human skeletal muscle *Am J Physiol* **268**, E75–E84

Bonadonna, RC, Saccomani, MP, Cobelli, C, DeFronzo, RA (1993) Effect of insulin on system A amino acid transport in human skeletal muscle *J Clin Invest* **91**, 514–521

Brand, WA (1996) High precision isotope ratio monitoring techniques in mass spectrometry *J Mass Spectrom* **31**, 225–235

Calloway, DH, Odell, AC, Margen, S (1971) Sweat and miscellaneous nitrogen losses in human balance studies *J Nutr* **101**, 775–786

Caso, G, Ford, GC, Nair, KS et al. (2002) Aminoacyl-tRNA enrichment after a flood of labeled phenylalanine: insulin effect on muscle protein synthesis *Am J Physiol Endocrinol Metab* **282**, E1029–E1038

Chevalier, S, Marliss, EB, Morais, JA et al. (2005) Whole-body protein anabolic response is resistant to the action of insulin in obese women *Am J Clin Nutr* **82**, 355–365

Ciechanover, A (2005) Intracellular protein degradation: from a vague idea thru the lysosome and the ubiquitin-proteasome system and onto human diseases and drug targeting *Cell Death Differ* **12**, 1178–1190

Cobelli, C, Foster, DM, Toffolo, G (2000) *Tracer kinetics in biomedical research: From data to model* Kluwer Academic/Plenum Publishers, New York

Cobelli, C, Saccomani, MP, Tessari, P et al. (1991) Compartmental model of leucine kinetics in humans *Am J Physiol* **261**, E539–E550

Commerford, SL, Carsten, AL, Cronkite, EP (1983) The distribution of tritium among the amino acids of proteins obtained from mice exposed to tritiated water *Radiat Res* **94**, 151–155

Corso, TN and Brenna, JT (1997) High-precision position-specific isotope analysis *Proc Natl Acad Sci USA* **94**, 1049–1053

D'Erasmo, E, Pisani, D, Ragno, A et al. (1997) Serum albumin level at admission: mortality and clinical outcome in geriatric patients *Am J Med Sci* **314**, 17–20

Darmaun, D, Manary, MJ, Matthews, DE (1985) A method for measuring both glutamine and glutamate levels and stable isotopic enrichments *Anal Biochem* **147**, 92–102

Darmaun, D, Rongier, M, Koziet, J, Robert, JJ (1991) Glutamine nitrogen kinetics in insulin-dependent diabetic humans *Am J Physiol* **261**, E713–E718

De Feo, P, Horber, FF, Haymond, MW (1992) Meal stimulation of albumin synthesis: a significant contributor to whole body protein synthesis in humans *Am J Physiol* **263**, E794–E799

Doherty, MK, Whitehead, C, McCormack, H et al. (2005) Proteome dynamics in complex organisms: using stable isotopes to monitor individual protein turnover rates *Proteomics* **5**, 522–533

Downey, RS, Mellone, A, Matthews, DE (1986) Effect of tracer infusion site on measurement of bicarbonate-carbon dioxide metabolism in dogs *J Appl Physiol* **60**, 1248–1253

Dufner, DA, Bederman, IR, Brunengraber, DZ et al. (2005) Using 2H2O to study the influence of feeding on protein synthesis: effect of isotope equilibration in vivo vs in cell culture *Am J Physiol Endocrinol Metab* **288**, E1277–E1283

Duggleby, SL and Waterlow, JC (2005) The end-product method of measuring whole-body protein turnover: a review of published results and a comparison with those obtained by leucine infusion *Br J Nutr* **94**, 141–153

Elia, M, Carter, A, Bacon, S, Smith, R (1980) The effect of 3-methylhistidine in food on its urinary excretion in man *Clin Sci (Lond)* **59**, 509–511

Felig, P, Wahren, J, Raf, L (1973) Evidence of inter-organ amino-acid transport by blood cells in humans *Proc Natl Acad Sci USA* **70**, 1775–1779

Fern, EB, Garlick, PJ, Waterlow, JC (1985) Apparent compartmentation of body nitrogen in one human subject: its consequences in measuring the rate of whole-body protein synthesis with 15N *Clin Sci (Lond)* **68**, 271–282

Gariballa, SE, Parker, SG, Taub, N, Castleden, CM (1998) Influence of nutritional status on clinical outcome after acute stroke *Am J Clin Nutr* **68**, 275–281

Gelfand, RA and Barrett, EJ (1987) Effect of physiologic hyperinsulinemia on skeletal muscle protein synthesis and breakdown in man *J Clin Invest* **80**, 1–6

Gersovitz, M, Munro, HN, Udall, J, Young, VR (1980) Albumin synthesis in young and elderly subjects using a new stable isotope methodology: response to level of protein intake *Metabolism* **29**, 1075–1086

Gougeon, R, Marliss, EB, Jones, PJ et al. (1998) Effect of exogenous insulin on protein metabolism with differing nonprotein energy intakes in Type 2 diabetes mellitus *Int J Obes Relat Metab Disord* **22**, 250–261

Gougeon, R, Pencharz, PB, Marliss, EB (1994) Effect of NIDDM on the kinetics of whole-body protein metabolism *Diabetes* **43**, 318–328

Gougeon, R, Pencharz, PB, Sigal, RJ (1997) Effect of glycemic control on the kinetics of whole-body protein metabolism in obese subjects with non-insulin-dependent diabetes mellitus during iso- and hypoenergetic feeding *Am J Clin Nutr* **65**, 861–870

Gougeon, R, Styhler, K, Morais, JA et al. (2000) Effects of oral hypoglycemic agents and diet on protein metabolism in type 2 diabetes *Diabetes Care* **23**, 1–8

Hamadeh, MJ and Hoffer, LJ (1998) Tracer methods underestimate short-term variations in urea production in humans *Am J Physiol* **274**, E547–E553

Hegsted, DM (1978) Assessment of nitrogen requirements *Am J Clin Nutr* **31**, 1669–1677

Hibbert, JM, Forrester, T, Jackson, AA (1992) Urea kinetics: comparison of oral and intravenous dose regimens *Eur J Clin Nutr* **46**, 405–409

Hoffer, LJ, Yang, RD, Matthews, DE et al. (1988) Alanine flux in obese and healthy humans as evaluated by 15N- and 2H3–labeled alanines *Am J Clin Nutr* **48**, 1010–1014

Hofmann, D, Gehre, M, Jung, K (2003) Sample preparation techniques for the determination of natural 15N/14N variations in amino acids by gas chromatography-combustion-isotope ratio mass spectrometry (GC-C-IRMS) *Isotopes Environ Health Stud* **39**, 233–244

Horber, FF, Horber-Feyder, CM, Krayer, S et al. (1989) Plasma reciprocal pool specific activity predicts that of intracellular free leucine for protein synthesis *Am J Physiol* **257**, E385–E399

Jeejeebhoy, K N, Bruce-Robertson, A, Ho, J Sodtke V (1973) The comparative effects of nutritional and hormonal factors on the synthesis of albumin, fibrinogen and transferrin *Protein Turnover* Elsevier, New York 217–247

Jones, CII, Newstead, CG, Wills, EJ, Davison, AM (1997) Serum albumin and survival in CAPD patients: the implications of concentration trends over time *Nephrol Dial Transplant* **12**, 554–558

Julka, S and Regnier, FE (2005) Recent advancements in differential proteomics based on stable isotope coding *Brief Funct Genomic Proteomic* **4**, 158–177

Kalhan, SC (1993) Rates of urea synthesis in the human newborn: effect of maternal diabetes and small size for gestational age *Pediatr Res* **34**, 801–804

Kalhan, SC, Tserng, KY, Gilfillan, C, Dierker, LJ (1982) Metabolism of urea and glucose in normal and diabetic pregnancy *Metabolism* **31**, 824–833

Katanik, J, McCabe, BJ, Brunengraber, DZ et al. (2003) Measuring gluconeogenesis using a low dose of 2H2O: advantage of isotope fractionation during gas chromatography *Am J Physiol Endocrinol Metab* **284**, E1043–E1048

Katz, J (1992) On the determination of turnover in vivo with tracers *Am J Physiol* **263**, E417–E424

Khairallah, EA and Mortimore, GE (1976) Assessment of protein turnover in perfused rat liver Evidence for amino acid compartmentation from differential labeling of free and tRNA-gound valine *J Biol Chem* **251**, 1375–1384

Kulik, W, Oosterveld, MJ, Kok, RM, de Meer, K (2003) Determination of 13C and 15N enrichments of urea in plasma by gas chromatography-combustion isotope ratio mass spectrometry and gas chromatography-mass spectrometry using the 2–methoxypyrimidine derivative *J ChromatogrB Analyt Technol Biomed Life Sci* **791**, 399–405

Lariviere, F, Kupranycz, DB, Chiasson, JL, Hoffer, LJ (1992) Plasma leucine kinetics and urinary nitrogen excretion in intensively treated diabetes mellitus *Am J Physiol* **263**, E173–E179

Lattuada, G, Sereni, LP, Ruggieri, D et al. (2004) Postabsorptive and insulin-stimulated energy homeostasis and leucine turnover in offspring of type 2 diabetic patients *Diabetes Care* **27**, 2716–2722

Layman, DK and Wolfe, RR (1987) Sample site selection for tracer studies applying a unidirectional circulatory approach *Am J Physiol* **253**, E173–E178

Lecker, SH, Solomon, V, Price, SR et al. (1999) Ubiquitin conjugation by the N-end rule pathway and mRNAs for its components increase in muscles of diabetic rats *J Clin Invest* **104**, 1411–1420

Leverton, RM and Gram, MR (1949) Nitrogen excretion of women related to the distribution of animal protein in daily meals *J Nutr* **39**, 57–65

Luzi, L, Castellino, P, Simonson, DC et al. (1990) Leucine metabolism in IDDM Role of insulin and substrate availability *Diabetes* **39**, 38–48

Luzi, L, Petrides, AS, De Fronzo, RA (1993) Different sensitivity of glucose and amino acid metabolism to insulin in NIDDM *Diabetes* **42**, 1868–1877

MacCoss, MJ, Wu, CC, Matthews, DE, Yates, JR, III (2005) Measurement of the Isotope Enrichment of Stable Isotope-Labeled Proteins Using High-Resolution Mass Spectra of Peptides *Anal Chem* **77**, 7646–7653

Mackenzie, TA, Clark, NG, Bistrian, BR et al. (1985) A simple method for estimating nitrogen balance in hospitalized patients: a review and supporting data for a previously proposed technique *J Am Coll Nutr* **4**, 575–581

Marchesini, G, Forlani, G, Zoli, M et al. (1982) Muscle protein breakdown in uncontrolled diabetes as assessed by urinary 3-methylhistidine excretion *Diabetologia* **23**, 456–458

Matthews, DE, Ben Galim, E, Bier, DM (1979) Determination of stable isotopic enrichment in individual plasma amino acids by chemical ionization mass spectrometry *Anal Chem* **51**, 80–84

Matthews, DE, Conway, JM, Young, VR, Bier, DM (1981) Glycine nitrogen metabolism in man *Metabolism* **30**, 886–893

Matthews, DE and Downey, RS (1984) Measurement of urea kinetics in humans: a validation of stable isotope tracer methods *Am J Physiol* **246**, E519–E527

Matthews, DE, Motil, KJ, Rohrbaugh, DK et al. (1980) Measurement of leucine metabolism in man from a primed, continuous infusion of L-[1–3C]leucine *Am J Physiol* **238**, E473–E479

Matthews, DE, Schwarz, HP, Yang, RD et al. (1982) Relationship of plasma leucine and alpha-ketoisocaproate during a L-[1–13C]leucine infusion in man: a method for measuring human intra-cellular leucine tracer enrichment *Metabolism* **31**, 1105–1112

Meier-Augenstein, W (1999) Applied gas chromatography coupled to isotope ratio mass spectrometry *J Chromatogr A* **842**, 351–371

Nair, KS, Ford, GC, Ekberg, K et al. (1995) Protein dynamics in whole body and in splanchnic and leg tissues in type I diabetic patients *J Clin Invest* **95**, 2926–2937

Nair, KS, Garrow, JS, Ford, C et al. (1983) Effect of poor diabetic control and obesity on whole body protein metabolism in man *Diabetologia* **25**, 400–403

Papageorgopoulos, C, Caldwell, K, Shackleton, C et al. (1999) Measuring protein synthesis by mass isotopomer distribution analysis (MIDA) *Anal Biochem* **267**, 1–16

Patterson, BW (1997) Use of stable isotopically labeled tracers for studies of metabolic kinetics: an overview *Metabolism* **46**, 322–329

Patterson, BW, Carraro, F, Wolfe, RR (1993) Measurement of 15N enrichment in multiple amino acids and urea in a single analysis by gas chromatography/mass spectrometry *Biol Mass Spectrom* **22**, 518–523

Peavy, DE, Taylor, JM, Jefferson, LS (1978) Correlation of albumin production rates and albumin mRNA levels in livers of normal, diabetic, insulin-treated diabetic rats *Proc Natl Acad Sci USA* **75**, 5879–5883

Peavy, DE, Taylor, JM, Jefferson, LS (1985) Time course of changes in albumin synthesis and mRNA in diabetic and insulin-treated diabetic rats *Am J Physiol* **248**, E656–E663

Preston, T and McMillan, DC (1988) Rapid sample throughput for biomedical stable isotope tracer studies *Biomed Environ Mass Spectrom* **16**, 229–235

Previs, SF, Fatica, R, Chandramouli, V et al. (2004) Quantifying rates of protein synthesis in humans by use of 2H2O: application to patients with end-stage renal disease *Am J Physiol Endocrinol Metab* **286**, E665–E672

Prod'homme, M, Rieu, I, Balage, M et al. (2004) Insulin and amino acids both strongly participate to the regulation of protein metabolism *Curr Opin Clin Nutr Metab Care* **7**, 71–77

Reeds, PJ, Hachey, DL, Patterson, BW et al. (1992) VLDL apolipoprotein B-100, a potential indicator of the isotopic labeling of the hepatic protein synthetic precursor pool in humans: studies with multiple stable isotopically labeled amino acids *J Nutr* **122**, 457–466

Reiter, AK, Crozier, SJ, Kimball, SR, Jefferson, LS (2005) Meal feeding alters translational control of gene expression in rat liver *J Nutr* **135**, 367–375

Rennie, MJ, Edwards, RH, Halliday, D et al. (1982) Muscle protein synthesis measured by stable isotope techniques in man: the effects of feeding and fasting *Clin Sci (Lond)* **63**, 519–523

Rennie, MJ, Smith, K, Watt, PW (1994) Measurement of human tissue protein synthesis: an optimal approach *Am J Physiol* **266**, E298–E307

Sacca, L, Toffolo, G, Cobelli, C (1992) V-A and A-V modes in whole body and regional kinetics: domain of validity from a physiological model *Am J Physiol* **263**, E597–E606

San Pietro, A and Rittenberg, D (1953) A study of the rate of protein synthesis in humans: II Measurement of the metabolic pool and the rate of protein synthesis *J Biol Chem* **201**, 457–473

Schoenheimer, R and Rittenberg, R (1940) The study of intermediary metabolism of animals with the aid of isotopes *Physiol Rev* **20**, 218–248

Selby, PL, Shearing, PA, Marshall, SM (1995) Hydroxyproline excretion is increased in diabetes mellitus and related to the presence of microalbuminuria *Diabet Med* **12**, 240–243

Shipley, RA and Clark, RE (1972) *Tracer methods for* in vivo *kinetics: Theory and application* Academic Press, New York

Smith, K, Reynolds, N, Downie, S et al. (1998) Effects of flooding amino acids on incorporation of labeled amino acids into human muscle protein *Am J Physiol* **275**, E73–E78

Stein, TP, Leskiw, MJ, Buzby, GP et al. (1980) Measurement of protein synthesis rates with [15N]glycine *Am J Physiol* **239**, E294–E300

Sun, G, Wang, B, Previs, SF, Anderson, VE (2004) Simultaneous determination of multiple protein synthesis rates by in vivo deuterium labeling *J Am Soc Mass Spec* **15**, 92S

Thompson, GN, Pacy, PJ, Merritt, H et al. (1989) Rapid measurement of whole body and forearm protein turnover using a [2H5]phenylalanine model *Am J Physiol* **256**, E631–E639

Toth, MJ, MacCoss, MJ, Poehlman, ET, Matthews, DE (2001) Recovery of (13)CO(2) from infused [1–(13)C]leucine and [1,2–(13)C(2)]leucine in healthy humans *Am J Physiol Endocrinol Metab* **281**, E233–E241

Ussing, HH (1941) The rate of protein renewal in mice and rats studied by means of heavy hydrogen *Acta Physiol Scand* **2**, 209–221

van Eijk, HM and Deutz, NE (2003) Plasma protein synthesis measurements using a proteomics strategy *J Nutr* **133**, 2084S-2089S

van Noorden, CJ (1991) Assessment of lysosomal function by quantitative histochemical and cyto-chemical methods *Histochem J* **23**, 429–435

Wahren, J, Felig, P, Hagenfeldt, L (1976) Effect of protein ingestion on splanchnic and leg metabolism in normal man and in patients with diabetes mellitus *J Clin Invest* **57**, 987–999

Wahren, J, Hagenfeldt, L, Felig, P (1975) Splanchnic and leg exchange of glucose, amino acids, free fatty acids during exercise in diabetes mellitus *J Clin Invest* **55**, 1303–1314

Waterlow, JC (1995) Whole-body protein turnover in humans–past, present, future *Annu Rev Nutr* **15**, 57–92

Watt, PW, Lindsay, Y, Scrimgeour, CM et al. (1991) Isolation of aminoacyl-tRNA and its labeling with stable-isotope tracers: Use in studies of human tissue protein synthesis *Proc Natl Acad Sci USA* **88**, 5892–5896

Wolfe, RR (1981) Measurement of urea kinetics in vivo by means of a constant tracer infusion of di-15N-urea *Am J Physiol* **240**, E428–E434

Wolfe, RR and Chinkes, DL (2004) *Isotope tracers in metabolic research: Principles and practice of kinetic analyses* Wiley-Liss, New York

Wu, CC, MacCoss, MJ, Howell, KE et al. (2004) Metabolic labeling of mammalian organisms with stable isotopes for quantitative proteomic analysis *Anal Chem* **76**, 4951–4959

Yang, RD, Matthews, DE, Bier, DM et al. (1984) Alanine kinetics in humans: influence of different isotopic tracers *Am J Physiol* **247**, E634–E638

Yang, RD, Matthews, DE, Bier, DM et al. (1986) Response of alanine metabolism in humans to manipulation of dietary protein and energy intakes *Am J Physiol* **250**, E39–E46

11

Assessment of Metabolic Fluxes by *In Vivo* MR Spectroscopy

Martin Krššák and **Michael Roden**

Phenomena of nuclear magnetic resonance – imaging and spectroscopy

Magnetic resonance a is noninvasive technique that allows the investigation of internal organs for their anatomy and morphology (imaging) as well as for their biochemical composition (spectroscopy). Magnetic resonance imaging (MRI) provides us with cross sectional or 3D images of the human body, where contrast is based on the local water and fat concentrations and the magnetic properties of soft tissue. With magnetic resonance spectroscopy (MRS), different chemical entities give their own characteristic signals, the amplitudes of which are mainly based on their concentration in the observed volume. Despite these differences in the outcome, both techniques are based on the same phenomenon of nuclear magnetism, which forces every nucleus with non-zero magnetic moment (spin) to precess in the direction of the external magnetic field (B_0) (Figure 11.1A). The phase of precession of individual nuclei occurs in random order, which results in cancellation of the magnetic moment in the plane perpendicular to the direction of the external magnetic field. On the other hand, components of the nuclear magnetic moments parallel with the external field form a non-zero macroscopic quantity – magnetisation (Figure 11.1B). To create the homogeneous external field, superconductive magnets with field strengths up to 3 tesla are used for clinical routine scanners. For experimental studies on humans, up to 9 tesla are used, while magnets with field strength of 11.75–14 Tesla can nowadays be used for pre-clinical experiments on small rodents. The angular frequency of the nuclei with non-zero spin is directly proportional to the magnetic field strength (B_0) and to the magnetic properties of these nuclei (γ – gyromagnetic ratio). This frequency is called the Larmor frequency.

To change the alignment of the magnetisation, we need to apply an external RF magnetic field (B_1) at Larmor frequency (Figure 11.1C). Any other frequencies will have no effect. For the purpose of metabolic investigation, the most important nuclei are proton (hydrogen-1), carbon-13 and phosporus-31. These nuclei have magnetic propertiess which make them

Clinical Diabetes Research: Methods and Techniques   Edited by Michael Roden
© 2007 John Wiley & Sons, Ltd   ISBN 978-0-470-01728-9

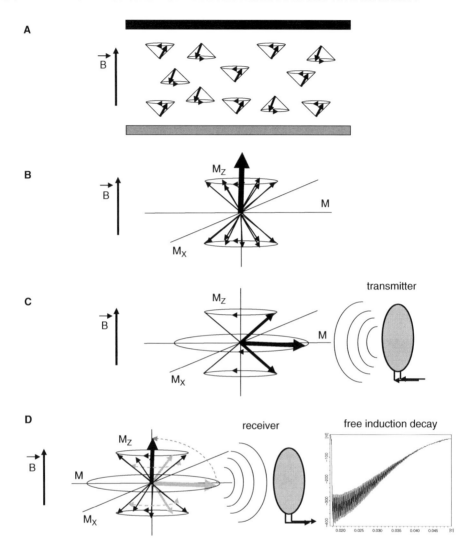

Figure 11.1 Detection of NMR Signal A) placement of the rotating spins into homogeneous magnetic field (B_0) forces them to align parallel or anti-parallel to the direction of the magnetic field and precess around this direction with Larmor frequency $\omega_L = \gamma \cdot B_0$, where γ is the gyromagnetic ratio characterising the magnetic properties of the nuclei; B) slight difference in the distribution between parallel and anti-parallel states create macroscopic magnetisation along the z-axis, M_z. Random phase of precession leaves no observable macroscopic magnetisation in the M_{xy}; C) transmission of radiowaves at Larmor frequency disturbs the thermodynamic equilibrium in favour of anti-parallel spin alignment, decreasing the magnetisation along the z-axis and forcing the spin to precess with the same phase. Both processes contribute to the generation of the observable magnetisation in the xy-plane, M_{xy}; D) after switching off the radio-frequency, the spin system strives to obtain the previous equilibrium. Changes in the M_{xy} induce an electric signal in the receiver coil – free induction decay (FID).

Table 11.1   Resonance Frequencies, Natural Abundance and Relative Sensitivity of Nuclei of Interest

Nucleus	Resonance frequency @3T [MHz]	Natural abundance [%]	Relative sensitivity
Proton – 1	125.5	99.98	100.0
Carbon – 13	31.4	1.1	$18*10^{-2}$
Nitrogen – 15	12.6	0.37	$3.8*10^{-4}$
Fluorine – 19	117.5	100.00	83.0
Phosphorus – 31	50.6	100.00	6.6

'resonate' at different frequencies (resonance frequencies at 3T for ^{1}H, ^{13}C and ^{31}P are summarised in Table 11.1). A practical consequence of the differences between the magnetic properties of the nuclei is that, in addition to usual clinical settings, an MR system has to be equipped with broad band radio frequency (RF) electronics (transmitter/amplifier/receiver). In addition, dedicated MR probes are necessary for observing signals originating not only from protons, but also from phosphorus and/or carbon (X-nuclei).

After applying the RF magnetic field, the magnetisation is no longer aligned with the external magnetic field and precession of its components is detected by the receiver. The MR signal corresponds to a superposition of oscillating magnetisation components attenuated in time, formed by different nuclei of the same isotope (free induction decay, FID) (Figure 11.1D). Fourier transformation translates the FID into a display of signal intensities vs frequency.

The distribution of the resonance frequencies in the spectrum is due to additional magnetic fields produced by the electron cloud of the molecule. These additional magnetic fields cause a very small change in the resonance frequency, which can serve as a chemical fingerprint of each molecule (Figure 11.2). The frequency change is usually expressed as a fraction of the resonance frequency and is called chemical shift. This parameter does not depend on the strength of the external magnetic field B_0 and is usually expressed in parts per million (ppm).

Well-defined magnetic field gradients are used to create position-dependent magnetic fields, which can be used to localise the signal. Information that is then encoded into the frequency or the phase of the signal can thereafter be transformed to localise it (Figure 11.3B). Based on the hardware performance and accessible length of the acquisition time, a sub-millimetre localisation of water signal, and hence geometrical resolution of the anatomical images, can be achieved. As the signal amplitude corresponds to the number of nuclei observed, lower concentration of metabolites limits the best achievable localisation of proton spectra to a cubic centimetre range. This resolution is sufficient to detect compounds in 0.1–1 mmol/l tissue concentration.

Spatial resolution of ^{31}P and ^{13}C experiments is hampered by low intrinsic sensitivity and, in the case of carbon, with low natural abundance of the isotope (Table 11.1). To overcome these problems, a volume of interest of hundreds of cubic centimetres is used (Figure 11.3A). Using this approach, the detection limit of ^{31}P MR spectra is about 0.1 mmol/l tissue, whereas it is about 20–50 mmol/l tissue in the case of ^{13}C MRS without artificial enrichment of the observed metabolite pool.

Additional measures for increasing the signal-to-noise ratio of non-proton spectra include: 1) the use of special ^{1}H (decoupling) coils to eliminate the interaction between X-nuclei and

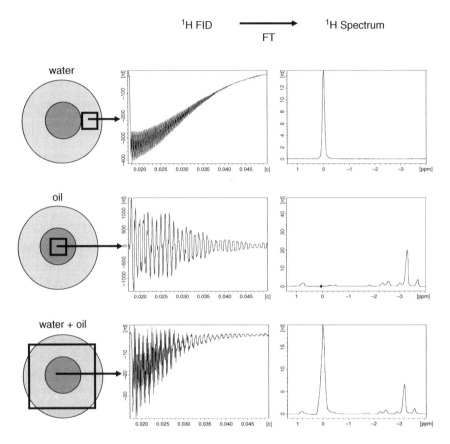

Figure 11.2 Spectral Dispersion and Superimposition of Different Frequencies The same isotope in different chemical entities, represented here by protons bound in water and fatty acids (oil), resonate at different frequency, yielding different forms of free induction decay (FID). Fourier Transformation (FT) of superimposed FID can depict and quantitate signal contributions of different frequencies.

their surrounding protons; 2) shimming procedures to increase the homogeneity of the static magnetic field, 3) increasing the field strength of whole body MR systems; 4) repeating the excitation many times and accumulating the MR signal prior to Fourier transformation; 5) selective suppression of unwanted signals; 6) design and construction of special dedicated X-nuclei MR coils; and 7) increasing the abundance of isotopes of interest, by systemic infusion of substrate metabolites in the case of ^{13}C MRS.

Once a spectrum with sufficient signal-to-noise ratio is acquired from the living tissue, another very important methodological issue has to be dealt with. Problems of quantification of spectroscopic information can be divided into two categories. First, the intensity of the resonance line, which is linearly dependent on the concentration of observed nuclei, has to be assessed. This task can be complicated in the *in vivo* situation, since many resonance lines tend to overlap, especially in the proton spectroscopy at lower magnetic fields. Several strategies of signal fitting in the time (e.g. AMARES) (Vanhamme & Van Huffel 1997; Mierisova et al. 1998; Vanhamme et al. 1999) and frequency domains, recently reviewed

A

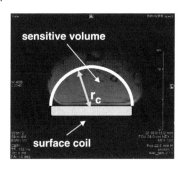
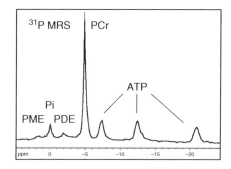

B

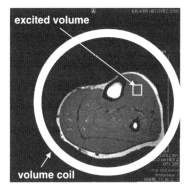
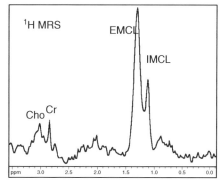

Figure 11.3 Localisation of MR Signal A) surface coils are mostly used for excitation of whole sensitive volume, which reaches up to ~r_c (the radius of the coil) into the tissue. As can be seen on the MR image of the calf muscle (left panel), muscle signal intensity decreases with increasing distance from the coil. The right panel shows a ^{31}P MR spectrum of skeletal muscle, acquired in this experimental set-up; B) volume resonators can be used for homogeneous excitations of measured samples, as can be seen from the MR image of the calf muscle within the volume MR coil (left panel). White square in the image depicts the volume of interest, which was selectively excited for the acquisition of ^{1}H MR spectra of muscle tibialis anterior (right panel).

by Mierisova & Ala-Korpela (2001), as well as linear combination of pre-acquired model spectra, (Provencher 1993, 2001) have been developed and lead to satisfactorily results.

The second issue is conversion of the signal intensity into molar concentration units. Different approaches here range from using the spectra of external phantom solution with known concentrations (Taylor et al. 1992; Gruetter et al. 1994), through linear combination of pre-acquired spectra (LC Model) (Provencher 1993, 2001), to using an internal concentration reference from a metabolite known for its stable concentration under given conditions (Rothman et al. 1992; Krššák et al. 1999; Anderwald et al. 2002).

There are two critical issues related to MR applications that could lead to safety hazards. First, the presence of a strong magnetic field and the switching of the magnetic field gradients makes metallic objects (splinters, tattoos, coloured contact lenses, piercings, uterus coils), different medical devices (pace makers, cardiac valves, clips, electrodes, neuro-stimulators), implants, prosthetics, shunts and stents contraindication for the MR examination. The ongoing search for new non-metallic materials might bring some improvement to this issue. Nevertheless, for every examination the physicist or radiologist should be consulted and the patient has to be well informed about the risks.

The second safety related issue is the application of an external pulsed electromagnetic field. In addition to magnetic excitation, the non-specific interaction between electromagnetic fields and the body can heat up tissue. Maximal values of the specific absorption rate (SAR), defined as energy per tissue mass per period of time in Watts per kg per min, have been set for different parts of the human body. All clinical and most experimental MR systems have integrated electronic tools to estimate SAR during given radiofrequency pulse sequences and prohibit experiments that are of potential danger to the patient. Among MRS experiments, these are for the most part so-called proton decoupled ^{13}C pulse sequences, which can reach the limits of allowed SAR. Values over the limit can usually be avoided by allowing tissue to cool down between radiofrequency pulses, by using longer repetition times or by applying weaker and shorter pulses.

More detailed and very well written introductions to the phenomena and techniques of magnetic resonance with respect to the *in vivo* situation can be found in Freeman (2003) and Gadian (1995). Recent developments in hardware engineering have emphasised the importance of this non-invasive, non-destructive and repeatable technology. State of the art versatile systems, from small animal to human body scanners allow for on-line *in vivo* monitoring of metabolism and the translation of knowledge from experimental animal studies to clinical patient investigation and vice versa.

Diabetes research was advanced with the advent and dissemination of MR methods. Skeletal muscle, liver and fat tissue, in which metabolism plays a major role in developing insulin resistance, as well as the brain, are now easily accessible for investigation. Skeletal muscle and liver biopsies have been replaced by ^{13}C/^{31}P MR spectroscopy in measuring glucose fluxes. Basal and stimulated intracellular energy metabolism can be monitored by ^{31}P MRS, and a combination of spectroscopic and imaging examinations of brain function and energetic metabolism can help in studies on perception and contra-regulation of hypoglycaemia. All of these issues, with respect to specific organs, historic perspective and research, as well as clinical applications, will be discussed in the rest of the chapter.

Skeletal muscle

Glucose fluxes

Radioactive tracer and stable isotope dilution techniques from 1960s to 1980s identified skeletal muscle as one of the major organs responsible for whole body insulin resistance under insulin stimulated conditions (DeFronzo 1988). *In vitro* studies on cellular suspensions, *in vivo* studies measuring arterio-venous isotope balance, and studies using skeletal muscle biopsies or freeze clamps of animal tissue all tried to identify the rate-controlling step in the glycogenic and glycolytic pathways that was responsible for the development of insulin resistance. The coordinated regulation of the activity of several enzymes on these pathways by insulin has complicated attempts to assign the conventional rate-limiting step

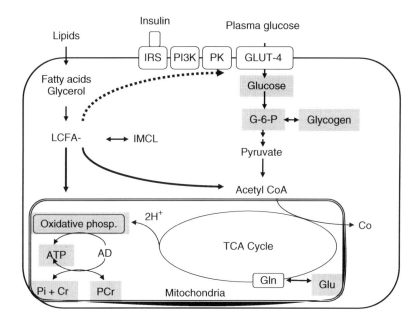

Figure 11.4 Metabolic Fluxes in Skeletal Muscle Schematic chart of the metabolic fluxes in the skeletal muscle discussed within this chapter. Shaded rectangles highlight the MR observable metabolites: i)^{13}C MRS – glucose, glycogen, glutamate; ii) ^{31}P MRS – glucose-6-phosphate (G6P), phosphocreatine (PCr), adenosine-triphosphate (ATP), inorganic phosphate (Pi); iii) ^{1}H MRS – intramyocellular lipids (IMCL).

for glycogen synthesis. Several candidates, including expression and translocation of the glucose transporter Glut-4, glucose phosphorylation by hexokinase II, glycogen synthase, as well as different enzymes of glycolysis were suggested, but none of these could sufficiently explain the *in vivo* conditions prevailing in type 2 diabetes mellitus (Figure 11.4).

Discovery of 100 % skeletal muscle and liver glycogen *in vivo* visibility by ^{13}C MR spectroscopy (Zang et al. 1990; Gruetter et al. 1991; Borgs et al. 1993) and later validation of this method (Taylor et al. 1992; Gruetter et al. 1994; Overloop et al. 1996) enabled the measurement of *in vivo* concentration and monitoring of glycogen synthesis under various conditions. Applying infusion of ^{13}C-labeled glucose as a substrate under steady state conditions increased the accuracy of the method (Jue et al. 1989) and skeletal muscle glycogen synthesis in gastrocnemius muscle (Figure 11.5A) could be correlated with whole body carbohydrate consumption (Shulman et al. 1990). Even though the latter conclusion was questioned by a recent study (Serlie et al. 2005), ^{13}C MR spectroscopy remains the non-invasive method of choice for assessing local skeletal muscle glycogen synthesis.

At the same time, ^{31}P MR spectroscopy was found to be able to detect and quantify skeletal muscle glucose-6-phosphate concentration and its changes in response to insulin stimulated conditions (Rothman et al. 1992) (Figure 11.5B). For the absolute quantification of this substrate of glycogen synthesis and glycolysis, the ^{31}P MRS resonance line of β-ATP is taken as an internal reference. Under hyperinsulinaemic-euglycaemic conditions, concentration of G6P in healthy skeletal muscle doubles to ∼200 μmol·l^{-1}.

A sophisticated experiment combining *in vivo* ^{13}C and ^{31}P MRS and microdialysis, using intravenously infused ^{13}C-labeled glucose as a substrate, i.v. infused ^{13}C-labeled mannitol

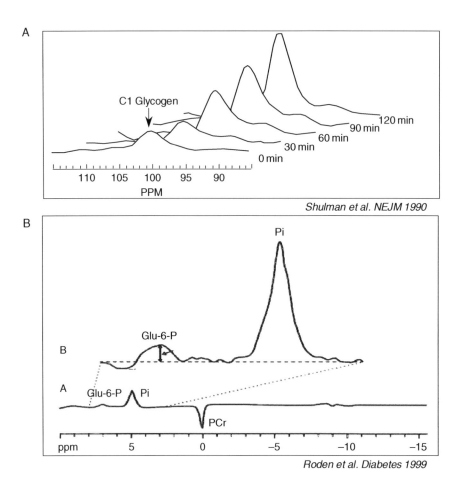

Shulman et al. NEJM 1990

Roden et al. Diabetes 1999

Figure 11.5   [13]C and ^{31}P MR Spectroscopy of Skeletal Muscle A) skeletal muscle glycogen synthesis under euglycemic-hyperinsulinemic condition in young healthy man. Increasing area under the curve corresponds to increasing incorporation of [1-^{13}C]glucose into skeletal muscle glycogen. Reproduced with permission from Shulman G I et al. (1990) *N Eng J Med* **322** (4), 223–228; B) Increase of glucose transport and phosphorylation in the skeletal muscle during euglycemic-hyperinsulinemic conditions can be observed by ^{31}P MR spectroscopy. Difference between the signals obtained from young healthy man in the basal and stimulated periods clearly shows the resonance of glucose-6-phosphate. Reproduced with permission from Roden M et al. (1999) *Diabetes* **48** (2), 358–364; C) ^{13}C MR spectra of blood plasma (lower trace) and skeletal muscle (upper trace) during simultaneous infusion of [1-^{13}C]glucose and [1-^{13}C]mannitol. Natural abundance signal of creatine serves as an indicator of intracellular volume and [1-^{13}C]mannitol as an indicator of extracellular volume of skeletal muscle tissue. Subtracting extracellular-(blood plasma and extrastitium) and G-6-P (measured simultaneously by ^{31}P MRS) contributions from total glucose signal yields free intracellular glucose concentration. Reproduced with permission from Cline G. W. et al. (1999) *N Eng J Med* **341** (4), 240–246.

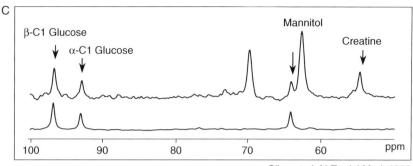

Cline et al, N Engl J Med. 1999

Figure 11.5 Continued.

as a marker for extracellular volume, ^{13}C creatine MRS signal as the intracellular marker and ^{31}P MRS signal of glucose-6-phosphate (Cline et al. 1998, 1999) was able to quantify the intracellular free glucose concentration (Figure 11.5C). This and alternative ^{13}C MRS methods (Roussel et al. 1996, 1997, 1998) have found that, under hyperinsulinaemic conditions, intracellular muscle glucose is lower than 1 mmol.l^{-1}, and it is even lower in T2DM, revealing the defect of glucose transport into the muscle cell which proceeds from the defects in phosphorylation and glycogen synthesis in T2DM patients (Cline et al. 1999) and thus identifying a crucial step in the development of insulin resistance.

Re-analysing the results of the first MRS studies (Shulman et al. 1990; Rothman et al. 1992) by means of metabolic control analysis (Kacser & Burns 1973) further supported the hypothesis that glycogenic flux in human skeletal muscle is not controlled solely by glycogen synthase, but rather by glucose transport and phosphorylation (Shulman 1996). This re-analysis also concluded that the activity of glycogen synthase is most probably controlled allosterically by glucose-6-phosphate concentration (Shulman 1996).

Defects of skeletal muscle glucose metabolism in insulin resistant states

Using the above mentioned methods, studies on skeletal muscle glycogen synthesis in insulin resistant populations revealed ~60 % decrease of insulin stimulated glycogen synthesis in overt T2DM patients (Shulman et al. 1990) (Figure 11.6) as well as ~70 % decrease in their lean insulin resistant offspring (Rothman et al. 1995). The same defect was found in obese non-diabetic insulin resistant volunteers (Petersen et al. 1998a). Further, defects in the insulin dependent phase of glycogen resynthesis that follows the depletion of glycogen stores by exhausting exercise were found in the insulin resistant offspring of T2DM patients (Price et al. 1996); decreased postprandial skeletal muscle glycogen synthesis in normal physiological conditions after a mixed meal was found in T2DM patients by the same method (Carey et al. 2003).

Increase of glucose-6-phosphate concentration during hyperinsulinaemic-euglycaemic clamp is blunted according to the extent of insulin resistance in all insulin resistant populations (Rothman et al. 1991, 1995; Perseghin et al. 1996; Petersen et al. 1998a) (Figure 11.6) and measurements of intracellular glucose concentration under hyperisulinaemic conditions in T2DM revealed a direct defect of glucose transport in this population (Roussel et al. 1996; Cline et al. 1999). Thus the impairment of glucose transport into muscle cells leads to defects in phosphorylation and glycogen synthesis in T2DM patients and represents a crucial step in the development of insulin resistance.

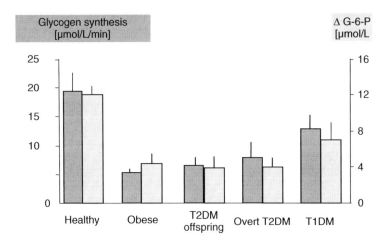

Figure 11.6 Glycogen Synthesis and Glucose Transport/Phosphorylation in Human Skeletal Muscle Rates of insulin stimulated glycogen synthesis (dark grey, left axis) and increase of intracellular concentration of glucose-6-phosphate (light grey, right axis) as a measure of glucose transport/phosphorylation in human skeletal muscle in various states of insulin resistance. Decrease of $\sim$60–70% was observed in both fluxes in obese, insulin resistant offsprings of type 2 diabetic patients and overt type 2 diabetic patient. Type 1 diabetic patients present with $\sim$50% decrease in both measures. (Data compiled from Shulman et al. 1990; Rothman et al. 1992, 1995; Petersen et al. 1998.)

Different combinations of these MRS methods were also used to monitor the effects of life style change or pharmacological insulin sensitising therapy on skeletal muscle glucose metabolism. One bout of aerobic exercise normalised insulin stimulated glucose transport/phosphorylation and glycogen synthesis, along with the normalisation of whole body insulin sensitivity in insulin resistant offspring of T2DM patients (Perseghin et al. 1996). Troglitazone treatment could improve insulin sensitivity in the skeletal muscle of patients with type 2 diabetes by improving glucose transport, phosphorylation activity and glycogen synthesis (Petersen et al. 2000; Van Den Bergh et al. 2000).

In summary, we can say that the combination ^{13}C and ^{31}P MR spectroscopic techniques 1) was able to measure glycogenic substrate flux in the human skeletal muscle under various conditions; 2) enabled metabolic control analysis of this metabolic pathway; and 3) helped find the defects of this pathway in insulin resistant conditions.

Perturbation of metabolic flux control – the role of substrate overabundance

It is well known that increased circulating triglycerides and FFA are frequently associated with pathophysiology of insulin resistance and diabetes mellitus. Searching for the mechanism of their action on glucose metabolism, Sir Randle et al. (1963) observed that elevated circulating free fatty acids (FFA) impair skeletal muscle glucose uptake. The results of his studies allowed him to postulate the hypothesis that substrate competition for mitochondrial oxidation is the major mechanism involved in this action. According to this hypothesis, experimental challenge by FFA would first increase the intracellular glucose-6-phosphate

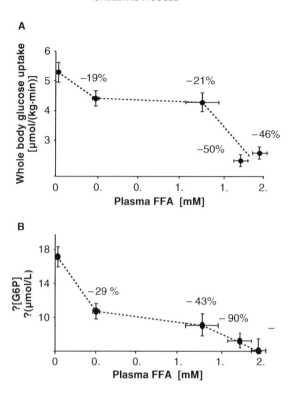

Figure 11.7 Insulin Sensitivity and Glucose Transport/Phosphorylation are Decreased by Elevated Free Fatty Acids (FFA) A) Gradual decrease of whole body glucose uptake during euglycemic-hyperinsulinemia as a measure of insulin sensitivity, with increasing experimental elevation of plasma FFA by Intralipid® infusion in young healthy men; B) Corresponding dose-dependent decrease in glucose transport/phosphorylation assessed by ^{31}P MRS measurement of glucose-6-phosphate (G6P) (Data compiled from Roden et al. 1996, 1999; Dresner et al. 1999).

and glycogen concentrations, then allosterically inhibit glucose transport into the muscle cell. Recent studies applying the above mentioned ^{13}C and ^{31}P MRS methods showed FFA inducing the decrease of glucose transport/phosphorylation (Figure 11.7) (Roden et al. 1996b, 1999; Krebs et al. 2001) and impairement of glycogen synthesis (Roden et al. 1996b) that precede the decrease of whole body glucose uptake in dose-depending manner (Roden et al. 1999), indicating a direct impairment of insulin signaling (Griffin et al. 1999) and therefore of glucose transport (Dresner et al. 1999) and phosphorylation. This mechanism holds true in various conditions of steady state hypersinsulinaemia (Roden et al. 1996b, 1999), hypoinsulinaemia (Krebs et al. 2001) and depleted skeletal muscle glycogen (Delmas-Beauvieux et al. 1999), showing the direct effect of circulating FFA on glucose metabolism.

Similarly, the results of several studies have suggested that increased protein intake, and therefore increased circulating plasma amino acids, can cause insulin resistance by affecting skeletal muscle and hepatic metabolism (Felig et al. 1969; Linn et al. 2000). Measuring skeletal glucose transport/phosphorylation (Figure 11.8A) and glycogen synthesis (Figure 11.8B) in the skeletal muscle of young, healthy men during experimental AA challenge confirmed this suspicion and showed the direct effects of amino acids on glucose transport/phosphorylation (Krebs et al. 2002). Analysis of biopsies taken from the skeletal muscle of young, healthy men under these conditions showed that overactivation of the mammalian target of the rapamycin/S6 kinase 1 pathway and inhibitory serine phosphorylation of insulin receptor substrate-1 underlie this impairment of insulin action in amino acid-infused humans (Tremblay et al. 2005).

Substrate overabundance and defects in lipid oxidation can lead to increased lipid accumulation inside the skeletal muscle. The link between intramyocellular lipid accumulation and skeletal muscle glucose uptake/oxidation has recently been established (Jacob et al. 1999; Krššák et al. 1999; Perseghin et al. 1999) and extensively studied in different states of insulin resistance and physical fitness (Thamer et al. 2003). This complex issue is discussed, together with hepatic and adipose fat accumulation, in Chapter 13.

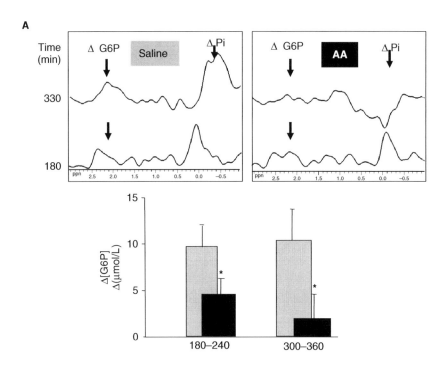

Figure 11.8 Amino Acid Induced Inhibition of Skeletal Muscle Glucose Transport/Phosphorylation and Glycogen Synthesis A) increase in glucose-6-phosphate (G6P) concentration in different periods of experimental euglycaaemic-hyperinsulinaemia in the skeletal muscle of young, healthy men (upper left panel) and its inhibition by the elevation of plasma amino acid concentration (upper right panel). Intravenous infusion of Aminoplasmal® inhibits glucose transport/phosphorylation by ∼50 % in the early period and ∼80 % in the later period of euglycaaemic-hyperinsulinaemia; B) skeletal muscle glycogen synthesis during experimental euglycaaemic-hyperinsulinaemia in the skeletal muscle of young, healthy men (upper left panel) and its inhibition by the elevation of plasma amino acid concentration (upper right panel). Intravenous infusion of Aminoplasmal® inhibits glucose transport/ phosphorylation by ∼40 % in the early period and ∼60 % in the later period of euglycaemic-hyperinsulinaemia (Krebs et al. 2002).

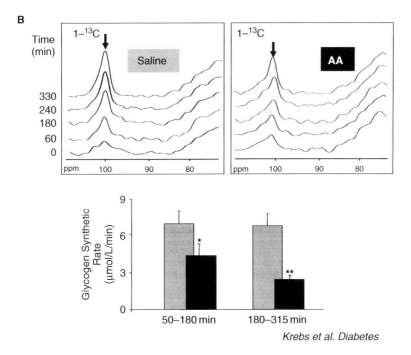

Krebs et al. Diabetes

Figure 11.8 Continued.

Mitochondrial function in insulin resistant states

Shifting the focus down the metabolic pathways to the point where lipid and glucose oxidation meet in cell, it was hypothesised that mitochondrial oxidative and phosphorylation capacity might be a contributing factor to insulin resistance and increased intracellular lipid storage: intramyocellular lipid (IMCL) content (Shulman 1999). One of the key intermediate metabolites of lipid oxidation long-chain acyl-CoA was found to be involved in the regulation of glycogen synthase (Wititsuwannakul & Kim 1977) and glucokinase (Tippett & Neet 1982) reactions and in the modulation of PCK isoforms (Faergeman & Knudsen 1997), and correlated with whole body insulin sensitivity (Ellis et al. 2000).

In accordance with previous results, recent MRS studies have found that skeletal muscle mitochondrial oxidative and phosphorylation capacity is associated with a decrease of peripheral insulin sensitivity and an increas in intramyocellular lipid content in elderly sedentary individuals (Petersen et al. 2003) and the insulin resistant offspring of T2DM patients (Petersen et al. 2005). In these experiments, skeletal muscle ATP synthesis was measured by means of a saturation transfer experiment. This method measures the flux of inorganic phosphate (Pi) in ATP synthesis, and the ATP synthesis rate, by magnetic labeling of the γ-ATP skeletal muscle pool and the decrease in the Pi pool (Figure 11.9A).

Alternative ^{31}P MRS methods can assess the mitochondrial function by measuring the recovery of the skeletal muscle phosphocreatine (PCr) pool following its depletion by well defined isometric exercise (Arnold et al. 1984; Kemp & Radda 1994; Radda et al. 1995; Newcomer & Boska 1997). This process is coupled with recovery of basal skeletal

A

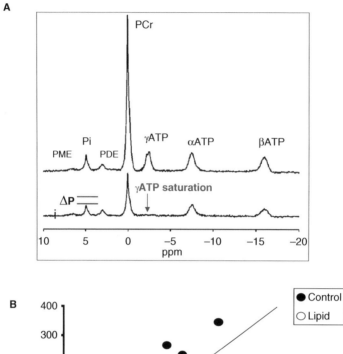

B

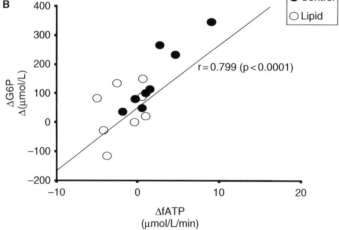

Figure 11.9 Assessment of Flux Through ATP Synthase by ^{31}P MR SpectroscopyA) ^{31}P MR spectra illustrate the saturation transfer method of ATP synthesis measurement. Frequency-selective saturation of γ-ATP resonance leads to decrease of the inorganic phosphate (Pi) resonace (lower trace). Comparing the Pi intensity with and without saturation (upper trace) yields enables us to calculate flux through ATP synthase; B) Experimental elevation of plasma FFA decreases simultaneously insulin-stimulated glucose transport/phosphorylation (glucose-6-phosphate, ΔG6P) and insulin-stimulated flux through ATP synthase (ΔfATP) show linear correlation between these two measures. (Copyright © 2006 American Diabetes Association. Reproduced with permission from Brehm A et al. (2006) *Diabetes* **55** (1), 135–140.

muscle ADP concentration, which can also be calculated from these measurements by using established models (Kemp & Radda 1994; Argov et al. 1996). These measurements were introduced in fields of exercise physiology and neuromuscular disorders (Radda et al. 1995) but defects in PCr and/or ADP recovery after one bout of isometric exercise have been recently linked to insulin resistance in T2DM patients (Scheuermann-Freestone et al. 2003), in Afro-American women (Sirikul et al. 2006) and in obese and overweight populations (Larson-Meyer et al. 2000; Newcomer et al. 2001). Even though this method cannot access basal resting mitochondrial function, it allows us to measure the mitochondrial capacity of activated muscle, and a cross-correlative link to insulin sensitivity agrees with the results of saturation transfer measurements (Figure 11.9B) (Petersen et al. 2003, 2004, 2005; Brehm et al. 2006).

The role of skeletal muscle oxidative capacity in the genesis of insulin resistance was further highlighted when it was identified as a better predictor of insulin sensitivity than either IMCL concentration or long-chain fatty acyl CoA content in a population spanning from older T2DM patients to young, well-trained athletes (Bruce et al. 2003). Impaired bioenergetic capacity of the mitochondria (Kelley et al. 2002), especially in the subsarcolemmal compartment (Ritov et al. 2005), was measured in biopsies from the skeletal muscle of T2DM patients. It was shown that experimental elevation of circulating FFA diminishes the effect of insulin stimulation on skeletal muscle ATP synthesis in parallel with the effects on glucose transport and phosphorylation (Figure 11.9B) (Brehm et al. 2006). Physical activity induced enhancement of lipid oxidation is also associated with improvements in insulin sensitivity in various study populations (Newcomer et al. 2001; Gan et al. 2003; Goodpaster et al. 2003; Menshikova et al. 2005, 2006; Larson-Meyer et al. 2006).

We can conclude that focused implementation of ^{31}P and ^{13}C MR spectroscopic techniques helped find the link between defects in mitochondrial activity/capacity, lipid oxidation and defects in whole body and/or skeletal muscle glucose metabolism.

Liver

Metabolic fluxes in healthy liver

Hepatic glucose fluxes play a pivotal role in maintaining normal glucose homeostasis in the liver. Hepatocytes can store large amounts of glucose in the form of glycogen, and rapidly release this glucose from its glycogen stores into the circulation by glycogenolysis. In addition, the liver and, to a minor extent, the kidney take up lactate, glycerol and amino acids and convert these substrates to glucose by gluconeogenesis, which also contributes to glucose production. The simultaneous nature of these processes presents a methodological obstacle, with the consequence that prior to the use of MR techniques, the relative contributions of gluconeogenesis and glycogenolysis to glucose production in humans were unknown (Figure 11.10).

Despite its low natural abundance of 1.1 %, ^{13}C can be used to measure hepatic glycogen (Rothman et al. 1991; Gruetter et al. 1994). Healthy liver usually presents with a glycogen concentration in the range of 200–400 mmol/l tissue. A large homogenous tissue volume close to the body surface can be well covered by an appropriate MR surface coil. Hepatocytes, which primarily account for glycogen metabolism, are distributed isotropically and represent ~80 % of the parenchymal volume of the liver. The rib cage, abdominal muscles and subcutaneous fat layers present anatomical obstacles that can lead to contamination of the MR signal. To overcome this, a suitable localisation technique has to be chosen. Traditionally, adapted one-dimensional inversion based or one-dimensional chemical shift imaging techniques, combined with use of surface MR probes, are applied to either suppress unwanted

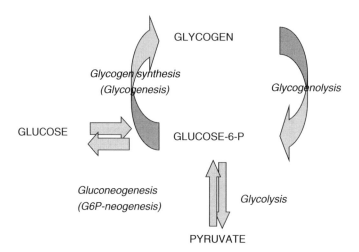

Figure 11.10 Schematic Presentation of Hepatic Glucose Metabolism The simultaneous nature of katalylic (glycogenolysis, glycolysis) and synthetic fluxes (glycogen synthesis, gluconeogenesis) provides an additional obstacle for the simple assessment of hepatic metabolism.

overlaying signals (Rothman et al. 1991) or excite and receive only liver-based MR signals (Kishore et al. 2006). Either of these techniques can be applied for a non-invasive and repetitive measurement of hepatic glycogen concentrations in real-time mode, allowing us to calculate rates of net glycogen synthesis and glycogenolysis *in vivo*.

In addition to quantification of natural abundance of ^{13}C glycogen, tracing ^{13}C incorporation into glycogen during infusion or ingestion of [1-^{13}C] enriched glucose (10–99 %) increases the sensitivity of the method by up to 100-fold. Sequential infusions of ^{13}C enriched and unlabeled glucose – so-called ^{13}C pulse-^{12}C chase experiments (Shulman et al. 1988) – allow us to assess rates of glycogen synthesis and simultaneous glycogenolysis in humans (Magnusson et al. 1994; Roden et al. 1996a; Petersen et al. 1998b; Krššák et al. 2004). In these experiments, the increment in total hepatic glycogen over time during infusion of [1-^{13}C]glucose gives the flux through glycogen synthase. To obtain an estimate of simultaneous glycogenolysis, the change in [1-^{13}C]glycogen concentration is compared with the predicted increment assuming constant flux through glycogen synthase and no glycogen breakdown. From the difference between predicted and observed glycogen concentrations, we can make a minimum estimate of simultaneous glycogenolysis, i.e. of only the glycogen that is broken down and escapes the hexose-1-phosphate pool (Figure 11.11).

In a pioneering study by Rothman et al. (1991), hepatic glucose fluxes have been monitored and quantified by combination of ^{13}C MR spectroscopy to determine glycogen concentration, magnetic resonance imaging to determine liver volume, and infusion of [3-^{3}H]glucose to determine, for the first time, glucose production over 68 hours of fasting. Initially, almost linear liver glycogen decrease, at a rate of $\sim$ 4.3 gμmol.kg bodyweight^{-1}.min^{-1}, accounted for 36 % of whole body glucose. Production proceeded overnight and hepatic glycogen reached a concentration of $\sim$250 mmol.l^{-1} at 15 h of fasting. This fasting concentration was in agreement with that of $\sim$270 mmol.l^{-1} obtained by needle biopsy (Nilsson & Hultman 1973) and was also confirmed by another group employing ^{13}C NMR spectroscopy (Beckmann et al. 1993). Thereafter, the consumption of hepatic glycogen flattened out to only about 10 %

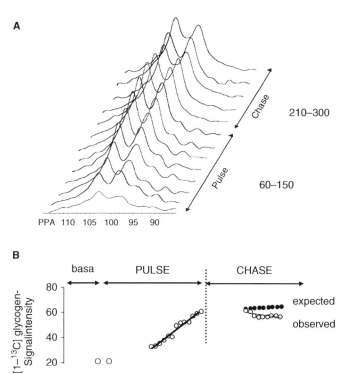

Figure 11.11 Measurements of Net Hepatic Glycogen Synthesis During Pulse-Chase ExperimentA) [1-^{13}C] MR spectra of human liver during [1-^{13}C]glucose pulse-[1-^{12}C]glucose chase experiment. A steep increase of the [1-^{13}C]glycogen signal during the infusion of labeled glucose is followed by stagnation or decrease caused by label wash-out during the infusion of unlabeled glucose; B) time course of the [1-^{13}C] glycogen signal intensity during pulse-chase experiment. The difference between expected (as without glycogenolysis) and observed (label wash-out due to glycogenolysis) signal aids in the estimation of hepatic glycogenolysis under hyperglycaemic-hyperinsulinaemic conditions.

of initial rate, between 46 h and 64 h. After 64 h, liver glycogen and volume had decreased by 83 % and 23 % respectively, and gluconeogenesis was almost exclusively (~96 %) responsible for endogenous glucose production. The high contribution of gluconeogenesis (~65 %) to glucose production, even after 22 h of fasting, is in contrast to earlier studies, which reported less than 38 % after a fast of 12–14 h (Wahren et al. 1972; Nilsson et al. 1973; Consoli et al. 1987). A later study by Petersen et al. (1999), which quantified the contribution of glycogenolysis to glucose production during the earliest hours (5–12 h) of an overnight fast following a large 1,000-kcal meal, confirmed these results, showing that net hepatic glycogenolysis (~5.8 μ mol.kg bw^{-1}.min^{-1}) contributed only ~45 % to whole body glucose production, implying that gluconeogenesis typically contributes ~50 % to the rate of whole body glucose metabolism during the early hours following a mixed meal. Studies in the postprandial state showed that ingestion of a liquid 650 kcal meal in glycogen depleted conditions after a 68 h fast increases hepatic glycogen from ~40 mmol.l^{-1} to almost 190 mmol.l^{-1}

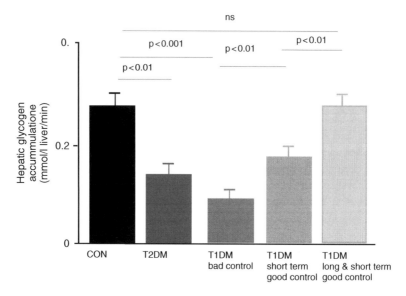

Figure 11.12   Hepatic Glycogen Accumulation in Healthy and Diabetic Patients Rates of postprandial hepatic glycogen accumulation as measured in healthy men [CON (Krššák et al. 2004)] and patients with type 2- and type 1 diabetes mellitus [T2DM (Krššák et al. 2004); T1DM (Bischof et al. 2001, 2002)]. A 50–60 % decrease in this measure was observed by natural abundance ^{13}C MR spectroscopy in both pathologies. Partial improvement was observed in type 1 diabetic patients after short term blood glucose normalisation by adjusted 24 h infusion of insulin. Combination of long and short term good metabolic control was able to restore the ability to accumulate glycogen in the liver in type 1 diabetic patients.

within three hours, yielding a net glycogenic rate of $\sim$0.8 mmol.l liver^{-1}.min^{-1} (Rothman et al. 1991). Monitoring the liver glycogen concentrations more closely after a normal overnight fast following an identically composed meal, liver glycogen increased from $\sim$200 mmol.l^{-1} to peak values of $\sim$315 mmol.l^{-1} at $\sim$5 h, giving a net rate of glycogen synthesis of 0.34 mmol.l liver^{-1}.min^{-1} (Taylor et al. 1996). Similar rates of hepatic glycogen synthesis (0.38 mmol.l liver^{-1}.min^{-1}) were observed by Krššák et al. (2004) following a test dinner (Figure 11.12). It can be calculated that $\sim$20 % of meal glucose was deposited as glycogen in the liver (Taylor et al. 1996; Krššák et al. 2004). These data are consistent with estimates of $\sim$25 % obtained after an oral 150 g glucose load by double tracer studies (Radziuk et al. 1978), splanchnic balance techniques (Katz et al. 1983) and another NMR study (Beckmann et al. 1993). A study by Hwang et al. (1995) which examined changes in hepatic glycogen content following normal eating behaviour in non-diabetic subjects observed steady step increases of hepatic glycogen stores, indicating negligible hepatic glycogenolysis. During the day, meals were ingested 5 h apart. Thus, glucose absorption from meals and gluconeogenesis account for the major part of whole body glucose appearance during daytime, while net hepatic glycogenolysis contributes to whole body glucose production only during the nighttime period.

^{13}C MR spectroscopy alone is able to quantify hepatic glycogen synthesis and glycogenolysis and thus, in combination with stable isotope dilution techniques, helps to non-invasively assess hepatic glucose fluxes in healthy liver under various conditions.

Defects of hepatic glucose metabolism in diabetes mellitus

Turning our attention to hepatic glucose fluxes following a normal meal in type 1 and type 2 diabetic patients, studies have revealed significant alterations of hepatic glycogen storage (Figure 11.12), glycogen release and gluconeogenesis in both patient groups (Taylor et al.1996; Hundal et al. 2000; Bischof et al. 2001, 2002; Singhal et al. 2002; Krššák et al. 2004). A defect in hepatic glycogen storage was observed in glucokinase deficient maturity-onset diabetes of the young 2 (MODY-2) patients, in whom the impaired hepatic glucokinase activity is held responsible for a reduction in the contribution of glucose (the direct pathway) to hepatic glycogen synthesis (Velho et al. 1996). Lower glycogen synthesis (Bischof et al. 2001, 2002; Krššák et al. 2004) and unsatisfactory suppression of endogenous glucose production (Sinha et al. 2002; Krššák et al. 2004) contribute to postprandial hyperglycaemia in both pathologies. Increased gluconeogenesis is the key to postabsorptive hyperglycaemia in T2DM (Hundal et al. 2000). Therapeutic interventions by metformin in T2DM (Hundal et al. 2000) or by insulin controlled long-term near normoglycaemia in T1DM (Bischof et al. 2002) were able to at least partially eliminate these defects and restore normal hepatic glucose fluxes.

Hormonal regulation of hepatic glucose metabolism

Hormones like insulin and glucagon are known to affect the enzymes involved in glycogen metabolism. The $[1-^{13}C]$-labeled glucose-$[1-^{12}C]$glucose chase technique was used to assess flux rates through glycogen phosphorylase in healthy humans, showing that rate of hepatic glycogen synthesis depends on portal vein insulin, requiring portal vein insulin concentration in the range of 130–170 pmol.l^{-1} for half-maximal stimulation of glycogen synthesis (Roden et al. 1996a) (Figure 11.13), which is good agreement with that for suppression of glucose production by insulin (Rizza et al.1981). Further study (Petersen et al. 1998b) trying to sort out the effects of hyperglycaemia and hyperinsulinaemia per se on hepatic glycogen metabolism showed that promotion of hepatic glycogen cycling may be the mechanism by which insulin decreases glycogenolysis and glucose production during euglycaemia. Additional stimulation of hepatic glycogen synthesis by low dose fructose infusion ($\sim$3.5 μmol.kg^{-1}.min^{-1}) during maximal insulin stimulation in healthy volunteers was measured by Petersen et al. (2001) in another pulse chase study, providing another possible therapeutic concept in both types of diabetes. The role of glucagon on hepatic glycogen cycling was studied using the $[1-^{13}C]$glucose-$[1-^{12}C]$glucose chase technique by Roden et al. (1996a) (Figure 11.13), showing that small changes in portal vein concentrations of insulin and glucagon independently affect hepatic glycogen synthesis and glycogenolysis.

Taking the above mentioned into account, differences in the postprandial hepatic glycogen metabolism in diabetic populations (Hundal et al. 2000; Bischof et al. 2001; Krššák et al. 2004) could have been caused by a decreased response in the portal insulin:glucagon ratio. In order to evaluate hepatic glucose metabolism independently of these T2DM associated alterations in postprandial metabolic and hormonal responses, we have assessed glycogen metabolism, as well as rates of EGP and whole body glucose disposal-matched conditions of hyperglycaemia, portal vein insulin:glucagon ratios and similar plasma FFA concentrations (Krššák et al. 2004). Nevertheless, $\sim$54 % reduced rates of net hepatic glycogen synthesis were still observed in T2DM (Figure 11.13). Detailed analysis of the responsive fluxes

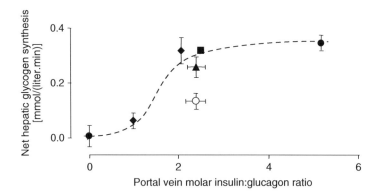

Figure 11.13 Hormonal Regulation of Hepatic Glucose Metabolism Dependence of net hepatic glycogen synthesis on the estimated molar insulin:glucagon ratio in the portal vein in type 2 diabetic (open circle) and nondiabetic humans (filled symbols: triangle: Krššák et al. 2004; diamond: Roden et al. 1996; circle: Petersen et al.; square: Cline et al. 1994) measured during hyperglycaemic-somatostatin clamp tests. T2DM presents with defect net hepatic glycogen synthesis despite comparable insulin:glucagon ratio applied in the experimental clamp study.

identified the flux through glycogen synthase as a major cause of diminished glycogen accumulation in T2DM under these conditions. During the hyperglycaemic-hyperinsulinaemic pancreatic clamp test, rates of EGP remained higher in T2DM, which is in line with persistent decreased insulin sensitivity at the level of the liver (Firth et al. 1986). On the other hand, long-term normalisation of glucose homeostasis combined with short-term tight insulin control was able to normalise rates of hepatic glycogen synthesis but not the contribution of gluconeogenesis to glycogen synthesis in type 1 diabetes (Bischof et al. 2002).

Perturbation of hepatic metabolic fluxes by substrate overabundance

Elevated circulating free fatty acids are associated with increased fasting EGP in type 2 diabetes (Hundal et al. 2000); furthermore, diminished postprandial hormonal response is not able to suppress FFA concentration to the same extent as in non-diabetic populations (Krššák et al. 2004), which again may contribute to higher postprandial EGP in T2DM (Singhal et al. 2002; Krššák et al. 2004). Studies in young, healthy volunteers have shown that an experimentally elevated FFA concentration increased gluconeogenesis (Roden et al. 2000), which led to a lower rate of hepatic glycogen breakdown (Stingl et al. 2001). However, matching insulin, glucagon, glucose and FFA concentrations during the clamp protocol in T2DM (Krššák et al. 2004) did not fully restore hepatic glycogen synthesis, indicating an additional defect besides the effects of metabolic and hormonal differences. But study focused on the effects of amino acids on hepatic glucose fluxes have shown that experimental amino acid challenge did not effect hepatic glycogenolysis but did increase gluconeogenesis, resulting in increased total endogenous glucose production (Krebs et al. 2003). In recent years the relationship between hepatic fat accumulation and whole body as well as hepatic glucose fluxes has been under detailed investigation (Krššák & Roden 2004). This issue is discussed in Chapter 13.

Brain

It is generally believed that changes in brain glucose metabolism are not directly linked to genesis of insulin resistance and type 2 diabetes mellitus, but rather that changes in brain tissue glucose uptake are due to an imbalance in glucose homeostasis. Under nonfasting conditions almost all of the energy produced and consumed by the brain derives from the catalysis of glucose (Siesjo 1978). Thus defects in glucose delivery caused by hypoglycaemia or decreased tissue perfusion and changes in glucose transport across the blood-brain barrier caused by chronic hyperglycaemia could both deteriorate brain activity, leading ultimately to dementia. Adaptations in brain energy metabolism in response to frequent hypoglycaemia were proposed as contributing to hypoglycaemia unawareness in long-term normoglycaemic type 1 diabetics. Measurements of tissue perfusion by perfusion MR imaging, brain activation by blood oxygenation level dependent (BOLD) MR imaging and energy metabolism by different MR spectroscopic techniques could all help to answer many questions we have on this subject.

Brain activity, energy metabolism and neurotransmitter cycling

Epidemiological, cross-sectional and prospective associations between T2DM and moderate cognitive impairment of memory and executive functions have been discovered and were reviewed by Pasquier et al. (2006). Both vascular and non-vascular factors were found to be the reasons for dementia in diabetes (Stewart & Liolitsa 1999). Direct study using functional BOLD MRI of brain activation has shown that hypoglycaemia induced impairment of brain function is associated with task specific localised reduction in brain activation (Rosenthal et al. 2001). Higher increase of deoxygenation, depicted as higher BOLD signal in active brain areas, can help to overcome the energy shortage caused by hypoglycaemia (Rosenthal et al. 2001) or micovascular damage in type 1 diabetic patients (Wessels et al. 2006) with retinopathy. Certain overcompensation mechanisms can be observed in ^{31}P and ^{1}H MR spectroscopic observation of energy metabolism in type 1 diabetic patients, where, in contrast to healthy volunteers, no decrease of energy buffer – phosphocreatine (Bischof et al. 2004) – and neurotransmitter – glutamine (Bischof et al. 2006) – has been observed in acute hypoglycaemia. In a similar population of type 1 diabetic patients with unawareness of hypoglycaemia, increased transport of glucose between plasma and brain tissue was detected in controlled conditions of hyperglycaemia by direct ^{1}H MR spectroscopic measurement of brain glucose (Criego et al. 2005a,b). These studies were based on previous results in which a linear relationship between plasma and brain glucose was established and validated (Gruetter et al. 1998; Choi et al. 2001; Seaquist et al. 2001). In order to increase glucose transport, in vivo studies in rat brain suggested that a mechanism of hypoglycaemia induced brain glycogen overcompensation could protect brain tissue from acute energy shortage during and following hypoglycaemia (Choi et al. 1999, 2003; Choi & Gruetter 2003). These measurements apply a robust ^{13}C MR signal localisation technique (Choi et al. 2000; Gruetter et al. 2003) that enables brain glycogen quantification, which was recently validated against biochemical measurements (Morgenthaler et al. 2006). First study in human brain (Oz et al. 2006) confirmed that brain glycogen stores exceed those of free glucose and that brain glycogen metabolism is very slow under normal conditions.

Several studies on healthy volunteers have characterised and measured fluxes in the glutamate/glutamine neurotransmitter cycle, which is critical to normal brain function and protection against excitotoxicity (Rothman 2001; de Graaf et al. 2003; Shulman et al. 2004). Using ^{13}C NMR measurements to follow ^{13}C-labeled glucose molecules into the glutamine and glutamate pool of neurons and glia (Shen et al. 1999; Gruetter et al. 2001; Lebon et al. 2002), the rates of neuronal and astroglial TCA cycle and glutamine synthesis anaplerosis could have been quantified. Most of these studies have been conducted using MR systems with higher magnetic field strengths (>2 T) and steady state physiological conditions, as well as steady state isotopic enrichment of blood plasma (Shen et al. 1999; Gruetter et al. 2001; Lebon et al. 2002), but a clinical approach using simple infusion of [1-^{13}C]glucose (Bluml et al. 2001; Moreno et al. 2001) and/or [1-^{13}C]acetate solution (Bluml et al. 2002) and a clinically available 1.5 T MR system also successfully assessed brain glucose metabolism (Bluml et al. 2001; Moreno et al. 2001) and astroglial TCA cycle (Bluml et al. 2002). Using this simpler approach, defect abnormalities in the ^{13}C enrichment pattern of brain metabolites were observed in pediatric patients with leukodystrophies and mitochondrial disorders (Bluml et al. 2001) and disturbed neurotransmitter glutamate/glutamine cycling in chronic hepatic encephalopathy (Bluml et al. 2001). Even though direct ^{13}C MRS provides excellent spectral resolution, allowing for detailed ^{13}C enrichment analysis, its inherent low sensitivity limits the signal detection to relatively large volumes. Several combined [1]H-^{13}C MR techniques, which take advantage of magnetisation transfer between highly abundant and highly sensitive protons and ^{13}C nuclei in specific ^{13}C-labeled chemical bounds, provide tissue specific localisation of neurotrasmitter studies (Mason et al. 1999, 2003; Shen et al. 1999; Chen et al. 2001; Gruetter et al. 2001; Lebon et al. 2002; Pan et al. 2002). Using this approach in functional studies, some experiments have been designed and performed to measure TCA cycle activity in healthy cortex during visual stimulation (Chen et al. 2001; Chhina et al. 2001). These experiments provided evidence for almost 50 % increase of oxidative glucose consumption in the visual cortex during activation. However, none of these elaborate techniques have been applied in human studies focusing on acute or chronic effects of hypo- or hyperglycaemia.

Conclusion

Modern methods of magnetic resonance imaging and spectroscopy have been able to open an *in vivo* window on skeletal muscle and hepatic glucose uptake and homeostasis, as well as on skeletal muscle mitochondrial activity. The results of these elaborate studies could quantify defects of glucose metabolism in both skeletal muscle and liver. This knowledge is proving helpful in phenotyping the metabolic syndrome, type 2 and type 1 diabetes, and these measurements enable us to monitor the response to insulin sensitising and/or lipid reduction therapies. Meanwhile, pilot studies suggest that overcompensating mechanisms are operative in the brain tissue of diabetic patients.

References

Anderwald, C, Bernroider, E, Krššák, M, Stingl, H, Brehm, A, Bischof, M G, Nowotny, P, Roden, M, Waldhausl, W (2002) Effects of insulin treatment in type 2 diabetic patients on intracellular lipid content in liver and skeletal muscle, *Diabetes*, **51**, 10, 3025–3032

Argov, Z, De Stefano, N, Arnold, D L (1996) ADP recovery after a brief ischemic exercise in normal and diseased human muscle – a 31P MRS study, *NMR Biomed*, **9**, 4, 165–172

Arnold, D L, Matthews, P M, Radda, G K (1984) Metabolic recovery after exercise and the assessment of mitochondrial function in vivo in human skeletal muscle by means of 31P NMR, *Magn Reson Med*, **1**, 3, 307–315

Beckmann, N, Fried, R, Turkalj, I, Seelig, J, Keller, U, Stalder, G (1993) Noninvasive observation of hepatic glycogen formation in man by 13C MRS after oral and intravenous glucose administration, *Magn Reson Med*, **29**, 5, 583–590

Bischof, M G, Bernroider, E, Krššák, M, Krebs, M, Stingl, H, Nowotny, P, Yu, C, Shulman, G I, Waldhausl, W, Roden, M (2002) Hepatic glycogen metabolism in type 1 diabetes after long-term near normoglycemia, *Diabetes*, **51**, 1, 49–54

Bischof, M G, Brehm, A, Bernroider, E, Krššák, M, Mlynarik, V, Krebs, M, Roden, M (2006) Cerebral glutamate metabolism during hypoglycaemia in healthy and type 1 diabetic humans, *Eur J Clin Invest*, **36**, 3, 164–169

Bischof, M G, Krššák, M, Krebs, M, Bernroider, E, Stingl, H, Waldhausl, W, Roden, M (2001) Effects of short-term improvement of insulin treatment and glycemia on hepatic glycogen metabolism in type 1 diabetes, *Diabetes*, **50**, 2, 392–398

Bischof, M G, Mlynarik, V, Brehm, A, Bernroider, E, Krššák, M, Bauer, E, Madl, C, Bayerle-Eder, M, Waldhausl, W, Roden, M (2004) Brain energy metabolism during hypoglycaemia in healthy and type 1 diabetic subjects, *Diabetologia*, **47**, 4, 648–651

Bluml, S, Moreno, A, Hwang, J H, Ross, B D (2001) 1-(13)C glucose magnetic resonance spectroscopy of pediatric and adult brain disorders, *NMR Biomed*, **14**, 1, 19–32

Bluml, S, Moreno-Torres, A, Ross, B D (2001) [1–13C]glucose MRS in chronic hepatic encephalopathy in man, *Magn ResonMed*, **45**, 6, 981–993

Bluml, S, Moreno-Torres, A, Shic, F, Nguy, C H, Ross, B D (2002) Tricarboxylic acid cycle of glia in the in vivo human brain, *NMR Biomed*, **15**, 1, 1–5

Borgs, M, Van Hecke, P, Overloop, K, Decanniere, C, Van Huffel, S, Stalmans, W, Vanstapel, F (1993) In situ 13C NMR quantification of hepatic glycogen, *NMR Biomed*, **6**, 6, 371–376

Brehm, A, Krššák, M, Schmid, A I, Nowotny, P, Waldhausl, W, Roden, M (2006) Increased lipid availability impairs insulin-stimulated ATP synthesis in human skeletal muscle, *Diabetes*, **55**, 1, 136–140

Bruce, C R, Anderson, M J, Carey, A L, Newman, D G, Bonen, A, Kriketos, A D, Cooney, G J, Hawley, J A (2003) Muscle oxidative capacity is a better predictor of insulin sensitivity than lipid status, *J Clin Endocrinol Metab*, **88**, 11, 5444–5451

Carey, P E, Halliday, J, Snaar, J E, Morris, P G, Taylor, R (2003) Direct assessment of muscle glycogen storage after mixed meals in normal and type 2 diabetic subjects, *Am J Physiol Endocrinol Metab*, **284**, 4, E688–E694

Chen, W, Zhu, X H, Gruetter, R, Seaquist, E R, Adriany, G, Ugurbil, K (2001) Study of tricarboxylic acid cycle flux changes in human visual cortex during hemifield visual stimulation using (1)H-[(13)C] MRS and fMRI, *Magn Reson Med*, **45**, 3, 349–355

Chhina, N, Kuestermann, E, Halliday, J, Simpson, L J, Macdonald, I A, Bachelard, H S, Morris, P G (2001) Measurement of human tricarboxylic acid cycle rates during visual activation by (13)C magnetic resonance spectroscopy, *J Neurosci Res*, **66**, 5, 737–746

Choi, I Y Gruetter, R (2003) In vivo 13C NMR assessment of brain glycogen concentration and turnover in the awake rat, *Neurochem Int*, **43**, 4–5, 317–322

Choi, I Y, Lee, S P, Kim, S G, Gruetter, R (2001) In vivo measurements of brain glucose transport using the reversible Michaelis-Menten model and simultaneous measurements of cerebral blood flow changes during hypoglycemia, *J Cereb Blood Flow Metab*, **21**, 6, 653–663

Choi, I Y, Seaquist, E R, Gruetter, R (2003) Effect of hypoglycemia on brain glycogen metabolism in vivo, *J Neurosci Res*, **72**, 1, 25–32

Choi, I Y, Tkac, I, Gruetter, R (2000) Single-shot, three-dimensional non-echo localization method for in vivo NMR spectroscopy, *Magn Reson Med*, **44**, 3, 387–394

Choi, I Y, Tkac, I, Ugurbil, K, Gruetter, R (1999) Noninvasive measurements of [1–(13)C]glycogen concentrations and metabolism in rat brain in vivo, *J Neurochem*, **73**, 3, 1300–1308

Cline, G W, Jucker, B M, Trajanoski, Z, Rennings, A J, Shulman, G I (1998) A novel 13C NMR method to assess intracellular glucose concentration in muscle, in vivo, *Am J Physiol*, **274**, 2 Pt 1, E381–E389

Cline, G W, Petersen, K F, Krššák, M, Shen, J, Hundal, R S, Trajanoski, Z, Inzucchi, S, Dresner, A, Rothman, D L, Shulman, G I (1999) Impaired glucose transport as a cause of decreased insulin-stimulated muscle glycogen synthesis in type 2 diabetes, *N Engl J Med*, **341**, 4, 240–246

Consoli, A, Kennedy, F, Miles, J, Gerich, J (1987) Determination of Krebs cycle metabolic carbon exchange in vivo and its use to estimate the individual contributions of gluconeogenesis and glycogenolysis to overall glucose output in man, *J Clin Invest*, **80**, 5, 1303–1310

Criego, A B, Tkac, I, Kumar, A, Thomas, W, Gruetter, R, Seaquist, E R (2005a) Brain glucose concentrations in healthy humans subjected to recurrent hypoglycemia, *J Neurosci Res*, **82**, 4, 525–530

Criego, A B, Tkac, I, Kumar, A, Thomas, W, Gruetter, R, Seaquist, E R (2005b) Brain glucose concentrations in patients with type 1 diabetes and hypoglycemia unawareness, *J Neurosci Res*, **79**, 1–2, 42–47

de Graaf, R A, Mason, G F, Patel, A B, Behar, K L, Rothman, D L (2003) In vivo 1H-[13C]-NMR spectroscopy of cerebral metabolism, *NMR Biomed*, **16**, 6–7, 339–357

Defronzo, R A (1988) Lilly lecture 1987 The triumvirate: beta-cell, muscle, liver A collusion responsible for NIDDM, *Diabetes*, **37**, 6, 667–687

Delmas-Beauvieux, M C, Quesson, B, Thiaudiere, E, Gallis, J L, Canioni, P, Gin, H (1999) 13C nuclear magnetic resonance study of glycogen resynthesis in muscle after glycogen-depleting exercise in healthy men receiving an infusion of lipid emulsion, *Diabetes*, **48**, 2, 327–333

Dresner, A, Laurent, D, Marcucci, M, Griffin, M E, Dufour, S, Cline, G W, Slezak, L A, Andersen, D K, Hundal, R S, Rothman, D L, Petersen, K F, Shulman, G I (1999) Effects of free fatty acids on glucose transport and IRS-1-associated phosphatidylinositol 3-kinase activity, *J Clin Invest*, **103**, 2, 253–259

Ellis, B A, Poynten, A, Lowy, A J, Furler, S M, Chisholm, D J, Kraegen, E W, Cooney, G J (2000) Long-chain acyl-CoA esters as indicators of lipid metabolism and insulin sensitivity in rat and human muscle, *Am J Physiol Endocrinol Metab*, **279**, 3, pp E554–E560

Faergeman, N J Knudsen, J (1997) Role of long-chain fatty acyl-CoA esters in the regulation of metabolism and in cell signalling, *BiochemJ*, **323** (Pt 1), 1–12

Felig, P, Marliss, E, Cahill, G F, Jr (1969) Plasma amiacid levels and insulin secretion in obesity, *N Engl J Med*, **281**, 15, 811–816

Firth, R G, Bell, P M, Marsh, H M, Hansen, I, Rizza, R A (1986) Postprandial hyperglycemia in patients with noninsulin-dependent diabetes mellitus Role of hepatic and extrahepatic tissues, *J Clin Invest*, **77**, 5, 1525–1532

Freeman, R (2003) *Magnetic resonance in chemistry and medicine*, first edn, Oxford University Press Inc, New York

Gadian, D G (1995) *NMR and its applications to living systems* Oxford University Press Inc, New York

Gan, S K, Kriketos, A D, Ellis, B A, Thompson, C H, Kraegen, E W, Chisholm, D J (2003) Changes in aerobic capacity and visceral fat but not myocyte lipid levels predict increased insulin action after exercise in overweight and obese men, *Diabetes Care*, **26**, 6, 1706–1713

Goodpaster, B H, Katsiaras, A, Kelley, D E (2003) Enhanced fat oxidation through physical activity is associated with improvements in insulin sensitivity in obesity, *Diabetes*, **52**, 9, 2191–2197

Griffin, M E, Marcucci, M J, Cline, G W, Bell, K, Barucci, N, Lee, D, Goodyear, L J, Kraegen, E W, White, M F, Shulman, G I (1999) Free fatty acid-induced insulin resistance is associated with activation of protein kinase C theta and alterations in the insulin signaling cascade, *Diabetes*, **48**, 6, 1270–1274

Gruetter, R, Adriany, G, Choi, I Y, Henry, P G, Lei, H, Oz, G (2003) Localized in vivo 13C NMR spectroscopy of the brain, *NMR Bio med*, **16**, 6–7, 313–338

Gruetter, R, Magnusson, I, Rothman, D L, Avison, M J, Shulman, R G, Shulman, G I (1994) Validation of 13C NMR measurements of liver glycogen in vivo, *Magn Reson Med*, **31**, 6, 583–588

Gruetter, R, Prolla, T A, Shulman, R G (1991) 13C NMR visibility of rabbit muscle glycogen in vivo, *Magn Reson Med*, **20**, 2, 327–332

Gruetter, R, Seaquist, E R, Ugurbil, K (2001) A mathematical model of compartmentalized neuro-transmitter metabolism in the human brain, *Am J Physiol Endocrinol Metab*, **281**, 1, E100–E112

Gruetter, R, Ugurbil, K, Seaquist, E R (1998) Steady-state cerebral glucose concentrations and transport in the human brain, *J Neurochem*, **70**, 1, 397–408

Hundal, R S, Krššák, M, Dufour, S, Laurent, D, Lebon, V, Chandramouli, V, Inzucchi, S E, Schumann, W C, Petersen, K F, Landau, B R, Shulman, G I (2000) Mechanism by which metformin reduces glucose production in type 2 diabetes, *Diabetes*, **49**, 12, 2063–2069

Hwang, J H, Perseghin, G, Rothman, D L, Cline, G W, Magnusson, I, Petersen, K F, Shulman, G I (1995) Impaired net hepatic glycogen synthesis in insulin-dependent diabetic subjects during mixed meal ingestion A 13C nuclear magnetic resonance spectroscopy study, *J Clin Invest*, **95**, 2, 783–787

Jacob, S, Machann, J, Rett, K, Brechtel, K, Volk, A, Renn, W, Maerker, E, Matthaei, S, Schick, F, Claussen, C D, Haring, H U (1999) Association of increased intramyocellular lipid content with insulin resistance in lean nondiabetic offspring of type 2 diabetic subjects, *Diabetes*, **48**, 5, 1113–1119

Jue, T, Rothman, D L, Shulman, G I, Tavitian, B A, Defronzo, R A, Shulman, R G (1989) Direct observation of glycogen synthesis in human muscle with 13C NMR, *Proc Natl Acad Sci USA*, **86**, 12, 4489–4491

Kacser, H Burns, J A (1973) The control of flux, *Symp Soc Exp Biol*, **27**, 65–104

Katz, L D, Glickman, M G, Rapoport, S, Ferrannini, E, Defronzo, R A (1983) Splanchnic and peripheral disposal of oral glucose in man, *Diabetes*, **32**, 7, 675–679

Kelley, D E, He, J, Menshikova, E V, Ritov, V B (2002) Dysfunction of mitochondria in human skeletal muscle in type 2 diabetes, *Diabetes*, **51**, 10, 2944–2950

Kemp, G J Radda, G K (1994) Quantitative interpretation of bioenergetic data from 31P and 1H magnetic resonance spectroscopic studies of skeletal muscle: an analytical review, *Magn Reson Q*, **10**, 1, 43–63

Kishore, P, Gabriely, I, Cui, M H, Di Vito, J, Gajavelli, S, Hwang, J H, Shamoon, H (2006) Role of hepatic glycogen breakdown in defective counterregulation of hypoglycemia in intensively treated type 1 diabetes, *Diabetes*, **55**, 3, 659–666

Krebs, M, Brehm, A, Krššák, M, Anderwald, C, Bernroider, E, Nowotny, P, Roth, E, Chandramouli, V, Landau, B R, Waldhausl, W, Roden, M (2003) Direct and indirect effects of amiacids on hepatic glucose metabolism in humans, *Diabetologia*, **46**, 7, 917–925

Krebs, M, Krššák, M, Bernroider, E, Anderwald, C, Brehm, A, Meyerspeer, M, Nowotny, P, Roth, E, Waldhausl, W, Roden, M (2002) Mechanism of amiacid-induced skeletal muscle insulin resistance in humans, *Diabetes*, **51**, 3, 599–605

Krebs, M, Krššák, M, Nowotny, P, Weghuber, D, Gruber, S, Mlynarik, V, Bischof, M, Stingl, H, Furnsinn, C, Waldhausl, W, Roden, M (2001) Free fatty acids inhibit the glucose-stimulated increase of intramuscular glucose-6-phosphate concentration in humans, *J Clin Endocrinol Metab*, **86**, 5, 2153–2160

Krššák, M, Brehm, A, Bernroider, E, Anderwald, C, Nowotny, P, Dalla, M C, Cobelli, C, Cline, G W, Shulman, G I, Waldhausl, W, Roden, M (2004) Alterations in postprandial hepatic glycogen metabolism in type 2 diabetes, *Diabetes*, **53**, 12, 3048–3056

Krššák, M, Falk, P K, Dresner, A, DiPietro, L, Vogel, S M, Rothman, D L, Roden, M, Shulman, G I (1999) Intramyocellular lipid concentrations are correlated with insulin sensitivity in humans: a 1H NMR spectroscopy study, *Diabetologia*, **42**, 1, 113–116

Krššák, M Roden, M (2004) The role of lipid accumulation in liver and muscle for insulin resistance and type 2 diabetes mellitus in humans, *Rev Endocr Metab Disord*, **5**, 2, 127–134

Larson-Meyer, D E, Heilbronn, L K, Redman, L M, Newcomer, B R, Frisard, M I, Anton, S, Smith, S R, Alfonso, A, Ravussin, E (2006) Effect of calorie restriction with or without exercise on insulin sensitivity, beta-cell function, fat cell size, and ectopic lipid in overweight subjects, *Diabetes Care*, **29**, 6, 1337–1344

Larson-Meyer, D E, Newcomer, B R, Hunter, G R, McLean, J E, Hetherington, H P, Weinsier, R L (2000) Effect of weight reduction, obesity predisposition, and aerobic fitness on skeletal muscle mitochondrial function, *Am J Physiol Endocrinol Metab*, **278**, 1, p E153–E161

Lebon, V, Petersen, K F, Cline, G W, Shen, J, Mason, G F, Dufour, S, Behar, K L, Shulman, G I, Rothman, D L (2002) Astroglial contribution to brain energy metabolism in humans revealed by 13C nuclear magnetic resonance spectroscopy: elucidation of the dominant pathway for neurotransmitter glutamate repletion and measurement of astrocytic oxidative metabolism, *J Neurosci*, **22**, 5, 1523–1531

Linn, T, Santosa, B, Gronemeyer, D, Aygen, S, Scholz, N, Busch, M, Bretzel, R G (2000) Effect of long-term dietary protein intake on glucose metabolism in humans, *Diabetologia*, **43**, 10, 1257–1265

Magnusson, I, Rothman, D L, Jucker, B, Cline, G W, Shulman, R G, Shulman, G I (1994) Liver glycogen turnover in fed and fasted humans, *Am J Physiol*, **266**, 5 Pt 1, p E796–E803

Mason, G F, Falk, P K, de Graaf, R A, Kanamatsu, T, Otsuki, T, Shulman, G I, Rothman, D L (2003) A comparison of (13)C NMR measurements of the rates of glutamine synthesis and the tricarboxylic acid cycle during oral and intravenous administration of [1-(13)C]glucose, *Brain Res Brain Res Protoc*, **10**, 3, 181–190

Mason, G F, Pan, J W, Chu, W J, Newcomer, B R, Zhang, Y, Orr, R, Hetherington, H P (1999) Measurement of the tricarboxylic acid cycle rate in human grey and white matter in vivo by 1H-[13C] magnetic resonance spectroscopy at 41T, *J Cereb Blood Flow Metab*, **19**, 11, 1179–1188

Menshikova, E V, Ritov, V B, Fairfull, L, Ferrell, R E, Kelley, D E, Goodpaster, B H (2006) Effects of exercise on mitochondrial content and function in aging human skeletal muscle, *J Gerontol A Biol Sci Med Sci*, **61**, 6, 534–540

Menshikova, E V, Ritov, V B, Toledo, F G, Ferrell, R E, Goodpaster, B H, Kelley, D E (2005) Effects of weight loss and physical activity on skeletal muscle mitochondrial function in obesity, *Am J Physiol Endocrinol Metab*, **288**, 4, E818–E825

Mierisova, S Ala-Korpela, M (2001) MR spectroscopy quantitation: a review of frequency domain methods, *NMR Biomed*, **14**, 4, 247–259

Mierisova, S, van den, B A, Tkac, I, Van Hecke, P, Vanhamme, L, Liptaj, T (1998) New approach for quantitation of short echo time in vivo 1H MR spectra of brain using AMARES, *NMR Biomed*, **11**, 1, 32–39

Moreno, A, Bluml, S, Hwang, J H, Ross, B D (2001) Alternative 1-(13)C glucose infusion protocols for clinical (13)C MRS examinations of the brain, *Magn Reson Med*, **46**, 1, 39–48

Morgenthaler, F D, Koski, D M, Kraftsik, R, Henry, P G, Gruetter, R (2006) Biochemical quantification of total brain glycogen concentration in rats under different glycemic states, *Neurochem Int*, **48**, 6–7, 616–622

Newcomer, B R Boska, M D (1997) Adenosine triphosphate production rates, metabolic economy calculations, pH, phosphomonoesters, phosphodiesters, and force output during short-duration maximal isometric plantar flexion exercises and repeated maximal isometric plantar flexion exercises, *Muscle Nerve*, **20**, 3, 336–346

Newcomer, B R, Larson-Meyer, D E, Hunter, G R, Weinsier, R L (2001) Skeletal muscle metabolism in overweight and post-overweight women: an isometric exercise study using (31)P magnetic resonance spectroscopy, *Int J Obes Relat Metab Disord*, **25**, 9, 1309–1315

Nilsson, L H, Furst, P, Hultman, E (1973) Carbohydrate metabolism of the liver in normal man under varying dietary conditions, *Scand J Clin Lab Invest*, **32**, 4, 331–337

Nilsson, L H Hultman, E (1973) Liver glycogen in man – the effect of total starvation or a carbohydrate-poor diet followed by carbohydrate refeeding, *Scand J Clin Lab Invest*, **32**, 4, 325–330

Overloop, K, Vanstapel, F, Van Hecke, P (1996) 13C-NMR relaxation in glycogen, *Magn Reson Med*, **36**, 1, 45–51

Oz, G, Seaquist, E R, Kumar, A, Criego, A B, Benedict, L E, Rao, J P, Henry, P G, Van de Moortele, P F, Gruetter, R (2006) Human Brain Glycogen Content and Metabolism: Implications on its Role in Brain Energy Metabolism, *Am J Physiol Endocrinol Metab*

Pan, J W, de Graaf, R A, Petersen, K F, Shulman, G I, Hetherington, H P, Rothman, D L (2002) [2,4-13 C2]-beta-Hydroxybutyrate metabolism in human brain, *J Cereb Blood Flow Metab*, **22**, 7, 890–898

Pasquier, F, Boulogne, A, Leys, D, Fontaine, P (2006) Diabetes mellitus and dementia, *Diabetes Metab*, **32**, 5 Pt 1, 403–414

Perseghin, G, Price, T B, Petersen, K F, Roden, M, Cline, G W, Gerow, K, Rothman, D L, Shulman, G I (1996) Increased glucose transport-phosphorylation and muscle glycogen synthesis after exercise training in insulin-resistant subjects, *N Engl J Med*, **335**, 18, 1357–1362

Perseghin, G, Scifo, P, De Cobelli, F, Pagliato, E, Battezzati, A, Arcelloni, C, Vanzulli, A, Testolin, G, Pozza, G, Del Maschio, A, Luzi, L (1999) Intramyocellular triglyceride content is a determinant of in vivo insulin resistance in humans: a 1H-13C nuclear magnetic resonance spectroscopy assessment in offspring of type 2 diabetic parents, *Diabetes*, **48**, 8, 1600–1606

Petersen, K F, Befroy, D, Dufour, S, Dziura, J, Ariyan, C, Rothman, D L, DiPietro, L, Cline, G W, Shulman, G I (2003) Mitochondrial dysfunction in the elderly: possible role in insulin resistance, *Science*, **300**, 5622, 1140–1142

Petersen, K F, Dufour, S, Befroy, D, Garcia, R, Shulman, G I (2004) Impaired mitochondrial activity in the insulin-resistant offspring of patients with type 2 diabetes, *N Engl J Med*, **350**, 7, 664–671

Petersen, K F, Dufour, S, Shulman, G I (2005) Decreased insulin-stimulated ATP synthesis and phosphate transport in muscle of insulin-resistant offspring of type 2 diabetic parents, *PLoS Med*, **2**, 9, E233

Petersen, K F, Hendler, R, Price, T, Perseghin, G, Rothman, D L, Held, N, Amatruda, J M, Shulman, G I (1998a) 13C/31P NMR studies on the mechanism of insulin resistance in obesity, *Diabetes*, **47**, 3, 381–386

Petersen, K F, Krššák, M, Inzucchi, S, Cline, G W, Dufour, S, Shulman, G I (2000) Mechanism of troglitazone action in type 2 diabetes, *Diabetes*, **49**, 5, 827–831

Petersen, K F, Krššák, M, Navarro, V, Chandramouli, V, Hundal, R, Schumann, W C, Landau, B R, Shulman, G I (1999) Contributions of net hepatic glycogenolysis and gluconeogenesis to glucose production in cirrhosis, *Am J Physiol*, **276**, 3 Pt 1, p E529–E535

Petersen, K F, Laurent, D, Rothman, D L, Cline, G W, Shulman, G I (1998b) Mechanism by which glucose and insulin inhibit net hepatic glycogenolysis in humans, *J Clin Invest*, **101**, 6, 1203–1209

Petersen, K F, Laurent, D, Yu, C, Cline, G W, Shulman, G I (2001) Stimulating effects of low-dose fructose on insulin-stimulated hepatic glycogen synthesis in humans, *Diabetes*, **50**, 6, 1263–1268

Price, T B, Perseghin, G, Duleba, A, Chen, W, Chase, J, Rothman, D L, Shulman, R G, Shulman, G I (1996) NMR studies of muscle glycogen synthesis in insulin-resistant offspring of parents with non-insulin-dependent diabetes mellitus immediately after glycogen-depleting exercise, *Proc Natl Acad Sci USA*, **93**, 11, 5329–5334

Provencher, S W (1993) Estimation of metabolite concentrations from localized in vivo proton NMR spectra, *Magn Reson Med*, **30**, 6, 672–679

Provencher, S W (2001) Automatic quantitation of localized in vivo 1H spectra with LCModel, *NMR Bio med*, **14**, 4, 260–264

Radda, G K, Odoom, J, Kemp, G, Taylor, D J, Thompson, C, Styles, P (1995) Assessment of mitochondrial function and control in normal and diseased states, *Biochim Biophys Acta*, **1271**, 1, 15–19

Radziuk, J, McDonald, T J, Rubenstein, D, Dupre, J (1978) Initial splanchnic extraction of ingested glucose in normal man, *Metabolism*, **27**, 6, 657–669

Randle, P J, Garland, P B, Hales, C N, Newsholme, E A (1963) The glucose fatty-acid cycle Its role in insulin sensitivity and the metabolic disturbances of diabetes mellitus, *Lancet*, **1**, 785–789

Ritov, V B, Menshikova, E V, He, J, Ferrell, R E, Goodpaster, B H, Kelley, D E (2005) Deficiency of subsarcolemmal mitochondria in obesity and type 2 diabetes, *Diabetes*, **54**, 1, 8–14

Rizza, R A, Mandarino, L J, Gerich, J E (1981) Dose-response characteristics for effects of insulin on production and utilization of glucose in man, *Am J Physiol*, **240**, 6, E630–E639

Roden, M, Krššák, M, Stingl, H, Gruber, S, Hofer, A, Furnsinn, C, Moser, E, Waldhausl, W (1999) Rapid impairment of skeletal muscle glucose transport/phosphorylation by free fatty acids in humans, *Diabetes*, **48**, 2, 358–364

Roden, M, Perseghin, G, Petersen, K F, Hwang, J H, Cline, G W, Gerow, K, Rothman, D L, Shulman, G I (1996a) The roles of insulin and glucagon in the regulation of hepatic glycogen synthesis and turnover in humans, *J Clin Invest*, **97**, 3, 642–648

Roden, M, Price, T B, Perseghin, G, Petersen, K F, Rothman, D L, Cline, G W, Shulman, G I (1996b) Mechanism of free fatty acid-induced insulin resistance in humans, *J Clin Invest*, **97**, 12, 2859–2865

Roden, M, Stingl, H, Chandramouli, V, Schumann, W C, Hofer, A, Landau, B R, Nowotny, P, Waldhausl, W, Shulman, G I (2000) Effects of free fatty acid elevation on postabsorptive endogenous glucose production and gluconeogenesis in humans, *Diabetes*, **49**, 5, 701–707

Rosenthal, J M, Amiel, S A, Yaguez, L, Bullmore, E, Hopkins, D, Evans, M, Pernet, A, Reid, H, Giampietro, V, Andrew, C M, Suckling, J, Simmons, A, Williams, S C (2001) The effect of acute hypoglycemia on brain function and activation: a functional magnetic resonance imaging study, *Diabetes*, **50**, 7, 1618–1626

Rothman, D L (2001) Studies of metabolic compartmentation and glucose transport using in vivo MRS, *NMR Bio med*, **14**, 2, 149–160

Rothman, D L, Magnusson, I, Cline, G, Gerard, D, Kahn, C R, Shulman, R G, Shulman, G I (1995) Decreased muscle glucose transport/phosphorylation is an early defect in the pathogenesis of non-insulin-dependent diabetes mellitus, *Proc Natl Acad Sci USA*, **92**, 4, 983–987

Rothman, D L, Magnusson, I, Katz, L D, Shulman, R G, Shulman, G I (1991) Quantitation of hepatic glycogenolysis and gluconeogenesis in fasting humans with 13C NMR, *Science*, **254**, 5031, 573–576

Rothman, D L, Shulman, R G, Shulman, G I (1991) Nmr studies of muscle glycogen synthesis in normal and non-insulin-dependent diabetic subjects, *Bio Chem Soc Trans*, **19**, 4, 992–994

Rothman, D L, Shulman, R G, Shulman, G I (1992) 31P nuclear magnetic resonance measurements of muscle glucose-6-phosphate Evidence for reduced insulin-dependent muscle glucose transport or phosphorylation activity in non-insulin-dependent diabetes mellitus, *J Clin Invest*, **89**, 4, 1069–1075

Roussel, R, Carlier, P G, Robert, J J, Velho, G, Bloch, G (1998) 13C/31P NMR studies of glucose transport in human skeletal muscle, *Proc Natl Acad Sci USA*, **95**, 3, 1313–1318

Roussel, R, Carlier, P G, Wary, C, Velho, G, Bloch, G (1997) Evidence for 100 % 13C NMR visibility of glucose in human skeletal muscle, *Magn Reson Med*, **37**, 6, 821–824

Roussel, R, Velho, G, Carlier, P G, Jouvensal, L, Bloch, G (1996) In vivo NMR evidence for moderate glucose accumulation in human skeletal muscle during hyperglycemia, *Am J Physiol*, **271**, 3 Pt 1, E434–E438

Scheuermann-Freestone, M, Madsen, P L, Manners, D, Blamire, A M, Buckingham, R E, Styles, P, Radda, G K, Neubauer, S, Clarke, K (2003) Abnormal cardiac and skeletal muscle energy metabolism in patients with type 2 diabetes, *Circulation*, **107**, 24, 3040–3046

Seaquist, E R, Damberg, G S, Tkac, I, Gruetter, R (2001) The effect of insulin on in vivo cerebral glucose concentrations and rates of glucose transport/metabolism in humans, *Diabetes*, **50**, 10, 2203–2209

Serlie, M J, De Haan, J H, Tack, C J, Verberne, H J, Ackermans, M T, Heerschap, A, Sauerwein, H P (2005) Glycogen synthesis in human gastrocnemius muscle is not representative of whole-body muscle glycogen synthesis, *Diabetes*, **54**, 5, 1277–1282

Shen, J, Petersen, K F, Behar, K L, Brown, P, Nixon, T W, Mason, G F, Petroff, O A, Shulman, G I, Shulman, R G, Rothman, D L (1999) Determination of the rate of the glutamate/glutamine cycle in the human brain by in vivo 13C NMR, *Proc Natl Acad Sci USA*, **96**, 14, 8235–8240

Shulman, G I (1999) Cellular mechanisms of insulin resistance in humans, *Am J Cardiol*, **84**, 1A, 3J–10J

Shulman, G I, Rothman, D L, Chung, Y, Rossetti, L, Petit, W A, Jr, Barrett, E J, Shulman, R G (1988) 13C NMR studies of glycogen turnover in the perfused rat liver, *J Biol Chem*, **263**, 11, 5027–5029

Shulman, G I, Rothman, D L, Jue, T, Stein, P, Defronzo, R A, Shulman, R G (1990) Quantitation of muscle glycogen synthesis in normal subjects and subjects with non-insulin-dependent diabetes by 13C nuclear magnetic resonance spectroscopy, *N Engl J Med*, **322**, 4, 223–228

Shulman, R G (1996) Nuclear magnetic resonance studies of glucose metabolism in non-insulin-dependent diabetes mellitus subjects, *Mol Med*, **2**, 5, 533–540

Shulman, R G, Rothman, D L, Behar, K L, Hyder, F (2004) Energetic basis of brain activity: implications for neuroimaging, *Trends Neurosci*, **27**, 8, 489–495

Siesjo, B K (1978) *Brain energy metabolism* Wiley, New York

Singhal, P, Caumo, A, Carey, P E, Cobelli, C, Taylor, R (2002) Regulation of endogenous glucose production after a mixed meal in type 2 diabetes, *Am J Physiol Endocrinol Metab*, **283**, 2, E275–E283

Sinha, R, Dufour, S, Petersen, K F, Lebon, V, Enoksson, S, Ma, Y Z, Savoye, M, Rothman, D L, Shulman, G I, Caprio, S (2002) Assessment of skeletal muscle triglyceride content by (1)H nuclear magnetic resonance spectroscopy in lean and obese adolescents: relationships to insulin sensitivity, total body fat, and central adiposity, *Diabetes*, **51**, 4, 1022–1027

Sirikul, B, Gower, B A, Hunter, G R, Larson-Meyer, D E, Newcomer, B R (2006) Relationship between insulin sensitivity and in vivo mitochondrial function in skeletal muscle, *Am J Physiol Endocrinol Metab*, **291**, 4, E724–E728

Stewart, R Liolitsa, D (1999) Type 2 diabetes mellitus, cognitive impairment and dementia, *Diabet Med*, **16**, 2, 93–112

Stingl, H, Krššák, M, Krebs, M, Bischof, M G, Nowotny, P, Furnsinn, C, Shulman, G I, Waldhausl, W, Roden, M (2001) Lipid-dependent control of hepatic glycogen stores in healthy humans, *Diabetologia*, **44**, 1, 48–54

Taylor, R, Magnusson, I, Rothman, D L, Cline, G W, Caumo, A, Cobelli, C, Shulman, G I (1996) Direct assessment of liver glycogen storage by 13C nuclear magnetic resonance spectroscopy and regulation of glucose homeostasis after a mixed meal in normal subjects, *J Clin Invest*, **97**, 1, 126–132

Taylor, R, Price, T B, Rothman, D L, Shulman, R G, Shulman, G I (1992) Validation of 13C NMR measurement of human skeletal muscle glycogen by direct biochemical assay of needle biopsy samples, *Magn Reson Med*, **27**, 1, 13–20

Thamer, C, Machann, J, Bachmann, O, Haap, M, Dahl, D, Wietek, B, Tschritter, O, Niess, A, Brechtel, K, Fritsche, A, Claussen, C, Jacob, S, Schick, F, Haring, H U, Stumvoll, M (2003) Intramyocellular lipids: anthropometric determinants and relationships with maximal aerobic capacity and insulin sensitivity, *J Clin Endocrinol Metab*, **88**, 4, 1785–1791

Tippett, P S Neet, K E (1982) An allosteric model for the inhibition of glucokinase by long chain acyl coenzyme A, *J Biol Chem*, **257**, 21, 12846–12852

Tremblay, F, Krebs, M, Dombrowski, L, Brehm, A, Bernroider, E, Roth, E, Nowotny, P, Waldhausl, W, Marette, A, Roden, M (2005) Overactivation of S6 kinase 1 as a cause of human insulin resistance during increased amiacid availability, *Diabetes*, **54**, 9, 2674–2684

Van Den Bergh, A J, Tack, C J, Van Den Boogert, H J, Vervoort, G, Smits, P, Heerschap, A (2000) Assessment of human muscle glycogen synthesis and total glucose content by in vivo 13C MRS, *Eur J Clin Invest*, **30**, 2, 122–128

Vanhamme, L, van den, B A, Van Huffel, S (1997) Improved method for accurate and efficient quantification of MRS data with use of prior knowledge, *J Magn Reson*, **129**, 1, 35–43

Vanhamme, L, Van Huffel, S, Van Hecke, P, van Ormondt, D (1999) Time-domain quantification of series of biomedical magnetic resonance spectroscopy signals, *J Magn Reson*, **140**, 1, 120–130

Velho, G, Petersen, K F, Perseghin, G, Hwang, J H, Rothman, D L, Pueyo, M E, Cline, G W, Froguel, P, Shulman, G I (1996) Impaired hepatic glycogen synthesis in glucokinase-deficient (MODY-2) subjects, *J Clin Invest*, **98**, 8, 1755–1761

Wahren, J, Felig, P, Cerasi, E, Luft, R (1972) Splanchnic and peripheral glucose and amiacid metabolism in diabetes mellitus, *J Clin Invest*, **51**, 7, 1870–1878

Wessels, A M, Rombouts, S A, Simsek, S, Kuijer, J P, Kostense, P J, Barkhof, F, Scheltens, P, Snoek, F J, Heine, R J (2006) Microvascular disease in type 1 diabetes alters brain activation: a functional magnetic resonance imaging study, *Diabetes*, **55**, 2, 334–340

Wititsuwannakul, D Kim, K H (1977) Mechanism of palmityl coenzyme A inhibition of liver glycogen synthase, *J Biol Chem*, **252**, 21, 7812–7817

Zang, L H, Laughlin, M R, Rothman, D L, Shulman, R G (1990) 13C NMR relaxation times of hepatic glycogen in vitro and in vivo, *Biochemistry*, **29**, 29, 6815–6820

12

Positron Emission Tomography in Metabolic Research

Pirjo Nuutila, Patricia Iozzo and **Juhani Knuuti**

Introduction

Positron emission tomography (PET) is a quantitative *in vivo* functional imaging method that can generate information on human physiology and pathophysiology at a molecular level currently unobtainable with other methods. PET is based on the use of short-lived positron emitting radioisotopes such as carbon-11 (half life = 20 min), nitrogen-13 (half life = 10 min), oxygen-15 (half life = 2 min) and fluorine-18 (half life = 110 min). Nearly any substrate and drugs can be labeled without changing their physicochemical or pharmacological properties (Phelps et al. 1975). Due to rapid decay of the positron emitters, most PET tracers have to be synthesised on site. The tracer is injected intravenously into the subject or inhaled as a gas. It distributes throughout the body via bloodstream and enters into organs. In tissue, positrons emitted from the tracer nucleus collide with their counterparts, electrons, and the masses of the two colliding particles are converted into two photons emitted simultaneously in opposite directions. PET imaging is based on the detection of these paired photons in coincidence. PET can thus measure the anatomical and temporal distribution of the radiolabeled molecules in the body since the site of collision is registered by the detector system. Physiological and pharmacological phenomena and biological parameters can be estimated *in vivo* by mathematical modeling of the tissue and blood time-activity curves obtained. PET is an extremely sensitive and specific imaging tool which allows reliable detection of even subpicomolar concentrations of compounds.

Anatomic information from computerised tomography (CT) and magnetic resonance imaging (MRI) add to the functional information obtained with PET, and these three 3D imaging modalities can be seen as complementary to each other. Image correlation can be facilitated by sophisticated software allowing co-registration of CT or MRI images with PET. PET scanners combined with CT have been shown to be superior in diagnostics and are widely available. The recent development of high-resolution micro-PET cameras will open entirely new perspectives for studying genetically engineered small animals. The goal is to

Clinical Diabetes Research: Methods and Techniques   Edited by Michael Roden
© 2007 John Wiley & Sons, Ltd   ISBN 978-0-470-01728-9

provide a similar *in vivo* molecular imaging capability in mouse, rat, monkey and human. The devices are being designed to provide high throughput *in vivo* differential screening of biological responses in transgenics rodents for monitoring of drug effects.

Tracers for metabolic imaging

The rapid and efficient labeling of organic molecules is a very special challenge. As molecules can be labeled to very high specific radioactivity, an intravenous injection of less than one microgram is often sufficient for the performing of a PET study. Thus 'tracer doses', i.e. doses without any pharmacological effects, can be used. Useful radionuclides for this purpose are carbon-11, nitrogen-13, oxygen-15 and fluorine-18. Because of the short half lives of these radionuclides, the radioactivity production must occur on-site with a cyclotron. Carbon-11 is especially useful as almost every compound of the living systems contains carbon. The rationale for using fluorine-18 is that in many molecules a hydrogen atom or a hydroxyl group can be substituted for a fluorine without altering its behaviour in the human body. Some fluorine labeled analogues are designed to be trapped into tissues and not further metabolised (e.g. FDG). The short half lives of nitrogen-13 and oxygen-15 limit the applications in radiochemical synthesis but both nuclides appear as perfusion agents in the form of nitrogen-13-ammonia ($[^{13}N]NH_3$) and oxygen-15-water ($[^{15}O]H_2O$).

The quantitation of glucose utilisation, fatty acid uptake and oxidation, perfusion and oxygen consumption is possible with PET (Table 12.1). This allows us to study the effects of nutritional interventions, hormonal and neural activity, as well as disease processes, on the metabolism and function of human organs.

Table 12.1 Positron emission tomography tracers used in human subjects in metabolic studies

	Tracer	Half-life (min)
Perfusion	$[^{15}O]H_2O$	2
	$[^{82}Rb]$rubidium	1.2
	$[^{13}N]$ammonia	10
Glucose uptake	$[^{18}F]FDG$	109
Free fatty acid metabolism	$[^{11}C]$glucose	20
	$[^{18}F]FTHA$	109
Oxidative metabolism	$[^{11}C]$palmitate	20
	$[^{15}O]O_2$	2
	$[^{11}C]$acetate	20
Hypoxia	$[^{18}F]$misonidasole	109
Amino acid uptake	$[^{11}C]$metionine	20
	$[^{11}C]$MeAIb	20

$[^{18}F]FDG$: fluorine-18-labelled 2-fluoro-2-deoxy-D-glucose;

$[^{18}F]FMISO$: $[^{18}F]$fluoromisonidazole;

$[^{18}F]FTHA$: fluorine-18-labelled 6-thia-hepta-decanoic acid.

Principles of modeling

PET tracer kinetics and modeling

Analysis of the radiation emitted by an organ allows us to estimate its functional parameters. PET is currently the only technique that permits noninvasive quantification of regional tissue perfusion, glucose and fatty acid metabolism, protein synthesis and oxygen consumption. Sequential images are acquired after tracer injection, monitoring the distribution of the tracer in the system of interest. Regions are drawn over the organ under study to obtain tissue-specific time-activity curves. These curves, together with corresponding radioactivity levels in plasma (input into the system), are used in tracer kinetic modeling – a mathematical description of the movement of a tracer within the system – which translates a biochemical process into a numeric value. The shape and magnitude of a time-activity curve depends on the properties of the radiopharmaceutical and of the biochemical process under investigation. Depending on tracer kinetics, compartmental, graphical or exponential curve analyses have mostly been applied in the quantification of tissue perfusion and metabolism.

Tracer kinetics

The perfusion tracers $[^{15}O]H_2O$ and $[^{13}N]NH_3$ have both been validated experimentally and clinically (Bergman et al. 1984; Bellina et al. 1990). $[^{15}O]H_2O$ is an ideal tracer for the measurement of blood flow as it is chemically inert and freely diffusible. $[^{13}N]NH_3$ is first extracted in proportion to blood flow. $[^{18}F]FDG$ is a fluorine-18 labeled glucose analogue, which is transported into the cell and phosphorylated (Sokoloff et al. 1977; Phelps et al. 1978). In contrast to glucose, it cannot enter glycolysis, being trapped for the duration of most PET studies; thus, initial steps in glucose uptake and metabolism can be traced with this radio-pharmaceutical. $[^{18}F]FTHA$ is a long-chain fatty acid analogue and inhibitor of fatty acid metabolism; after transport into the mitochondria it undergoes the initial steps of β-oxidation and is thereafter trapped in the cell (DeGrado et al. 1991; Ebert et al. 1994). The natural tracers $[1-^{11}C]$acetate and $[^{15}O]O_2$ $[1-^{11}C]$palmitate and $[1-^{11}C]$glucose have been used with PET in humans for measuring oxygen consumption, fatty acid metabolism and glucose metabolism, respectively (Grover-McKay et al. 1986; Ukkonen et al. 2001; Herrero et al. 2002; Knuuti et al. 2004). Unlike their analogues, and similar to their endogenous isotope counterparts, these tracers enter a multitude of metabolic pathways and generate breakdown-metabolites and products, which are released in blood and need to be taken into account when determining the input function.

Compartmental modeling

Compartmental modeling involves the concept of a finite number of compartments, representing distinct physical spaces or chemical forms (e.g. FDG vs FDG-6-phosphate). Rate-constants regulating the transfer of tracer between compartments are estimated by setting up a number of differential equations describing the changing concentration of the radio-tracer in each compartment as a function of time. Usually, compartmental modeling requires knowledge of the number and configuration of the compartments representing the biological system to be described. One-tissue compartment models are used in the quantification of organ perfusion with H_2O. A three-compartment model has been most commonly adopted to describe the kinetics of FDG in the brain, skeletal muscle, heart and liver (Phelps et al. 1978, 1979; Sokoloff et al. 1978; Choi et al. 1994); more articulate models have been used to account for the complex metabolic fate of acetate, glucose and palmitate (Bergman et al. 2001; Herrero et al. 2002; Chen et al. 2004).

Graphical methods

Graphical methods have the advantage of being independent of compartment number and configuration. Gjedde-Patlak analysis (Figure 12.1) was first developed for the assessment of irreversible tracer transfer (Patlak et al. 1983). A graph is generated by plotting:

$$[C_t(t)/C_p(t)] \, vs \, [\textstyle\int_o^t C_p(t)dt/C_p(t)]$$

where C_t is tissue radioactivity at each sampling time point (t) and C_p is plasma radioactivity. When irreversible influx of tracer occurs, the two variables describe a linear relationship after a few minutes of equilibration. The influx constant is then given by the slope of the linear fit of the data, excluding the first few values. If reversible uptake occurs, metabolite loss can be corrected for by using the linearisation method described by Patlak & Blasberg

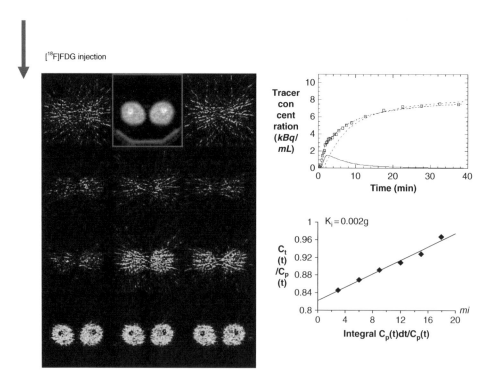

Figure 12.1 Example of dynamic femoral images after [18F]FDG injection (on the left); tissue time activity curves (upper panel on the right); the graphical analyses from the same study (lower panel on the right).

(1985). Logan analysis (Logan 2000) was introduced for the evaluation of reversible tracers. In this case a graph is obtained by plotting:

$$[\textstyle\int_o^t C_t(t)dt/C_t(t)] \, vs \, [\int_o^t C_p(t)dt/C_t(t)]$$

yielding a curve that becomes linear for a reversible uptake. The slope of the linear portion of the curve represents the distribution volume of tracer in the organ, and should be inversely proportional to the efflux of the tracer.

The outflow of labeled products from an organ has been also evaluated by its wash-out curve (Grover-McKay et al. 1986); this approach is commonly used in the estimation of oxidative metabolism from $[1\text{-}^{11}C]$-labeled acetate and palmitate, which lose their label in carbon-dioxide.

Lumped constant

The quantification of the fate of a natural compound, e.g. glucose or fatty acid, by use of its analogue, e.g. FDG or FTHA, requires the introduction of a conversion term, denominated 'lumped constant', representing the ratio of the metabolic rate of the tracer to that of the tracee (Sokoloff et al. 1977). Relative to FDG, this numerical value has been shown to approximate unity in skeletal muscle (Peltoniemi et al. 2000), myocardium (Ng et al. 1998) and adipose tissue (Virtanen et al. 2001), and to hold constant across metabolic disease states.

Systemic substrate turnover

Together with regional image data, the plasma kinetics of metabolic PET tracers can be used to estimate the turnover of substrates, namely glucose and fatty acids, providing complementary information on systemic substrate clearance, consumption and production (e.g. lipolysis, endogenous glucose production) (Guiducci et al. 2006; Iozzo et al. 2006).

Applications of PET for the assessment of skeletal muscle metabolism

By combining PET and the glucose-insulin clamp technique, insulin resistance for glucose was shown to localise in skeletal muscle in type 1 and type 2 diabetes (Nuutila et al. 1993; Utriainen et al. 1998). Using compartmental modeling, insulin is shown to affect transport and phosphorylation but not extracellular kinetics, with the transport step becoming the main site of control (Kelley et al. 1999; Bertoldo et al. 2001). Skeletal muscle free fatty acid uptake measured using 18-F-FTHA under fasting conditions has been shown to be decreased with insulin use, but myocardial free fatty acid uptake is similar in both patients with impaired glucose tolerance and normal patients (Turpeinen et al. 1999), suggesting that not only glucose but also lipid metabolism is defective in type 2 diabetes.

Perfusion regulates muscle oxygen and nutrient supply at rest and during exercise and is distributed heterogeneously between and within skeletal muscles in humans (Kalliokoski et al. 2001). In addition, muscle glucose uptake is more heterogeneous in obese subjects than in lean ones (Peltoniemi et al. 2001). Because regional perfusion and glucose uptake can be measured independently with PET, the relationship between metabolism and perfusion has been assessed in different insulin-resistant populations. Although impaired muscle vasodilatation capacity has been observed in subjects with impaired insulin sensitivity, no evidence has been found to support direct causality between perfusion and metabolism insulin-resistant conditions. If muscle blood flow was increased by 60 % in one leg by bradykinin, an endothelium-dependent vasodilatator, insulin stimulated glucose uptake was increased neither in non-obese nor in obese subjects (Laine et al. 1998). Exercise increases cardiac output and the total number of perfused capillaries, resulting in a 15–20-fold increase in blood flow. The synergic effects of exercise and insulin action have been found to be impaired in patients with type 1 diabetes as compared to healthy subjects (Peltoniemi et al. 2001). In a placebo controlled intervention study with rosiglitazone and metformin, sequential scanning of different tissues was performed (Figure 12.2). When the effect of rosiglitazone was compared to that of the placebo, insulin-estimated muscle glucose uptake was increased by 39 % in the resting muscle but the increment induced by exercise was doubled (Figure 12.3) (Hällsten et al. 2002). PET is a powerful tool for the assessment of the mode of action of drugs affecting peripheral vasculature and metabolism.

Adipose glucose uptake

The FDG-PET method provides direct depot-specific measurements of insulin-stimulated glucose uptake in subcutaneous and intra-abdominal adipose tissues (Virtanen et al. 2001) (Figure 12.4). To evaluate the role of adipose tissue insulin resistance in obesity and T2DM, we applied FDG-PET to measure insulin-stimulated glucose uptake in non-obese and moderately obese men who were either normoglycaemic or had a recent diagnosis of T2DM (Virtanen et al. 2005). Adipose tissue depots were quantified by magnetic resonance imaging. Insulin stimulated glucose uptake per unit tissue weight was higher in visceral (20.5 ± 1.4 μmol/min^{-1}/kg^{-1}) than in abdominal (9.8 ± 0.9 μmol/min^{-1}/kg^{-1}, $p < 0.001$) or femoral subcutaneous tissue (12.3 ± 0.6 μmol/min^{-1}/kg^{-1}, $p < 0.001$), and ~40 % lower than in skeletal muscle (33.1 ± 2.5 μmol/min^{-1}/kg^{-1}, $p < 0.0001$). Abdominal obesity was found to be associated with a marked reduction in glucose uptake per unit tissue weight in all fat depots and in skeletal muscle ($p < 0.001$ for all regions). However, when regional glucose uptake was multiplied by tissue mass, total glucose uptake per fat depot was similar irrespective of abdominal obesity or T2DM. This study showed that an expanded fat mass (especially

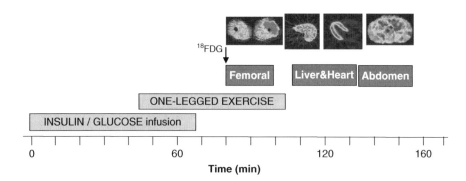

Figure 12.2 An example of sequential scanning of the femoral, hepatic and thoracic and abdominal regions after [^{18}F]FDG injection during glucose-insulin infusion and one-legged exercise (Hällsten et al. 2002).

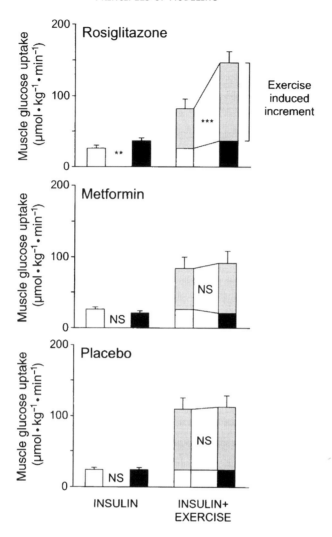

Figure 12.3 Rates of skeletal muscle glucose uptake during hyperinsulinaemia at baseline (open bars) and after 26 weeks of treatment with rosiglitazone, metformin and placebo (black bars). Grey areas show exercise-induced increments in glucose uptake. ***$P < 0.001$, **$P < 0.01$ compared with baseline (Hällsten et al. 2002).

subcutaneous) provides a sink for glucose, resulting in a compensatory attenuation of insulin resistance at the whole-body level.

Liver

New and better probes and models for investigating liver metabolism by PET imaging are being developed reflecting the important role of this tissue in the regulation of whole-body homeostasis. Extrapolating our mean liver and skeletal muscle uptake data to the average 75 kg man, with muscle mass of 30 kg and liver volume of 1.5 l, hepatic glucose

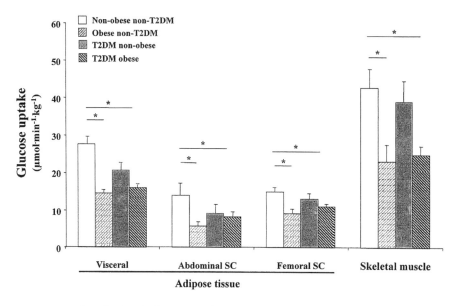

Figure 12.4 Insulin-stimulated glucose uptake rate per unit tissue weight in adipose tissue and skeletal muscle as measured directly by [^{18}F]FDG-PET. Bars denote means ± SE. *P < 0.01 (Virtanen et al. 2005).

uptake is $\sim$23 and 35 µmol/min^{-1} and liver fatty acid disposal is $\sim$302 and 41 µmol/min^{-1} in the fasting and insulinised states, respectively (Iozzo et al. 2003a, 2004a); corresponding figures in muscle are 570 and 1380 (glucose disposal) (Nuutila et al. 1994; Peltoniemi et al. 2000) or $\sim$132 and 40 µmol/min^{-1} (FFA uptake). Thus, each ml of liver takes up an amount of FFA which is around 25–50 times higher than that taken up by 1 g of muscle, but shows similar glucose disposal, underscoring the central contribution of the liver in disposing of fatty acids. The remarkable metabolic shift occurring between fasted and insulin stimulated conditions highlights the important role of nutritional and hormonal regulation in combating diabetes.

Insulin was shown to increase hepatic glucose uptake by 50–70 % over fasting values in non-diabetic individuals, regardless of mild insulin resistance (Iozzo et al. 2003b). In patients with type 2 diabetes, but not in age and BMI matched non-diabetic insulin-resistant individuals, insulin-mediated glucose uptake was impaired in proportion with fasting glucose levels (Iozzo et al. 2003c). During fasting conditions, the ability of the liver to extract FFA was impaired and reciprocally related with glucose and lactate levels in healthy and glucose intolerant subjects, suggesting inverse substrate competition (Iozzo et al. 2004). Altogether, these findings indicate that chronic hyperglycaemia may obstruct liver provision of its principal energy source, namely fatty acid in the fasting state, or glucose in the insulin stimulated state; in the latter condition, the relationship is mutual, such that a high liver FFA exposure reduces hepatic glucose utilisation (Iozzo et al. 2004). This reciprocal interaction is supported by studies in which two hypoglycaemic agents, with different molecular targets but nearly comparable outcome on glucose control, promoted hepatic insulin sensitivity to a similar extent; the change was significantly related to the decrease in HbA$_{1c}$ and to the enhancement in insulin-mediated suppression of FFA release (Iozzo et al. 2003d). The evidence that endurance training concertedly increased insulin-mediated glucose and FFA disposal in skeletal muscle, while lowering hepatic FFA uptake, is in line with the concept that higher insulin sensitivity reduces substrate competition in the liver.

The quantification of liver metabolism by PET imaging has to account for the dual (arterial and portal venous) input of tracer to the organ. Though the use of a single arterial input may influence the rate of rapid delivery of tracer to the organ, the available animal data have shown that the quantified glucose uptake in the organ is not different from that obtained by using a dual input function (Munk et al. 2001). In evaluating fatty acid metabolism by FTHA, caution should be adopted in extrapolating findings from this analogue to any endogenous FFA until the equivalence is proven.

PET in cardiac studies

The tracers $[^{11}C]$acetate and $[^{15}O]O_2$ have been used for measuring myocardial oxygen consumption with PET in humans (Iida et. al. 1996; Sun et al. 1998). The myocardial kinetics of the $[^{11}C]$acetate correlate closely and directly with myocardial oxygen consumption over a wide range of conditions. The model employed with $[^{15}O]O_2$ requires additional measurements of myocardial blood volume and flow, which makes it more demanding.

The $[^{18}F]$FDG method has been also widely used to study myocardial glucose metabolism in various conditions, such as in coronary heart disease, diabetes, hypertension and cardiac failure. Although $[^{11}C]$glucose has been in use for a long time, it has been applied in studies of cardiac metabolism only recently (Herrero et al. 2002). It has recently been shown to provide accurate quantitation of myocardial glucose uptake (Herrero et al. 2002) and has been successfully applied in humans (Davila-Roman et al. 2002).

The natural tracer $[^{11}C]$palmitic acid has traditionally been used to assess myocardial FFA metabolism by PET. The retention of the tracer serves as an index of FFA uptake and the rapid washout of the tracer is assumed to be associated with the oxidative metabolism of fatty acids, while the slower washout is associated with the incorporation to the myocardial triglyceride pool (Selbert et al. 1986; Taegtmeyer 1994).

The tracer analogue ^{18}F-labeled 6-thia-hepta-decanoicacid ($[^{18}F]$FTHA) has also been used to study fatty acid metabolism in human heart (DeGrado et al. 1991). $[^{18}F]$FTHA is a 'false' long-chain fatty acid substrate and inhibitor of fatty acid metabolism (DeGrado et al. 1999). After transport into the mitochondria it undergoes initial steps of β-oxidation and is thereafter trapped in the cell, because further β-oxidation is blocked by sulphur heteroatom. It has been suggested that an accumulation of $[^{18}F]$FTHA indicates FFA-oxidation in the heart (DeGrado et al. 1999). Indeed, 80 % of the tracer is entering and trapped in the mitochondria of myocytes (Takala et al. 2002). A similar graphical analysis to that used with $[^{18}F]$FDG has been successfully applied in quantitation of $[^{18}F]$FTHA uptake in the heart.

Lactate has been also labeled with $[^{11}C]$ and human studies have been successfully performed. The label must be attached to 3-carbon of lactate to provide myocardial image, since in $[1-^{11}C]$-lactate, label is metabolised rapidly (personal information, Bengt Langstrom, Uppsala PET Centre). Some studies of cardiac amino acid metabolism have been reported, but uptake of these tracers has been found low. Imaging of tissue hypoxia is an attractive approach in cardiology. Although hypoxia tracers have been widely used in oncology, the imaging window in cardiology has limited their use in the heart. Recently, copper-ATSM has been successfully used to image cardiac hypoxia in canine heart.

The most common cardiac PET study has been the measurement of glucose uptake and myocardial viability. In the detection of myocardial viability, [^{18}F]FDG PET has been regarded as a gold standard. The assessment of myocardial viability, distinguishing reversible from irreversible damage to cardiac tissue, is a clinically important issue for the management of patients with coronary artery disease and severe impairment of cardiac pump function. The PET method is based on the biochemical principle that glucose is a protective substrate for generating ATP in oxygen-limited states and maintaining the viability of tissue, even though local cardiac work is lost. In addition, PET imaging is able to identify patients at increased risk of an adverse cardiac event or death.

Hyperinsulinaemia stimulates uptake of both glucose and FDG, in the myocardium and in skeletal muscle, and yields images of consistently high diagnostic quality, even in patients with diabetes (Knuuti et al. 1992). Myocardial insulin sensitivity has been either normal (Nuutila et al. 1993; Utriainen et al. 1998) or impaired (Iozzo et al. 2002; Lautamäki et al. 2005) in patients with type 1 or type 2 diabetes and peripheral insulin resistance. Similar myocardial glucose uptake has been observed in subjects who were younger and without diabetic complications (Nuutila et al. 1993; Utriainen et al. 1998). If patients with type 2 diabetes were older and had simultaneous coronary heart disease, there was a direct relationship between myocardial glucose uptake and whole-body insulin sensitivity (Iozzo et al. 2002; Lautamäki et al. 2005).

Combined with the measurement of tissue perfusion, oxygen consumption and mechanical function, the knowledge of substrate metabolism provides a more comprehensive picture of myocardial physiology and pathophysiology. Since preserved myocardial utilisation of glucose has been suggested to be beneficial for myocardial injury during ischemia and reperfusion, attempts have been made to develop drugs to modify myocardial energy metabolism towards glucolysis and glucose oxidation and to decrease fatty acid oxidation rates.

Future perspectives

Information which traditionally was obtained from molecular biology and from *in vitro* microscopic studies can now be gathered in humans by *in vivo* molecular imaging. Molecular *in vivo* imaging using PET allows the study of pathogenesis in intact micro-environments of living systems. Diabetes and pre-diabetes are associated with increased systemic inflammation and accumulation of lipids in and around normally lean organs. The study of lipid metabolism and its early aberrations, by using molecular imaging of lipid tracers, may clarify the association between diabetes and cardiovascular disease and reveal important targets for pharmacological intervention. Not only the organs discussed above, but all human tissues can be studied using PET. When information from cerebral and pancreatic metabolism and perfusion is included, interactions and links between different tissues can be evaluated. Recently, printng of data about imaging of β-cell mass has been reported (Souza et al. 2006). Molecular imaging reveals the 'microscopic' dynamic characteristics of the disease, and it does so in a noninvasive fashion; for this reason, it is suitable for large scale application, and is the only tool for routine earliest detection of disease in humans *in vivo*. In addition, PET can gather information on the distribution, accumulation (toxicology) and kinetics of novel compounds. This is achieved through radiolabeling (*in vivo* administration of drugs in tracer amounts) at the earliest stage of drug development.

References

Bellina CR, Parodi O, Camici P, Salvadori PA, Taddei L, Fusani L et al. (1990) Simultaneous in vitro and in vivo validation of nitrogen–13–ammonia for the assessment of regional myocardial blood flow *J Nucl Med*, **31**(8), 1335–43

Bergmann SR, Fox KA, Rand AL, McElvany KD, Welch MJ, Markham J et al. (1984 Oct) Quantification of regional myocardial blood flow in vivo with H215O *Circulation*, **70**(4), 724–33

Bergmann SR, Herrero P, Sciacca R, Hartman JJ, Rubin PJ, Hickey KT et al. (2001) Characterization of altered myocardial fatty acid metabolism in patients with inherited cardiomyopathy *J Inherit Metab Dis*, **24**(6), 657–74

Bertoldo A, Peltoniemi P, Oikonen V, Knuuti J, Nuutila P, Cobelli C (2001 Sep) Kinetic modeling of [18F]FDG in skeletal muscle by PET, a four-compartment five-rate-constant model *Am J Physiol Endocrinol Metab*, **281**(3), E524–36

Chen S, Ho C, Feng D, Chi Z (2004) Tracer kinetic modeling of 11C-acetate applied in the liver with positron emission tomography IEEE *Trans Med Imaging*, **23**(4), 426–32

Choi Y, Hawkins RA, Huang SC, Brunken RC, Hoh CK, Messa C et al. (1994) Evaluation of the effect of glucose ingestion and kinetic model configurations of FDG in the normal liver *J Nucl Med*, **35**, 818–823

Davila-Roman VG, Vedala G, Herrero P, et al. (2002 Jul 17) Altered myocardial fatty acid and glucose metabolism in idiopathic dilated cardiomyopathy *J Am Coll Cardiol*, **40**(2), 271–7

DeGrado TR, Coenen HH, Stöcklin G (1991) 14(R, S)-[¹⁸F]fluoro-6-thiaheptadecanoic acid (FTHA), evaluation in mouse of a new probe of myocardial utilization of long-chain fatty acids *J Nucl Med*, **32**, 1888–1896

Ebert A, Herzog H, Stöcklin GL, Henrich MM, DeGrado TR, Coenen HH, Feinendegen LE (1994) Kinetics of 14(R, S)-fluorine-18-fluoro-6-thiaheptadecanoic acid in normal human hearts at rest, during exercise and after dipyridamole injection *J Nucl Med*, **35**, 51–56

Grover–McKay M, Schelbert HR, Schwaiger M, Sochor H, Guzy PM, Krivokapich J et al. (1986 Aug) Identification of impaired metabolic reserve by atrial pacing in patients with significant coronary artery stenosis *Circulation*, **74**(2), 281–92

Giducci L , Kiss J, Jarvisalo M, Nagren K, Viljanen A, Buzzigoli E et al. (2006) Metabolism of circulating palmitate across the liver, kinetics in arterial, portal, and hepatic venous plasma and release of labeled triglycerides during fasting and euglycemic hyperinsulinemia *Nucl Med Biol*, in press

Hällsten K, Virtanen KA, Lönnqvist F, Sipilä H, Oksanen A, Viljanen T et al. (2002 Dec) Rosiglitazone but not metformin enhances insulin- and exercise-stimulated skeletal muscle glucose uptake in patients with newly diagnosed type 2 diabetes *Diabetes*, **51**(12), 3479–85

Herrero P, Sharp TL, Dence C et al. (2002 Nov) Comparison of 1-(11)C-glucose and (18)F–FDG for quantifying myocardial glucose use with PET *J Nucl Med*, **43**(11), 1530–41

Iida H, Rhodes CG, Araujo LI, et al. (1996) Noninvasive quantification of regional myocardial metabolic rate for oxygen by use of 15O2 inhalation and positron emission tomography Theory, error analysis, and application in humans *Circulation*, **94**, 792 807

Iozzo P, Oikonen V, Turpeinen AK , Takala T, Solin O, Ferrannini E, Nuutila P, Knuuti J (2003a) Liver uptake of free fatty acids in vivo in humans with 14(R,S)-¹⁸F-6-heptadecanoic acid and PET *Eur J Nucl Med Mol Imaging*, **30**(8), 1160–1164

Iozzo P, Chareonthaitawee P, Dutka D, Betteridge DJ, Ferrannini E, Camici PG (2002) Independent association of type 2 diabetes and coronary artery disease with myocardial insulin resistance *Diabetes*, **51**(10), 3020–3024

Iozzo P, Gastaldelli A, Jarvisalo M, Kiss J, Borra R, Viljanen A et al. (2006) Assessment of glucose turnover and endogenous production by 18F-fluorodeoxyglucose A validation study *J Nucl Med*, in press

Iozzo P, Geisler F, Oikonen V, Mäki M, Takala T, Solin O et al. (2003b) Insulin Stimulates Liver Glucose Uptake in Man, a ¹⁸F-fluoro-2-Deoxy-Glucose Positron-Emission Tomography Study *J Nucl Med*, **44**, 682–689

Iozzo P, Hallsten K, Oikonen V, Virtanen KA, Kemppainen J, Solin O et al. (2003c) Insulin-mediated hepatic glucose uptake is impaired in type 2 diabetes Evidence for a relationship with glycemic control *J Clin Endocrinol Metab*, **88**(5), 2055–2060

Iozzo P, Hallsten K, Oikonen V, Virtanen KA, Kemppainen J, Solin O et al. (2003d) Effect of metformin and rosiglitazone monotherapy on insulin–mediated hepatic glucose uptake and its relation with visceral fat metabolism in human type 2 diabetes *Diabetes Care*, **26**, 2069–2074

Iozzo P, Lautamaki R, Geisler F, Virtanen K, Oikonen V, Haaparanta M et al. (2004c) Nonesterified fatty acids impair insulin-mediated glucose uptake and disposition in the liver *Diabetologia*, **47**(7), 1149–1156

Iozzo P, Takala T, Oikonen V, Bergman J, Grönroos T, Ferrannini E et al. (2004a) Effect of training status on regional disposal of circulating free fatty acids in the liver and in skeletal muscle during physiological hyperinsulinemia *Diabetes Care*, **27**(9), 2172–2177

Iozzo P, Turpeinen AT, Takala T, Oikonen V, Bergman J, Grönroos T et al. (2004b) Defective liver disposal of free fatty acids in patients with impaired glucose tolerance *J Clin Endocrinol Metab*, **89**(7), 3496–3502

Kalliokoski KK, Oikonen V, Takala TO, Sipilä H, Knuuti J, Nuutila P (2001) Enhanced oxygen extraction and reduced flow heterogeneity in exercising muscle in endurance–trained men *Am J Physiol Endocrinol Metab*, **280**, E1015–E1021

Kelley DE, Williams K, Price JC (1999) Insulin regulation on glucose transport and phosphorylation in skeletal muscle asessed by PET *Am J Physiol*, **277**, E361–E369

Knuuti J, Nuutila P, Ruotsalainen U, Saraste M, Härkönen R, Ahonen A et al. (1992) Euglycemic hyperinsulinemic clamp and oral glucose load in stimulating myocardial glucose utilization during positron emission tomography *J Nucl Med*, **33**, 1255–1262

Knuuti J, Sundell J, Naum A, Engblom E, Koistinen J, Ylitalo A et al. (2004 Dec) Assessment of right ventricular oxidative metabolism by PET in patients with idiopathic dilated cardiomyopathy undergoing cardiac resynchronization therapy *Eur J Nucl Med Mol Imaging*, **31**(12), 1592–8

Laine H, Yki-Järvinen H, Kirvelä O, Tolvanen T, Raitakari M, Solin O et al. (1998) Insulin ressitance of glucose uptake in skeletal muscle cannot not be ameliorated by enhancing endothelium-dependent blood flow in obesity *J Clin Invest*, **101**, 1156–1162

Lautamaki R, Airaksinen KE, Seppanen M, Toikka J, Luotolahti M, Ball E et al. (2005 Sep) Rosiglitazone improves myocardial glucose uptake in patients with type 2 diabetes and coronary artery disease, a 16-week randomized, double-blind, placebo-controlled study *Diabetes*, **54**(9), 2787–94

Logan J (2000) Graphical analysis of PET data applied to reversible and irreversible tracers *Nucl Med Biol*, **27**(7), 661–70

Munk OL, Bass L, Roelsgaard K, Bender D, Hansen SB, Keiding S (2001 May) Liver kinetics of glucose analogs measured in pigs by PET, importance of dual-input blood sampling *J Nucl Med*, **42**(5), 795–801

Ng CK, Soufer R, McNulty PH (1998) Effect of hyperinsulinemia on myocardial fluorine-18-FDG uptake *J Nucl Med*, **39**, 379–383

Nuutila P, Knuuti J, Ruotsalainen U, Koivisto VA, Ruotsalainen U, Eronen E et al. (1993) Insulin resistance is localized to skeletal but not heart muscle in type 1 diabetes *Am J Physiol*, **264**(*Endocrinol Metab* 27), E756–62

Nuutila P, Knuuti MJ, Raitakari M, Ruotsalainen U, Teras M, Voipio-Pulkki LM et al. (1994 Dec) Effect of antilipolysis on heart and skeletal muscle glucose uptake in overnight fasted humans *Am J Physiol*, **267**(6 Pt 1), E941–6

Opie LH (1998) Fuels, Aerobic and anaerobic metabolism In: Opie LH (Ed) *The Heart Physiology, from cell to circulation* Philadelphia, Lippincott-Raven, pp. 295–341

Patlak CS, Blasberg RG (1985) Graphical evaluation of blood-to-brain transfer constants from multiple-time uptake data Generalizations *J Cereb Blood Flow Metab*, **5**, 584–590

Peltoniemi P, Lonnroth P, Laine H, Oikonen V, Tolvanen T, Gronroos T et al. (2000) Lumped constant for [(18)F]fluorodeoxyglucose in skeletal muscles of obese and nonobese humans *Am J Physiol Endocrinol Metab*, **279**(5), E1122–30

Peltoniemi P, Yki-Järvinen H, Laine H, Oikonen V, Rönnemaa T, Kalliokoski K et al. (2001) Evidence for spatial heterogeneity in insulin- and exercise induced increases in glucose uptake Studies in normal subjects and patients with type 1 diabetes *J Clin Endocr Metab*, **86**, 5525–33

Phelps ME, Hoffman EJ, Mullani NA, Ter-Pogossian MM (1975) Application of annihilation coincidence detection to transaxial reconstruction tomography *J Nucl Med*, **16**, 210–224

Phelps ME, Huang SC, Hoffman EJ, Selin CJ, Khul DE (1979) Tomographic measurement of local cerebral glucose metabolic rate in humans with (F-18)2-fluoro-d-deoxy-D-glucose, validation of method *Ann Neurol*, **6**, 371–388

Schelbert H, Schwaiger M (1986) PET studies of the heart: Positron emission tomography and autoradiography, principles and applications for the brain and heart (Edited by Phelps, Marizziotta MJ, Schelbert H) New York, Raven Press, p 599

Sokoloff L, Reivich M, Kennedy C, Des Rosiers MH, Patlak CS, Pettigrew KD et al. (1977) The [14C]deoxyglucose method for the measurement of local cerebral glucose utilization, theory, procedure, and normal values in the conscious and anesthetized albino rat *J Neurochem*, **28**, 897–916

Souza F, Simpson N, Raffo A, Saxena C, Maffei A, Hardy M, Kilbourn M, Goland R, Leibel R, Mann JJ, Van Heertum R, Harris PE (2006). Longitudinal noninvasive PET-based β cell mass estimates in a spontaneous diabietes rat model *J. Clin. Invest.*, **116**, 1506–13

Sun KT, Yeatman LA, Buxton DB et al. (1998) Simultaneous measurement of myocardial oxygen consumption and blood flow using [1-carbon-11]acetate *J Nucl Med*, **39**, 272–280

Taegtmeyer H (1994) Energy metabolism of the heart, from basic concepts to clinical applications *Curr Probl Cardiol*, **19**, 59–113

Takala TO, Nuutila P, Pulkki K, et al. (2002) 14(R,S)-[18F]Fluoro-6-thia-heptadecanoic acid as a tracer of free fatty acid uptake and oxidation in myocardium and skeletal muscle *Eur J Nucl Med*, **29**, 1617–1622

Turpeinen A, Takala TO, Nuutila P, Luotolahti M, Haaparanta M, Bergman J et al. (1999) Impaired free fatty acid uptake in skeletal muscle but not in myocardium in patients with impaired glucose tolerance, Studies with PET and 14(R,S)-[18F]fluoro-6-thia-heptadecanoic acid *Diabetes*, **48**, 1245–1250

Ukkonen H, Knuuti J, Katoh C, Iida H, Sipila H, Lehikoinen P et al. (2001) Use of [11C]acetate and [15O]O2 PET for the assessment of myocardial oxygen utilization in patients with chronic myocardial infarction *Eur J Nucl Med*, **28**, 334–9

Utriainen T, Takala T, Luotolahti M, Rönnemaa T, Laine H, Ruotsalainen U et al. (1998) Insulin resistance characterizes glucose uptake in skeletal muscle but not the heart in non-insulin-dependent diabetes mellitus *Diabetologia*, **41**, 555–559

Virtanen KA, Iozzo P, Hällsten K, Huupponen R, Parkkola R, Janatuinen T et al. (2005 Sep) Increased fat mass compensates for insulin resistance in abdominal obesity and type 2 diabetes, a positron-emitting tomography study *Diabetes*, **54**(9), 2720–6

Virtanen KA, Peltoniemi P, Marjamaki P, Asola M, Strindberg L, Parkkola R et al. (2001) Human adipose tissue glucose uptake determined using [(18)F]-fluoro-deoxy-glucose ([(18)F]FDG) and PET in combination with microdialysis *Diabetologia*, **44**(12), 2171–9

13

Assessment of Body Fat Content and Distribution

Martin Krššák

Introduction

Disorders of lipid metabolism, increased concentrations of plasma free fatty acids, increased fat ingestion and obesity are closely related to both features of insulin resistance: 1) reduced skeletal muscle glucose uptake and 2) insufficient hormonal suppression of endogenous glucose production upon carbohydrate challenge (McGarry 2002). Thus the assessment of whole body fat content and distribution is crucial for the modern diagnosis of metabolic syndrome. Furthermore, there is substantial evidence of different metabolic activities of subcutaneous, visceral and intracellular triglyceride pools, some of which cannot be assessed by conventional anthropomorphic (Wang et al. 2000), volume displacement (Dempster & Aitkens 1995) or stable isotope dilution (Schoeller et al. 1980) measurement techniques. To this end, this chapter will discuss the role and the contribution of modern diagnostic techniques to the assessment of size and metabolic activity of various triglyceride pools in the diagnosis and therapy assessment of patients with different features of metabolic syndrome and type 2 diabetes mellitus.

Measurement techniques

Besides to antropometric methods of subcutaneous fat tissue assessment (Heymsfield et al. 2000) and volume displacement measurement (Fields et al. 2002) there are techniques of assessment of whole body fat distribution which are based on the physical properties of tissue water and fat and their interaction with ionising and non-ionising radiation. Differences in water and fat interaction with electric current (bioelectrical impedance analysis – BIA), ultrasound waves (ultrasound – US) or X-rays (double energy X-ray absorption – DXA; computed tomography – CT) and the different electromagnetic properties of water and fat molecules (magnetic resonance – MR) enable us to characterise both compartments. Some of these methods can be used at the bedside (BIA, US); others need a special diagnostic

Clinical Diabetes Research: Methods and Techniques   Edited by Michael Roden
© 2007 John Wiley & Sons, Ltd   ISBN 978-0-470-01728-9

Table 13.1 Overview of Methods for the Assessment of Body Fat Content and Distribution

Measuring Method	Mechanism of Action	Fat Compartmentation	2D/3D Resolution	Ionising Radiation	Cost
Bioelectrical Impedance Analysis	Body electric resistance	Body segment average population dependent	N/A	No	Low
Ultrasonography	Reflection of ultrasound waves	Adipose tissue layers volume extrapolation	> 1 mm	No	Low
Dual Energy X-ray Absorption	X-ray absorption by tissue	Body segments average	$\sim$2 mm planar projection	Low	Low
Computed Tomography	X-ray absorption by tissue	Adipose tissue volume/ Tissue specific fat accumulation	< 1 mm in plane	High	Middle
Magnetic Resonance Imaging	Magnetic relaxation properties of fat and water	Adipose tissue volume/Tissue specific fat accumulation	< 1 mm in plane	No	High
Magnetic Resonance Spectroscopy	Spectral dispersion of water and fat resonance frequencies	Tissue specific fat accumulation/ intra and extramyocellular compartment	$< 1\ cm^3$ volume of interest	High	

suite (DXA, CT, MR). The methods also differ in terms of cost, body measures accessible and accuracy achievable (Table 13.1), limiting the employment of each particular method to a specific diagnostic task and/or specific study design.

Bioelectrical Impedance Analysis (Bia)

Bioelectrical impedance analysis applies indirect measurement of total body (or body segment) water volume by measuring the body resistance to electrical current at a defined frequency. The calculated weight of body water can then be subtracted from whole body weight, yielding body fat amount. The method applies various population and multi-compartment model-based equations for the calculation of total body water (TBW) and fat free mass (FFM) from measured values of electrical impedance. Due to its underlying mechanism, changes of body impedance are closely related to changes of FFM volume and hydration, and the contribution of the trunk and abdominal compartment can be strongly underestimated due to its geometry (Kyle et al. 2004a,b). Investigators are reminded that diverse leg lengths, frame sizes and body builds are responsible for ethnic differences in the body mass index (BMI) to percentage body fat relationship. Differences in subject hydration and electrolyte abnormalities can increase the coefficient of variation of whole body BIA TBW and FFM measurement. With vast numbers of studies conducted in healthy populations (recently reviewed by Kyle et al. 2004a), the measurement of whole body composition using BIA has been validated. The bioimpedance equation has therefore been proposed for diabetic (Leiter et al. 1994) and obese or overweight (Jakicic et al. 1998; De Lorenzo et al. 1999; Cox-Reijven & Soeters 2000) populations. Localised BIA measurement has been applied in the prediction of abdominal subcutaneous fat layers (Scharfetter et al. 2001). Nevertheless, despite the advantage of low cost and bedside applicability, methodological limitations and a higher coefficient of variation restrict the measurement to epidemiologic cross-sectional studies on large populations.

Ultrasonography (US)

Differences in the ultrasonic reflection and transmission coefficient between water and fat tissue enables us to visualise fat layer accumulation in the subcutaneous regions. Even though the imaging ability of the method can be limited by human anatomy and the depth of observed regions, US measurement has made its way to broad clinical applicability. Measurement schemes for the assessment of visceral fat volumes have been introduced (Armellini et al. 1990; Abe et al. 1995) and validated against measurements by computed tomography (Ribeiro-Filho et al. 2003; Hirooka et al. 2005). Using US, the distances between anatomical landmarks in the subcutaneous area and abdominal cavity (Hirooka et al. 2005) or the lower back region (Ribeiro-Filho et al. 2003) are measured, and the volume of intra-abdominal fat is calculated by empirical model equations (Figure 13.1).

Fat accumulation in the liver is assessed from the bright echo appearance and the loss of the typical liver structure in the image (Quinn & Gosink 1985). Qualitative staging was introduced by Saadeh et al. (2002), leaving fat amount assessment to pattern recognition by the operator rather than specific quantitative measurement. But clear diagnosis of fatty liver is hampered by the fact that fibrosis, often associated with fat accumulation, has a similar bright echo appearance (Needleman et al. 1986; Celle et al. 1988). Nevertheless, despite its

A

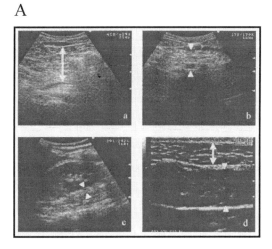

B

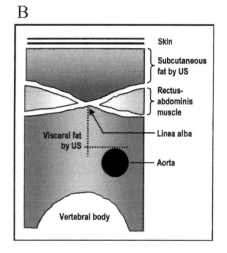

Figure 13.1 Assessment and Quantitation of Abdominal Fat by Ultrasonography A) the a) distance between abdominal muscle and splenic vein; b) distance between abdominal muscle and aorta; c) thickness of the fat layer of the posterior right renal wall; and d) thickness of the subcutaneous and preperitoneal fat layers are measured and abdominal fat volume is calculated (Copyright © 2005 Japanese Society of Internal Medicine, All rights reserved. Reproduced with permission from Hirooka, M. et al. *Intern. Med.*, vol. 44, no. 8, pp. 794–799); B) illustration of abdominal adipose tissue and anatomical landmarks used for ultrasonographic measurements, according to Ribeiro-Filho A) Reproduced from Hirooka M et al. (2005) *Intern Med* **44** (8), 794–799. Courtesy of the Japanese Society of Internal Medicine. B) Reproduced form Ribeiro-Filho F F et al. (2003) *Obes Res.*, **11** (12), 1488–1494. Courtesy of NAASO The Obestity Society.

lower sensitivity (Fontana & Lok 2002) and diagnostic accuracy (Aube et al. 1999) compared to CT or MR, its broad availability and low costs have established US measurement as a leading clinical tool for the assessment of fatty liver (Joy et al. 2003; Bedogni et al. 2006).

Dual Energy X-ray Absorptiometry (DXA)

Measurement of body composition by dual energy X-ray absorptiometry is based on differences in the absorption of X-rays by various atoms. The different molecular compositions of fat, lean tissue and bone material result in different X-ray absorption in these tissues. X-rays of 40 keV and 70 keV, produced by tungsten X-ray tubes and filtered by rare-earth material filters, are used for the measurement of localised tissue X-ray attenuation in planar projection. The fat and lean mass composition of soft tissue pixels is than calculated by linear decomposition of measured attenuation according to calibration measurement with fat and lean tissue samples (Pietrobelli et al. 1996). Specific additional assumptions for fat and lean mass distribution have to be made for the signal from bone-containing pixels (Tothill & Nord 1995).

Several studies have shown some correlation between DXA and CT measurements of body compositions and abdominal obesity (Kelley et al. 2000; Park et al. 2002; Snijder et al. 2002). But methodological limitations linked to the effect of hydration on X-ray attenuation (Pietrobelli et al. 1996, 1998; Lohman et al. 2000) and distortions of planar projections when scanning the thicker tissue of obese or overweight patients (Roubenoff et al. 1993; Brownbill & Ilich 2005) (Figure 13.2) make DXA model dependent and less accurate than CT or MRI.

Computed Tomography (CT)

Signal intensity in the CT images corresponds to the linear attenuation coefficient, which depends on physical properties (including density) of tissue within the volume of interest. Signal intensity is expressed in so-called computed tomography numbers or Hounsfield units (HU), which range from −1,000 to +3,095 (4,096 values). Based on their density and the resulting differences in X-ray attenuation, muscle and fat tissue display different ranges of intensity (−190 to −30 HU for fat and 0 to 100 HU for muscle), resulting in muscle/fat contrast on the CT image (Figure 13.3). Recorded fat accumulation (for subcutaneous and visceral fat depots) is thus based on volumetric measurements (Dixon 1983; Tokunaga et al. 1983; Busetto et al. 1992). For ectopic (intrahepatic, intramyocellular) lipid accumulation, measurements are based on comparison of X-ray attenuation in liver tissue and spleen (Figure 13.4) or in muscle and fat tissue (bone marrow or external phantom (Goodpaster et al. 2000a)). These measurements have been validated against histological and biochemical measurement from biopsy (Ricci et al. 1997; Goodpaster et al. 2000a), yielding satisfactory correlation and showing an X-ray attenuation of 1.6 HU per mg tissue fat content.

The main advantage of imaging methods (CT and MRI) is the ability to quantitate localised adipose tissue or intracellular (ectopic) fat (Figure 13.3). The need for localised information can to some extent be met by DXA measurement, where images of specific body segments can be separated for the analysis, but DXA cannot provide the differentiation of subcutaneous and deeper fat or intracellular fat depots found in CT and MRI. Studies focusing on the measurement of abdominal distribution of fat tissue concluded that both

A

B

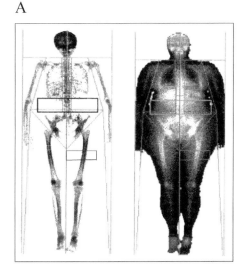
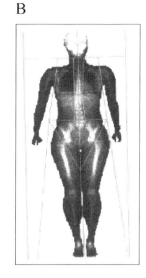

Figure 13.2 Assessment of Body Composition by Dual Energy X-ray Absorptiometry (DXA) DXA scans of strongly overweight and normal weight women: A) total body scan, with bones only (left) and with soft tissue (right), of a 104 kg woman (BMI = 34.1 kg/m^2). Portions of the arms fell out of the scan area and there is overlapping tissue in the chest, arm and hip regions. The abdominal and thigh regions of interest can be defined manually, while regions of interest in other parts of the body are determined by computer software (although the results can be manually changed); B) total body scan of a 59 kg woman (BMI = 22.6 kg/m^2) showing proper positioning on the scan table and no overlapping regions. Reprinted from Brownbill and Ilich, *BMC. Med. Imaging*, **5** (1), 1 Courtesy of BioMed Central.

CT and DXA measurement can successfully measure total abdominal fat mass (Jensen et al. 1995; Kelley et al. 2000) (Figure 13.2, 13.3) but only CT or MRI scans can predict intrabdominal (visceral) fat amount (Jensen et al. 1995). Early CT and MRI measurements of abdominal fat distribution were often limited to a single-slice scan in the L4–L5 level, but later studies identified this procedure as the source of an under-sampling error, increasing the variation of the results (Greenfield et al. 2002; Thomas & Bell 2003). For correct assessment of fat distribution, investigators are strongly advised to apply multi-slice or whole-body CT or MRI scans (Figure 13.5). However, this proposal highlights the safety limitation of CT scans: the relatively high radiation dose applied during whole-body measurements, which should restrict the use of CT, particularly in children.

Magnetic Resonance Imaging (MRI) and spectroscopy

Positioning of measured samples in strong homogeneous magnetic fields forces protons within the sample to align according to the direction of the magnetic field and thus create a macroscopic magnetisation of the sample. Interaction of spins with externally applied radiofrequency (RF) waves at the resonant frequency changes the magnitude and direction

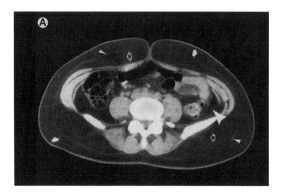

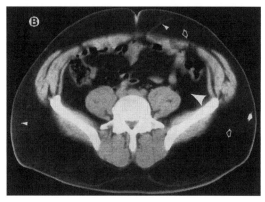

Figure 13.3 Assessment of Abdominal Fat Storage by Computed Tomography (CT) Representative cross-sectional abdominal CT scans of a lean (A) and an obese (B) research volunteer, demonstrating the fat/muscle CT contrast shown with demarcations of visceral (large arrowheads), deep subcutaneous (open arrows) and superficial subcutaneous (closed arrows) adipose tissue (AT) depots. The fascia (small arrowhead) within subcutaneous abdominal AT was used to distinguish superficial from deep depot. In the two CT scans shown, the area of superficial subcutaneous AT was similar (144 vs 141 cm^2), whereas areas of deep subcutaneous (126 vs 273 cm^2) and visceral (84 vs 153 cm^2) AT were quite different. Insulin-stimulated glucose metabolism was 6.1 and 4.0 mg/min^{-1}/kg FFM-1 in lean and obese volunteers, respectively (FFM: fat-free mass). Reproduced from Kelley D E et al. (2000) *Am J Physiol Endocrinol Metab* **278** (5) E941–E948. Courtesy of the American Physiological Society.

of this macroscopic magnetisation, in a process called excitation. After switching off the RF waves, magnetisation returns to the thermal equilibrium in a time and direction dependent manner. This process is called relaxation and the changing macroscopic magnetisation induces an electrical signal in the receiver coil. Signal intensity in MRI is dependent not only on the proton density in the volume of interest, but also on the interaction between tissue protons and externally applied RF waves during the excitation, and on the interaction between nuclei within the tissue during the relaxation. The different physical properties of protons within water and fatty acid molecules result in strong differences in the time and phase dependent behaviours of these nuclei during the relaxation, producing a relaxation and phase dependent contrast for magnetic resonance imaging.

A   B

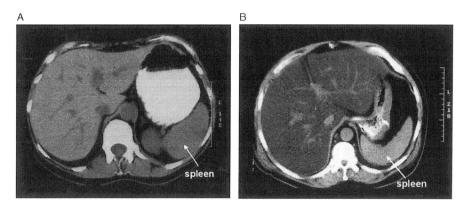

Figure 13.4 Assessment of Liver Fat Accumulation by CT A) CT scan of normal liver. The liver is denser (brighter) than the spleen; B) CT scan of a fatty liver. The liver is less dense (darker) than the spleen. Reproduced with permission from Joy D et al. (2003) *Eur J Gastroenterol Hepatol* **15** (5), 539–543.

T_1-relaxation based contrast can be used for volumetric measurements of subcutaneous and intra-abdominal fat accumulation. Multi-segment multi-slice 2D images or real 3D data sets are acquired (Thomas et al. 1998) and areas of fat volume can be segmented and divided into separate compartments in more or less automated fashion (Thomas & Bell 2003; Positano et al. 2004) (Figure 13.5). The acquisition of multi-segment multi-slice 2D data sets once required about 30 minutes, but the development of MRI hardware, data acquisition and reconstruction now allow for continuous whole body data acquisition during the defined movement of the patient table in the magnet (Kruger et al. 2002, 2005; Aldefeld et al. 2006; Sommer et al. 2006) (Figure 13.6). This improvement can reduce scanning time to less than three minutes and will make whole-body MRI measurement of fat distribution highly desirable and affordable, even for clinical praxis.

Phase-behaviour based contrast can be used for the quantitation of intrahepatic fat accumulation. Images with water and fat signal contributions 'in phase' and 'out of phase' are added or subtracted in order to obtain pure water and pure fat images (Dixon 1984; Reeder et al. 2004). Recently an iterative decomposition method yielding water and fat images from a single image acquisition was presented (Reeder et al. 2005; Fuller et al. 2006) and its feasibility for dynamic imaging was proven (Yu et al. 2006). Spatial resolution of MR images is given by system hardware performance and can be lower than 1 mm in plane.

In addition to imaging techniques, magnetic resonance can be applied in a spectroscopic fashion. Different electron clouds within the molecule result in a different resonance frequency of protons in water and fatty acid. This effect is called chemical shift of resonant frequencies and it does not depend on the magnetic field strength applied. In praxis it is given in relative units – parts per million (ppm). Localisation of the spectroscopic signal can be achieved in single voxel (volume pixel) (Figure 13.7) or in matrix-based multi voxel fashion. In the latter case, the method is called chemical shift imaging (CSI) or spectroscopic imaging (SI). The signal intensities of different chemical entities can be used to produce distribution maps of metabolites of interest. Current best achievable geometric resolution is $\sim$1 cm^3 for the ^{1}H single voxel spectroscopy (Anderwald et al. 2002) and $\sim$0.5 cm^3 for spectroscopic imaging (Hwang et al. 2001; Vermathen et al. 2004) (Figure 13.8). The main

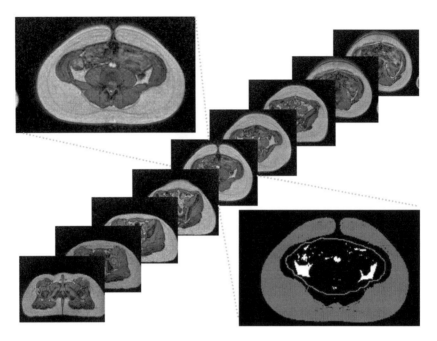

Figure 13.5 Assessment and Quantitation of Subcutaneous and Visceral Fat Amount by Multi-Slice MRI of Abdomen Selected representative MRI images acquired from the lower abdomen (lower left corner) up to the level of the liver (upper right corner) of a young overweight patient depict the T1 weighted MRI fat/muscle contrast. Middle slice in the belly region is enlarged (left) and the semi-automatic segmentation of different fat contributions (right; subcutaneous layer: grey; visceral fat: white) preceding the quantitation of fat volume is illustrated. Image data were kindly provided by M. Chmelík, Medical University of Vienna.

advantage of spectroscopic measurement is the direct separation and quantitation of water and fat fractions of diverse soft tissues. ^{13}C MRS, even though not so sensitive regarding the spectroscopic volume of interest, can also easily distinguish saturated and unsaturated tissue fat contributions (Beckmann et al. 1992; Petersen et al. 1996; Thomas et al. 1997). Absolute fat quantitation by MRS has been validated against gold standard histological and biochemical measures or CT measurements for liver (Longo et al. 1993; Thomsen et al. 1994; Petersen et al. 1996; Szczepaniak et al. 1999) and myocardial lipid measurements (Szczepaniak et al. 2003).

Differences in the magnetic properties of bulk cylinders like extramyocellular lipids (EMCL) and spherical vesicle-accumulated intramyocellular lipids (IMCL) give the potential to separate these two compartments. This phenomenon was observed for the first time in the early 1990s (Schick et al. 1993) and confirmed by theory (Boesch et al. 1997; Boesch & Kreis 2001) and model experiments (Szczepaniak et al. 2002) later on (Figure 13.7). Successful validation by histological and biochemical analysis of biopsies (Howald et al. 2002) and the increasing accessibility of MR equipment have led to numerous metabolic studies ever since (Krššák & Roden 2004; Boesch et al. 2006). For quantification purposes, the signal of tissue water (Boesch et al. 1997; Szczepaniak et al. 1999) or skeletal muscle creatine (Rico-Sanz et al. 1999) is taken as the internal reference. Lipid concentration can be given in these relative units (Krššák et al. 1999) or, assuming certain hydration or creatine concentration in

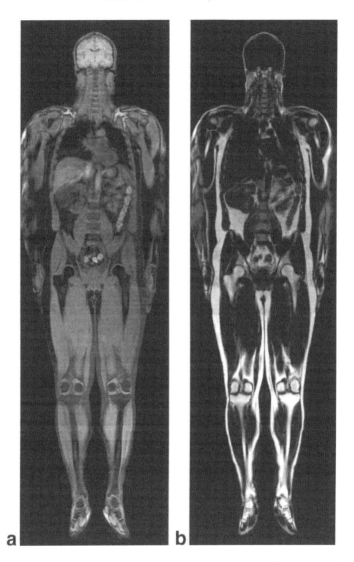

Figure 13.6 Whole Body Fat Distribution by Continuous Moving Table MRI Head-to-toe images acquired in two 3D MRI scans, with water-selective (a) and fat-selective (b) presaturation pulses. Each image shows one coronal plane from a 3D data set. The total scan time was 6 min per run. Reproduced with permission from Aldefeld B et al. (2006) *Magn Reson Med* **55** (5), 1210a–1216.

the tissue, fatty acid chain length and saturation distribution, and the specific weight of the water and fat compartment, calculated into normal concentration units ($mmol/l^{-1}$; mg/kg^{-1}) (Szczepaniak et al. 1999).

Another MR technique using conventional imaging technology, but exciting only the fat fraction of the tissue – based on its specific resonance frequency – is the recently introduced fat-selective MRI (Schick et al. 2002) (Figure 13.7). This method can produce fat distribution maps of liver and muscle with excellent spatial resolution (< 1 mm in plane)

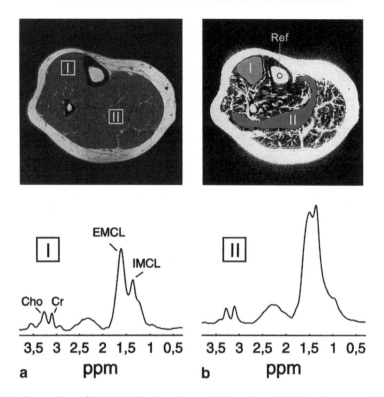

Figure 13.7 Comparison of Fat-Selective Imaging and Volume Localised Spectroscopy of Lipids Upper left panel shows a traditional T1 weighted MRI image, which guides the localisation of spectrum acquisition. Two volume elements of 12 mm X 12 mm X 20 mm were examined by a single-voxel STEAM technique. The spectra were recorded from representative regions of the tibialis anterior muscle (ROI I) and the soleus muscle (ROI II). The lipid signals in the spectra show a composition of EMCL and IMCL components. The water signal in spectra without water suppression (not shown) serves as reference for the assessment of total fat content. Upper right panel: analysis of the muscular lipid content in fat-selective images with 10 mm thickness was performed by the mean SI in selected ROIs (ROI I in the tibialis anterior muscle and ROI II in the soleus muscle). The borders of the ROIs can interactively be chosen during data processing in order to avoid undesired contributions from fatty material in the septa. Tibial bone marrow (Ref) serves as an internal reference with nearly 100 % fat content. Reproduced with permission from Schick F et al. (2005) *Magn Reson Med* **47** (4), 720–727.

(Machann et al. 2003; Goodpaster et al. 2004) but cannot separate extramyocellular and intramyocellular signal contributions. A similar disadvantage is found in CT quantification of muscle fat by overall signal attenuation. A recent study found that CT measurement was correlated with total intramuscular lipid concentration measured by MR spectroscopy (EMCL & IMCL) (Larson-Meyer et al. 2006b). Splitting the MRS measure into extra- and intra-cellular compartments yielded greater CT prediction of EMCL in the tibialis anterior muscle and of IMCL in the soleus muscle (Larson-Meyer et al. 2006b). This observation can be explained by the prevailing amount of EMCL and IMCL in the respective muscle group (Jacob et al. 1999; Anderwald et al. 2002; Kautzky-Willer et al. 2003).

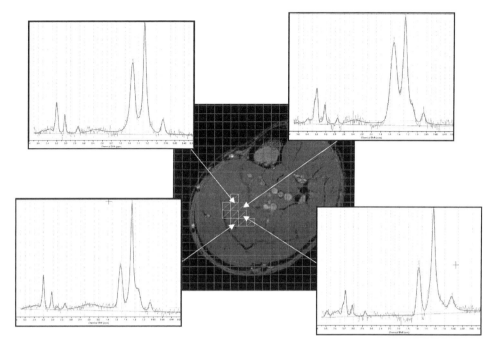

Figure 13.8 Assesment of Intramyocellular Fat Distribution by Proton Chemical Shift Imaging (CSI) Superb localisation ($\sim$0.33 cm^3) of spectral information and resulting excellent spectral resolution (separation between EMCL and IMCL contribution) achieved by ^{1}H CSI at higher field strength (3T). ^{1}H MR spectra are simultaneously obtained from the volumes of interest in soleus muscle as depicted on the image. Particular spectra can be added, yielding higher signal-to-noise ratio and anatomically matched voxel distribution. Image data were kindly provided by S. Gruber & M. Chmelík, Medical University of Vienna.

From a safety point of view, magnetic resonance techniques represent no radiation risk, but as discussed in Chapter 11, the presence of a strong magnetic field and the switching of magnetic field gradients make metallic objects (splinters, tattoos, coloured contact lenses, piercings, uterus coils), other medical devices (pace makers, cardiac valves, clips, electrodes, neuro-stimulators), implants, prosthetics, shunts and stents contraindication for the MR examination. Another practical consideration is the restricted space in the clear bore of the magnet. The usual clear diameter of $\sim$60–70 cm can exclude morbidly obese patients from the examination. Nevertheless, the advantages and the versatility of the method as well as the wider spread of clinical MR systems predetermine broad application in future clinical praxis.

Body fat distribution and insulin resistance

Skeletal muscle – intramyocellular lipids

Overabundance of plasma triglycerides and free fatty acids entering the circulation by lipolysis from adipose tissue or by ingestion from food is frequently associated with pathophysiology of insulin resistance and diabetes mellitus (Defronzo 2004). Results of radioactive tracer and stable isotope dilution studies have suggested that both hepatic and peripheral muscle tissues are involved in the development of insulin resistance (Defronzo 1988). Focusing on glucose uptake in skeletal muscle, based on the results of his experimental studies series, Sir Randle (Randle et al. 1963) postulated the hypothesis that the substrate competition for mitochondrial oxidation is the major mechanism involved in the impairment of glucose uptake into skeletal muscle. Recent studies applying ^{13}C and ^{31}P MRS methods (reviewed in Chapter 11 of this book) and analysis of skeletal muscle biopsy have shown that direct impairment of insulin signalling cascade (Griffin et al. 1999), and therefore direct impairment of glucose transport (Cline et al. 1999), phosphorylation (Roden et al. 1996, 1999; Krebs et al. 2001) and glycogen synthesis (Roden et al. 1996; Delmas-Beauvieux et al. 1999) are the effect of circulating FFA on the glucose metabolism. These and other studies (Boden & Chen 1995; Boden et al. 1995) have shown that experimental elevation of free fatty acids causes similar defects in the skeletal muscle glucose metabolism as those found in various pathologically insulin-resistant states – T2DM, offspring, IR (Shulman et al. 1990; Rothman et al. 1991, 1992; Perseghin et al. 1996; Petersen et al. 1998). On the other hand, it is still under debate whether or not – and why – persistent suppression of plasma FFA concentration is necessary to improve skeletal muscle insulin sensitivity (Bajaj et al. 2004, 2005; Johnson et al. 2006; Santomauro et al. 1999).

Another metabolically active source of triglycerides that could influence cellular glucose uptake is the lipids stored in the cytosol of non-adipose tissue. Such lipid vesicles can be found in the skeletal muscle, myocardum, liver and pancreatic β-cells. These fat depots are not released into the circulation, but may influence glucose utilisation directly. Early evidence from histological and biochemical skeletal muscle biopsy analysis have shown a correlation between skeletal muscle triglyceride aggregation and insulin resistance (Phillips et al. 1996; Pan et al. 1997; Ebeling et al. 1998). These techniques, however, could not sufficiently discriminate between intramyocellular (IMCL) and extramyocellular (EMCL) lipid stores and so the question about the direct effect of intracellular lipids remained open. Consequent correlative studies, using localised ^{1}H MRS of skeletal muscle, have shown increased IMCL content in different insulin resistant – lean, obese, adolescent, type 1 and type 2 diabetic – populations (Jacob et al. 1999; Krššák et al. 1999; Perseghin et al. 1999, 2003; Sinha et al. 2002; Larson-Meyer et al. 2006a) (Figure 13.9). These findings are supported by the results of studies using CT measurement of skeletal muscle fat content (Goodpaster et al. 2000a,b). Further experiments have revealed differences in IMCL content in different muscle groups (Jacob et al. 1999; Perseghin et al. 1999; Hwang et al. 2001; Anderwald et al. 2002; Schick et al. 2002; Kautzky-Willer et al. 2003; Vermathen et al. 2004) (Figure 13.7), highlighting the different relationships between insulin sensitivity and IMCL content in predominantly oxidative or predominantly glycolytic muscles. These studies showed lower IMCL content in glycolytic, fibre type II – tibialis anterior muscle, as compared to the oxidative fibre type I – soleus muscle (Jacob et al.1999; Perseghin et al. 1999; Hwang et al. 2001; Anderwald et al. 2002; Kautzky-Willer et al. 2003; Vermathen et al. 2004). These results (Jacob et al. 1999; Anderwald et al. 2002; Kautzky-Willer et al. 2003) could also show that IMCL content in tibialis anterior muscle is a better predictor of peripheral insulin resistance than IMCL content in soleus muscle, which is more tightly associated with the indexes of whole body adiposity such as body mass index (BMI). Taken together, these studies suggested the hypothesis that IMCLs, especially in glycolytic tibialis anterior muscle, influence directly skeletal muscle glucose uptake and therefore that its content is a good marker of insulin resistance. However, increased IMCL content was also observed in endurance-

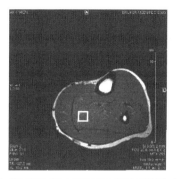

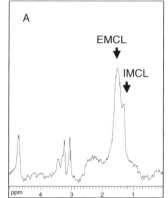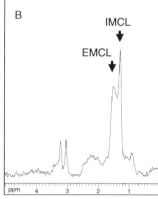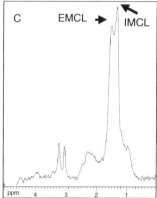

Figure 13.9 Differences in Intramyocellular Fat Accumulation Single voxel ^{1}H MR spectra of the soleus muscle obtained at magnetic field strength of 3T in three different subjects. Spectrum A is from the solues muscle, with low IMCL content (0.70 % of water resonance); spectrum B is from muscle with average IMCL content (1.47 %); and spectrum C is from muscle with high IMCL content (1.94 %). EMCL denotes extramyocellular lipids. Upper panel shows cross-sectional image of human calf muscle, with a typical volume of the area of interest for single voxel localised MR spectroscopy of soleus muscle.

trained athletes (Goodpaster et al. 2001; Thamer et al. 2003), who are also highly insulin sensitive.

Revealing this paradox demanded systematic explanation. Recent papers using histo-chemical analysis of muscle biopsies focusing on muscle fibre type specific triglyceride content and fibre type distribution in insulin sensitive, insulin resistant and endurance trained states, show a shift in muscle fibre distribution towards oxidative type 1 muscle fibres (Hickey et al. 1995; Anderson et al. 1997; Nyholm et al. 1997; Clore et al. 1998), increased type 1 fibre specific IMCL content in trained individuals and increased skeletal muscle and whole-body oxidative capacity in those with endurance training (Essen & Haggmark 1975; He et al. 2001; Goodpaster et al. 2003). The observation of IMCL depletion during prolonged sub-maximal exercise (Krššák et al. 2000; Brechtel et al. 2001; Larson-Meyer et al. 2002; White et al. 2003), suggesting the idea that increased IMCL stores could be of substantial benefit for endurance runners, sparked the question of whether the increased muscular triglyceride concentrations are the cause of insulin resistance or rather the result of impaired oxidative capacity in the skeletal muscle of insulin-resistant individuals.

Further studies were designed to assess the regulation of IMCL stores in various conditions. First of all it was hypothesised that experimental elevation of IMCL content would cause or at least would be associated with increased insulin resistance. At the same time, diet or pharmacologically introduced increase in insulin sensitivity should be mirrored by a decrease in IMCL content.

The first part was shown to be true in the case of a three days (Bachmann et al. 2001) high fat diet and intravenous intralipid/heparin infusion induced peripheral insulin resistance (Bachmann et al. 2001; Boden et al. 2001). Researchers could observe a parallel increase of IMCL content, relatively more pronounced in the tibialis anterior muscle of young healthy humans (Bachmann et al. 2001; Boden et al. 2001). Similar results, accompanied by molecular adaptations favouring fat storage in muscle, were found in another study after one week of high fat diet (Schrauwen-Hinderling et al. 2005). Inducing insulin resistance by i.v. amino acid infusion during euglycaemic-hyperinsulinaemia (Krebs et al. 2001) was met by a subtle increase of IMCL content in soleus muscle. IMCL content decreased with increasing insulin sensitivity due to 8–10 months of leptin replacement in patients generalised lipodystrophy (Simha et al. 2003) and 6 months of caloric restriction with or without exercise in an overweight population (Larson-Meyer et al. 2006a).

On the other hand, similar (Bachmann et al. 2001; Boden et al. 2001) but shorter intralipid infusion in young healthy men decreased the glucose uptake but did not increase the IMCL content in the soleus muscle (Brehm et al. 2006). Another study showed that increased plasma FFA elevated by three days of fasting induced increase of IMCL level in the vastus lateralis muscle (Stannard et al. 2002) of young healthy males. Prolonged tight glycaemic control by i.v. insulin infusion did not improve peripheral insulin sensitivity in T2DM, and increased IMCL content in soleus but not tibialis anterior muscle (Anderwald et al. 2002). IMCL stores also increased with the endurance exercise training programme, despite obvious increase of insulin sensitivity (Schrauwen-Hinderling et al. 2003), and remained stable despite improving insulin sensitivity by diet intervention in young healthy humans (Frost et al. 2003), or three months of glitazone treatment in T2DM (Mayerson et al. 2002).

These, to some extent controversial, findings shifted the focus back to the skeletal muscle lipid oxidation pathway, as it was hypothesised that mitochondrial oxidative and phosphorylation capacity might be a contributing factor to insulin resistance and increased IMCL content (Shulman 2000). One of the key intermediate metabolites of lipid oxidation long-chain acyl-CoA was found to be involved in the regulation of skeletal muscle glucose transport and utilisation (Wititsuwannakul & Kim 1977; Faergeman & Knudsen 1997; Tippett & Neet 1982), and its intracellular content was negatively correlated with whole-body insulin sensitivity (Ellis et al. 2000). in vitro studies also found that accelerated beta-oxidation in muscle cells exerts an insulin-sensitising effect independently of changes in intracellular lipid content (Perdomo et al. 2004) and that increased stearoyl-CoA desaturase 1 activity protects against fatty acid induced skeletal muscle insulin resistance (Pinnamaneni et al. 2006). Recent studies found that skeletal muscle mitochondrial phosphorylation capacity and/or ATP demand is associated with decrease of peripheral insulin sensitivity and increased IMCL content in elderly sedentary individuals (Petersen et al. 2003) and insulin-resistant offspring of T2DM patients (Petersen et al. 2005). Skeletal muscle oxidative capacity was identified as a better predictor of insulin sensitivity than either IMCL concentration or long-chain fatty acyl-CoA content in a population spanning from older T2DM to young, well trained athletes (Bruce et al. 2003), and in another, slightly overweight (BMI ~ 29 kg/m^{-2}) type 2 diabetic population (Schrauwen-Hinderling et al. 2006). It was also shown that experimental elevation of circulating FFA diminishes the effect of insulin stimulation on skeletal muscle ATP synthesis in the parallel, with the effect on glucose transport and phosphorylation but without an influence on IMCL content in skeletal muscle (Brehm et al. 2006). Physical activity induced enhancement of lipid oxidation is also associated with improvements in insulin sensitivity in overweight and obese sedentary humans (Gan et al. 2003; Goodpaster et al. 2003; Larson-Meyer et al. 2006a).

To summarise, recent studies have revealed increased IMCL content in sedentary and insulin-resistant individuals. However, the result also supports the hypothesis that increased intramyocellular fat accumulation is a result of defects in lipid oxidation and/or lipid oversupply, rather than a direct cause of insulin resistance, and that IMCL stores are an efficient energy storage pool, which is increased in endurance trained individuals.

Liver – intrahepatic lipids

As with skeletal muscle, elevated circulating free fatty acids (FFA) are associated with hepatic features of insulin resistance: increased fasting endogenous glucose production (EGP;Hundal et al. 2000), insufficient suppression of EGP in the postprandial state (Singhal et al. 2002; Krššák et al. 2004) and defects in hepatic glycogen synthesis (Krššák et al. 2004) in type 2 diabetes. Studies in young healthy volunteers have shown that experimentally elevated FFA concentration increased gluconeogenesis (Roden et al. 2000), which then led to a lower rate of hepatic glycogen breakdown (Stingl et al. 2001). Besides direct effects on hepatic glucose metabolism, chronically increased circulating FFA favours intrahepatic lipid accumulation (Krššák & Roden 2004; Roden 2006), which relationship to whole-body and hepatic glucose fluxes can effectively be studied only using modern imaging techniques.

The invasiveness of the biopsy procedure and non-quantitative nature of ultrasound measurement made it very difficult to assess liver fat accumulation in different populations, but MRI (Dixon 1984), localised ^{1}H (Thomsen et al. 1994) and ^{13}C MRS (Petersen et al. 1996) and computed tomography (Longo et al. 1993; Ricci et al. 1997) can provide a direct quantitative estimate of intrahepatic lipid content. Application of the noninvasive method enabled studies on larger populations, showing that almost one third of the population ($n = 2{,}287$) of Dallas County, Texas, has hepatic steatosis (Browning et al. 2004).

As in the skeletal muscle, the first studies were designed to find an association between hepatic fat content and features of insulin resistance in various populations. Increased hepatic fat content was found and associated with various measures of insulin resistance in T2DM (Figure 13.10) (Ryysy et al. 2000; Anderwald et al. 2002; Mayerson et al. 2002; Kelley et al. 2003; Krššák et al. 2004), in women with previous gestational diabetes (Seppala-Lindroos et al. 2002; Tiikkainen et al. 2002; Larson-Meyer et al. 2006a) as well as in insulin resistant lipodystrophic patients (Petersen et al. 2002; Sutinen et al. 2002). It was also linked with hepatic insulin resistance (Marchesini et al. 2001) and impaired whole-body reaction to oral glucose test challenge (Sargin et al. 2003) in non-alcoholic fatty liver disease.

Pharmacological and lifestyle intervention studies successfully found the association between improved insulin sensitivity or splanchnic glucose uptake and decreased hepatocellular fat content in T2DM after glitazone treatment (Katoh et al. 2001; Carey et al. 2002; Mayerson et al. 2002; Bajaj et al. 2003), in lipodystrophic patients due to the leptin treatment

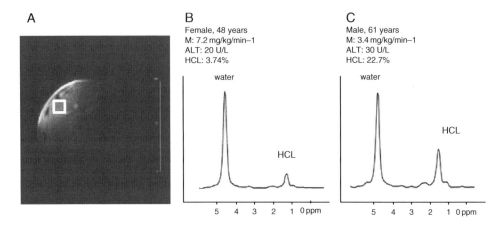

Figure 13.10 Localised [1] H MR Spectroscopy for the Quantification of Hepatocellular Lipid Concentrations A) Liver image guides the localisation of the region of interest within the liver; B) ^{1}H MR spectrum obtained from the liver of an insulin-sensitive woman with low hepatocellular lipid levels; C) ^{1}H MR spectrum obtained from the liver of an insulin-resistant man with increased aminotransferase and hepatocellular lipid levels. ALT: aminotransferase; HCL: hepatocellular lipid; M: M value is a measure of whole-body insulin sensitivity and denominates the glucose infusion rate per bodyweight and time required to maintain normoglycaemia during the hyperinsulinaemic clamp (Copyright © 2006 Nature Publishing Group. All rights reserved. Reproduced with permission from Roden M. *Nat. Clin. Pract. Endocrinol. Metab.* vol. 2, pp. 335–348).

(Petersen et al. 2002; Simha et al. 2003) and after six months of calorie restriction with or without exercise in overweight populations (Larson-Meyer et al. 2006a). However, the 72 h of tight glycaemic control in T2DM using manually adjusted intravenous insulin infusion induced an increase in hepatocellular lipid content despite a subtle improvement of insulin induced suppression of EGP (Anderwald et al. 2002).

Whole body fat distribution – subcutaneous and visceral fat

Along with the fat ingestion in the postprandial state, the lipolysis from different adipose tissues within the human body is the main source of circulating FFA in fasting conditions.

Even though the total fat mass determines the plasma pool of FFA and thereby the FFA flux from adipose to non-adipose tissue (Lewis et al. 2002), there are differences in the relationship of subcutaneous and visceral fat depots to features of peripheral and hepatic insulin sensitivity (Misra et al. 1997). Visceral fat cells are more sensitive than subcutaneous fat cells to the lipolytic effect of catecholamines and less sensitive to the antilipolytic and fatty acid re-esterification effects of insulin (Kahn & Flier 2000). Furthermore, the venous effluent of visceral fat depots leads directly into the portal vein, resulting in greater FFA flux to the liver. This makes the visceral fat depots more efficient than subcutaneous fat in influencing the carbohydrate metabolism in the human body (Kissebah 1996).

Whole-body MRI and CT are the methods of choice for the quantitation of visceral fat accumulation and whole-body fat distribution. Their noninvasive nature and easy-to-follow clinical measurement protocols enable broad usage of this measurement (Dixon 1983;

Tokunaga et al. 1983; Busetto et al. 1992; Thomas & Bell 2003; Positano et al. 2004; Machann et al. 2005;). Using these methods, total amount of visceral fat was linked to different measures of insulin resistance in T2DM (Kohrt et al. 1993; Anderson et al. 1997; Gautier et al. 1998; Gastaldelli et al. 2002; Miyazaki et al. 2002a; Kelley et al. 2003), obese childrens and adolescents (Caprio et al. 1995; Caprio 1999; Weiss et al. 2003), HIV protease inhibitor-related lipodystrophy patients (Gan et al. 2002), obese Hispanic children with a family history of type 2 diabetes (Goodfriend et al. 1999; Cruz et al. 2002) and Caucasian men (Seidell et al. 1989; Forouhi et al. 1999; Kelley et al. 2000). Some studies also suggested a major role for deep subcutaneous adipose tissue in the genesis of insulin resistance (Kelley et al. 2000). It was found that the amount of visceral fat is a good predictor of intrahepatic fat accumulation (Thamer et al. 2004).

In the intervention studies, decrease of visceral fat content with concomitant increase of insulin sensitivity was observed after glitazone therapy in T2DM (Carey et al. 2002; Miyazaki et al. 2002b; Gastaldelli et al. 2006) and non-diabetic obesity (Shadid & Jensen 2003), and preferential decrease of visceral and/or intrahepatic fat was observed after weight reduction following lifestyle change in healthy, T2DM-risk patients (Machann et al. 2006) and also in obese (Goodpaster et al. 1999; Ross et al. 2004) and non-obese (Thomas et al. 2000) study populations. Another study found that weight loss by diet restriction alone does not yield a decreased visceral adiposity; however, the addition of exercise to diet regimen is necessary for visceral adipose tissue loss (Giannopoulou et al. 2005) in women with type 2 diabetes.

To conclude, there is strong evidence that, together with intramyocellular lipids, visceral and hepatic fat accumulation is a very good indicator of peripheral and hepatic insulin resistance in sedentary population and type 2 diabetic patients. The more uniform response of hepatic and visceral fat content to lifestyle intervention and pharmacological therapies makes it a better marker of changes of insulin sensitivity in insulin resistant and T2DM individuals. Further studies are, however, needed to fully explain the mechanism of the interaction between intracellular lipids and insulin action in the human tissue. More understanding, widespread and intensive use of noninvasive quantitative methods – such as magnetic resonance imaging and spectroscopy, as well as computed tomography – will enable even larger scale cross-sectional and interventional studies of this issue.

References

Abe, T, Kawakami, Y, Sugita, M, Yoshikawa, K, Fukunaga, T (1995) Use of B–mode ultrasound for visceral fat mass evaluation: comparisons with magnetic resonance imaging, *Appl Human Sci*, **14**, 3, 133–139

Aldefeld, B, Bornert, P, Keupp, J (2006) Continuously moving table 3D MRI with lateral frequency-encoding direction, *Magn Reson Med*, **55**, 5, 1210–1216

Anderson, P J, Chan, J C, Chan, Y L, Tomlinson, B, Young, R P, Lee, Z S, Lee, K K, Metreweli, C, Cockram, C S, Critchley, J A (1997) Visceral fat and cardiovascular risk factors in Chinese NIDDM patients, *Diabetes Care*, **20**, 12, 1854–1858

Anderwald, C, Bernroider, E, Krššák, M, Stingl, H, Brehm, A, Bischof, M G et al. (2002) Effects of insulin treatment in type 2 diabetic patients on intracellular lipid content in liver and skeletal muscle, *Diabetes*, **51**, 10, 3025–3032

Armellini, F, Zamboni, M, Rigo, L, Todesco, T, Bergamo-Andreis, I A, Procacci, C, Bosello, O (1990) The contribution of sonography to the measurement of intra-abdominal fat, *J Clin Ultrasound*, **18**, 7, 563–567

Aube, C, Oberti, F, Korali, N, Namour, M A, Loisel, D, Tanguy, J Y et al. (1999) Ultrasonographic diagnosis of hepatic fibrosis or cirrhosis, *J Hepatol*, **30**, 3, 472–478

Bachmann, O P, Dahl, D B, Brechtel, K, Machann, J, Haap, M, Maier et al. (2001) Effects of intravenous and dietary lipid challenge on intramyocellular lipid content and the relation with insulin sensitivity in humans, *Diabetes*, **50**, 11, 2579–2584

Bajaj, M, Suraamornkul, S, Kashyap, S, Cusi, K, Mandarino, L, Defronzo, R A (2004) Sustained reduction in plasma free fatty acid concentration improves insulin action without altering plasma adipocytokine levels in subjects with strong family history of type 2 diabetes, *J Clin Endocrinol Metab*, **89**, 9, 4649–4655

Bajaj, M, Suraamornkul, S, Pratipanawatr, T, Hardies, L J, Pratipanawatr, W, Glass, L, Cersosimo, E, Miyazaki, Y, Defronzo, R A (2003) Pioglitazone reduces hepatic fat content and augments splanchnic glucose uptake in patients with type 2 diabetes, *Diabetes*, **52**, 6, 1364–1370

Bajaj, M, Suraamornkul, S, Romanelli, A, Cline, G W, Mandarino, L J, Shulman, G I, Defronzo, R A (2005) Effect of a sustained reduction in plasma free fatty acid concentration on intramuscular long-chain fatty Acyl-CoAs and insulin action in type 2 diabetic patients, *Diabetes*, **54**, 11, 3148–3153

Beckmann, N, Brocard, J-J, Keller, U, Seelig, J (1992) Relationship between the degree of unsaturation of dietary fatty acids and adipose tissue fatty acids assessed by natural-abundance 13C magnetic resonance spectroscopy in man, *Magn Reson Med*, **27**, 97–106

Bedogni, G, Bellentani, S, Miglioli, L, Masutti, F, Passalacqua, M, Castiglione, A, Tiribelli, C (2006) The Fatty Liver Index: a simple and accurate predictor of hepatic steatosis in the general population, *BMCG astroenterol*, **6**, 33

Boden, G Chen, X (1995) Effects of fat on glucose uptake and utilization in patients with non–insulin-dependent diabetes, *J Clin Invest*, **96**, 3, 1261–1268

Boden, G, Chen, X, Rosner, J, Barton, M (1995) Effects of a 48-h fat infusion on insulin secretion and glucose utilization, *Diabetes*, **44**, 10, 1239–1242

Boden, G, Lebed, B, Schatz, M, Homko, C, Lemieux, S (2001) Effects of acute changes of plasma free fatty acids on intramyocellular fat content and insulin resistance in healthy subjects, *Diabetes*, **50**, 7, 1612–1617

Boesch, C Kreis, R (2001) Dipolar coupling and ordering effects observed in magnetic resonance spectra of skeletal muscle, *NMR Biomed*, **14**, 2, 140–148

Boesch, C, Machann, J, Vermathen, P, Schick, F (2006) Role of proton MR fort he study of muscle lipid metabolism, *NMR Biomed*, **19**, 968–988

Boesch, C, Slotboom, J, Hoppeler, H, Kreis, R (1997) In vivo determination of intra–myocellular lipids in human muscle by means of localized 1H–MR–spectroscopy, *Magn Reson Med*, **37**, 4, 484–493

Brechtel, K, Niess, A M, Machann, J, Rett, K, Schick, F, Claussen, C D, Dickhuth, H H, Haering, H U, Jacob, S (2001) Utilisation of intramyocellular lipids (IMCLs) during exercise as assessed by proton magnetic resonance spectroscopy (1H-MRS), *Horm Metab Res*, **33**, 2, 63–66

Brehm, A, Krššák, M, Schmid, A I, Nowotny, P, Waldhausl, W, Roden, M (2006) Increased lipid availability impairs insulin–stimulated ATP synthesis in human skeletal muscle, *Diabetes*, **55**, 1, 136–140

Brownbill, R A Ilich, J Z (2005) Measuring body composition in overweight individuals by dual energy x-ray absorptiometry, *BMC Med Imaging*, **5**, 1, 1

Browning, J D, Szczepaniak, L S, Dobbins, R, Nuremberg, P, Horton, J D, Cohen, J C, Grundy, S M, Hobbs, H H (2004) Prevalence of hepatic steatosis in an urban population in the United States: impact of ethnicity, *Hepatology*, **40**, 6, 1387–1395

Bruce, C R, Anderson, M J, Carey, A L, Newman, D G, Bonen, A, Kriketos, A D, Cooney, G J, Hawley, J A (2003) Muscle oxidative capacity is a better predictor of insulin sensitivity than lipid status, *J Clin Endocrinol Metab*, **88**, 11, 5444–5451

Busetto, L, Baggio, M B, Zurlo, F, Carraro, R, Digito, M, Enzi, G (1992) Assessment of abdominal fat distribution in obese patients: anthropometry versus computerized tomography, *Int J Obes Relat Metab Disord*, **16**, 10, 731–736

Caprio, S (1999) Relationship between abdominal visceral fat and metabolic risk factors in obese adolescents, *Am J Human Biol*, **11**, 2, 259–266

Caprio, S, Hyman, L D, Limb, C, McCarthy, S, Lange, R, Sherwin, R S, Shulman, G, Tamborlane, W V (1995) Central adiposity and its metabolic correlates in obese adolescent girls, *Am J Physiol*, **269**, 1, E118–E126

Carey, D G, Cowin, G J, Galloway, G J, Jones, N P, Richards, J C, Biswas, N, Doddrell, D M (2002) Effect of rosiglitazone on insulin sensitivity and body composition in type 2 diabetic patients [corrected], *Obes Res*, **10**, 10, 1008–1015

Celle, G, Savarino, V, Picciotto, A, Magnolia, M R, Scalabrini, P, Dodero, M (1988) Is hepatic ultrasonography a valid alternative tool to liver biopsy? Report on 507 cases studied with both techniques, *Dig Dis Sci*, **33**, 4, 467–471

Cline, G W, Petersen, K F, Krššák, M, Shen, J, Hundal, R S, Trajanoski, Z, Inzucchi, S, Dresner, A, Rothman, D L, Shulman, G I (1999) Impaired glucose transport as a cause of decreased insulin–stimulated muscle glycogen synthesis in type 2 diabetes, *N Engl J Med*, **341**, 4, 240–246

Clore, J N, Li, J, Gill, R, Gupta, S, Spencer, R, Azzam, A, Zuelzer, W, Rizzo, W B, Blackard, W G (1998) Skeletal muscle phosphatidylcholine fatty acids and insulin sensitivity in normal humans, *Am J Physiol*, **275**, 4 Pt 1, E665–E670

Cox-Reijven, P L Soeters, P B (2000) Validation of bio–impedance spectroscopy: effects of degree of obesity and ways of calculating volumes from measured resistance values, *Int J Obes Relat Metab Disord*, **24**, 3, 271–280

Cruz, M L, Bergman, R N, Goran, M I (2002) Unique effect of visceral fat on insulin sensitivity in obese Hispanic children with a family history of type 2 diabetes, *Diabetes Care*, **25**, 9, 1631–1636

De Lorenzo, A, Sorge, R P, Candeloro, N, Di Campli, C, Sesti, G, Lauro, R (1999) New insights into body composition assessment in obese women, *Can J Physiol Pharmacol*, **77**, 1, 17–21

Defronzo, R A 1988, Lilly lecture (1987) The triumvirate: beta-cell, muscle, liver A collusion responsible for NIDDM, *Diabetes*, **37**, 6, 667–687

Defronzo, R A (2004) Pathogenesis of type 2 diabetes mellitus, *Med Clin North Am*, **88**, 4, 787–835, ix

Delmas-Beauvieux, M C, Quesson, B, Thiaudiere, E, Gallis, J L, Canioni, P, Gin, H (1999) 13C nuclear magnetic resonance study of glycogen resynthesis in muscle after glycogen-depleting exercise in healthy men receiving an infusion of lipid emulsion, *Diabetes*, **48**, 2, 327–333

Dempster, P Aitkens, S (1995) A new air displacement method for the determination of human body composition, *Med Sci Sports Exerc*, **27**, 12, 1692–1697

Dixon, A K (1983) Abdominal fat assessed by computed tomography: sex difference in distribution, *Clin Radiol*, **34**, 2, 189–191

Dixon, W T (1984) Simple proton spectroscopic imaging, *Radiology*, **153**, 1, 189–194

Ebeling, P, Essen-Gustavsson, B, Tuominen, J A, Koivisto, V A (1998) Intramuscular triglyceride content is increased in IDDM, *Diabetologia*, **41**, 1, 111–115

Ellis, B A, Poynten, A, Lowy, A J, Furler, S M, Chisholm, D J, Kraegen, E W, Cooney, G J (2000) Long-chain acyl-CoA esters as indicators of lipid metabolism and insulin sensitivity in rat and human muscle, *Am J Physiol Endocrinol Metab*, **279**, 3, p E554–E560

Essen, B Haggmark, T (1975) Lactate concentration in type I and II muscle fibres during muscular contraction in man, *Acta Physiol Scand*, **95**, 3, 344–346

Faergeman, N J Knudsen, J (1997) Role of long-chain fatty acyl–CoA esters in the regulation of metabolism and in cell signalling, *BiochemJ*, **323**, 1, 1–12

Fields, D A, Goran, M I, McCrory, M A (2002) Body-composition assessment via air-displacement plethysmography in adults and children: a review, *Am J ClinNutr*, **75**, 3, 453–467

Fontana, R J Lok, A S (2002) Noninvasive monitoring of patients with chronic hepatitis C, *Hepatology*, **36**, 5, Suppl. 1, S57–S64

Forouhi, N G, Jenkinson, G, Thomas, E L, Mullick, S, Mierisova, S, Bhonsle, U, McKeigue, P M, Bell, J D (1999) Relation of triglyceride stores in skeletal muscle cells to central obesity and insulin sensitivity in European and South Asian men, *Diabetologia*, **42**, 8, 932–935

Frost, G S, Goff, L M, Hamilton, G, Thomas, E L, Dhillo, W S, Dornhorst, A, Bell, J D (2003) Carbohydrate-induced manipulation of insulin sensitivity independently of intramyocellular lipids, *Br J Nutr*, **89**, 3, 365–375

Fuller, S, Reeder, S, Shimakawa, A, Yu, H, Johnson, J, Beaulieu, C, Gold, G E (2006) Iterative decomposition of water and fat with echo asymmetry and least-squares estimation (IDEAL) fast spin-echo imaging of the ankle: initial clinical experience, *AJR Am J Roentgenol*, **187**, 6, 1442–1447

Gan, S K, Kriketos, A D, Ellis, B A, Thompson, C H, Kraegen, E W, Chisholm, D J (2003) Changes in aerobic capacity and visceral fat but not myocyte lipid levels predict increased insulin action after exercise in overweight and obese men, *Diabetes Care*, **26**, 6, 1706–1713

Gan, S K, Samaras, K, Thompson, C H, Kraegen, E W, Carr, A, Cooper, D A, Chisholm, D J (2002) Altered myocellular and abdominal fat partitioning predict disturbance in insulin action in HIV protease inhibitor–related lipodystrophy, *Diabetes*, **51**, 11, 3163–3169

Gastaldelli, A, Miyazaki, Y, Pettiti, M, Matsuda, M, Mahankali, S, Santini, E, Defronzo, R A, Ferrannini, E (2002) Metabolic effects of visceral fat accumulation in type 2 diabetes, *J Clin Endocrinol Metab*, **87**, 11, 5098–5103

Gastaldelli, A, Miyazaki, Y, Pettiti, M, Santini, E, Ciociaro, D, Defronzo, R A, Ferrannini, E (2006) The effect of rosiglitazone on the liver: decreased gluconeogenesis in patients with type 2 diabetes, *J Clin Endocrinol Metab*, **91**, 3, 806–812

Gautier, J F, Mourier, A, de Kerviler, E, Tarentola, A, Bigard, A X, Villette, J M, Guezennec, C Y, Cathelineau, G (1998) Evaluation of abdominal fat distribution in noninsulin-dependent diabetes mellitus: relationship to insulin resistance, *J Clin Endocrinol Metab*, **83**, 4, 1306–1311

Giannopoulou, I, Fernhall, B, Carhart, R, Weinstock, R S, Baynard, T, Figueroa, A, Kanaley, J A (2005) Effects of diet and/or exercise on the adipocytokine and inflammatory cytokine levels of postmenopausal women with type 2 diabetes, *Metabolism*, **54**, 7, 866–875

Goodfriend, T L, Kelley, D E, Goodpaster, B H, Winters, S J (1999) Visceral obesity and insulin resistance are associated with plasma aldosterone levels in women, *Obes Res*, **7**, 4, 355–362

Goodpaster, B H, He, J, Watkins, S, Kelley, D E (2001) Skeletal muscle lipid content and insulin resistance: evidence for a paradox in endurance-trained athletes, *J Clin Endocrinol Metab*, **86**, 12, 5755–5761

Goodpaster, B H, Katsiaras, A, Kelley, D E (2003) Enhanced fat oxidation through physical activity is associated with improvements in insulin sensitivity in obesity, *Diabetes*, **52**, 9, 2191–2197

Goodpaster, B H, Kelley, D E, Thaete, F L, He, J, Ross, R (2000a) Skeletal muscle attenuation determined by computed tomography is associated with skeletal muscle lipid content, *J Appl Physiol*, **89**, 1, 104–110

Goodpaster, B H, Kelley, D E, Wing, R R, Meier, A, Thaete, F L (1999) Effects of weight loss on regional fat distribution and insulin sensitivity in obesity, *Diabetes*, **48**, 4, 839–847

Goodpaster, B H, Stenger, V A, Boada, F, McKolanis, T, Davis, D, Ross, R, Kelley, D E (2004) Skeletal muscle lipid concentration quantified by magnetic resonance imaging, *Am J Clin Nutr*, **79**, 5, 748–754

Goodpaster, B H, Theriault, R, Watkins, S C, Kelley, D E (2000b) Intramuscular lipid content is increased in obesity and decreased by weight loss, *Metabolism*, **49**, 4, 467–472

Greenfield, J R, Samaras, K, Chisholm, D J, Campbell, L V (2002) Regional intra-subject variability in abdominal adiposity limits usefulness of computed tomography, *Obes Res*, **10**, 4, 260–265

Griffin, M E, Marcucci, M J, Cline, G W, Bell, K, Barucci, N, Lee, D, Goodyear, L J, Kraegen, E W, White, M F, Shulman, G I (1999) Free fatty acid-induced insulin resistance is associated with activation of protein kinase C theta and alterations in the insulin signaling cascade, *Diabetes*, **48**, 6, 1270–1274

He, J, Watkins, S, Kelley, D E (2001) Skeletal muscle lipid content and oxidative enzyme activity in relation to muscle fiber type in type 2 diabetes and obesity, *Diabetes*, **50**, 4, 817–823

Heymsfield, S B, Nunez, C, Testolin, C, Gallagher, D (2000) Anthropometry and methods of body composition measurement for research and field application in the elderly, *Eur J Clin Nutr*, **54**, Suppl. 3, S26–S32

Hickey, M S, Weidner, M D, Gavigan, K E, Zheng, D, Tyndall, G L, Houmard, J A (1995) The insulin action–fiber type relationship in humans is muscle group specific, *Am J Physiol*, **269**, 1, E150–E154

Hirooka, M, Kumagi, T, Kurose, K, Nakanishi, S, Michitaka, K, Matsuura, B, Horiike, N, Onji, M (2005) A technique for the measurement of visceral fat by ultrasonography: comparison of measurements by ultrasonography and computed tomography, *Intern Med*, **44**, 8, 794–799

Howald, H, Boesch, C, Kreis, R, Matter, S, Billeter, R, Essen-Gustavsson, B, Hoppeler, H (2002) Content of intramyocellular lipids derived by electron microscopy, biochemical assays, and (1)H-MR spectroscopy, *J Appl Physiol*, **92**, 6, 2264–2272

Hundal, R S, Kršśák, M, Dufour, S, Laurent, D, Lebon, V, Chandramouli, V et al. (2000) Mechanism by which metformin reduces glucose production in type 2 diabetes, *Diabetes*, **49**, 12, 2063–2069

Hwang, J H, Pan, J W, Heydari, S, Hetherington, H P, Stein, D T (2001) Regional differences in intramyocellular lipids in humans observed by in vivo 1H-MR spectroscopic imaging, *J Appl Physiol*, **90**, 4, 1267–1274

Jacob, S, Machann, J, Rett, K, Brechtel, K, Volk, A, Renn, W, Maerker, E, Matthaei, S, Schick, F, Claussen, C D, Haring, H U (1999) Association of increased intramyocellular lipid content with insulin resistance in lean nondiabetic offspring of type 2 diabetic subjects, *Diabetes*, **48**, 5, 1113–1119

Jakicic, J M, Wing, R R, Lang, W (1998) Bioelectrical impedance analysis to assess body composition in obese adult women: the effect of ethnicity, *Int J Obes Relat Metab Disord*, **22**, 3, 243–249

Jensen, M D, Kanaley, J A, Reed, J E, Sheedy, P F (1995) Measurement of abdominal and visceral fat with computed tomography and dual-energy x-ray absorptiometry, *Am J Clin Nutr*, **61**, 2, 274–278

Johnson, N A, Stannard, S R, Rowlands, D S, Chapman, P G, Thompson, C H, Sachinwalla, T, Thompson, M W (2006) Short-term suppression of plasma free fatty acids fails to improve insulin sensitivity when intramyocellular lipid is elevated, *Diabet Med*, **23**, 10, 1061–1068

Joy, D, Thava, V R, Scott, B B (2003) Diagnosis of fatty liver disease: is biopsy necessary?, *Eur J Gastroenterol Hepatol*, **15**, 5, 539–543

Kahn, B B Flier, J S (2000) Obesity and insulin resistance, *J Clin Invest*, **106**, 4, 473–481

Katoh, S, Hata, S, Matsushima, M, Ikemoto, S, Inoue, Y, Yokoyama, J, Tajima, N (2001) Troglitazone prevents the rise in visceral adiposity and improves fatty liver associated with sulfonylurea therapy – a randomized controlled trial, *Metabolism*, **50**, 4, 414–417

Kautzky-Willer, A, Kršśák, M, Winzer, C, Pacini, G, Tura, A, Farhan, S, Wagner, O, Brabant, G, Horn, R, Stingl, H, Schneider, B, Waldhausl, W, Roden, M (2003) Increased intramyocellular lipid concentration identifies impaired glucose metabolism in women with previous gestational diabetes, *Diabetes*, **52**, 2, 244–251

Kelley, D E, McKolanis, T M, Hegazi, R A, Kuller, L H, Kalhan, S C (2003) Fatty liver in type 2 diabetes mellitus: relation to regional adiposity, fatty acids, and insulin resistance, *Am J Physiol Endocrinol Metab*, **285**, 4, E906–E916

Kelley, D E, Thaete, F L, Troost, F, Huwe, T, Goodpaster, B H (2000) Subdivisions of subcutaneous abdominal adipose tissue and insulin resistance, *Am J Physiol Endocrinol Metab*, **278**, 5, E941–E948

Kissebah, A H (1996) Intra-abdominal fat: is it a major factor in developing diabetes and coronary artery disease?, *Diabetes Res Clin Pract*, **30**, Suppl., 25–30

Kohrt, W M, Kirwan, J P, Staten, M A, Bourey, R E, King, D S, Holloszy, J O (1993) Insulin resistance in aging is related to abdominal obesity, *Diabetes*, **42**, 2, 273–281

Krebs, M, Kršśák, M, Nowotny, P, Weghuber, D, Gruber, S, Mlynarik, V et al. (2001) Free fatty acids inhibit the glucose-stimulated increase of intramuscular glucose-6-phosphate concentration in humans, *J Clin Endocrinol Metab*, **86**, 5, 2153–2160

Kršśák, M, Brehm, A, Bernroider, E, Anderwald, C, Nowotny, P, Dalla, M C et al. (2004) Alterations in postprandial hepatic glycogen metabolism in type 2 diabetes, *Diabetes*, **53**, 12, 3048–3056

Krššák, M, Falk, P K, Dresner, A, DiPietro, L, Vogel, S M, Rothman, D L, Roden, M, Shulman, G I (1999) Intramyocellular lipid concentrations are correlated with insulin sensitivity in humans: a 1H NMR spectroscopy study, *Diabetologia*, **42**, 1, 113–116

Krššák, M, Petersen, K F, Bergeron, R, Price, T, Laurent, D, Rothman, D L, Roden, M, Shulman, G I (2000) Intramuscular glycogen and intramyocellular lipid utilization during prolonged exercise and recovery in man: a 13C and 1H nuclear magnetic resonance spectroscopy study, *J Clin Endocrinol Metab*, **85**, 2, 748–754

Krššák, M, Roden, M (2004) The role of lipid accumulation in liver and muscle for insulin resistance and type 2 diabetes mellitus in humans, *Rev Endocrin Metab Disorders*, **5**, 127–134

Kruger, D G, Riederer, S J, Grimm, R C, Rossman, P J (2002) Continuously moving table data acquisition method for long FOV contrast-enhanced MRA and whole-body MRI, *Magn Reson Med*, **47**, 2, 224–231

Kruger, D G, Riederer, S J, Polzin, J A, Madhuranthakam, A J, Hu, H H, Glockner, J F (2005) Dual-velocity continuously moving table acquisition for contrast-enhanced peripheral magnetic resonance angiography, *Magn Reson Med*, **53**, 1, 110–117

Kyle, U G, Bosaeus, I, De Lorenzo, A D, Deurenberg, P, Elia, M, Gomez, J M et al. (2004a) Bioelectrical impedance analysis – part I: review of principles and methods, *Clin Nutr*, **23**, 5, 1226–1243

Kyle, U G, Bosaeus, I, De Lorenzo, A D, Deurenberg, P, Elia, M, Manuel, G J et al. (2004b) Bioelectrical impedance analysis – part II: utilization in clinical practice, *Clin Nutr*, **23**, 6, 1430–1453

Larson-Meyer, D E, Heilbronn, L K, Redman, L M, Newcomer, B R, Frisard, M I, Anton, S et al. (2006a) Effect of calorie restriction with or without exercise on insulin sensitivity, beta-cell function, fat cell size, and ectopic lipid in overweight subjects, *Diabetes Care*, **29**, 6, 1337–1344

Larson-Meyer, D E, Newcomer, B R, Hunter, G R (2002) Influence of endurance running and recovery diet on intramyocellular lipid content in women: a 1H NMR study, *Am J Physiol Endocrinol Metab*, **282**, 1, E95–E106

Larson-Meyer, D E, Smith, S R, Heilbronn, L K, Kelley, D E, Ravussin, E, Newcomer, B R (2006b) Muscle-associated triglyceride measured by computed tomography and magnetic resonance spectroscopy, *Obesity(SilverSpring)*, **14**, 1, 73–87

Leiter, L A, Lukaski, H C, Kenny, D J, Barnie, A, Camelon, K, Ferguson, R S et al. (1994) The use of bioelectrical impedance analysis (BIA) to estimate body composition in the Diabetes Control and Complications Trial (DCCT), *Int J Obes Relat Metab Disord*, **18**, 12, 829–835

Lewis, G F, Carpentier, A, Adeli, K, Giacca, A (2002) Disordered fat storage and mobilization in the pathogenesis of insulin resistance and type 2 diabetes, *Endocr Rev*, **23**, 2, 201–229

Lohman, T G, Harris, M, Teixeira, P J, Weiss, L (2000) Assessing body composition and changes in body composition Another look at dual-energy X-ray absorptiometry, *Ann NY AcadSci*, **904**, 45–54

Longo, R, Ricci, C, Masutti, F, Vidimari, R, Croce, L S, Bercich, L, Tiribelli, C, Dalla, P L (1993) Fatty infiltration of the liver Quantification by 1H localized magnetic resonance spectroscopy and comparison with computed tomography, *Invest Radiol*, **28**, 4, 297–302

Machann, J, Bachmann, O P, Brechtel, K, Dahl, D B, Wietek, B, Klumpp, B, Haring, H U, Claussen, C D, Jacob, S, Schick, F (2003) Lipid content in the musculature of the lower leg assessed by fat selective MRI: intra– and interindividual differences and correlation with anthropometric and metabolic data, *J Magn ResonImaging*, **17**, 3, 350–357

Machann, J, Thamer, C, Schnoedt, B, Haap, M, Haring, H U, Claussen, C D, Stumvoll, M, Fritsche, A, Schick, F (2005) Standardized assessment of whole body adipose tissue topography by MRI, *J Magn ResonImaging*, **21**, 4, 455–462

Marchesini, G, Brizi, M, Bianchi, G, Tomassetti, S, Bugianesi, E, Lenzi, M, McCullough, A J, Natale, S, Forlani, G, Melchionda, N (2001) Nonalcoholic fatty liver disease: a feature of the metabolic syndrome, *Diabetes*, **50**, 8, 1844–1850

Mayerson, A B, Hundal, R S, Dufour, S, Lebon, V, Befroy, D, Cline, G W, Enocksson, S, Inzucchi, S E, Shulman, G I, Petersen, K F (2002) The effects of rosiglitazone on insulin sensitivity, lipolysis, and hepatic and skeletal muscle triglyceride content in patients with type 2 diabetes, *Diabetes*, **51**, 3, 797–802

McGarry, J D (2002) Banting lecture 2001: dysregulation of fatty acid metabolism in the etiology of type 2 diabetes, *Diabetes*, **51**, 1, 7–18

Misra, A, Garg, A, Abate, N, Peshock, R M, Stray–Gundersen, J, Grundy, S M (1997) Relationship of anterior and posterior subcutaneous abdominal fat to insulin sensitivity in nondiabetic men, *Obes Res*, **5**, 2, 93–99

Miyazaki, Y, Glass, L, Triplitt, C, Wajcberg, E, Mandarino, L J, Defronzo, R A (2002a) Abdominal fat distribution and peripheral and hepatic insulin resistance in type 2 diabetes mellitus, *Am J Physiol Endocrinol Metab*, **283**, 6, E1135–E1143

Miyazaki, Y, Mahankali, A, Matsuda, M, Mahankali, S, Hardies, J, Cusi, K, Mandarino, L J, Defronzo, R A (2002b) Effect of pioglitazone on abdominal fat distribution and insulin sensitivity in type 2 diabetic patients, *J Clin Endocrinol Metab*, **87**, 6, 2784–2791

Needleman, L, Kurtz, A B, Rifkin, M D, Cooper, H S, Pasto, M E, Goldberg, B B (1986) Sonography of diffuse benign liver disease: accuracy of pattern recognition and grading, *AJR AmJRoentgenol*, **146**, 5, 1011–1015

Nyholm, B, Qu, Z, Kaal, A, Pedersen, S B, Gravholt, C H, Andersen, J L, Saltin, B, Schmitz, O (1997) Evidence of an increased number of type IIb muscle fibers in insulin-resistant first-degree relatives of patients with NIDDM, *Diabetes*, **46**, 11, 1822–1828

Pan, D A, Lillioja, S, Kriketos, A D, Milner, M R, Baur, L A, Bogardus, C, Jenkins, A B, Storlien, L H (1997) Skeletal muscle triglyceride levels are inversely related to insulin action, *Diabetes*, **46**, 6, 983–988

Park, Y W, Heymsfield, S B, Gallagher, D (2002) Are dual-energy X-ray absorptiometry regional estimates associated with visceral adipose tissue mass?, *Int J ObesRelat Metab Disord*, **26**, 7, 978–983

Perdomo, G, Commerford, S R, Richard, A M, Adams, S H, Corkey, B E, ODoherty, R M, Brown, N F (2004) Increased beta-oxidation in muscle cells enhances insulin-stimulated glucose metabolism and protects against fatty acid-induced insulin resistance despite intramyocellular lipid accumulation, *J Biol Chem*, **279**, 26, 27177–27186

Perseghin, G, Lattuada, G, Danna, M, Sereni, L P, Maffi, P, De Cobelli, F, Battezzati, A, Secchi, A, Del Maschio, A, Luzi, L (2003) Insulin resistance, intramyocellular lipid content, and plasma adiponectin in patients with type 1 diabetes, *Am J Physiol Endocrinol Metab*, **285**, 6, E1174–E1181

Perseghin, G, Price, T B, Petersen, K F, Roden, M, Cline, G W, Gerow, K, Rothman, D L, Shulman, G I (1996) Increased glucose transport–phosphorylation and muscle glycogen synthesis after exercise training in insulin–resistant subjects, *N Engl J Med*, **335**, 18, 1357–1362

Perseghin, G, Scifo, P, De Cobelli, F, Pagliato, E, Battezzati, A, Arcelloni, C, Vanzulli, A, Testolin, G, Pozza, G, Del Maschio, A, Luzi, L (1999) Intramyocellular triglyceride content is a determinant of in vivo insulin resistance in humans: a 1H-13C nuclear magnetic resonance spectroscopy assessment in offspring of type 2 diabetic parents, *Diabetes*, **48**, 8, 1600–1606

Petersen, K F, Befroy, D, Dufour, S, Dziura, J, Ariyan, C, Rothman, D L, DiPietro, L, Cline, G W, Shulman, G I (2003) Mitochondrial dysfunction in the elderly: possible role in insulin resistance, *Science*, **300**, 5622, 1140–1142

Petersen, K F, Dufour, S, Shulman, G I (2005) Decreased insulin–stimulated ATP synthesis and phosphate transport in muscle of insulin-resistant offspring of type 2 diabetic parents, *PLoS Med*, **2**, 9, E233

Petersen, K F, Hendler, R, Price, T, Perseghin, G, Rothman, D L, Held, N, Amatruda, J M, Shulman, G I (1998) 13C/31P NMR studies on the mechanism of insulin resistance in obesity, *Diabetes*, **47**, 3, 381–386

Petersen, K F, Oral, E A, Dufour, S, Befroy, D, Ariyan, C, Yu, C, Cline, G W, DePaoli, A M, Taylor, S I, Gorden, P, Shulman, G I (2002) Leptin reverses insulin resistance and hepatic steatosis in patients with severe lipodystrophy, *J Clin Invest*, **109**, 10, 1345–1350

Petersen, K F, West, AB, Reuben, A, Rothman, DL, Shulman, GI (1996) Non–invasive assessment of hepatic triglyceride content in humans with 13C nuclear magnetic resonance spectroscopy, *Hepatology*, **24**, 114–117

Phillips, D I, Caddy, S, Ilic, V, Fielding, B A, Frayn, K N, Borthwick, A C, Taylor, R (1996) Intramuscular triglyceride and muscle insulin sensitivity: evidence for a relationship in nondiabetic subjects, *Metabolism*, **45**, 8, 947–950

Pietrobelli, A, Formica, C, Wang, Z, Heymsfield, S B (1996) Dual-energy X-ray absorptiometry body composition model: review of physical concepts, *Am J Physiol*, **271**, 6 Pt 1, p E941–E951

Pietrobelli, A, Wang, Z, Formica, C, Heymsfield, S B (1998) Dual-energy X-ray absorptiometry: fat estimation errors due to variation in soft tissue hydration, *Am J Physiol*, **274**, 5, E808–E816

Pinnamaneni, S K, Southgate, R J, Febbraio, M A, Watt, M J (2006) Stearoyl CoA desaturase 1 is elevated in obesity but protects against fatty acid-induced skeletal muscle insulin resistance in vitro, *Diabetologia*, **49**, 12, 3027–3037

Positano, V, Gastaldelli, A, Sironi, A M, Santarelli, M F, Lombardi, M, Landini, L (2004) An accurate and robust method for unsupervised assessment of abdominal fat by MRI, *J Magn Reson Imaging*, **20**, 4, 684–689

Quinn, S F Gosink, B B (1985) Characteristic sonographic signs of hepatic fatty infiltration, *AJR Am J Roentgenol*, **145**, 4, 753–755

Randle, P J, Garland, P B, Hales, C N, Newsholme, E A (1963) The glucose fatty-acid cycle Its role in insulin sensitivity and the metabolic disturbances of diabetes mellitus, *Lancet*, **1**, 785–789

Reeder, S B, Pineda, A R, Wen, Z, Shimakawa, A, Yu, H, Brittain, J H, Gold, G E, Beaulieu, C H, Pelc, N J (2005) Iterative decomposition of water and fat with echo asymmetry and least-squares estimation (IDEAL): application with fast spin-echo imaging, *Magn ResonMed*, **54**, 3, 636–644

Reeder, S B, Wen, Z, Yu, H, Pineda, A R, Gold, G E, Markl, M, Pelc, N J (2004) Multicoil Dixon chemical species separation with an iterative least–squares estimation method, *Magn Reson Med*, **51**, 1, 35–45

Ribeiro-Filho, F F, Faria, A N, Azjen, S, Zanella, M T, Ferreira, S R (2003) Methods of estimation of visceral fat: advantages of ultrasonography, *Obes Res*, **11**, 12, 1488–1494

Ricci, C, Longo, R, Gioulis, E, Bosco, M, Pollesello, P, Masutti, F, Croce, L S, Paoletti, S, de Bernard, B, Tiribelli, C, Dalla, P L (1997) Noninvasive in vivo quantitative assessment of fat content in human liver, *J Hepatol*, **27**, 1, 108–113

Rico-Sanz, J, Thomas, E L, Jenkinson, G, Mierisova, S, Iles, R, Bell, J D (1999) Diversity in levels of intracellular total creatine and triglycerides in human skeletal muscles observed by (1)H-MRS, *J Appl Physiol*, **87**, 6, 2068–2072

Roden, M (2006) Mechanisms of Disease: hepatic steatosis in type 2 diabetes – pathogenesis and clinical relevance, *Nat Clin Pract Endocrinol Metab*, **2**, 335–48

Roden, M, Krššák, M, Stingl, H, Gruber, S, Hofer, A, Furnsinn, C, Moser, E, Waldhausl, W (1999) Rapid impairment of skeletal muscle glucose transport/phosphorylation by free fatty acids in humans, *Diabetes*, **48**, 2, 358–364

Roden, M, Price, T B, Perseghin, G, Petersen, K F, Rothman, D L, Cline, G W, Shulman, G I (1996) Mechanism of free fatty acid-induced insulin resistance in humans, *J Clin Invest*, **97**, 12, 2859–2865

Roden, M, Stingl, H, Chandramouli, V, Schumann, W C, Hofer, A, Landau, B R, Nowotny, P, Waldhausl, W, Shulman, G I (2000) Effects of free fatty acid elevation on postabsorptive endogenous glucose production and gluconeogenesis in humans, *Diabetes*, **49**, 5, 701–707

Ross, R, Janssen, I, Dawson, J, Kungl, A M, Kuk, J L, Wong, S L, Nguyen-Duy, T B, Lee, S, Kilpatrick, K, Hudson, R (2004) Exercise-induced reduction in obesity and insulin resistance in women: a randomized controlled trial, *Obes Res*, **12**, 5, 789–798

Rothman, D L, Shulman, R G, Shulman, G I (1991) Nmr studies of muscle glycogen synthesis in normal and non-insulin-dependent diabetic subjects, *Biochem Soc Trans*, **19**, 4, 992–994

Rothman, D L, Shulman, R G, Shulman, G I (1992) 31P nuclear magnetic resonance measurements of muscle glucose-6-phosphate Evidence for reduced insulin-dependent muscle glucose transport or phosphorylation activity in non-insulin-dependent diabetes mellitus, *J Clin Invest*, **89**, 4, 1069–1075

Roubenoff, R, Kehayias, J J, Dawson-Hughes, B, Heymsfield, S B (1993) Use of dual-energy x-ray absorptiometry in body-composition studies: not yet a gold standard, *Am J Clin Nutr*, **58**, 5, 589–591

Ryysy, L, Hakkinen, A M, Goto, T, Vehkavaara, S, Westerbacka, J, Halavaara, J, Yki-Jarvinen, H (2000) Hepatic fat content and insulin action on free fatty acids and glucose metabolism rather than insulin absorption are associated with insulin requirements during insulin therapy in type 2 diabetic patients, *Diabetes*, **49**, 5, 749–758

Saadeh, S, Younossi, Z M, Remer, E M, Gramlich, T, Ong, J P, Hurley, M, Mullen, K D, Cooper, J N, Sheridan, M J (2002) The utility of radiological imaging in nonalcoholic fatty liver disease, *Gastroenterology*, **123**, 3, 745–750

Santomauro, A T, Boden, G, Silva, M E, Rocha, D M, Santos, R F, Ursich, M J, Strassmann, P G, Wajchenberg, B L (1999) Overnight lowering of free fatty acids with Acipimox improves insulin resistance and glucose tolerance in obese diabetic and nondiabetic subjects, *Diabetes*, **48**, 9, 1836–1841

Sargin, M, Uygur-Bayramicli, O, Sargin, H, Orbay, E, Yayla, A (2003) Association of nonalcoholic fatty liver disease with insulin resistance: is OGTT indicated in nonalcoholic fatty liver disease?, *J Clin Gastroenterol*, **37**, 5, 399–402

Scharfetter, H, Schlager, T, Stollberger, R, Felsberger, R, Hutten, H, Hinghofer–Szalkay, H (2001) Assessing abdominal fatness with local bioimpedance analysis: basics and experimental findings, *Int J Obes Relat Metab Disord*, **25**, 4, 502–511

Schick, F, Eismann, B, Jung, W I, Bongers, H, Bunse, M, Lutz, O (1993) Comparison of localized proton NMR signals of skeletal muscle and fat tissue in vivo: two lipid compartments in muscle tissue, *Magn Reson Med*, **29**, 2, 158–167

Schick, F, Machann, J, Brechtel, K, Strempfer, A, Klumpp, B, Stein, D T, Jacob, S (2002) MRI of muscular fat, *Magn Reson Med*, **47**, 4, 720–727

Schoeller, D A, van Santen, E, Peterson, D W, Dietz, W, Jaspan, J, Klein, P D (1980) Total body water measurement in humans with 18O and 2H labeled water, *Am J Clin Nutr*, **33**, 12, 2686–2693

Schrauwen-Hinderling, V B, Kooi, M E, Hesselink, M K, Jeneson, J A, Backes, W H, van Echteld, C J, van Engelshoven, J M, Mensink, M, Schrauwen, P (2006) Impaired in vivo mitochondrial function but similar intramyocellular lipid content in patients with type 2 diabetes mellitus and BMI-matched control subjects, *Diabetologia*

Schrauwen-Hinderling, V B, Kooi, M E, Hesselink, M K, Moonen-Kornips, E, Schaart, G, Mustard, K J, Hardie, D G, Saris, W H, Nicolay, K, Schrauwen, P (2005) Intramyocellular lipid content and molecular adaptations in response to a 1-week high-fat diet, *Obes Res*, **13**, 12, 2088–2094

Schrauwen-Hinderling, V B, van Loon, L J, Koopman, R, Nicolay, K, Saris, W H, Kooi, M E (2003) Intramyocellular lipid content is increased after exercise in nonexercising human skeletal muscle, *J Appl Physiol*, **95**, 6, 2328–2332

Seidell, J C, Bjorntorp, P, Sjostrom, L, Sannerstedt, R, Krotkiewski, M, Kvist, H (1989) Regional distribution of muscle and fat mass in men – new insight into the risk of abdominal obesity using computed tomography, *Int J Obes*, **13**, 3, 289–303

Seppala-Lindroos, A, Vehkavaara, S, Hakkinen, A M, Goto, T, Westerbacka, J, Sovijarvi, A, Halavaara, J, Yki-Jarvinen, H (2002) Fat accumulation in the liver is associated with defects in insulin suppression of glucose production and serum free fatty acids independent of obesity in normal men, *J Clin Endocrinol Metab*, **87**, 7, 3023–3028

Shadid, S Jensen, M D (2003) Effects of pioglitazone versus diet and exercise on metabolic health and fat distribution in upper body obesity, *Diabetes Care*, **26**, 11, 3148–3152

Shulman, G I (2000) Cellular mechanisms of insulin resistance, *J Clin Invest*, **106**, 2, 171–176

Shulman, G I, Rothman, D L, Jue, T, Stein, P, Defronzo, R A, Shulman, R G (1990) Quantitation of muscle glycogen synthesis in normal subjects and subjects with non-insulin-dependent diabetes by 13C nuclear magnetic resonance spectroscopy, *N Engl J Med*, **322**, 4, 223–228

Simha, V, Szczepaniak, L S, Wagner, A J, DePaoli, A M, Garg, A (2003) Effect of leptin replacement on intrahepatic and intramyocellular lipid content in patients with generalized lipodystrophy, *Diabetes Care*, **26**, 1, 30–35

Singhal, P, Caumo, A, Carey, P E, Cobelli, C, Taylor, R (2002) Regulation of endogenous glucose production after a mixed meal in type 2 diabetes, *Am J Physiol Endocrinol Metab*, **283**, 2, E275–E283

Sinha, R, Dufour, S, Petersen, K F, Lebon, V, Enoksson, S, Ma, Y Z, Savoye, M, Rothman, D L, Shulman, G I, Caprio, S (2002) Assessment of skeletal muscle triglyceride content by (1)H nuclear magnetic resonance spectroscopy in lean and obese adolescents: relationships to insulin sensitivity, total body fat, and central adiposity, *Diabetes*, **51**, 4, 1022–1027

Snijder, M B, Visser, M, Dekker, J M, Seidell, J C, Fuerst, T, Tylavsky, F, Cauley, J, Lang, T, Nevitt, M, Harris, T B (2002) The prediction of visceral fat by dual-energy X-ray absorptiometry in the elderly: a comparison with computed tomography and anthropometry, *Int J Obes Relat Metab Disord*, **26**, 7, 984–993

Sommer, G, Fautz, H P, Ludwig, U, Hennig, J (2006) Multicontrast sequences with continuous table motion: a novel acquisition technique for extended field of view imaging, *Magn Reson Med*, **55**, 4, 918–922

Stannard, S R, Thompson, M W, Fairbairn, K, Huard, B, Sachinwalla, T, Thompson, C H (2002) Fasting for 72 h increases intramyocellular lipid content in nondiabetic, physically fit men, *Am J Physiol Endocrinol Metab*, **283**, 6, E1185–E1191

Stingl, H, Krššák, M, Krebs, M, Bischof, M G, Nowotny, P, Furnsinn, C, Shulman, G I, Waldhausl, W, Roden, M (2001) Lipid-dependent control of hepatic glycogen stores in healthy humans, *Diabetologia*, **44**, 1, 48–54

Sutinen, J, Hakkinen, A M, Westerbacka, J, Seppala-Lindroos, A, Vehkavaara, S, Halavaara, J, Jarvinen, A, Ristola, M, Yki-Jarvinen, H (2002) Increased fat accumulation in the liver in HIV-infected patients with antiretroviral therapy-associated lipodystrophy, *AIDS*, **16**, 16, 2183–2193

Szczepaniak, L S, Babcock, E E, Schick, F, Dobbins, R L, Garg, A, Burns, D K, McGarry, J D, Stein, D T (1999) Measurement of intracellular triglyceride stores by H spectroscopy: validation in vivo, *Am J Physiol*, **276**, 5, E977–E989

Szczepaniak, L S, Dobbins, R L, Metzger, G J, Sartoni-DAmbrosia, G, Arbique, D, Vongpatanasin, W, Unger, R, Victor, R G (2003) Myocardial triglycerides and systolic function in humans: in vivo evaluation by localized proton spectroscopy and cardiac imaging, *Magn Reson Med*, **49**, 3, 417–423

Szczepaniak, L S, Dobbins, R L, Stein, D T, McGarry, J D (2002) Bulk magnetic susceptibility effects on the assessment of intra– and extramyocellular lipids in vivo, *Magn Reson Med*, **47**, 3, 607–610

Thamer, C, Machann, J, Bachmann, O, Haap, M, Dahl, D, Wietek, B, Tschritter, O, Niess, A, Brechtel, K, Fritsche, A, Claussen, C, Jacob, S, Schick, F, Haring, H U, Stumvoll, M (2003) Intramyocellular lipids: anthropometric determinants and relationships with maximal aerobic capacity and insulin sensitivity, *J Clin Endocrinol Metab*, **88**, 4, 1785–1791

Thamer, C, Machann, J, Haap, M, Stefan, N, Heller, E, Schnodt, B, Stumvoll, M, Claussen, C, Fritsche, A, Schick, F, Haring, H (2004) Intrahepatic lipids are predicted by visceral adipose tissue mass in healthy subjects, *Diabetes Care*, **27**, 11, 2726–2729

Thomas, E L Bell, J D (2003) Influence of undersampling on magnetic resonance imaging measurements of intra-abdominal adipose tissue, *Int J Obes Relat Metab Disord*, **27**, 2, 211–218

Thomas, E L, Brynes, A E, McCarthy, J, Goldstone, A P, Hajnal, J V, Saeed, N, Frost, G, Bell, J D (2000) Preferential loss of visceral fat following aerobic exercise, measured by magnetic resonance imaging, *Lipids*, **35**, 7, 769–776

Thomas, E L, Saeed, N, Hajnal, J V, Brynes, A, Goldstone, A P, Frost, G, Bell, J D (1998) Magnetic resonance imaging of total body fat, *J Appl Physiol*, **85**, 5, 1778–1785

Thomas, E L, Taylor-Robinson, SD, Barnard, ML, Frost, G, Sargetoni, J, Davidson, BR, Cunnane, SC, Bell, JD (1997) Changes in adipose tissue composition in malnourished patients before and after liver transplantation: A carbon-13 magnetic resonance spectroscopy and gas–liquid chromatography study, *Hepatology*, **25**, 178–183

Thomsen, C, Becker, U, Winkler, K, Christoffersen, P, Jensen, M, Henriksen, O (1994) Quantification of liver fat using magnetic resonance spectroscopy, *Magn Reson Imaging*, **12**, 3, 487–495

Tiikkainen, M, Tamminen, M, Hakkinen, A M, Bergholm, R, Vehkavaara, S, Halavaara, J, Teramo, K, Rissanen, A, Yki-Jarvinen, H (2002) Liver-fat accumulation and insulin resistance in obese women with previous gestational diabetes, *Obes Res*, **10**, 9, 859–867

Tippett, P S Neet, K E (1982) An allosteric model for the inhibition of glucokinase by long chain acyl coenzyme A, *J Biol Chem*, **257**, 21, 12846–12852

Tokunaga, K, Matsuzawa, Y, Ishikawa, K, Tarui, S (1983) A novel technique for the determination of body fat by computed tomography, *Int J Obes*, **7**, 5, 437–445

Tothill, P Nord, R H (1995) Limitations of dual-energy x-ray absorptiometry, *Am J Clin Nutr*, **61**, 2, 398–400

Vermathen, P, Kreis, R, Boesch, C (2004) Distribution of intramyocellular lipids in human calf muscles as determined by MR spectroscopic imaging, *Magn Reson Med*, **51**, 2, 253–262

Wang, J, Thornron, JC, Kolesnick, S, Pierson, RJ (2000) Anthropometry in body composition, *Ann NY Acad Sci*, **905**, 317–326

Weiss, R, Dufour, S, Taksali, S E, Tamborlane, W V, Petersen, K F, Bonadonna, R C et al. (2003) Prediabetes in obese youth: a syndrome of impaired glucose tolerance, severe insulin resistance, and altered myocellular and abdominal fat partitioning, *Lancet*, **362**, 9388, 951–957

White, LJ, Ferguson, MA, McCoy, SC, Kim, H (2003) Intramyocellular Lipid changes in men and women during aerobic exercise: A 1H-magnetic resonance spectroscopy study, *J Clin Endocrinol Metab*, **88**, 5638–5643

Wititsuwannakul, D Kim, K H (1977) Mechanism of palmityl coenzyme A inhibition of liver glycogen synthase, *J Biol Chem*, **252**, 21, 7812–7817

Yu, H, Reeder, S B, McKenzie, C A, Brau, A C, Shimakawa, A, Brittain, J H, Pelc, N J (2006) Single acquisition water-fat separation: feasibility study for dynamic imaging, *Magn Reson Med*, **55**, 2, 413–422

14

Tissue Biopsies in Diabetes Research

Kurt Højlund, Michael Gaster and **Henning Beck-Nielsen**

Introduction

Type 2 diabetes is characterised by insulin resistance in major metabolic tissues such as skeletal muscle, liver and fat cells, and failure of the pancreatic β-cells to compensate for this abnormality (Beck-Nielsen & Groop 1994; Beck-Nielsen 1998). Skeletal muscle is the major site of glucose disposal in response to insulin, and insulin resistance of glucose disposal and glycogen synthesis in this tissue are hallmark features of type 2 diabetes in humans (Beck-Nielsen 1998; Beck-Nielsen et al. 2003). During the past two decades, we have carried out more than 1,200 needle biopsies of skeletal muscle to study the cellular mechanisms underlying insulin resistance in type 2 diabetes. Together with morphological studies, measurement of energy stores and metabolites, enzyme activity and phosphorylation, gene and protein expression in skeletal muscle biopsies have revealed a variety of cellular abnormalities in patients with type 2 diabetes and prediabetes. The possibility of establishing human muscle cell cultures from muscle biopsies of diabetic subjects has further extended our ability to study the cellular mechanisms of insulin resistance and potentially distinguish between primary and secondary defects (Beck-Nielsen et al. 2003). More recently, the application of global approaches such as proteomics and gene expression profiling on skeletal muscle biopsies has pointed to abnormalities in mitochondrial oxidative phosphorylation in type 2 diabetes. These novel insights will inevitably cause a renewed interest in studying skeletal muscle. This chapter reviews our experience to date and gives a thorough description of the technique of percutaneous needle biopsy of skeletal muscle and the establishment of human muscle cell cultures, together with a discussion of the advantages and limitations of the methods in diabetes research.

Clinical Diabetes Research: Methods and Techniques   Edited by Michael Roden
© 2007 John Wiley & Sons, Ltd   ISBN 978-0-470-01728-9

Percutaneous needle biopsy of skeletal muscle

Extensive investigation of the metabolism of normal and abnormal tissue requires a simple method for tissue sampling. The percutaneous muscle biopsy technique developed and introduced by Bergström in the 1960s provides a simple and repeatable sampling method (Bergström 1962, 1975), which has made skeletal muscle one of the few tissues suitable for direct studies of structure and metabolic functions in human subjects. The percutaneous muscle biopsy procedure has been used widely to study many aspects of human muscle metabolism, in particular changes caused by exercise, insulin resistance and type 2 diabetes. As reviewed by others, this method of sampling is rapid and relatively atraumatic (Goldberger et al. 1978; Edwards et al. 1980, 1983). It carries a very low complication rate and repeated biopsies are well tolerated, allowing follow-up studies after treatment.

The Bergström needle – with a facility for suction – is the biopsy needle that we currently use (Figure 14.1). This needle is available with external diameters ranging from 4–6.5 mm, and it consists of a sharp-tipped hollow outer needle with a small opening (window) near the tip. A sharp-edged inner cutting cylinder fits tightly into the needle. A stylet is used to eject muscle samples from the cylinder (Bergström 1975; Goldberger et al. 1978). Generally the biopsy should be carried out under aseptic conditions and done under local anaesthesia. In most studies, the biopsy is taken from the vastus lateralis muscle 10–15 cm above the patella. This part of the lateral quadriceps muscle is well clear of the major vessels and nerves of the thigh, rendering the procedure relatively safe. Moreover, it is the major extensor of the knee joint and thus particularly suitable for studies in which structure or chemistry are to be

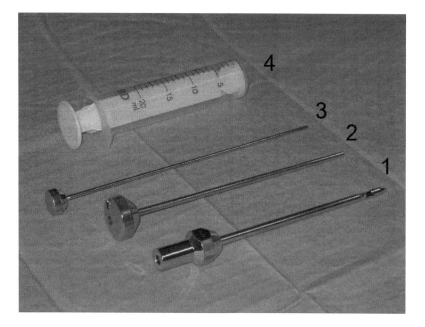

Figure 14.1 Bergström Needle The modified Bergström needle consists of 1) a sharp-tipped hollow outer needle with a small opening; 2) a sharp-edged inner cutting cylinder; 3) a stylet; 4) a 20 ml syringe fitting to the top of the inner cutting cylinder.

related to function (Edwards et al. 1980, 1983). In particular, the application of suction to the biopsy needle has improved the technique by increasing the reliability of the amount of tissue obtained and the average size of the muscle samples, while still allowing the procedure to be safe and simple (Greig et al. 1985).

Developments in analytical methods have greatly extended the usefulness of the technique in the investigation of muscle cell structure and metabolism. The muscle specimens are easily prepared for different purposes, e.g. 1) snap-frozen in liquid nitrogen for measurements of metabolites, enzyme activity and phosphorylation, gene and protein expression; 2) fixed for histological, histochemical and electronic microscopic studies; or 3) stored in medium for studies of isolated mitochondria or human muscle cell cultures established from isolated satellite cells. In fact, only our imagination limits the potential usefulness of skeletal muscle biopsies.

Biopsy procedure and sample handling

All research involving skeletal muscle biopsies must be approved by an institutional review board/ethics committee. The subject must be fully informed about the study and the potential risk and discomfort – this includes information about the potential establishment of muscle cell cultures and the long-term storage and use of the obtained biological material. For subjects undergoing skeletal muscle biopsies, we recommend careful history-taking and physical examination to exclude current infection and any disease which could interfere with the results of the study. Also avoid muscle that has recently suffered trauma. All medications should be discontinued at least one weak prior to biopsy. This is particularly important in subjects taking oral anticoagulants or other drugs interfering with haemostasis. Volunteers are usually admitted to the research centre after a standardised 12 h overnight fast and instructed to refrain from strenuous physical activity for a period of 48 h before the experiment.

1) Mark the biopsy site 10–15 cm above the patella on the vastus lateralis muscle and wash the skin with antiseptic solution (alcohol swaps).

2) Using a thin s.c. needle (0.6 × 30 mm), the skin and subcutaneous tissues down to the fascia are infiltrated with 4–10 ml of 2 % lidocaine, depending on the thickness of subcutis. It is important to avoid lidocaine in muscle. Try to locate the fascia by the tip of the needle. Otherwise, push the needle through the fascia, bend it against the fascia while slowly pulling it back, and sense the unbending of the needle as it passes back through the fascia.

3) Wait ~10 min before a skin incision is made. Prepare the biopsy table, as shown in Figure 14.2, and a sample handling table, which should include sterile gloves, IV needles for dissection of muscle samples, liquid nitrogen in a small container (200 ml), dry ice to pre-cool three vials with screw caps for the frozen muscle samples, small metal forceps for sample handling during freezing-procedure, Tissue-Tek (Sakura, Torrance, CA), glutaraldehyde and tubes with transport medium for the part of the muscle specimen that is used for isolation of satellite cells or mitochondria.

4) Using sterile gloves, disinfect the skin with chlorhexidine and drape the thigh, with the hole surrounding the biopsy site. Wash again and prick the skin with the tip of the

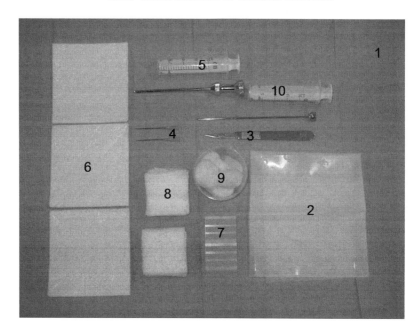

Figure 14.2 Biopsy Table The biopsy table, which is covered by 1) a utility drape (Klinidrape® 45 × 75 cm; Mölnlycke Health Care, Göteborg, Sweden); contains 2) a small drape with adhesive aperture (Steri-Drape™ 40 × 40 cm, hole 6.3 cm in diameter; 3M Health Care, Borken, Germany); 3) a sterile scalpel (blade size 11); 4) two IV needles (1.2 × 40 mm); 5) one extra 20 ml syringe; 6) three low adherent adsorbent dressing (Melolin 10 × 10 cm; Smith & Nephew, Hull, England); 7) Steri-Strips™ (3M Health Care, Borken, Germany); 8) four gauze swabs, 8 ply (Multisorb® Cotton 5 × 5 cm; BSN medical GmbH & Co, Hamburg, Germany); 9) five cotton soaked in chlorhexidine placed in a sterile container 60 ml; and 10) a modified Bergström needle (4 mm) connected to a 20 ml syringe.

scalpel to ensure proper anaesthesia. Make a 3–5 mm skin incision with the scalpel, continue in one slow move through the subcutis, and penetrate the underlying fascia with the tip of the scalpel. Avoid making the incision in the fascia too large as this can make it difficult to achieve proper vacuum during suction.

5) Using sterile gauze swaps, apply firm pressure over the incision to halt any oozing of blood, which may otherwise coat the needle, contaminate the muscle specimen and cause freezing artifact in morphological studies and error in chemical analysis.

6) With the window closed, introduce the Bergström needle – attached to a 20 ml syringe, fitted to the top of the inner cutting cylinder – through the incisions in the skin and the fascia and insert it into the muscle so that the window of the needle is in the belly of the muscle, to a depth of approximately 2–5 cm below the level of the skin.

7) After applying suction to the needle using the syringe, rapidly pull the inner cutting cylinder back >1 cm, allowing muscle to be drawn into the open window of the needle. Then quickly push the inner cylinder down again, cutting the muscle specimen. In this way the sample is guillotined. Several cuts can be made in quick succession by rotating

the needle while in the muscle, but the procedure should not exceed 30 seconds. The window must be closed upon withdrawal of the needle from the muscle. A second sample can be taken through the same incision to provide additional material e.g. for establishment of cell cultures. In this way samples weighing 200–300 mg are easily obtained.

8) Quickly remove muscle tissue from the inner cutting cylinder of the needle and place the syringe on the shiny film side of a low adherent adsorbent (Melolin) dressing. The sample should be inspected by another person, and all visible blood, fat and connective tissue should be rapidly removed by rolling the tissue on the shiny surface of the adsorbent dressing using an IV needle.

9) Snap freeze pieces of ~50 mg muscle in liquid nitrogen within 30 sec of excision. For measurements of metabolites, protein expression, activity and phosphorylation, and gene expression, it is essential that the samples are frozen as quickly as possible.

10) Place small pieces of ~5 mg in a small folio vial and mount them in cryo embedding medium (Tissue-Tek), then rapidly freeze in isopentane, cooled to –160 °C in liquid nitrogen, for histochemistry/immunohistochemistry. Pre-fix small cubes of muscle (1mm^3) in buffered (0.1 M cacodylate) 2–6 % glutaraldehyde for electron microscopy. Put the remaining muscle tissue into a tube containing medium for isolation of satellite cells (see later). If muscle is to be used for isolation of mitochondria, this part is done first (Table 14.1).

11) Upon withdrawal of the needle, apply firm pressure to the biopsy site, using sterile gauze swaps, for 5 min to assure haemostasis and prevent subsequent haematoma formation. Aseptic precautions should be maintained throughout the biopsy procedure. Oppose the edges of the small skin wound with one sterile tape (Steri-Strip), and cover the wound with a Melonin dressing and a plaster. The subject should wear a compression bandage for at least 3 h or until bedtime. Volunteers should be informed about potential complications and given the ability to get in touch with a doctor if they are concerned about anything.

12) It is important to keep the needle sharp. The cutting edge should be examined after each biopsy and sharpened if necessary (regularly).

Discomfort and complications of needle biopsy

In general, most subjects experience only minimal discomfort with a few seconds' sensation of pressure or pain during the procedure. The pain experienced during biopsy is greater if the fascia is caught in the needle or if a nerve is touched or damaged. The response of subjects to biopsy is, however, somewhat variable, as is their account of subsequent feelings of discomfort. Muscle function is usually little impaired, and patients need not restrict their activities after biopsy, although a sensation of muscle stiffness may persist for 48 h or more. Complications of the needle biopsy procedure are rare but include infection, haematoma and denervation (Goldberger et al. 1978; Edwards et al. 1980, 1983). In our experience with ~1,200 biopsies, haematoma formation at the biopsy site occurred on three occasions, but they were all resorbed spontaneously. Until now we have experienced no case of infection at the biopsy site. All wounds healed with a minimal visible scar.

Advantages and limitations of needle biopsy

The needle biopsy circumvents many of the disadvantages of the open muscle biopsy, which include higher costs, the need for general anaesthetic, increased scarring and the inconvenience of repeated biopsies (Goldberger et al. 1978; Edwards et al. 1980, 1983). The fact that many of our patients and control subjects have participated in several studies involving muscle biopsies emphasises that this technique is easy to learn, repeatable and relatively atraumatic. It is a safe procedure that is almost free of complication. As repeated biopsies are generally well tolerated, biopsies can be taken before, during and after acute or chronic intervention, e.g. insulin stimulation, lipid infusion, exercise, treatment with drugs, training etc.

There is always a slight delay in freezing the specimen. This can lead to inaccuracy in the determination of some muscle metabolites and cause areas of artifact formation, making morphological studies troublesome. Nevertheless, most analytical methods are probably not influenced by this slight delay in freezing (Bergström 1975; Edwards et al. 1980, 1983). On the other hand, we have observed that non-muscle contaminants of skeletal muscle samples create considerable variation in assays, including measurement of insulin signaling events. Freeze-drying of muscle specimens allows dissection and purification of the muscle from non-muscle contaminants. This may reduce within-biopsy variation and hence the sample size needed, and improve analytical precision. Prior to freeze-drying and purification, biopsies of human vastus lateralis muscle have been shown to contain between 1 % and 40 % non-muscle contaminants (Korsheninnikova et al. 2002). Insulin signaling events can be reliably assessed in freeze-dried muscle specimens that are free of non-muscle contaminants.

Application of muscle biopsy in diabetes

Insulin resistance in skeletal muscle is a major hallmark of type 2 diabetes (Beck-Nielsen & Groop 1994; Beck-Nielsen 1998; Beck-Nielsen et al. 2003). During the past two decades, skeletal muscle biopsies have been increasingly applied in the search for biochemical and molecular abnormalities responsible for insulin resistance. It is evident that type 2 diabetes is caused by a complex interplay between genetic and environmental factors. The latter include intrauterine malnutrition and postnatal factors such as obesity, physical inactivity and modern Western lifestyle, as well as the metabolic milieu associated with type 2 diabetes and prediabetes, including glucose intolerance, hyperglycaemia, hyperlipidaemia and hyperinsulinaemia (Beck-Nielsen & Groop 1994; Beck-Nielsen 1998; Beck-Nielsen et al. 2003). The choice of study design is therefore extremely important for the interpretation of data obtained (Table 14.1).

Novel potential markers of insulin resistance and type 2 diabetes are usually studied first in muscle samples obtained from type 2 diabetic subjects and matched non-diabetic control subjects, preferably including both an obese and a lean control group. If abnormalities are found in these studies, the next step is to test for these defects in glucose-tolerant non-obese subjects with prediabetes such as first degree relatives of patients with type 2 diabetes (Vaag et al. 1992), or glucose-tolerant non-diabetic co-twins of monozygotic twin-pairs discordant for type 2 diabetes (Vaag et al. 1996). Abnormalities confirmed in prediabetic subjects are less likely to be due to environmental factors and provide support for early defects having genetic origin. It is possible to study *in vivo* abnormalities in cultured skeletal muscle cells (myotubes) from patients with type 2 diabetes, which are assumed to provide evidence for early defects (see later).

Studies of the biochemical and molecular mechanisms of skeletal muscle insulin resistance in the fasting basal and insulin-stimulated states have been performed with or without intervention (such as endurance-training, treatment with drugs, lipid infusion etc.). Some methodological aspects may affect the data obtained. It is often useful to combine muscle sampling with the euglycaemic-hyperinsulinaemic clamp technique and indirect calorimetry (Table 14.1). Combined with tracer-technology, these techniques allow assessment of rates of glucose disposal, glycolytic flux, glucose storage, non-oxidative glucose metabolism and glucose and lipid oxidation, and hence allow us to investigate the relationship of these parameters to biochemical and molecular findings in muscle biopsies (Vaag et al. 1992, 1996; Højlund et al. 2003). Drawing conclusions from such experiments, it should be recognised that whole-body indirect calorimetry only reflects glucose metabolism in skeletal muscle during insulin stimulation (Kelley & Mandarino 2000). It is possible to circumvent this problem by using limb-balance techniques, which allow assessment of substrate metabolism (indirect calorimetry) across a large bed of muscle (Kelley & Simoneau 1994; Mandarino et al. 1996).

Another important aspect to consider when studying the effects of insulin on muscle enzymes, genes and metabolites, is whether to stimulate with physiological (200–800 pmol/l) or supraphysiological (3,000–6,000 pmol/l) concentrations of insulin (Højlund et al. 2003; Kim et al. 2003), and whether insulin-stimulated muscle samples should be obtained in the steady-state period of a clamp after hours of insulin stimulation (Højlund et al. 2003; Kim et al. 2003), or after 30–40 min of insulin stimulation before euglycaemia or steady-state are obtained (Cusi et al. 2000). Sometimes insulin activation of enzymes reported in rodent muscle or cell lines using extreme insulin levels cannot be confirmed in human muscle biopsies using physiological concentrations of insulin. Moreover, in rodent muscle the response of enzymes to insulin may be transient, whereas in human skeletal muscle the effects of insulin on signaling enzymes are sustained for several hours (Wojtaszewski et al. 2000; Grimmsmann et al. 2002; Kim et al. 2003).

Using a diversity of study designs (Table 14.1), we have studied a number of enzymes, genes and metabolites in skeletal muscle samples obtained by the percutaneous needle biopsy technique. This includes biochemical determination of 1) glucose, glucose-6-phosphate, lactate and glycogen in muscle cells (Damsbo et al. 1991; Vaag et al. 1991, 1992); 2) activity, phosphorylation and/or protein content of insulin signaling enzymes including insulin receptor tyrosine kinase (IRTK), phosphotyrosine phosphatase (PTPase), insulin receptor substrate-1 and -2 (IRS-1 and -2), phosphoinositide-3-kinase (PI3K), phosphoinositide-dependent-kinase-1 (PDK-1), glucose transporter 4 (GLUT4), Akt/protein kinase B (PKB), glycogen synthase kinase-3 (GSK-3) and glycogen synthase (GS) (Mandarino et al. 1987; Wright et al. 1988; Handberg et al. 1990, 1993; Damsbo et al. 1991, 1998; Vaag et al. 1991, 1992a, 1992b, 1996; Worm et al. 1996; Meyer et al. 2002a, 2002b; Højlund et al. 2003; Levin et al. 2004); as well as 3) enzymes in other pathways regulating glucose and lipid metabolism, such as pyruvate dehydrogenase (PDH), phosphofructokinase (PFK), protein phosphatase 2A (PP2A), AMP-activated protein kinase (AMPK) and acetyl-carboxylase CoA (ACC) (Mandarino et al. 1987; Wright et al. 1988; Højlund et al. 2002, 2004). The most consistent abnormality associated with insulin resistance in subjects with type 2 diabetes and prediabetes is impaired insulin activation of GS (Wright et al. 1988; Vaag et al. 1992a; Damsbo et al. 1998; Højlund et al. 2003). A recent study suggests that this may involve

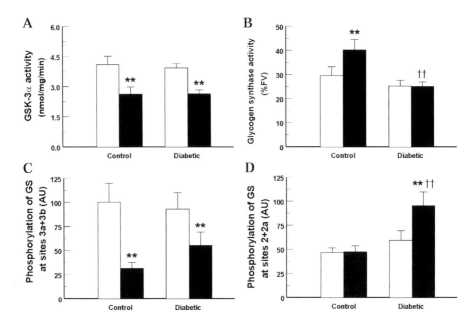

Figure 14.3 Impaired Insulin Activation of Muscle GS in Type 2 Diabetes The effect of insulin on: A) glycogen synthase kinase-3α (GSK-3α); B) glycogen synthase (GS) activity, given as fractional velocity; C) phosphorylation of GS at sites 3a+3b; and D) phosphorylation of GS at sites 2+2a in skeletal muscle biopsies from 10 obese type 2 diabetic patients and 10 obese non-diabetic control subjects. Muscle biopsies were obtained from the vastus lateralis muscle before (white bars) and after (black bars) a 4 h euglycaemic-hyperinsulinaemic clamp using insulin infusion rate of 40 mU/min/m^2. $**P < 0.01$ vs basal; $\dagger\dagger P < 0.01$ vs control.

hyperphosphorylation of GS at sites 2+2a. This seems to counteract a normal insulin-mediated dephosphorylation of GS at sites 3a+3b in patients with type 2 diabetes (Højlund et al. 2003) (Figure 14.3).

An increasing number of enzymes either directly involved in insulin signaling or working as modulators of insulin signaling, metabolic fuel regulators or nutrient sensors, have been suggested to be involved in the pathogenesis of skeletal muscle insulin resistance (Shulman 2000, 2004; Evans et al. 2002; Schmitz-Peiffer 2002; Wells et al. 2003; Krebs & Roden 2004; Pirola et al. 2004). Therefore, there has been a growing demand for global approaches capable of evaluating these multiple genes and proteins, and their modifications, simultaneously. Indeed, two such techniques – gene expression profiling using cDNA microarray and quantitative proteomics – emerged in the mid 90s. Recently, the application of these novel global approaches has revealed a coordinated down-regulation of genes and proteins involved in mitochondrial oxidative phosphorylation and increased cellular stress in skeletal muscle biopsies on subjects with type 2 diabetes and prediabetes (Sreekumar et al. 2002; Højlund et al. 2003; Mootha et al. 2003; Patti et al. 2003). Together with recent morphological studies of muscle mitochondria (see later) and the use of nuclear magnetic resonance spectroscopy, they have provided evidence for perturbations in skeletal muscle mitochondrial metabolism in the pathogenesis of type 2 diabetes (Petersen et al. 2004, 2005; Lowell & Shulman 2005). These abnormalities have been hypothesised to be responsible for lipid accumulation and increased oxidative stress, which may cause activation of lipid- and stress-activated serine/threonine protein kinases, with subsequent inhibitory modulation of insulin signaling (Kelley & Mandarino 2000; Evans et al. 2002; Schmitz-Peiffer 2002; Shulman 2004). Taken together, these novel insights into the molecular mechanisms underlying insulin resistance will inevitably cause an even higher interest in studying skeletal muscle biopsies in the future.

Morphology of skeletal muscle

Morphological studies of skeletal muscle are based on analysis of thin sections of muscle using either light microscopy for histological and histochemical studies or electron microscopy. Using a wide range of procedures, these techniques allow the assessment of changes in muscle structure, fibre type composition and ultrastructure associated with any disease affecting skeletal muscle. Moreover, morphological analysis is often used to clarify whether proteins verified in muscle tissue extracts originate from muscle or contaminating tissue types, and to determine the precise subcellular localisation of proteins and organelles within muscle cells. Combining these techniques with the principles of stereology, which is the field describing methods for counting and measuring morphological structures in an unbiased way (Gundersen et al. 1988), it is also possible to obtain quantitative measurements of abnormalities associated with e.g. insulin resistance and type 2 diabetes. There are numerous protocols for tissue fixation, processing in histology, visualisation by immunostaining, electron microscopy and application of stereology. Please refer to standard texts for further information.

The essential steps in morphological studies are the fixation of the muscle specimen and the preparation of thin muscle sections. The structure of muscle tissue will start to undergo alterations immediately after isolation. A rapid fixation of the muscle tissue ensures minimal artifact formation and optimal preservation of tissue architecture. In practice, we split muscle specimens into two minor parts, which are either cryopreserved (snap frozen) in Tissue-Tek for histological and histochemical studies or chemically fixed by cacodylate buffered glutaraldehyde, followed by post-fixation with 1 % osmium tetraoxide, for electron microscopy. Muscle tissue fixed in Tissue-Tek can be cut into thin sections directly, using a cryostat (5–10 μm sections), whereas muscle tissue chemically fixed for electron microscopy needs to be rigidly supported by dehydration in graded ethanol and subsequent embedding in epoxy resins (Epon) before thin sections can be cut by an ultramicrotome (80 nm section). Muscle fragments may be crushed when removed from the Bergström needle and insufficient freezing can result in freezing/ice crystal artifacts. To evaluate whether the muscle sections can be used for further analysis, we therefore recommend using traditional hematoxylin and eosin (HE) staining, which provides a good overview of the general tissue architecture and any areas of artifacts that may be present. In general, morphological analysis of muscle tissue sections should be based on the investigation of at least 200 muscle fibres in order to obtain reproducible observations.

Application of muscle morphology in type 2 diabetes

Insulin resistance and type 2 diabetes are associated with a number of morphological characteristics in skeletal muscle. In humans, muscle fibre composition is more mixed than in rodents (Johnson et al. 1973). This has implications for many biochemical and metabolic abnormalities observed in studies of crude muscle extracts, as the functional and metabolic properties of muscle are to a large extent determined by its fibre type composition. Using the myofibrillar ATPase histochemical staining procedure, muscle fibres can be divided into two major types: slow-twitch oxidative (red) type 1 fibres, and fast-twitch non-oxidative (white) type 2 fibres. The latter can be further subdivided into type 2a fibres and type 2b fibres.

In most (Marin et al. 1994; Gaster et al. 2001) but not all (Zierath et al. 1996) studies, a lower proportion of type 1 muscle fibres and a higher proportion of type 2 (particularly 2b) muscle fibres have been reported in type 2 diabetes. Furthermore, histochemical studies have shown a lower capillary density in skeletal muscle in type 2 diabetes (Marin et al. 1994). Using electron microscopy and stereology we have found an increased intramyocellular lipid content (IMCL) and a lower muscle glycogen content in type 2 diabetes (Levin et al. 2001) (Figure 14.4). In first degree relatives of patients with type 2 diabetes, an increased content of IMCL and type 2b muscle fibres has been confirmed, whereas muscle capillary density was normal (Nyholm et al. 1997). Nevertheless, IMCL content, proportion of type 2 muscle fibres and capillary density in muscle all correlate with insulin resistance in healthy, type 2 diabetic and prediabetic individuals (Lillioja et al. 1987; Jacob et al. 1999; Virkamaki et al. 2001). Moreover, the use of antidiabetic therapeutics in patients with type 2 diabetes has been demonstrated to increase capillary density and reduce IMCL content, whereas no changes in fibre type composition were seen (Mathieu-Costello et al. 2003).

It has been shown by electron microscopy that muscle mitochondria are smaller in type 2 diabetic and obese subjects than in lean non-diabetic subjects (Kelley et al. 2002). Mitochondria can be divided into subtypes according to their subcellular location, and it appears that subsarcolemmal and intermyofibrillar mitochondria display differential susceptibility to apoptotic stimuli such as reactive oxygen species (ROS) (Adhihetty et al. 2005) and play distinct roles in regulating skeletal muscle fatty acid metabolism (Koves et al. 2005). Recently, it was suggested that mitochondrial dysfunction in the muscle of patients with type 2 diabetes could be due to a specific reduction in subsarcolemmal mitochondria and electron transport chain activity within these mitochondria (Ritov et al. 2005).

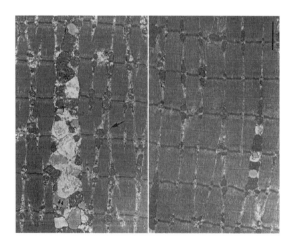

Figure 14.4 Increased Intramyocellular Lipid Content in Type 2 Diabetes Ultrastructure of longitudinally cut, striated muscle from a type 2 diabetic subject (left) and a normoglycaemic obese subject (right). Prominent lipid vacuoles are seen in the diabetic muscle. Mitochondria morphology in the two pictures is similar. Lipid droplets: double arrow; mitochondria: asterisk; area with glycogen granules: single arrow; 1.5 my-meter: line.

Fibre type dependent protein expression cannot be resolved by techniques using tissue homogenates due to the loss of protein origin information. The lack of significant differences in fibre type compositions in some studies indicates that not all abnormalities are explained by fibre types. In this regard, the ability to study fibre type specific changes in proteins or organelles is a powerful tool, which has already provided promising results. Combining a double immunolabeling technique with stereology (Figure 14.5), we examined fibre type specific expressions of GLUT4 in muscle specimens and showed that type 1 fibres contain a higher expression of GLUT4 (Gaster et al. 2000). In patients with type 2 diabetes (Figure 14.6), however, the GLUT4 expression in type 1 fibres was significantly reduced (Gaster et al. 2001). Moreover, by combining histochemical staining for fibre types with staining for oxidative enzyme activity, glycolytic enzyme activity and IMCL (Oil red staining), it has been shown that reduced oxidative capacity and increased IMCL are present

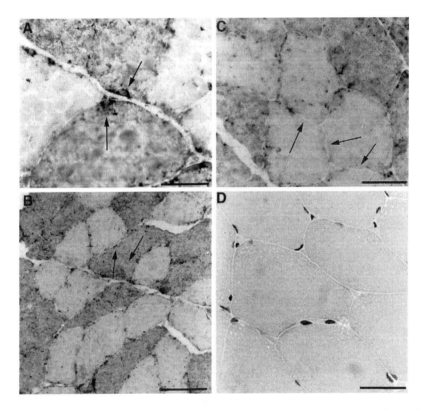

Figure 14.5 Double Immunostaining of Skeletal Muscle GLUT4 and Myosins Cryosections of muscle biopsies were double immunostained as described by Gaster et al. (2000). GLUT4 was visualised by an immunoperoxidase reaction and fibre type by an immunophosphatase reaction. A) GLUT4 immunoreactivity in the perinuclear region (arrows). Scale bar 25 μm; B) granular GLUT4 immunoreactivity is present in relation to sarcolemma and is visible in most appositions between unstained slow fibres, whereas several appositions between stained fast fibres are without GLUT4 immunoreactivity (arrowheads). Scale bar 100 μm; C) stained slow fibres present more GLUT4 than unstained fast fibres (arrows). Scale bar 50 μm; D) control section stained with detection system without primary antibody. Scale bar 50 μm.

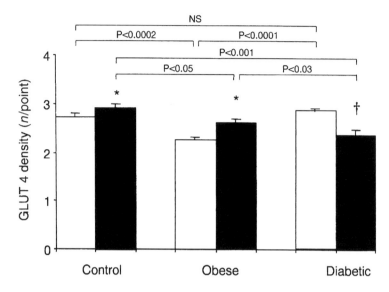

Figure 14.6 GLUT4 Density in Slow and Fast Fibres GLUT4 densities in slow and fast skeletal muscle fibres in control subjects, obese subjects and subjects with type 2 diabetes were determined as described by Gaster et al. (2001). GLUT4 densities in fast fibres (white bars) and slow fibres (black bars) are shown as means ± SE, $n = 9$ in the control subjects and $n = 8$ in the type 2 diabetic subjects and obese subjects. $*P < 0.05$ and $†P < 0.001$, slow vs fast fibres. GLUT4 is reduced in slow muscle fibres of type 2 diabetic patients: is insulin resistance in type 2 diabetes a slow, type 1 fiber disease: Reproduced courtesy of Diabetes **50**, 1324–1329, (2001).

in both type 1 and type 2 muscle fibres in type 2 diabetic and obese subjects, suggesting that these abnormalities are fibre type independent (He et al. 2001).

These data clearly demonstrate that morphological analyses are supplemental to biochemical and metabolic studies of skeletal muscle insulin resistance. Further improvements in these techniques allowing determination of function and translocation of proteins and organelles into different subcellular compartments will further increase our understanding of type 2 diabetes pathophysiology.

Human myotube cultures

Cultured myotubes offer a unique model for separating the genetic influence on insulin resistance and type 2 diabetes from environmental factors (Henry et al. 1996a,b; Nikoulina et al. 2001; Gaster et al. 2002, 2004a,b, 2005; Gaster & Beck-Nielsen 2004; McIntyre et al. 2004). As an *in vitro* model of skeletal muscle, they are devoid of extracellular influence and offer excellent material for performing studies under standardised conditions. The basis of this model system is satellite cells (quiescent multipotent cells) lying between the basal membrane and the sarcolemma of muscle fibres. They are isolated, scaled up and allowed to differentiate into multinuclear myotubes. The underlying idea is that cultured muscle cells express their genetic background only when precultured under physiological conditions and express adaptive traits when precultured under 'inducing' conditions. A genetic cause for a known *in vivo* pathophysiological abnormality will be evident if the abnormality is present *in vitro* under physiological conditions (Beck-Nielsen et al. 2003). The model is based on the assumption that preconditioning *in vivo* is not a serious problem, i.e. that acquired defects, as a consequence of e.g. chronic hyperglycaemia, dyslipidaemia and/or hyperinsulinaemia, will not be preserved after culturing under physiological conditions and after replication for weeks. Like the *in vivo* environment, this new environment will influence cell metabolism in a new way and thereby diminish previous metabolic influences. Moreover, the differentiation of myoblasts to myotubes changes the protein expression and metabolism to the direction of mature muscle fibres, further reducing the influence of the *in vivo* metabolic milieu. Human myotubes established from satellite cells are widely used. These cell cultures are the model of choice for the study of myogenesis and muscle regeneration, but they are also intensively used in metabolic studies.

Established myotubes express traits known from mature skeletal muscle, i.e. multinucleation, cross-striation, expression of most cytoskeletal proteins, increased creatine kinase (CK) activity and, occasionally, spontaneous contractions (Gaster et al. 2001a,b). Differentiated myotube cultures are metabolically stable for days when the differentiation-dependent changes have been finalised on day 4 after induction of differentiation (Gaster et al. 2001b). Myotubes express most of the proteins (enzymes and transporters) of the intermediate metabolism, and essential components of the insulin signaling cascade (Henry et al. 1996a,b; Nikoulina et al. 2001; Gaster et al. 2002, 2004a,b, 2005; Gaster & Beck-Nielsen 2004; McIntyre et al. 2004). Interestingly, in these cells the expression of the glucose transporter GLUT1 is about 10-fold higher than the expression of GLUT4 (Sarabia et al. 1992; Al-Khalili et al. 2003). Nevertheless, insulin stimulation of glucose uptake seems mediated solely by the translocation of GLUT4 to the plasma membrane, as shown by the photolabeling technique (Al-Khalili et al. 2003). Not only glucose uptake, but also glucose oxidation, glycogen synthesis and lipid uptake and storage have been demonstrated to exhibit insulin responsiveness in human myotubes that is similar to that observed *in vivo* (Henry et al. 1995, 1996a,b; Nikoulina et al. 2001; Gaster et al. 2001, 2002, 2004a,b, 2005; Gaster & Beck-Nielsen 2004; McIntyre et al. 2004, Ortenblad et al. 2005). Thus, myotube cultures seem suitable as models of skeletal muscle and for the study of insulin resistance.

The cell culture principle of human myotubes

Satellite cells can be isolated from muscle biopsy samples by enzymatic digestion (Yasin et al. 1977; Blau & Webster 1981) or by migration from muscle tissue explants (Askanas & Engel 1975). We and most other laboratories use the former principle. The initial myogenic purity after enzymatic digestion is high (>95 %) but it decreases easily through fibroblast overgrowth and as satellite cells differentiate into myotubes. The purity and the differentiation degree of obtained myotubes cultures can be increased by favouring conditions for myogenic growth and differentiation. We have previously described optimised conditions of growth and differentiation based on the presence of the serum substitute ultroser G (UG) and coating of the culturing surfaces by extracellular matrix gel (ECM) during growth (Gaster et al. 2001). Differentiation seems preferable at low foetal calf serum (FCS) concentration without UG (Gaster et al. 2001).

Pre-isolation: Muscle tissue fragments used for the isolation of satellite cells are immediately placed in a 10 ml test tube with Dulbecco's modified Eagle's medium

(DMEM), containing 10 % FCS, 50 U/ml penicillin, 50 μg/ml streptomycin, and 1.25 μg/ml amphotericin B at room temperature. If the isolation procedure is not initiated within an hour of obtaining the biopsy material, the tube is placed in the refrigerator at 5 ° C and can be stored for up to 48 hours. However, extended storage is associated with reduced cell gain.

1) Muscle biopsy tissue is rinsed in 20 ml sterile DMEM in a tube to get rid of blood and then transferred by a Pasteur pipette to a sterile Petri dish. 2 ml DMEM is added.

2) The muscle tissue is dissected free of fat, vessels and connective tissue, and subsequently chopped finely with crossed scalpels to obtain fragments smaller than 1 mm cubes.

3) The muscle fragments are transferred by a Pasteur pipette to a 50 ml sterile centrifuge tube and allowed to settle down. The supernatant is removed.

4) To remove residual cell debris, divalent ions and leaked enzymes, the muscle fragments are washed twice by adding 20 ml 0.05 % trypsin-EDTA to the tube and discharging the supernatant after the fragments have settled down.

5) The tissue fragments are then dissociated by three successive treatments (3 × steps 5 and 6) with 20 ml 0.05 % trypsin-EDTA, with the tube placed in a water bath at 37°C for 20 min with regular stirring.

6) After each treatment, the overlying cell suspension (supernatant) is transferred to a centrifuge tube and centrifuged at 500 g for 5 min. The resulting supernatant is discharged and the cell pellet is resuspended in 10 ml DMEM containing 10 % FCS, which terminates further protease activity. The obtained cell suspension after each treatment is transferred by a Pasteur pipette to a 50 ml sterile centrifuge tube (collecting tube).

7) Any cells remaining in the original tube after the three treatments are discharged.

8) The collected cell suspensions are pooled and centrifuged at 500 g for 5 min. The resulting supernatant is discharged and the pellet is resuspended in 10 ml DMEM containing 10 % FCS, 50 U/ml penicillin, 50 μg/ml streptomycin and 1.25 μg/ml amphotericin B. The final cell suspension is seed on uncoated sterile Petri dishes for 30 min (preplating) in order to reduce contamination with fibroblasts, which adhere faster to uncoated plastic surfaces than satellite cells.

9) After preplating, the cell suspension is transferred to ECM-gel coated dishes.

10) After 24 h, cell debris and non-adherent cells are removed by changing the growth medium to DMEM supplemented with 2 % FCS, 2 % UG, 50 U/ml penicillin, 50 μg/ml streptomycin and 1.25 μg/ml amphotericin B. Cells can be further subcultured (see below) before final seeding.

11) At 75 % confluence (evaluated by phase contrast microscopy), the growth medium is replaced by basal medium containing DMEM (glucose 5.5 mM) supplemented with 2 % FCS, 50 U/ml penicillin, 50 μg/ml streptomycin, 1.25 μg/ml amphotericin B and 25 pmol/l insulin in order to induce differentiation.

12) We recommend the use of differentiated myotubes in the period from day 4 to day 8 after induction of differentiation as only minor differentiation-related changes will take place during this period.

Samples of established satellite cultures (step 10) can be stored frozen in order to avoid total cell loss by infection, failure in laboratory facilities, senescence and insufficient designs, or to ensure further material for additional experiments. Trypsinated, proliferating satellite cells are frozen in suspension at high cell concentration added cryoprotective dimethyl sulfoxide at a rate of 1 °C per min and finally stored in liquid nitrogen. The cells are cultured in humidified 5 % CO_2 atmosphere at 37°C and the medium is changed every 2–3 days. DMEM (glucose 5.5 mM), FCS, UG, penicillin-streptomycin-amphotericin B and trypsin-EDTA can be obtained from Life Technology (Scotland). ECM-gel can be purchased from Sigma Chemical Co. (St Louis, USA).

Warning: Biopsy material carries a risk of infection, and muscle tissue has to be handled according to this risk. Therefore, we recommend that either the patients/volunteers or the muscle tissue are screened for infections such as HIV and hepatitis. Disposable material should be used where possible and all other utensils should be autoclaved or immersed in a suitable disinfectant after use.

Advantages of human myotubes

The extracellular environment can be controlled precisely and kept constant over time, which allows study of the importance of the genetic background and the impact of various compensatory mechanisms. The culture environment lacks systemic homeostatic regulatory components from the nervous and endocrine systems, promoting a more constant cellular metabolism. Contraction-induced changes do not seem to be a major problem either, as contractions are rarely seen in human myotubes. The muscle cell cultures are easily handled and experimental designs allow many variables and replicates. Myotubes are exposed directly to a reagent, with direct access to the cells. In contrast, human and animal studies are often limited by the number of subjects, due to a higher cost and ethical considerations. Muscle cell culture tissue is suitable for almost the same analysis as muscle biopsy tissue, and often the same assays and analyses can be directly applied to extracts from myotubes (Table 14.2). Muscle cell cultures have the advantage that they can be established in various culture dishes, allowing us to designate the right amount of tissue material for a specific analysis. In contrast to *in vivo* muscle biopsies, cultured myotubes allow studies on living muscle cell *in vitro*, i.e. testing the effects of a particular hormone, substrate, drug or compound on different metabolic and signaling pathways, including time-course and dose-response analyses, as well as assessment of substrate metabolism, thereby allowing investigation of causal relationships and the interactions of various pathways (Table 14.2).

Limitations of human myotubes

Cell culture techniques are dependent on aseptic conditions. The laboratory has to be equipped with the necessary cell culturing facilities and has to have good laboratory practice (GLP). Although the technique seems simple, success with cultures of human myotubes depends on technicians with appropriate aseptic skills and the ability to diagnose problems as they arise. It is important to realise that we are dealing with a primary culture system, with restrictions such as limited lifespan of established cultures. Experiments have to be carefully designed. Muscle phenotypic characteristics are lost by extensive propagation of the cells. This is based on overgrowth of undifferentiated cells of the same

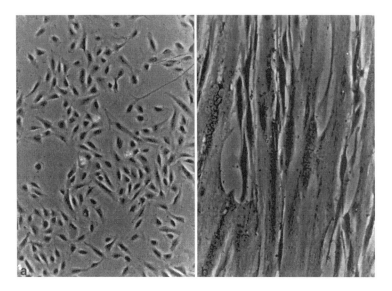

Figure 14.7 Phase Contrast Appearance of Human Satellite Cell Culture Human satellite cell cultures were established, grown, and differentiated as described by Gaster et al. (2001a,b). Morphological appearance was investigated by phase contrast microscopy. A) mononucleated cells under proliferation (X100); B) day 8 differentiated cultures, cultured under physiological conditions (5.0 mmol/l glucose and 25 pmol/l insulin). The cultures contain many multinucleated myofibres (×200).

lineage, rather then degeneration or dedifferentiation. Observation of morphology is the simplest and most direct technique used to follow the cultures of myotubes during proliferation, differentiation and various exposures (Figure 14.7). This can be done without increasing the risk of contamination of the established cultures. It is useful to keep a set of photographs for each cell exposure condition as documentation in case of morphological changes. A set of pictures from representative cultures of myotubes in each study group is recommended.

Working with cell culture models requires a strategy for verifying that obtained cultures have a high myogenic purity and a low contamination by fibroblasts, and that culture conditions ensure comparable cultures of myotubes from different patient subgroups and allow identification of transdifferentiation. The plasticity of satellite cells has previously been highlighted by showing that the presence of thiazolidinediones converted myogenic cells into more adipose-like cells (Kausch et al. 2001). We use immuno-histochemistry of muscle specific proteins and mRNA expression of myogenic (myogenin, tropomyosin, NCAM) and adipogenic (FABP4) markers (Gaster et al. 2001a,b; Abdallah et al. 2005; Kase et al. 2005). The risk of transdifferentiation can be reduced by waiting until the myotubes are fully differentiated (Gaster et al. 2001b).

Cell culturing has traditionally been regarded in a sceptical light. Indeed, cultured muscle cells do not retain all the features of adult skeletal muscle and as such, differences may occur that do not translate to the normal physiological state. Investigators should be cautious in their interpretation of data suggesting primary events in the myotube model system, particularly when extrapolating data of gene expression to protein levels. Without comparing the presence of a specific trait in myotubes to the mature adult skeletal muscle, authors cannot be sure that their findings are primary.

The human myotube model can, however, become a valuable tool in diabetes research as long as these limitations are appreciated and the model is used in a proper way.

Application of myotubes in diabetes research

In human myotubes established from skeletal muscle biopsies of both healthy subjects and patients with type 2 diabetes, we have used a variety of approaches to study possible mediators of insulin resistance under both physiological and so-called 'inducing' conditions (Table 14.2). This includes biochemical determination of 1) glucose, G6P, glycogen and triacylglycerol (TAG) (Gaster et al. 2001c, 2002, 2004; Kase et al. 2005); 2) activity, kinetics and/or protein expression of distal components of the insulin signaling cascade such as GS and GSK-3 (Gaster et al. 2001c, 2002, 2004); and 3) other enzymes essential for glucose and lipid metabolism such as hexokinase (HK), citrate synthase (CS), CK and 3-hydroxy-acyl-CoA dehydrogenase (HAD) (Gaster et al. 2001a,b; Ortenblad et al. 2005); as well as 4) gene expression analysis in myotubes using both the cDNA microarray technique and real time (RT)-PCR reactions (Hansen et al. 2004; Abdallah et al. 2005; Kase et al. 2005). Moreover, we have determined rates of substrate metabolism, including glucose uptake, glucose oxidation, glycogen synthesis, lipid uptake, oxidation, lipogenesis and the incorporation of fatty acids into different lipids under various conditions, as well as mitochondrial respiration in isolated myotubes' mitochondria (Gaster et al. 2002, 2004; Gaster & Beck-Nielsen 2004; Abdallah et al. 2005; Kase et al. 2005; Ortenblad et al. 2005). Taken together,

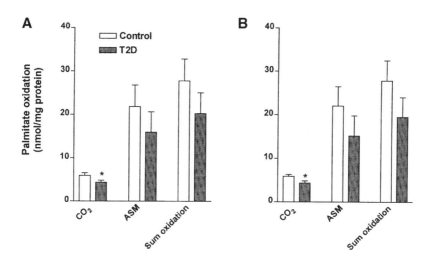

Figure 14.8 Oxidation of Palmitic Acid in Myotubes Established from Control and Type 2 Diabetic Subjects Differentiated myotubes (day 8) were exposed to [1-^{14}C]palmitic acid (2.0 μCi/ml, 0.6 mmol/l), 5.5 mmol/l glucose and 25 pmol/l or 1 μmol/l insulin in serum-free DMEM for 4 h to determine palmitate oxidation under basal conditions (A) and acute insulin stimulation (B). Data are means ±SE. $n = 9$ and 10 for control and diabetic myotubes, respectively. *$P \leq 0.05$ for type 2 diabetic vs control myotubes. Reduced lipid oxidation in skeletal muscle from type 2 diabetic subjects may be of genetic origin: evdence from cultured myotubes. Reproduced courtesy of Diabetes **53**, 542–548, (2004).

these studies have provided evidence that the myotube model is a strong tool for differentiating genes vs environment. For a number of abnormalities observed in skeletal muscle *in vivo*, the diabetic phenotype is conserved in diabetic myotubes. This includes a lower lipid oxidation in the basal state (Figure 14.8), reduced insulin-mediated glucose oxidation and impaired insulin activation of GS and CS in diabetic myotubes than in control myotubes (Gaster et al. 2002, 2004; Gaster & Beck-Nielsen 2004; Ortenblad et al. 2005). Cluster analysis further confirms that diabetic myotubes retain their phenotype. In addition, human myotubes are sensitive to induction of insulin resistance by high concentrations of insulin or palmitate, whereas exposure to oleate does not induce insulin resistance (Gaster et al. 2001, 2004, 2005; Gaster & Beck-Nielsen 2004). The presence of parameters of both primary and induced insulin resistance in myotubes provides the possibility of gaining further insight into the molecular mechanisms underlying skeletal muscle insulin resistance, e.g. by using a range of commercially available compounds inhibiting or stimulating enzymes in various signaling and metabolic pathways, but also of studying the effects of potential antidiabetic drugs (Table 14.2).

Taken together, the above characteristics demonstrate that the human myotube model system is a powerful tool in studies of metabolism under controlled experimental conditions and seems to be a good extension of traditional studies of human muscle biopsies in diabetes research.

Conclusion

The invention of the percutaneous muscle biopsy technique in combination with euglycaemic-hyperinsulinaemic clamp studies and indirect calorimetry has opened up the possibility of *in vivo* studies of intracellular metabolism in skeletal muscle. The development of human skeletal muscle cultures based on these biopsies has further provided the opportunity of differentiating between genetic and environmental etiologies to the abnormalities seen, as well as the possibility of *in vitro* manipulation of cell metabolism by the study of the influences of various hormones, lipids, drugs and chemical substances. Our detailed characterisation of the primary defects in glycogen metabolism as one major cause of insulin resistance in skeletal muscle has been based on these techniques. The finding of abnormalities in skeletal muscle in patients with type 2 diabetes and insulin resistance has opened up the possibility for new interventions based on this pathophysiological knowledge. Used carefully and with respect for their limitations, these tools may in the future let us understand the mechanisms underlying insulin resistance and therefore type 2 diabetes.

Table 14.1 Summary Box 1

Muscle biopsies in diabetes research

Study subjects
  Patients with type 2 diabetes
  Monozygotic twins discordant for type 2 diabetes
  Offspring of patients with type 2 diabetes
  Obese non-diabetic controls
  Lean non-diabetic controls

Intervention
None
Treatment with drugs
Exercise-training
Indirect calorimetry (local or systemic)
Follow-up

Metabolic characterisation
Fasting plasma glucose, insulin, lipid profile, etc.
Euglycaemic-hyperinsulinaemic clamp
Indirect calorimetry (local or systemic)

Percutaneous muscle biopsy (+/− insulin)
50 mg pieces frozen in liquid nitrogen
5 mg piece embedded in Tissue-Tek
1 mm cubes pre-fixed in glutaraldehyde
min 50 mg for isolation of mitochondria
min 50 mg for isolation of satelite cells

Biochemical analysis
Metabolites, energy stores
Enzyme activity, modification, expression
Gene expression, modification
Proteomics, genomics, lipidomics

Morphological and histochemical analysis
Fiber type composition
Staining for enzyme levels
Capillary density
Lipid, glycogen, mitochondria
Fiber-type specific studies

Table 14.2 Summary Box 2

Myotubes in diabetes research

Study subjects
As in summary box 1

Study design
Physiological vs. "inducing" conditions
Chronic (days) vs. acute (min to h) exposure
Time-course and dose-response studies

Stimuli/intervention
Hormones, peptides, cytokines
Substrates, (glucose, palmitate,etc)
Drugs (anti-diabetic, lipid lowering ect)
Enzyme modulators (kinase inhibitors, etc)
Electrical stimulation, heat, hypoxia
Gene transfection, RNA interference

Table 14.2   Continued

Metabolism
  Glucose and lipid uptake
  Glucose and lipid oxidation
  Glycogen synthesis

Biochemical analysis
  Metabolites, energy stores
  Enzyme activity, modification, expression
  Gene expression, modification
  Proteomics, genomics, lipidomics

Morphological and histochemical analysis
  Myotube/cell characteristics
  Ultrastructure (mitochondria, etc)
  Enzyme activity, expression and localisation
  Translocation of proteins, e.g. GLUT4
  Glycogen and TAG

References

Abdallah BM, Beck-Nielsen H, Gaster M (2005) Increased expression of 11beta-hydroxysteroid dehydrogenase type 1 in type 2 diabetic myotubes *Eur J Clin Invest* **35**, 627–634

Adhihetty PJ, Ljubicic V, Menzies KJ, Hood DA (2005) Differential susceptibility of subsarcolemmal and intermyofibrillar mitochondria to apoptotic stimuli*Am J Physiol Cell Physiol*, **289**, C994–C1001

Al-Khalili L, Chibalin AV, Kannisto K, Zhang BB, Permert J, Holman GD, Ehrenborg E, Ding VD, Zierath JR, Krook A (2003) Insulin action in cultured human skeletal muscle cells during differentiation, assessment of cell surface GLUT4 and GLUT1 content *Cell Mol Life Sci* **60**, 991–998

Askanas V, Engel WK (1975) A new program for investigating adult human skeletal muscle grown aneurally in tissue culture *Neurology* **25**, 58–67

Beck-Nielsen H, Groop LC (1994) Metabolic and genetic characterization of prediabetic states Sequence of events leading to non-insulin-dependent diabetes mellitus *J Clin Invest* **94**, 1714–1721

Beck-Nielsen H (1998) Mechanisms of insulin resistance in non-oxidative glucose metabolism, the role of glycogen synthase *J Basic Clin Physiol Pharmacol* **9**, 255–279

Beck-Nielsen H, Vaag A, Poulsen P, Gaster M (2003) Metabolic and genetic influence on glucose metabolism in type 2 diabetic subjects – experiences from relatives and twin studies *Best Pract Res Clin Endocrinol Metab* **17**, 445–467

Bergström J (1962) Muscle electrolytes in man, determined by neutron activation analysis on needle biopsy specimens, a study in normal subjects, kidney patients, and patients with chronic diarrhoea *Scand J Clin Lab Invest* **14**, Suppl. 68, 1–110

Bergström J (1975) Percutaneous needle biopsy of skeletal muscle in physiological and clinical research *Scand J Clin Lab Invest* **35**, 609–616

Blau HM, Webster C (1981) Isolation and characterization of human muscle cells *Proc Natl Acad Sci USA* **78**, 5623–5627

Cusi K, Maezono K, Osman A, Pendergrass M, Patti ME, Pratipanawatr T, DeFronzo RA, Kahn CR, Mandarino LJ (2000) Insulin resistance differentially affects the PI 3-kinase- and MAP kinase-mediated signaling in human muscle *J Clin Invest* **105**, 311–320

Damsbo P, Hermann LS, Vaag A, Hother-Nielsen O, Beck-Nielsen H (1998) Irreversibility of the defect in glycogen synthase activity in skeletal muscle from obese patients with NIDDM treated with diet and metformin *Diabetes Care* **21**, 1489–1494

Damsbo P, Vaag A, Hother-Nielsen O, Beck-Nielsen H (1991) Reduced glycogen synthase activity in skeletal muscle from obese patients with and without type 2 (non-insulin-dependent) diabetes mellitus *Diabetologia* **34**, 239–245

Edwards R, Young A, Wiles M (1980) Needle biopsy of skeletal muscle in the diagnosis of myopathy and the clinical study of muscle function and repair *N Engl J Med* **302**, 261–271

Edwards RH, Round JM, Jones DA (1983) Needle biopsy of skeletal muscle, a review of 10 years experience *Muscle Nerve* **6**, 676–683

Evans JL, Goldfine ID, Maddux BA, Grodsky GM (2002) Oxidative stress and stress–activated signaling pathways, a unifying hypothesis of type 2 diabetes *Endocr Rev* **23**, 599–622

Gaster M, Beck-Nielsen H (2004) The reduced insulin-mediated glucose oxidation in skeletal muscle from type 2 diabetic subjects may be of genetic origin – evidence from cultured myotubes *Biochim Biophys Acta* **1690**, 85–91

Gaster M, Beck-Nielsen H, Schroder HD (2001a) Proliferation conditions for human satellite cells The fractional content of satellite cells *APMIS* **109**, 726–734

Gaster M, Brusgaard K, Handberg A, Højlund K, Wojtaszewski JFP, Beck-Nielsen H (2004b) The primary defect in glycogen synthase activity is not based on increased glycogen synthase kinase-3α activity in diabetic myotubes *Biochem Biophys Res Com* **319**, 1235–1240

Gaster M, Kristensen SR, Beck-Nielsen H, Schroder HD (2001b) A cellular model system of differentiated human myotubes *APMIS* **109**, 735–744

Gaster M, Petersen I, Højlund K, Poulsen P, Beck-Nielsen H (2002) The diabetic phenotype is conserved in myotubes established from diabetic subjects, evidence for primary defects in glucose transport and glycogen synthase activity *Diabetes* **51**, 921–927

Gaster M, Poulsen P, Handberg A, Schroder HD, Beck-Nielsen H (2000) Direct evidence of fibre type-dependent GLUT-4 expression in human skeletal muscle *Am J Physiol Endocrinol Metab* **278**, E910–E916

Gaster M, Rustan AC, Aas V, Beck-Nielsen H (2004a) Reduced lipid oxidation in skeletal muscle from type 2 diabetic subjects may be of genetic origin, evidence from cultured myotubes *Diabetes* **53**, 542–548

Gaster M, Rustan A, Beck-Nielsen H (2005) Differential utilization of saturated palmitate and unsaturated oleate: Evidence from Cultured Myotubes *Diabetes* **54**, 648–656

Gaster M, Schroder HD, Handberg A, Beck-Nielsen H (2001c) The basal kinetic parameters of glycogen synthase in human myotube cultures are not affected by chronic high insulin exposure *Biochim Biophys Acta* **1537**, 211–221

Gaster M, Staehr P, Beck-Nielsen H, Schroder HD, Handberg A (2001) GLUT4 is reduced in slow muscle fibres of type 2 diabetic patients, is insulin resistance in type 2 diabetes a slow, type 1 fibre disease? *Diabetes* **50**, 1324–1329

Goldberger JH, Henry WL, Randall HT (1978) Percutaneous needle biopsy of skeletal muscle, technic and application *Am J Surg* **136**, 410–412

Greig PD, Askanazi J, Kinney JM (1985) Needle biopsy of skeletal muscle using suction *Surg Gynecol Obstet* **160**, 466–468

Grimmsmann T, Levin K, Meyer MM, Beck-Nielsen H, Klein HH (2002) Delays in insulin signaling towards glucose disposal in human skeletal muscle *J Endocrinol* **172**, 645–651

Gundersen HJ, Bendtsen TF, Korbo L, Marcussen N, Moller A, Nielsen K, Nyengaard JR, Pakkenberg B, Sorensen FB, Vesterby A (1988) and Some new, simple and efficient stereological methods and their use in pathological research and diagnosis *APMIS* **96**, 379–394

Handberg A, Vaag A, Vinten J, Beck-Nielsen H (1993) Decreased tyrosine kinase activity in partially purified insulin receptors from muscle of young, non-obese first degree relatives of patients with type 2 (non-insulin-dependent) diabetes mellitus *Diabetologia* **36**, 668–674

Handberg A, Vaag A, Damsbo P, Beck-Nielsen H, Vinten J (1990) Expression of insulin regulatable glucose transporters in skeletal muscle from type 2 (non-insulin-dependent) diabetic patients *Diabetologia* **33**, 625–627

Hansen L, Gaster M, Oakeley EJ, Brusgaard K, Damsgaard Nielsen EM, Beck-Nielsen H, Pedersen O, Hemmings BA (2004) Expression profiling of insulin action in human myotubes, induction of inflammatory and pro-angiogenic pathways in relationship with glycogen synthesis and type 2 diabetes *Biochem Biophys Res Commun* **323**, 685–695

He J, Watkins S, Kelley DE (2001) Skeletal muscle lipid content and oxidative enzyme activity in relation to muscle fibre type in type 2 diabetes and obesity *Diabetes* **50**, 817–823

Henry RR, Abrams L, Nikoulina S, Ciaraldi TP (1995) Insulin action and glucose metabolism in nondiabetic control and NIDDM subjects Comparison using human skeletal muscle cell cultures *Diabetes* **44**, 936–946

Henry RR, Ciaraldi TP, Abrams-Carter L, Mudaliar S, Park KS, Nikoulina SE (1996a) Glycogen synthase activity is reduced in cultured skeletal muscle cells of non-insulin-dependent diabetes mellitus subjects Biochemical and molecular mechanisms *J Clin Invest* **98**, 1231–1236

Henry RR, Ciaraldi TP, Mudaliar S, Abrams L, Nikoulina SE (1996b) Acquired defects of glycogen synthase activity in cultured human skeletal muscle cells, influence of high glucose and insulin levels *Diabetes* **45**, 400–407

Højlund K, Mustard KJ, Staehr P, Hardie DG, Beck-Nielsen H, Richter EA, Wojtaszewski JF (2004) AMPK activity and isoform protein expression are similar in muscle of obese subjects with and without type 2 diabetes *Am J Physiol Endocrinol Metab* **286**, E239–E244

Højlund K, Poulsen M, Staehr P, Brusgaard K, Beck-Nielsen H (2002) Effect of insulin on protein phosphatase 2A expression in muscle in type 2 diabetes *Eur J Clin Invest* **32**, 918–923

Højlund K, Staehr P, Hansen BF, Green KA, Hardie DG, Richter EA, Beck-Nielsen H, Wojtaszewski JF (2003) Increased phosphorylation of skeletal muscle glycogen synthase at NH2–terminal sites during physiological hyperinsulinemia in type 2 diabetes *Diabetes* **52**, 1393–1402

Højlund K, Wrzesinski K, Larsen PM, Fey SJ, Roepstorff P, Handberg A, Dela F, Vinten J, McCormack JG, Reynet C, Beck-Nielsen H (2003) Proteome analysis reveals phosphorylation of ATP synthase beta-subunit in human skeletal muscle and proteins with potential roles in type 2 diabetes *J Biol Chem* **278**, 10436–10442

Jacob S, Machann J, Rett K, Brechtel K, Volk A, Renn W, Maerker E, Matthaei S, Schick F, Claussen CD, Haring HU (1999) Association of increased intramyocellular lipid content with insulin resistance in lean nondiabetic offspring of type 2 diabetic subjects *Diabetes* **48**, 1113–1119

Johnson MA FAU, Polgar JF, Weightman DF, Appleton D (1973) Data on the distribution of fibre types in thirty-six human muscles An autopsy study *J Neurosci Res* **18**, 118–129

Kausch C, Krutzfeldt J, Witke A, Rettig A, Bachmann O, Rett K, Matthaei S, Machicao F, Haring HU, Stumvoll M (2001) Effects of troglitazone on cellular differentiation, insulin signaling, and glucose metabolism in cultured human skeletal muscle cells *Biochem Biophys Res Commun* **280**, 664–674

Kase ET, Wensaas AJ, Aas V, Højlund K, Levin K, Thoresen GH, Beck-Nielsen H, Rustan AC, Gaster M (2005) Skeletal muscle lipid accumulation in type 2 diabetes may involve the liver X receptor pathway *Diabetes* **54**, 1108–1115

Kelley DE, He J, Menshikova EV, Ritov VB (2002) Dysfunction of mitochondria in human skeletal muscle in type 2 diabetes *Diabetes* **51**, 2944–2950

Kelley DE, Mandarino LJ (2000) Fuel selection in human skeletal muscle in insulin resistance, a reexamination *Diabetes* **49**, 677–683

Kelley DE, Simoneau JA (1994) Impaired free fatty acid utilization by skeletal muscle in non–insulin–dependent diabetes mellitus *J Clin Invest* **94**, 2349–2356

Kim YB, Kotani K, Ciaraldi TP, Henry RR, Kahn BB (2003) Insulin-stimulated protein kinase C lambda/zeta activity is reduced in skeletal muscle of humans with obesity and type 2 diabetes, reversal with weight reduction *Diabetes* **52**, 1935–1942

Korsheninnikova E, Seppala-Lindroos A, Vehkavaara S, Goto T, Virkamaki A (2002) Elevated fasting insulin concentrations associate with impaired insulin signaling in skeletal muscle of healthy subjects independent of obesity *Diabetes Metab Res Rev* **18**, 209–216

Koves TR, Noland RC, Bates AL, Henes ST, Muoio DM, Cortright RN (2005) Subsarcolemmal and intermyofibrillar mitochondria play distinct roles in regulating skeletal muscle fatty acid metabolism *Am J Physiol Cell Physiol* **288**, C1074–1082

Krebs M, Roden M (2004) Nutrient–induced insulin resistance in human skeletal muscle *Curr Med Chem* **11**, 901–918

Levin K, Daa Schroeder H, Alford FP, Beck-Nielsen H (2001) Morphometric documentation of abnormal intramyocellular fat storage and reduced glycogen in obese patients with Type II diabetes *Diabetologia* **44**, 824–833

Levin K, Hother-Nielsen O, Henriksen JE, Beck-Nielsen H (2004) Effects of troglitazone in young first-degree relatives of patients with type 2 diabetes *Diabetes Care* **27**, 148–154

Lillioja S, Young AA, Culter CL, Ivy JL, Abbott WG, Zawadzki JK, Yki-Jarvinen H, Christin L, Secomb TW, Bogardus C (1987) Skeletal muscle capillary density and fibre type are possible determinants of in vivo insulin resistance in man *J Clin Invest* **80**, 415–424

Lowell BB, Shulman GI (2005) Mitochondrial dysfunction and type 2 diabetes *Science* **307**, 384–387

Mandarino LJ, Consoli A, Jain A, Kelley DE (1996) Interaction of carbohydrate and fat fuels in human skeletal muscle, impact of obesity and NIDDM *Am J Physiol* **270**, E463–E470

Mandarino LJ, Wright KS, Verity LS, Nichols J, Bell JM, Kolterman OG, Beck-Nielsen H (1987) Effects of insulin infusion on human skeletal muscle pyruvate dehydrogenase, phosphofructokinase, and glycogen synthase Evidence for their role in oxidative and nonoxidative glucose metabolism *J Clin Invest* **80**, 655–663

Mathieu-Costello O, Kong A, Ciaraldi TP, Cui L, Ju Y, Chu N, Kim D, Mudaliar S, Henry RR (2003) Regulation of skeletal muscle morphology in type 2 diabetic subjects by troglitazone and metformin, relationship to glucose disposal *Metabolism* **52**, 540–546

Marin P, Andersson B, Krotkiewski M, Bjorntorp P (1994) Muscle fibre composition and capillary density in women and men with NIDDM *Diabetes Care* **17**, 382–386

McIntyre EA, Halse R, Yeaman SJ, Walker M (2004) Cultured muscle cells from insulin-resistant type 2 diabetes patients have impaired insulin, but normal 5-amino-4-imidazolecarboxamide riboside-stimulated, glucose uptake *J Clin Endocrinol Metab* **89**, 3440–3448

Meyer MM, Levin K, Grimmsmann T, Beck-Nielsen H, Klein HH (2002a) Insulin signalling in skeletal muscle of subjects with or without Type II-diabetes and first degree relatives of patients with the disease *Diabetologia* **45**, 813–822

Meyer MM, Levin K, Grimmsmann T, Perwitz N, Eirich A, Beck-Nielsen H, Klein HH (2002b) Troglitazone treatment increases protein kinase B phosphorylation in skeletal muscle of normoglycaemic subjects at risk for the development of type 2 diabetes *Diabetes* **51**, 2691–2697

Mootha VK, Lindgren CM, Eriksson KF, Subramanian A, Sihag S, Lehar J et al. (2003) PGC-1alpha-responsive genes involved in oxidative phosphorylation are coordinately downregulated in human diabetes *Nat Genet* **34**, 267–273

Nikoulina SE, Ciaraldi TP, Carter L, Mudaliar S, Park KS, Henry RR (2001) Impaired muscle glycogen synthase in type 2 diabetes is associated with diminished phosphatidylinositol 3-kinase activation *J Clin Endocrinol Metab* **86**, 4307–4314

Nyholm B, Qu Z, Kaal A, Pedersen SB, Gravholt CH, Andersen JL, Saltin B, Schmitz O (1997) Evidence of an increased number of type IIb muscle fibres in insulin-resistant first-degree relatives of patients with NIDDM *Diabetes* **46**, 1822–1828

Ortenblad N, Mogensen M, Petersen I, Højlund K, Levin K, Sahlin K, Beck-Nielsen H, Gaster M (2005) Reduced Insulin-mediated Citrate Synthase Activity in cultured Skeletal Muscle cells from patients with Type 2 Diabetes; Evidence for an intrinsic oxidative enzyme defect *Biochim Biophys Acta* **1741**, 206–214

Patti ME, Butte AJ, Crunkhorn S, Cusi K, Berria R, Kashyap S, Miyazaki Y, Kohane I, Costello M, Saccone R, Landaker EJ, Goldfine AB, Mun E, DeFronzo R, Finlayson J, Kahn CR, Mandarino LJ (2003) Coordinated reduction of genes of oxidative metabolism in humans with insulin resistance and diabetes, Potential role of PGC1 and NRF1 *Proc Natl Acad Sci USA* **100**, 8466–8471

Petersen KF, Dufour S, Befroy D, Garcia R, Shulman GI (2004) Impaired mitochondrial activity in the insulin–resistant offspring of patients with type 2 diabetes *N Engl J Med* **350**, 664–671

Petersen KF, Dufour S, Shulman GI (2005) Decreased insulin-stimulated ATP synthesis and phosphate transport in muscle of insulin-resistant offspring of type 2 diabetic parents *PLoS Med* **2**(233)

Pirola L, Johnston AM, Van Obberghen E (2004) Modulation of insulin action *Diabetologia* **47**, 170–184

Ritov VB, Menshikova EV, He J, Ferrell RE, Goodpaster BH, Kelley DE (2005) Deficiency of subsarcolemmal mitochondria in obesity and type 2 diabetes *Diabetes* **54**, 8–14

Sarabia V, Lam L, Burdett E, Leiter LA, Klip A (1992) Glucose transport in human skeletal muscle cells in culture Stimulation by insulin and metformin *J Clin Invest* **90**, 1386–1395

Schmitz-Peiffer C (2002) Protein kinase C and lipid-induced insulin resistance in skeletal muscle *Ann NY Acad Sci* **967**, 146–157

Shulman GI (2000) Cellular mechanisms of insulin resistance *J Clin Invest* **106**, 171–176

Shulman GI (2004) Unraveling the cellular mechanism of insulin resistance in humans, new insights from magnetic resonance spectroscopy *Physiology* (Bethesda) **19**, 183–190

Sreekumar R, Halvatsiotis P, Schimke JC, Nair KS (2002) Gene expression profile in skeletal muscle of type 2 diabetes and the effect of insulin treatment *Diabetes* **51**, 1913–1920

Vaag A, Alford F, Beck-Nielsen H (1996) Intracellular glucose and fat metabolism in identical twins discordant for non-insulin-dependent diabetes mellitus (NIDDM), acquired versus genetic metabolic defects? *Diabet Med* **13**, 806–815

Vaag A, Damsbo P, Hother-Nielsen O, Beck-Nielsen H (1992b) Hyperglycaemia compensates for the defects in insulin–mediated glucose metabolism and in the activation of glycogen synthase in the skeletal muscle of patients with type 2 (non-insulin-dependent) diabetes mellitus *Diabetologia* **35**, 80–88

Vaag A, Henriksen JE, Beck-Nielsen H (1992a) Decreased insulin activation of glycogen synthase in skeletal muscles in young nonobese Caucasian first-degree relatives of patients with non-insulin-dependent diabetes mellitus *J Clin Invest* **89**, 782–788

Vaag A, Skott P, Damsbo P, Gall MA, Richter EA, Beck-Nielsen H (1991) Effect of the antilipolytic nicotinic acid analogue acipimox on whole–body and skeletal muscle glucose metabolism in patients with non–insulin–dependent diabetes mellitus *J Clin Invest* **88**, 1282–1290

Virkamaki A, Korsheninnikova E, Seppala-Lindroos A, Vehkavaara S, Goto T, Halavaara J, Hakkinen AM, Yki-Jarvinen H (2001) Intramyocellular lipid is associated with resistance to in vivo insulin actions on glucose uptake, antilipolysis, and early insulin signaling pathways in human skeletal muscle *Diabetes* **50**, 2337–2343

Wells L, Vosseller K, Hart GW (2003) A role for N-acetylglucosamine as a nutrient sensor and mediator of insulin resistance *Cell Mol Life Sci* **60**, 222–228

Wojtaszewski JF, Hansen BF, Gade, Kiens B, Markuns JF, Goodyear LJ, Richter EA (2000) Insulin signaling and insulin sensitivity after exercise in human skeletal muscle *Diabetes* **49**, 325–331

Worm D, Vinten J, Staehr P, Henriksen JE, Handberg A, Beck-Nielsen H (1996) Altered basal and insulin–stimulated phosphotyrosine phosphatase (PTPase) activity in skeletal muscle from NIDDM patients compared with control subjects *Diabetologia* **39**, 1208–1214

Wright KS, Beck-Nielsen H, Kolterman OG, Mandarino LJ (1988) Decreased activation of skeletal muscle glycogen synthase by mixed-meal ingestion in NIDDM *Diabetes* **37**, 436–440

Yasin R, Van BG, Nurse KC, Al-Ani S, Landon DN, Thompson EJ (1977) A quantitative technique for growing human adult skeletal muscle in culture starting from mononucleated cells *J Neurol Sci* **32**, 347–360

Zierath JR, He L, Guma A, Odegoard Wahlstrom E, Klip A, Wallberg-Henriksson H (1996) Insulin action on glucose transport and plasma membrane GLUT4 content in skeletal muscle from patients with NIDDM *Diabetologia* **39**, 1180–1189

15

Assessment of Vascular Function

Johannes Pleiner and **Michael Wolzt**

Basic theoretical concepts

It is known that the majority of diabetes-related deaths arise from cardiovascular complications such as myocardial infarction, stroke and peripheral artery disease.

Over the past decade, the concept that chronic vascular injury precedes development of structural atherosclerosis has been widely accepted. It includes the idea that a subclinical injury to the vasculature starts the atherosclerotic process (Ross 1996). Briefly, the different progressive steps of atherosclerosis can be classified as follows:

Type I: vascular injury involving functional changes in the endothelium with minimal structural changes (i.e. increased lipoprotein permeability and white blood cell adhesion).

Type II: vascular injury involving endothelial disruption with minimal thrombosis.

Type III: vascular injury involving damage to media, which may stimulate severe thrombosis, results in unstable coronary syndromes.

In this concept, the initial step is considered dysfunction of the endothelium, the innermost layer of the vasculature, by local disturbances of blood flow, along with metabolic and humoral risk factors (e.g. hyperglycemia, dyslipidemia, cigarette smoking, inflammation). These alterations of the endothelium perpetuate a series of events that culminate in the development of an atherosclerotic plaque.

The vascular endothelium

It has been known since the early 1980s that the endothelium is more than a wall separating the blood vessel and the inside cavity. The human vascular endothelium covers almost $700\,m^2$ and weighs about 1.5 kg. Acting as a paracrine organ, the endothelium constitutively secretes various vasoactive agents in response to different stimuli. Healthy endothelium maintains vascular tone and structure by regulating the balance between vasodilation and vasoconstriction, growth inhibition and growth promotion, antithrombosis and prothrombosis, antiinflammation and proinflammation, and also antioxidation and prooxidation (Vanhoutte 1989).

Clinical Diabetes Research: Methods and Techniques   Edited by Michael Roden
© 2007 John Wiley & Sons, Ltd   ISBN 978-0-470-01728-9

Early endothelial damage, which precedes structural changes of the vasculature, can be demonstrated in individuals with dyslipidemia, hypertension, advanced age, nicotine exposure and type 1 and type 2 diabetes mellitus. Endothelial damage may cause changes that are localised or generalised and transient or persistent, as follows:

- Increased permeability to lipoproteins
- Decreased nitric oxide production
- Increased leukocyte migration and adhesion
- Prothrombotic dominance
- Vascular growth stimulation
- Vasoactive substance release

Endothelial dysfunction is considered to be the initial step that allows diffusion of lipids and inflammatory cells (monocytes, T lymphocytes) into the endothelial and subendothelial interstitium (Ross 1986). Secretion of cytokines and growth factors promotes intimal migration, smooth muscle cell proliferation and accumulation of collagen matrix and peripheral blood mononuclear cells, forming an atheroma and thus leading to thrombosis and the development of advanced cardiovascular disease.

Several studies have shown that endothelial damage can be reversed if the underlying cause is attenuated (Bonetti et al. 2003). Early diagnosis is therefore pivotal, and assessment of endothelial function of importance in patients at risk.

Several methods for assessing early vascular changes have been introduced in experimental clinical medicine. Most of these methods utilise the assumption that clinically relevant endothelial dysfunction is not only present in vessels at risk for atherosclerosis, but detectable systemically (Benjamin et al. 1995). Assessment of vascular function in selected vascular beds is therefore extrapolated to reflect a systemic phenomenon.

Below we will introduce several methods that can be used for measuring vascular function in patients with diabetes, as follows:

- Strain gauge plethysmography
- Flow mediated dilation (FMD) of the brachial artery
- Intima media thickness of the carotid artery
- Assessment of arterial stiffness

Strain gauge plethysmography

Strain gauge plethysmography has been developed since the early 1990s for assessment of endothelial function. Since the advent of mercury-in-rubber strain gauges, venous occlusion plethysmography has been easy to perform, and measurement of forearm blood flow (FBF) is now widely used to probe the mechanisms of human vascular control. The underlying principle of venous occlusion plethysmography is straightforward: if venous return from the arm is obstructed and arterial inflow continues unimpeded, the forearm swells at a rate proportional to the rate of arterial inflow. The approach allows for the study of human vascular physiology, pharmacology and pathophysiology, and has the advantage that vessels are studied in their physiological environment under the influence of neuronal, circulating and local humoral mediators. Measurement of FBF response to vasoactive agents using strain gauge plethysmography can be considered the gold standard for assessing endothelial function in resistance arteries.

Practical description

Normally mercury-filled silatic strain gauges are used, connected to a plethysmograph. The strain gauge is attached to the upper part of the forearm and inflatable cuffs are placed on the upper arm and the wrist. The distance of the strain gauge from the elbow should be recorded if measurements are repeated at different time points. The forearm should be placed above the right atrium to allow venous emptying between measurement cycles. With the forearm placed above the level of the right atrium, rapid inflation of the upper arm venous occlusion cuff for 7–10 seconds to a supravenous pressure (40–50 mmHg) at every 15–30 seconds causes a linear increase in forearm volume, and the deflation period is usually long enough to allow emptying of the forearm veins before the next measurement is made. However, at high flow rates, it may be necessary to decrease the duration of the inflation period and increase the duration of the deflation period, to ensure adequate venous emptying and avoid a rise in venous pressure to 40 mmHg. When the upper arm congesting cuff is inflated, the FBF output signal is transmitted to a computer and traces are analysed by software. FBF is expressed as ml per minute per 100 ml of forearm tissue volume. Recordings spanning usually 4–10 cycles are averaged for analysis of FBF at baseline and during administration of drugs. Forearm vascular resistance is calculated as the mean arterial pressure divided by FBF.

Venous occlusion plethysmography measures total forearm blood flow, of which, under resting conditions, blood flow through skeletal muscle is the bulk (50 % to 70 % of total), the remainder being flow through skin (Barcroft 1943). The hands should therefore be excluded from circulation, as blood flow in the hand is predominantly through skin and there is a high proportion of arteriovenous shunts; hand blood flow has different pharmacology and physiology from forearm blood flow (Benjamin et al. 1995). A wrist cuff is consequently inflated to a pressure of 50 mmHg above systolic blood pressure, to exclude hand circulation from the measurements, at one minute before and throughout the measurement of FBF.

When FBF measurements are performed, subjects should be in fasting condition to prevent any dietary confounders. Fatty meals, for instance, were shown to impair endothelial function acutely (Steer et al. 2003). Subjects should be in supine position in a quiet, temperature-controlled room throughout the study. After 30 minutes of acclimatisation in supine position, stable conditions are generally established for FBF measurements.

The effects of vasoactive agents such as endothelium-dependent vasodilators acetylcholine, metacholine, bradykinin or histamine, and endothelium-independent vasodilators glycerol trinitrate, sodium nitroprusside or isosorbide dinitrate, on forearm haemodynamic responses can be assessed. To this end, a fine 27–30 gauge needle is inserted into the brachial artery of the non-dominant arm for infusion of vasoactive agents. Alternatively, a 23 gauge polyethylene catheter can be used, which allows recording of arterial pressure. Vasoactive drugs are infused intra-arterially for 3–5 minutes at escalating dosages, using a constant rate infusion pump. An appropriate washout period of at least 10 minutes between the infusion of vasoactive drugs should be considered to allow forearm blood flow to return to baseline. An example for an experimental arrangement for FBF measurements is given in Figure 15.1.

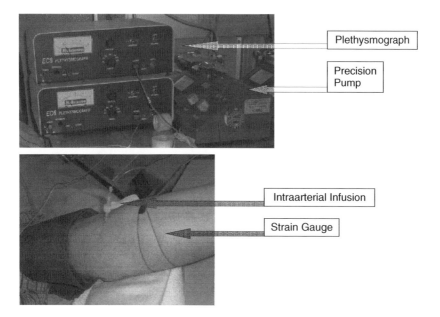

Figure 15.1 FBF measurements.

Acetylcholine is the most commonly used vasodilator for assessing endothelium-dependent vasodilation. It is believed that the vasodilatory effect of acetylcholine is to bind to the muscarine receptor and activate endothelial NO-synthase, resulting in vascular relaxation. Although acetylcholine-induced vasodilation is mainly caused by endothelial cell NO release, potassium-ATP channels also play a role in acetylcholine induced vasodilation (Higashi & Yoshizumi 2003).

The use of a nitric oxide (NO) synthase inhibitor, like N^G-monomethyl-$_L$-arginine (L-NMMA) or N^G-nitro-$_L$-arginine-methyl-ester (L-NAME) is useful for confirming the role of basal and stimulated NO release. After the administration of L-NMMA, the effect of endothelium-dependent vasodilation is inhibited for up to four hours in the peripheral circulation.

Confounding factors such as small alterations in blood pressure or sympathetic arousal can be compensated for by measuring FBF simultaneously in both arms (Benjamin et al. 1995). In the absence of intervention, the ratio of flow in the two arms is stable and stays constant even if blood flow alters markedly in response to changes in systemic arterial pressure or sympathetic arousal. If a physiological or pharmacological intervention is made in one arm only, any change in the ratio of blood flow between the two arms is a direct reflection of change in local vascular tone in the test arm. Expressing results in terms of the ratio of blood flow in the two arms provides an internal control, uses all the available data, minimises variation and gives consistent and reproducible results (Figure 15.2).

Major data and relevance to better understanding of diabetes

Endothelial dysfunction, evidenced by strain gauge plethysmography, has been described since the early 1990s in patients with diabetes. McVeigh et al. (1992) showed that endothelium dependent and independent vasodilation was attenuated in 29 patients with

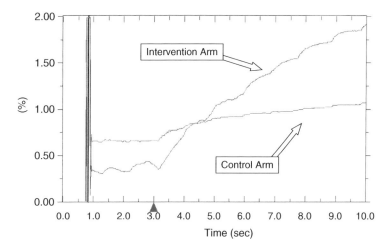

Figure 15.2   FBF responses to acetylcholine in the intervention arm, compared to FBF in a non-infused control arm.

non-insulin dependent diabetes mellitus. An impairment of endothelium dependent vasodilation was also detected in patients with type 1 diabetes (Johnstone et al. 1993). These studies were followed by numerous experiments focusing on possible treatment options for endothelium dysfunction in patients with diabetes.

As an example, forearm blood flow studies have helped to identify oxidative stress as one of the key factors in the development of vascular damage in diabetes. The generation of reactive oxygen species in diabetes occurs via several mechanisms and is initiated not only by glucose, but also by other substances that are found at elevated levels in diabetic patients. The resulting oxidative stress leads to a number of proatherogenic events (Jay et al. 2006).

Although there is no direct method available for assessing oxidative stress in humans, most studies utilised vitamin C, as a scavenger of free oxygen radicals, to assess the bioactivity of endogenous free oxygen radicals in biological systems (Jackson et al. 1998). In clinical studies, vitamin C increased endothelium-dependent dilatation in patients with insulin dependent (Timimi et al. 1998) and independent (Ting et al. 1997) diabetes mellitus.

In contrast to these studies, where vitamin C was given in high intra-arterial doses, oral vitamin C was not shown to reverse endothelial dysfunction in patients with diabetes (Chen et al. 2006).

However, as forearm blood flow studies are technically very elaborate to perform and significant changes can be seen in a small number of patients, no large scale trials have been performed and the prognostic value is not established.

Advantages and limitations

As already mentioned above, the response to intraarterial infusion of vasoactive substances is considered the gold standard in assessing endothelial function. The technique is reproducible and can detect small alterations in endothelial function. However, the invasive method is time consuming and burdensome for the subjects under study. Puncture of the brachial artery might be uncomfortable and carries the risk of arterial occlusion, bleeding or infection. Although no severe side effects, especially if using thin (27 G) needles, are reported in the literature, these drawbacks should always be considered before initiating a study.

As an alternative, the noninvasive method of measuring reactive hyperaemia with strain gauge plethysmography may be considered, as it does not cause any of the adverse effects of artery puncture. To obtain reactive hyperaemia, FBF is occluded by inflating of the cuff on the upper arm to suprasystolic pressures (usually >200 mmHg) for five minutes. After release of the ischemic occlusion, FBF is measured for 180 seconds. Nitroglycerine is administered sublingually to assess endothelium-independent vasodilation and FBF is measured for 300 seconds. Peak FBF response following ischemia strongly correlates with the FBF response to acetylcholine (Higashi & Yoshizumi 2003).

Practical example

The following example shows a typical measurement of FBF in response to the endothelium-dependent vasodilator acetylcholine and the endothelium-independent glyceroltrinitrate. The example given is taken from a protocol in which FBF was assessed in healthy volunteers (Pleiner et al. 2002) (Figure 15.3). A brief summary of advantages and disadvantages of this method is given in Table 15.1.

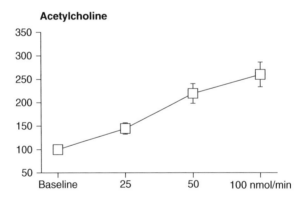

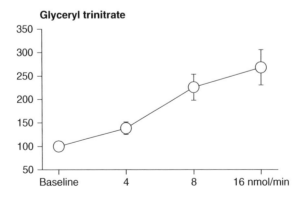

Figure 15.3 FBF responses to increasing doses of acetylcholine and glyceryltrinitrate in healthy volunteers ($n = 8$). Data presented as (100) change over baseline (100), as mean and SEM.

Table 15.1 Summary Box with Key Points

+	Strain gauge plethysmography is considered the gold standard for assessing endothelial function
+	Enables identification of early functional alterations, employing pharmacological model drugs
+	Well established in patients with diabetes
+	Differences between (treatment) groups can be achieved with a relatively small sample size
+	Observer independent measurement with 'off-line' analysis
−	Technicaly elaborate; special, relatively expensive devices are necessary
−	Demanding for patients; possible adverse effects of arterial puncture

A fine-bore needle (27 G needle Sterican; B. Braun, Melsungen, Germany) was inserted into the brachial artery of the non-dominant arm for the administration of vasodilators. After a 20 min resting period, in which physiological saline solution was infused to avoid clotting, baseline forearm blood flow was measured in response to the endothelium-dependent dilator, acetylcholine (ACh; 25, 50 and 100 nmol/min; each dose for three minutes; Clinalfa, Läufelfingen, Switzerland). After a 15 minute washout period to allow restoration of control blood flow, forearm blood flow was measured in response to the endothelium-independent dilator glyceryltrinitrate (GTN; 4, 8 and 16 nmol/min; each dose for three minutes; G. Pohl Boskamp GmbH, Hohenlockstedt, Germany). Forearm blood flow measurements were measured as ml/min/100 ml forearm volume and expressed as percentage change from baseline ratio. The effects of ACh and GTN were assessed by analysis of variance for repeated measurements (ANOVA) using the Statistica® software package (Release 4.5, StatSoft Inc., Tulsa, OK, USA).

Flow Mediated Dilation (FMD) of the brachial artery

As an alternative to invasive forearm blood flow measurements with strain gauge plethysmography and intra-arterial infusions of vasoactive agents, endothelial function can be assessed noninvasively by flow-mediated vasodilation (FMD) of the brachial artery. This method was first described by Celermajer et al. (1992).

Practical description

This method is based on the capacity of blood vessels to self-regulate tone and blood flow in response to changes in the local environment. Many blood vessels respond to an increase in flow, and therefore shear stress, by dilating. This phenomenon is called FMD.

Although the precise mechanisms for the vasculatures' ability to detect shear stress and subsequently modulate vascular tone are not fully understood, endothelium derived NO seems to be one of the principal mediators. Endothelial cells contains ion channels, such as calcium-activated potassium channels, that open in response to shear stress (Cooke et al. 1991; Miura et al. 2001). Open potassium channels hyperpolarise the endothelial cell and increase the driving force for calcium entry. Calcium activates endothelial nitric oxide synthase (eNOS). The subsequent generation of NO appears to account for FMD (Joannides et al. 1995). Indeed, removal of the endothelium or treatment with an (e)NOS inhibitor abolishes FMD. However, other factors like endothelium derived prostanoid formation are also able to act as a signal between endothelium and underlying smooth muscle and therefore mediate FMD (Sun et al. 1999).

Numerous factors affect FMD, including temperature, food, drugs and sympathetic stimuli. Therefore, subjects should fast for at least 8–12 h before the study. High-fat foods especially are known to ameliorate FMD. Subjects should be studied in a quiet, temperature-controlled room. If possible, all vasoactive medications should be withheld for at least four half lives. In addition, subjects should not exercise, should not ingest substances that might affect FMD such as caffeine and antioxidative substances (e.g. Vitamin C) and should not use tobacco for at least 4–6 h before the study. With female subjects, the investigator should be aware of the phase of the menstrual cycle, as it may affect FMD (Hashimoto et al. 1995). As usual, all possible confounding factors must be considered in studies that seek to determine the impact of a single intervention.

In most cases, FMD is measured in the brachial artery, although other sites such as the radial, axillary and femoral arteries might be considered. According to the International Brachial Artery Reactivity Task Force, an ultrasound system equipped with a high-frequency vascular transducer (minimum 7 Mhz), colour and spectral Doppler and an internal electro-cardiogram is required to obtain images with sufficient resolution for subsequent analysis (Corretti et al. 2002).

The subject should be supine, with the arm in a comfortable position for imaging the brachial artery. The brachial artery should be imaged distal of the antecubital fossa in the longitudinal plane. A segment with clear anterior and posterior intimal interfaces between the lumen and vessel wall is selected (Figure 15.4). Continuous 2D grey-scale imaging is prefered, although M and A mode (wall tracking) can be used to measure diameter (Stadler et al. 1997). Anatomical landmarks such as veins and fascial planes can serve as markers to maintain the image of the artery throughout the study. Alternatively, a probe-holding device can be helpful. Timing of image acquisition with respect to the cardiac cycle is determined with simultaneous ECG recording. Peak systolic diameter is larger than end systolic diameter, because the vessel expands during systole to accommodate the increase in

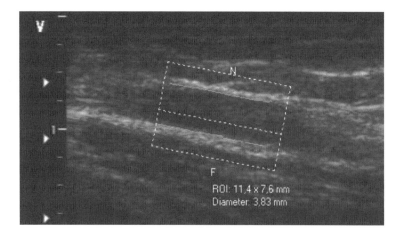

Figure 15.4 Segment of the brachial artery for FMD measurements using a wall tracking system.

pressure and volume. Brachial artery diameter should therefore always be measured at the same point in the cardiac cycle, ideally by ECG gating.

A blood pressure cuff is placed above the antecubital fossa to create a flow stimulus in the brachial artery. The cuff could also be placed on the forearm. However, the change in diameter is smaller with wrist cuff ischaemia than with that produced by placing the cuff on the upper arm. Baseline images are acquired and blood flow is measured. Thereafter, arterial occlusion is created by inflating the cuff to at least 50 mmHg above systolic pressure to occlude arterial inflow. Typically, four to five minutes of occlusion are used, since the change in brachial artery diameter after cuff release increases over 0.5–5 min of cuff inflation, but remains similar after 10 min. Subsequent cuff deflation induces a brief high-flow state through the brachial artery (reactive hyperaemia), resulting in increased shear stress and dilation of the brachial artery. FMD is expressed as percentage change of basal vessel diameter. Images should be acquired from 30 seconds before to two minutes after cuff deflation. Blood flow with the midartery Doppler signal should be measured immediately after cuff release.

At least 10 minutes of rest are needed after measurement of FMD to reestablish baseline conditions. Thereafter, endothelium-independent vasodilation reflecting vascular smooth muscle function should be assessed. Application of an exogenous NO donor, such as a single high dose of nitroglycerine (0.4–0.8 mg spray or sublingual tablet), causes maximum obtainable vasodilator response (Stadler et al. 1997). Continuous image acquisition should be performed three to four minutes after nitroglycerine administration, reflecting peak vasodilation. Caution is needed when administering nitroglycerine to patients with bradycardia or hypotension.

Major data and relevance to better understanding of diabetes and metabolism

Several studies in diabetic patients revealed the effects of lifestyle modification or physical exercise on endothelial function.

In insulin-resistant subjects, lifestyle modification with exercise and weight reduction over six months improved endothelial function (Hamdy et al. 2003). Interestingly, the relationship between percentage weight reduction and improved FMD was linear. A similar result was seen in patients with type 2 diabetes (Maiorana et al. 2001). Likewise, in patients with type 1 diabetes, FMD could be improved by four months of bicycle exercise (Fuchsjager-Mayrl et al. 2002). However, the positive training effect on endothelial function was not maintained after cessation of regular exercise (Figure 15.5). In all studies, GTN-mediated dilation was unaffected by exercise.

Another interesting study assessing FMD in 75 children with type 1 diabetes revealed that even children with diabetes have impaired endothelial function compared to healthy controls (Jarvisalo et al. 2004).

As this method is also predominantly assessing endothelial function, the relevance of data generated is comparable to vascular function testing with strain gauge plethysmography, with the limitation that vascular responses cannot be tested in response to vasoactive agents.

On the other hand, the non-invasive and less time consuming nature of this method makes it easier to perform studies in larger cohorts.

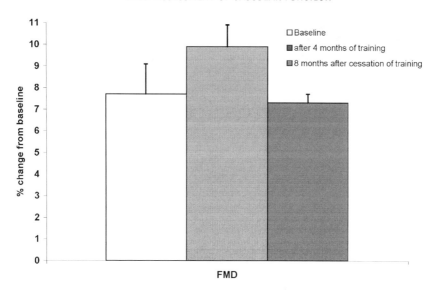

Figure 15.5 Flow mediated dilation in percentage change from baseline in type 1 diabetes patients before, during and after physical exercise training.

Advantages and limitations of the method

Measurement of FMD is a generally available non-invasive tool for assessing endothelial function. Early vascular impairment can be detected and the technique is able to detect results from short-term interventions.

However, despite its relatively simple appearance, ultrasonographic assessment of FMD is technically challenging. The technique has a significant learning curve. Ideally, an observer should be trained in the principles and technical aspects of 2D and Doppler ultrasonography. Several months of training, depending on the frequency with which the technique is performed, are necessary. Thorough training helps to establish high quality and consistency in the method and in the data generated. The International Brachial Artery Reactivity Task Force recommend at least 100 supervised scans and measurements be performed before independent scanning and reading are attempted (Corretti et al. 2002). 100 scans per year should be performed to maintain competency. Intraobserver and interobserver variability should be established periodically.

Expensive and specialised ultrasound equipment is necessary to perform technically sound FMD measurements. This might be a problem in small centres.

Placement of the cuff and ultrasound probe might become a problem in small subjects, children or obese patients, which could strongly influence the quality of the measurements. In addition, correct and stable placement of the ultrasound probe, if possible with a probe holding device, is very important.

Due to the observer-dependent nature of the technique and several other confounding factors, the sample size needed to observe significant changes in FMD is relatively high compared to that in invasive measurement of forearm blood flow. Approximately 20 subjects in a crossover design and 40 in a parallel-group design are recommended as a minimum requirement for detecting meaningful FMD changes. A brief summary of advantages and disadvantages of this method is given Table 15.2.

Table 15.2 Summary Box with Key Points

+	Noninvasive alternative to strain gauge plethysmography
+	Can be introduced in standard sonography labs
+	Generally applicable
+	No additional devices besides a high resolution ultrasound
−	Larger sample sizes needed
−	Observer dependent technique with limited reproducibility
−	Limited information on mechanism of functional changes
−	Expensive ultrasound equipment needed

Practical example for performance of the technique or for calculation of data

The most important thing to consider when measuring FMD is the quality of ultrasound images. Accurate detection and analysis of artery diameter is a prerequisite for obtaining reliable and reproducible results. Edge detecting software, such as the brachial analyser (Medical Imaging Applications LLC, Coralville, IA, USA), is a very helpful tool for improving the quality of FMD measurements.

The diameter of the brachial artery should be measured from longitudinal images in which the lumen-intima interface is visualised on the near and far walls. These boundaries are best seen when the angle of the ultrasound probe is perpendicular. Once the image for analysis is chosen, the boundaries for diameter measurements (lumen-intima or media-adventitia) are identified manually or by the edge detection software. Variability of readings can be decreased by determination of the diameter along a segment of the vessel, or by less robust manual point-to-point measurement of a single frame.

Maximal increase in brachial artery diameter occurs approximately 45–60 seconds after cuff release (Corretti et al. 1995). FMD is typically expressed as the percentage change in artery diameter from baseline (Corretti et al. 2002). However, percentage change might be influenced by baseline diameter, as smaller arteries tend to dilate relatively more than larger arteries. Absolute and percentage change in diameter should therefore both be reported.

Intima media thickness of the carotid artery

Measuring intima media thickness (IMT), mostly of the carotid artery, utilises the fact that early morphological abnormalities of arterial walls can be imaged by ultrasonography. This high-resolution, noninvasive technique has been introduced for detection of early stages of atherosclerotic disease because it demonstrates the wall structure with better resolution than currently available magnetic resonance angiography or conventional angiography. Increased IMT of the carotid artery is considered a surrogate marker of atherosclerosis (Grobbee & Bots 1994). IMT has repeatedly been shown to predict the occurrence of cardiovascular events such as stroke and myocardial infarction (Bots et al. 1997; O'Leary et al. 1999). Carotid IMT is significantly greater in patients with diabetes than in nondiabetic subjects, and baseline carotid IMT predicted the incidence of cardiovascular events in type 2 diabetic subjects (Yamasaki et al. 2000; Bernard et al. 2005). The pathophysiological concept behind IMT is that intimal thickening at the carotid artery may be an early stage of atherosclerotic disease in conduit arteries, representing macroangiopathy. The intimal thickening itself cannot be measured *in vivo* non-invasively, but the intima media complex can be measured by ultrasound.

Practical description of techniques and methods

In the absence of atherosclerotic plaque, B-mode ultrasound displays the vascular wall as a regular pattern that correlates with anatomical layers. The intima media portion of this pattern is represented by the area of tissue starting at the luminal edge of the artery and ending at the boundary between the media and the adventitia. This interface is well depicted by high resolution ultrasound.

However, increased IMT can be due to intimal and/or muscular thickening. In contrast to the more peripheral muscular arteries, the carotid artery is an elastic artery and the muscular media is relatively small. Therefore, increased carotid IMT is considered to represent mainly endothelial thickening (Grobbee & Bots 1994), which is assumed to explain the observed association between increased carotid IMT and cardiovascular events.

Measurement of IMT is most easily performed in a region free of plaque where the double-line pattern is observed – this is advantageous as measurements are more accurate, reproducible and can be standardised by computer analyses. IMT should be measured in the common carotid artery, at the bulb or the origin of the internal carotid artery.

When assessing IMT of the carotid artery, one should keep in mind that IMT is not constant. It continuously changes during the heart cycle. It decreases during systole, due to the larger vessel diameter, and increases during diastole. Although measurement of IMT at a fixed timepoint during the cardiac cycle will decrease variability between data, the maximal error due to IMT changes during the cardiac cycle is estimated to be 3.8 % and the difference between diastolic and mean IMT is 1.3 % (Van Bortel 2005). Therefore, IMT variation during the cardiac cycle is present but small and often negligible.

Major data relevance to better understanding of diabetes and metabolism

One of the advantages of IMT measurements is that they can be performed quickly and easily by an experienced observer. Thus, large trials can be performed. IMT measurements are suitable for assessing the incidence of early stages of atherosclerosis in patients with diabetes.

In a large trial in 5,858 subjects of 65 years or older without cardiovascular disease, IMT was used to assess cardiovascular risk (O'Leary et al. 1999). Cardiovascular events (new myocardial infarction or stroke) were defined as outcome variables and patients were observed over a median follow-up period of over six years. There was a positive association between carotid-artery intima media thickness and the incidence of new myocardial infarction and stroke in adults of 65 years or older who did not have a history of cardiovascular disease. The relative risk of myocardial infarction or stroke for the quintile with the highest IMT as compared with the quintile with the lowest IMT was 3.87 (95 % CI 2.72–5.51) (Figure 15.6). It was shown that IMT is a strong predictor of both myocardial infarction and stroke and that the risk gradients are similar. Even after statistical adjustment was made for traditional cardiovascular risk factors, carotid artery IMT remained a significant predictor

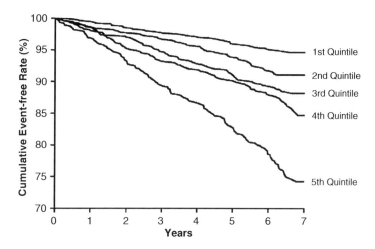

Figure 15.6 Unadjusted cumulative event-free rates for the combined end point of myocardial infarction or stroke, according to quintile of combined intima media thickness.

of cardiovascular events. The strength of the associations between IMT and outcome was at least the same as for the associations seen with traditional risk factors.

Accordingly, in a smaller study including 229 patients with type 2 diabetes, IMT was shown to be an independent predictor of cardiovascular events (Bernard et al. 2005). The odds ratio for cardiovascular events per SD increase in carotid IMT was 1.63 (95 % CI 1.01–2.63).

In contrast to the methods that estimate endothelial function, described above, IMT assesses a more advanced stage of atherosclerosis, in which structural changes of the vascular wall are already demonstrable. Nevertheless, therapeutic intervention studies have shown that enhanced IMT is at least partially reversible in patients with diabetes.

An example for such an intervention study is that by Langenfeld et al. (2005) in patients with type 2 diabetes. The effects of the insulin sensitiser pioglitazone (45 mg/d) were compared to glimepiride for 24 weeks on metabolic control (HbA1c) and carotid IMT in a randomised controlled study in 173 patients with type 2 diabetes. Despite similar improvements in HbA1c after 24 weeks, carotid IMT was significantly reduced only in the pioglitazone group. Reduction of IMT was independent of improvement in glycaemic control.

Advantages and limitations of the method

Provided that a high resolution ultrasound system is available, measurement of IMT is applicable in most patients, readily available, and demonstrates the wall structure with good resolution and quality. However, some issues arise when assessing IMT.

Most importantly, increased IMT reflects early, already visible atherosclerosis. In contrast to FBF and FMD, where functional alterations of the vessel wall are assessed, measurement of IMT only detects a more advanced stage of vascular impairment, namely morphological change. It is therefore unlikely that short term intervention leads to significant changes in IMT.

Although ultrasonographic assessment of IMT is easier than measurement of FMD, it is still an observer dependent technique. Therefore training is necessary and intraobserver and interobserver variability should be established periodically.

There are no generally accepted criteria for distinguishing atherosclerosis as seen in early plaque formation from thickening of the intima media complex. This is because IMT reflects not only early atherosclerosis, but also nonatherosclerotic intimal reactions such as intimal hyperplasia and intimal fibrocellular hypertrophy. Is, therefore, every intima media thickening a marker of atherosclerosis? The process of intima media thickening is complex. Intima media thickening can be reactive to a higher blood pressure and changes in shear stress pattern. The latter explains the prominent IMT changes at the carotid bifurcation where turbulent blood flow occurs. Reactive changes are not a marker of early atherosclerosis per se. The Rotterdam study supports the view that, at lower degrees of IMT, thickening reflects an equilibrium state in which the effects of pressure and flow on the arteries are in balance, given the characteristic relationship between shear stress and local transmural pressure (Bots et al. 1997). Beyond a certain level, IMT more likely represents atherosclerosis.

The Mannheim Intima Media Thickness Consensus recommends the following definitions for ultrasound characterisation of IMT and atherosclerotic plaque (Touboul et al. 2004):

- IMT is a double-line pattern visualised by echotomography on both walls of the common carotid arteries in a longitudinal image. It is formed by two parallel lines, which consist of the leading edges of two anatomical boundaries: the lumen-intima and media-adventitia interfaces.

- Plaque is a focal structure encroaching into the arterial lumen of at least 0.5 mm or 50 % of the surrounding IMT value, or demonstrates a thickness of 1.5 mm as measured from the media-adventitia interface to the intima-lumen interface.

- These definitions will allow classification of the great majority of the carotid lesions observed with ultrasound.

Practical example for performance of the technique or for calculation of data

The equipment necessary for IMT assessment includes a high-resolution ultrasound system with preferentially linear ultrasound transducers at frequencies above 7 MHz. Appropriate depth of focus (e.g. 30–40 mm), frame rate (> 15 Hz) and gain settings (minimal intraluminal artifacts) are recommended to obtain the best image quality. The arterial wall segments should be assessed in a longitudinal view, perpendicular to the ultrasound beam, with both walls clearly visualised in order to achieve diameter measurements. IMT measurements obtained from the far wall should be prefered, because measurements at the near wall are performed at the trailing edge of the ultrasound pulse (Van Bortel et al. 2001). As a result, these measurements are highly influenced by the gain settings and resolution characteristics of the ultrasound device. The near wall may represent only 80 % of the histological thickness, possibly leading to IMT values underestimating true IMT, making any comparison with studies using only far wall measurements less appropriate.

A minimum of 10 mm length of an arterial segment is required for reproducible measurements. Edge detection systems, like the Carotid analyser (Medical Imaging Applications LLC, Coralville, IA, USA), that are properly calibrated, provide more accurate measurements of IMT (Figure 15.7). Observations made by hand need to be controlled and are time

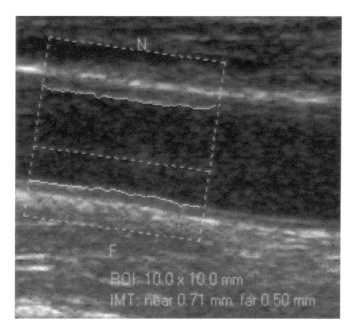

Figure 15.7 Measurement of IMT with edge detection software (Carotid analyser).

Table 15.3 Summary Box with Key Points

+ Measurements can be performed quickly by an experienced investigator
+ Available in standard sonography labs
+ Suitable for large clinical/epidemiology trials
− Changes in IMT reflect a more advanced step in atherosclerosis compared to endothelial function measurments
− Observer dependent; experienced investigator necessary
− Short term intervention studies are not likely to affect IMT
− Expensive ultrasound equipment required

consuming compared to automated systems, which can provide the mean maximal value of 150 measurements performed on 10 mm of common carotid artery in a very short time (<0.1 s). Interadventitial and lumen diameter measurements must be obtained as IMT is significantly correlated with the arterial diameter. A brief summary of advantages and disadvantages of this method is given in Table 15.3.

Assessment of arterial stiffness

Although the concept of arterial stiffness goes back to the 1880s (Roy 1880), it was only in recent years that attention was drawn to precise measurement of arterial stiffness (O'Rourke et al. 2002). Superficially the assessment of arterial stiffness seems simple, but actually the issue is rather complex.

The shape of the arterial pressure waveform provides an estimate of arterial stiffness and can be assessed noninvasively by using the technique of pulse-wave (contour) analysis (PWA). Simplified, the arterial system is like a tube, with one end representing the peripheral resistance and the other end receiving blood in spurts from the heart. A wave generated by cardiac activity travels along the tube toward the periphery and is reflected back from the periphery. The pressure wave at any point along the tube is a result of incident and reflected wave. When the tube is distensible, as in youth, the wave velocity is slow, therefore reflection returns late to the heart, in diastole. When the tube wall is stiffened, as in the elderly, wave travel is fast, and the reflected wave merges with the systolic part of the incident wave, causing a high pressure in systole and corresponding low pressure in diastole throughout the tube (Figure 15.8).

Arterial stiffness depends on vascular smooth muscle tone and the structure of the vessel wall. In addition, arterial stiffness depends on arterial pressure. A higher arterial pressure will increase arterial stiffness (Laurent et al. 1993). Arterial stiffness is also inversely related to arterial distensibility (D). Arterial distensibility and arterial volume (V) are related to arterial compliance (C) by the formula $C = D \cdot V$. Compliance (C) is defined as the change in volume (DV) for a given change in pressure (DP) i.e. C=DV/DP.

Within the arterial circulation, compliance relates to the changes in vessel diameter following left ventricular ejection, while distensibility is used to express compliance relative to the initial volume or diameter of a vessel. A loss of arterial elasticity leads to reduced arterial compliance and distensibility, which decreases non-linearly with increasing pressure, i.e. the pressure-volume (diameter) curve is nonlinear. Thus, as pressure increases, a transition point is eventually reached, with less distensibility occurring at higher pressures. This is the consequence of physical properties of the arterial media, which contains smooth muscle cells, elastin and collagen. The elastin fibres assume tension at low pressures, whereas tension is absorbed at higher pressures the by the more rigid collagen fibres and compliance consequently decreases. Changes in arterial compliance following intervention studies are therefore adjusted for changes in blood pressure. This can be achieved by a higher ventricular ejection, an increased heart rate, a higher vascular resistance, and by early wave reflections (Mangoni et al. 1996). As a consequence, *in vivo* arterial stiffness is not a static but a dynamic property. This means that standardisation of measurement conditions is

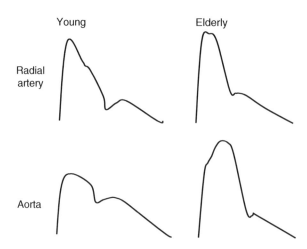

Figure 15.8 Schematic pulse waves of the aorta and the radial artery of a young and elderly person.

imperative. In addition, apart from the elastic properties obtained at the operating pressure, assessment of elastic properties under isobaric conditions may be important.

Practical description of techniques and methods

In general three types of arterial stiffness can be considered: systemic, regional or segmental, and local, which can be measured by different devices.

Systemic arterial stiffness

In the past, the ratio of pulse pressure (PP) and stroke volume has been used as a measure of systemic arterial stiffness. However, this method is considered a very crude approximation.

Pulse wave analysis can be performed with an applanation tonometer (Liang et al. 1998) or more advanced semiautomated devices (McVeigh et al. 1999). They make use of an arterial pressure sensor to provide an arterial pressure waveform at the radial artery, which is calibrated by an oscillometric upper arm BP measurement. The device analyses the pulse contour and aims to calculate large and small artery elasticity index independently. These data are calculated by an algorithm.

An optimal pressure wave signal is important as the amplitude of the pressure wave is critical to the analysis. This procedure can be facilitated by a dedicated wrist stabiliser.

Regional or segmental arterial stiffness

Regional arterial stiffness is measured indirectly by measuring pulse wave velocity over the arterial segment. Pulse wave velocity can be measured by various commercial and customised devices. All devices can measure PWV in different arterial segments. Pulse wave velocity is calculated by the formula: PWV = distance (m)/transit time (sec).

The accuracy of the method is expected to be better with a longer distance. Distance is usually measured with a tape measure. Distance can be estimated with acceptable accuracy by direct superficial measurement between the centres of the two pressure transducers in the cases of relatively straight arterial segments like the brachial radial segment. If arterial segments are not straight, measurement of the distance may be a weak point. This is for instance the case for the carotid femoral PWV measurement, an estimate of stiffness of mainly the aortic tract. Transit times are measured as the time delay between the feet of the recorded proximal and distal waves.

Some devices measure the time delay between the two ends of the arterial segment beat to beat, others measure the time between the R-wave of the electrocardiogram and the feet of the pressure and distension wave, respectively, at the site of measurement (Van Bortel et al. 2002). By measuring consecutively the two ends of the arterial segment under study, the transit time can be calculated, and PWV calculated manually. It is likely that simultaneous measurement on the two sites is more precise than consecutive measurement.

Local arterial stiffness

Local arterial stiffness of superficial arteries is measured using echo-tracking techniques. In addition, some researchers measure local arterial stiffness of deep arteries like the aorta using cine magnetic resonance imaging (MRI).

Local arterial compliance is expressed as compliance coefficient (CC) and is defined as the compliance per unit of length (L), which is the change in cross-sectional area (ΔA) per unit of pressure (ΔP). Likewise, local arterial distensibility is expressed as distensibility coefficient (DC), defined as the relative change in cross-sectional area ($\Delta A/A$) of the vessel per unit of pressure. PP is calculated as SBP – DBP. ΔP during the heart cycle equals PP.

From diameter (d), change in diameter during the heart cycle (distension, Δd) and ΔP, artery wall properties are calculated using the following equations (van der Heijden-Spek et al. 2000): $DC = (\Delta A/A)/\Delta P = (2\Delta d.d + \Delta d^2)/(\Delta P \cdot d^2)$ and $CC = (\Delta V/L)/\Delta P = \Delta A/\Delta P = \pi (2d \cdot \Delta d + \Delta d^2)/4\Delta P$, where V is arterial volume.

A major source of error with this method may be the accurate assessment of local PP. The PP should be measured at the site of the distension measurements. For the assessment of local PP, applanation tonometry has been proposed. Applanation tonometry allows noninvasive recording of the arterial pressure waveform and magnitude in both central and peripheral arteries (Benetos et al. 1993). Applanation tonometry requires a stiff or bony structure to flatten but not obstruct the artery wall and a lean skin to avoid cushioning of the pressure pulse. Applanation tonometry is a hand-held procedure at all arterial sites except for the radial artery, where a wristband can be used. In general, the signal showing the largest amplitude of the pressure waveform is the most reliable record, but it has been shown that overestimation of the PP is also possible.

Applanation tonometry cannot be applied to all subjects or at all arterial sites. In obese subjects for instance, applanation tonometry is often inaccurate at a majority of arterial sites. In lean subjects, good waveforms can easily be obtained at the radial artery, but in a substantial number of subjects applanation tonometry is not reliable at the femoral artery. In addition, in patients with atherosclerotic plaques or calcified arteries, this method may not be free from risk.

As the amplitude of the distension wave is critical, investigators have to be well trained. The most important aspects of training are the proper positioning of the probe perpendicular to the artery and the placement of the calipers with respect to the lumen wall boundaries. Placement of the calipers on the adventitia results in an overestimation of diameter and underestimation of distension.

Cine magnetic resonance imaging has been proposed by some investigators for measuring local arterial compliance (Resnick et al. 1997). It could be complementary to other devices because cine MRI can measure diameter and distension of deeper arteries like the aorta. However, accuracy of distension measurements should be improved and the problem of noninvasive assessment of local PP of the artery has not yet been resolved.

Major data or studies where the method was used successfully

The majority of clinical trials assessing arterial stiffness were focused on patients with hypertension. Although patients with diabetes often also suffer from hypertension, specific data for diabetic subjects is scarce.

Nevertheless, increased arterial stiffening has been demonstrated consistently in both type 1 and type 2 diabetes in a number of studies (Woodman & Watts 2003). Again, these data reflect a composite of functional and structural abnormalities of the vascular system.

Advantages and limitations of the method

While measurements of arterial stiffness are useful in large-scale studies, they are either limited or not practical for the clinical setting of small scale trials. Many different devices estimate arterial stiffness via various methods and various indices, which makes it almost impossible to compare the results of studies. In addition, inter-subject variation is often relatively small even between diseased states and healthy subjects and may therefore not be apparent except for with large-scale trials.

Some devices require considerable training before adequate measurements can be performed.

Practical example for performance of the technique or for calculation of data

There is a large variety of devices and methods available for the assessment of arterial stiffness and pulse wave analysis, with different device-specific procedures. General recommendations for the assessment of arterial stiffness are given by The Arterial Stiffness: Task Force III (Van Bortel et al. 2002).

To limit possible errors in measurement due to temporary changes in subject conditions or technical errors, at least two consecutive measurements should be performed. If the second varies much from the first, a third measurement is advised. To limit interobserver variation in measurements, these are preferably made by one observer, especially in studies with repeated measures.

As already mentioned, arterial stiffness is directly or indirectly influenced by many factors that influence blood pressure (BP). Therefore, subjects should rest for some time in a quiet room before starting a measurement.

For most methods/devices, the supine position of the subject is obligatory. With some devices, measurements can also be performed in sitting position. As BP differs between the sitting and the supine position, it is likely that arterial stiffness will also differ depending on the subject's position. Researchers should mention the position in which measurements have been performed.

After a meal, systemic vascular resistance decreases, accompanied by an increase in heart rate and cardiac output (Kelbaek et al. 1989). Measurements should therefore be performed early in the morning or 3–4 h after a light meal. Subjects should not drink beverages containing caffeine within three hours before assessments.

To minimise short-term influences on arterial stiffness, subjects should not speak during measurements and data should be reported as the mean or median of a 10 to 15 sec period, to cover at least one respiratory cycle. Another short-term variation in arterial stiffness is induced by spontaneous diameter and distension oscillations with a period ranging from 45 to 70 sec (Hayoz et al. 1993). These spontaneous oscillations are assumed more pronounced in muscular than in elastic arteries and at the radial artery are accompanied by a 1.5- to 2-fold change in distensibility (Hayoz et al. 1993). Due to the duration of one oscillation, it is often not practical or feasible to correct for these subtle variations.

Finally, arterial stiffness measurements may be disturbed or made technically inadequate in patients with arrhythmia such as atrial fibrillation or multiple extrasystolies. A brief summary of advantages and disadvantages of this method is given in Table 15.4.

Table 15.4 Summary Box with Key Points

+	Technique with the longest tradition and worldwide experience of assessing vascular function
+	Well described advantages and limitations
+	Useful in large studies
−	Very limited use in small studies or in a clinical setting
−	Multiple confounding cardiovascular factors
−	Different methods and sites of assessment make it difficult to compare studies

References

Benetos A, Laurent S, Hoeks AP, Boutouyrie PH, Safar ME (1993) Arterial alterations with aging and high blood pressure A noninvasive study of carotid and femoral arteries *Arterioscler Thromb* **13**, 90–7

Benjamin N, Calver A, Collier J, Robinson B, Vallance P, Webb D (1995) Measuring forearm blood flow and interpreting the responses to drugs and mediators *Hypertension* **25**, 918–23

Bernard S, Serusclat A, Targe F, Charriere S, Roth O, Beaune J et al. (2005) Incremental predictive value of carotid ultrasonography in the assessment of coronary risk in a cohort of asymptomatic type 2 diabetic subjects *Diabetes Care* **28**, 1158–62

Bonetti PO, Lerman LO, Lerman A (2003) Endothelial dysfunction: a marker of atherosclerotic risk *Arterioscler Thromb Vasc Biol* **23**, 168–75

Bots ML, Hoes AW, Koudstaal PJ, Hofman A, Grobbee DE (1997) Common carotid intima-media thickness and risk of stroke and myocardial infarction: the Rotterdam Study *Circulation* **96**, 1432–7

Celermajer DS, Sorensen KE, Gooch VM, Spiegelhalter DJ, Miller OI, Sullivan ID et al. (1992) Non-invasive detection of endothelial dysfunction in children and adults at risk of atherosclerosis *Lancet* **340**, 1111–5

Chen H, Karne RJ, Hall G, Campia U, Panza JA, Cannon RO 3rd et al. (2006) High-dose oral vitamin C partially replenishes vitamin C levels in patients with Type 2 diabetes and low vitamin C levels but does not improve endothelial dysfunction or insulin resistance *Am J Physiol Heart Circ Physiol* **290**, H137–45

Cooke JP, Rossitch E Jr, Andon NA, Loscalzo J, Dzau VJ (1991) Flow activates an endothelial potassium channel to release an endogenous nitrovasodilator *J Clin Invest* **88**, 1663–71

Corretti MC, Anderson TJ, Benjamin EJ, Celermajer D, Charbonneau F, Creager MA et al. (2002) Guidelines for the ultrasound assessment of endothelial-dependent flow-mediated vasodilation of the brachial artery: a report of the International Brachial Artery Reactivity Task Force *J Am Coll Cardiol* **39**, 257–65

Corretti MC, Plotnick GD, Vogel RA (1995) Correlation of cold pressor and flow-mediated brachial artery diameter responses with the presence of coronary artery disease *Am J Cardiol* **75**, 783–7

Fuchsjager-Maryl G, Pleiner J, Wiesinger GF, Sieder AE, Quittan M, Nuhr MJ et al. (2002) Exercise training improves vascular endothelial function in patients with type 1 diabetes *Diabetes Care* **25**, 1795–801

Grobbee DE, Bots ML (1994) Carotid artery intima-media thickness as an indicator of generalized atherosclerosis *J Intern Med* **236**, 567–73

Hamdy O, Ledbury S, Mullooly C, Jarema C, Porter S, Ovalle K et al. (2003) Lifestyle modification improves endothelial function in obese subjects with the insulin resistance syndrome *Diabetes Care* **26**, 2119–25

Hashimoto M, Akishita M, Eto M, Ishikawa M, Kozaki K, Toba K et al. (1995) Modulation of endothelium-dependent flow-mediated dilatation of the brachial artery by sex and menstrual cycle *Circulation* **92**, 3431–5

Hayoz D, Tardy Y, Rutschmann B, Mignot JP, Achakri H, Feihl F et al. (1993) Spontaneous diameter oscillations of the radial artery in humans *Am J Physiol* **264**, H2080–4

Higashi Y, Yoshizumi M (2003) New methods to evaluate endothelial function: method for assessing endothelial function in humans using a strain-gauge plethysmography: nitric oxide-dependent and -independent vasodilation *J Pharmacol Sci* **93**, 399–404

Jackson TS, Xu A, Vita JA, Keaney JF Jr (1998) Ascorbate prevents the interaction of superoxide and nitric oxide only at very high physiological concentrations *Circ Res* **83**, 916–22

Jarvisalo MJ, Raitakari M, Toikka JO, Putto-Laurila A, Rontu R, Laine S et al. (2004) Endothelial dysfunction and increased arterial intima-media thickness in children with type 1 diabetes *Circulation* **109**, 1750–5

Jay D, Hitomi H, Griendling KK (2006) Oxidative stress and diabetic cardiovascular complications *Free Radic Biol Med* **40**, 183–92

Joannides R, Haefeli WE, Linder L, Richard V, Bakkali EH, Thuillez C et al. (1995) Nitric oxide is responsible for flow-dependent dilatation of human peripheral conduit arteries in vivo *Circulation* **91**, 1314–9

Johnstone MT, Creager SJ, Scales KM, Cusco JA, Lee BK, Creager MA (1993) Impaired endothelium-dependent vasodilation in patients with insulin-dependent diabetes mellitus *Circulation* **88**, 2510–6

Kelbaek H, Munck O, Christensen NJ, Godtfredsen J (1989) Central haemodynamic changes after a meal *Br Heart J* **61**, 506–9

Langenfeld MR, Forst T, Hohberg C, Kann P, Lubben G, Konrad T et al. (2005) Pioglitazone decreases carotid intima-media thickness independently of glycemic control in patients with type 2 diabetes mellitus: results from a controlled randomized study *Circulation* **111**, 2525–31

Laurent S, Hayoz D, Trazzi S, Boutouyrie P, Waeber B, Omboni S et al. (1993) Isobaric compliance of the radial artery is increased in patients with essential hypertension *J Hypertens* **11**, 89–98

Liang YL, Teede H, Kotsopoulos D, Shiel L, Cameron JD, Dart AM et al. (1998) Non-invasive measurements of arterial structure and function: repeatability, interrelationships and trial sample size *Clin Sci* (London) **95**, 669–79

Maiorana A, O'Driscoll G, Cheetham C, Dembo L, Stanton K, Goodman C et al. (2001) The effect of combined aerobic and resistance exercise training on vascular function in type 2 diabetes *J Am Coll Cardiol* **38**, 860–6

Mangoni AA, Mircoli L, Giannattasio C, Ferrari AU, Mancia G (1996) Heart rate-dependence of arterial distensibility in vivo *J Hypertens* **14**, 897–901

McVeigh GE, Bratteli CW, Morgan DJ, Alinder CM, Glasser SP, Finkelstein SM et al. (1999) Age-related abnormalities in arterial compliance identified by pressure pulse contour analysis: aging and arterial compliance *Hypertension* **33**, 1392–8

McVeigh GE, Brennan GM, Johnston GD, McDermott BJ, McGrath LT, Henry WR (1992) Impaired endothelium-dependent and independent vasodilation in patients with type 2 (non-insulin-dependent) diabetes mellitus *Diabetologia* **35**, 771–6

Miura H, Wachtel RE, Liu Y, Loberiza FR Jr, Saito T, Miura M et al. (2001) Flow-induced dilation of human coronary arterioles: important role of $Ca(2+)$-activated $K(+)$ channels *Circulation* **103**, 1992–8

O'Leary DH, Polak JF, Kronmal RA, Manolio TA, Burke GL, Wolfson SK Jr (1999) Carotid-artery intima and media thickness as a risk factor for myocardial infarction and stroke in older adults Cardiovascular Health Study Collaborative Research Group *N Engl J Med* **340**, 14–22

O'Rourke MF, Staessen JA, Vlackopoulos C, Duprez D, Plante GE (2002) Clinical applications of arterial stiffness; definitions and reference values *Am J Hypertens* **15**, 426–44

Pleiner J, Mittermayer F, Schaller G, MacAllister RJ, Wolzt M (2002) High doses of vitamin C reverse Escherichia coli endotoxin-induced hyporeactivity to acetylcholine in the human forearm *Circulation* **106**, 1460–4

Resnick LM, Militianu D, Cunnings AJ, Pipe JG, Evelhoch JL, Soulen RL (1997) Direct magnetic resonance determination of aortic distensibility in essential hypertension: relation to age, abdominal visceral fat, and in situ intracellular free magnesium *Hypertension* **30**, 654–9

Ross R (1986) The pathogenesis of atherosclerosis – an update *N Engl J Med* **314**, 488–500

Ross R (1996) *The Pathogenesis of Atherosclerosis* Lippincott-Raven, Philadelphia

Stadler RW, Taylor JA, Lees RS (1997) Comparison of B-mode, M-mode and echo-tracking methods for measurement of the arterial distension waveform *Ultrasound Med Biol* **23**, 879–87

Steer P, Sarabi DM, Karlstrom B, Basu S, Berne C, Vessby B et al. (2003) The effect of a mixed meal on endothelium-dependent vasodilation is dependent on fat content in healthy humans *Clin Sci* (London) **105**, 81–7

Sun D, Huang A, Smith CJ, Stackpole CJ, Connetta JA, Shesely E et al. (1999) Enhanced release of prostaglandins contributes to flow-induced arteriolar dilation in eNOS knockout mice *Circ Res* **85**, 288–93

Timimi FK, Ting HH, Haley EA, Roddy MA, Ganz P, Creager MA (1998) Vitamin C improves endothelium-dependent vasodilation in patients with insulin-dependent diabetes mellitus *J Am Coll Cardiol* **31**, 552–7

Ting HH, Timimi FK, Haley EA, Roddy MA, Ganz P, Creager MA (1997) Vitamin C improves endothelium-dependent vasodilation in forearm resistance vessels of humans with hypercholesterolemia *Circulation* **95**, 2617–22

Touboul PJ, Hennerici MG, Meairs S, Adams H, Amarenco P, Desvarieux M et al. (2004) Mannheim intima-media thickness consensus *Cerebrovasc Dis* **18**, 346–9

Van Bortel LM (2005) What does intima-media thickness tell us? *J Hypertens* **23**, 37–9

Van Bortel LM, Duprez D, Starmans-Kool MJ, Safar ME, Giannattasio C, Cockcroft J (2002) Clinical applications of arterial stiffness, Task Force III: recommendations for user procedures *Am J Hypertens* **15**, 445–52

Van Bortel LM, Vanmolkot FH, Van der Heijden-Speak JJ, Bregu M, Staessen JA, Hoeks AP (2001) Does B-mode common carotid artery intima-media thickness differ from M-model? *Ultrasound Med Biol* **27**, 1333–6

Van der Heijden-Spek JJ, Staessen JA, Fagard RH, Hoeks AP, Boudier HA, Van Bortel LM (2000) Effect of age on brachial artery wall properties differs from the aorta and is gender dependent: a population study *Hypertension* **35**, 637–42

Vanhoutte PM (1989) Endothelium and control of vascular function State of the Art lecture *Hypertension* **13**, 658–67

Woodman RJ, Watts GF (2003) Measurement and application of arterial stiffness in clinical research: focus on new methodologies and diabetes mellitus *Med Sci Monit* **9**, RA81–9

Yamasaki Y, Kodama M, Nishizawa H, Sakamoto K, Matsuhisa M, Kajimoto Y et al. (2000) Carotid intima-media thickness in Japanese type 2 diabetic subjects: predictors of progression and relationship with incident coronary heart disease *Diabetes Care* **23**, 1310–5

16

Cardiovascular Autonomic Function Testing

Dan Ziegler

Introduction

Diabetic autonomic neuropathy (DAN) may affect any organ innervated by the autonomic nervous system. Although DAN has been appreciated as a clinical entity since the classic report by Rundles (1945), in the past it has received less attention than peripheral sensorimotor neuropathy. This is due on one hand to the fact that the onset of clinical features is insidious and severe clinical symptoms usually occur relatively late in the course of diabetes, and on the other hand, because non-invasive, quantitative and reliable methods for assessment of DAN have only been available for the last two decades. Asymptomatic involvement of the autonomic nervous system can be widespread but remains undetected without careful examination; at the same time, severe symptoms confined to a single organ can result in extensive diagnostic evaluation and intense therapeutic efforts. The late stages of DAN are associated with considerable morbidity and increased mortality (Ewing & Clarke 1986). Hence, early detection aimed at prevention of the advanced symptomatic stages of this complication is essential. Since the clinical symptoms of DAN may be ambiguous and the asymptomatic stages elude clinical examination, reliable, specific and sensitive diagnostic methods are required.

Cardiovascular autonomic neuropathy (CAN) is a serious complication of diabetes that is associated with a poor prognosis and may result in severe postural hypotension, exercise intolerance, enhanced intraoperative instability and, presumably, increased incidence of silent myocardial infarction and ischemia. After the introduction to clinical routine of cardiovascular reflex tests based on changes in heart rate variability (HRV) and blood pressure regulation, CAN was frequently detected in patients in the early stages of asymptomatic diabetes. CAN can be divided into: 1) subclinical, which is diagnosed only by tests and 2) clinical, which presents with symptoms or signs (San Antonio Conference 1988; Proceedings of a Consensus 1992; Ziegler 1999).

Clinical Diabetes Research: Methods and Techniques Edited by Michael Roden
© 2007 John Wiley & Sons, Ltd ISBN 978-0-470-01728-9

Prognosis

In one meta-analysis, the overall mortality rates over periods up to 10 years were 30.4 % in diabetic patients with CAN, detected by reduced heart rate variability (HRV), and only 13.4 % in those without evidence of CAN. The relative risk of mortality with 95 % CI from 15 studies (n = 2,900) was increased in patients with CAN by 2.14 (1.83–2.51) (Vinik et al. 2003). However, if CAN was defined adequately by the presence of at least two abnormal autonomic function tests (AFTs), this risk increased to 3.45 (CI: 2.66–4.47) (Maser et al. 2003). In the population-based MONICA/KORA cohort from the Augsburg region in southern Germany, we observed a significantly increased rate of mortality in diabetic patients with reduced HRV as compared to those with normal HRV (37.5 % vs 23.9 %) (Ziegler et al. 2004). The rates of sudden death tend to be higher among diabetic patients with CAN. However, it must be kept in mind that autonomic dysfunction may also be found in the absence of diabetes as a consequence of common cardiovascular diseases such as coronary artery disease, myocardial infarction and heart failure, and it has been shown an independent indicator of poor prognosis in these patients. Since cardiovascular diseases represent the major cause of death in diabetic patients, the impacts of diabetes and, for example, coronary sclerosis on ANS may overlap in some patients, to such a degree that CAN is at least potentially not the only factor responsible for the increased mortality.

The mechanisms by which CAN leads to increased mortality remain a matter of debate. A number of studies have shown an association between CAN and QT interval prolongation, and a meta-analysis revealed a 2.3-fold increased risk of CAN in diabetic patients with a prolonged QT interval (Whitsel et al. 2000). This led to the speculation that, much like the QT prolongation encountered in idiopathic long QT syndrome, which is characterised by recurrent episodes of syncope or cardiac arrest due to torsades de pointes, CAN may also predispose to malignant ventricular arrhythmias and sudden death. A five-year study in Italy showed a considerably increased risk of mortality in type 1 diabetic patients with QT prolongation (odds ratio: 24.6 [95 % CI: 6.5–92.9]); this requires further confirmation (Veglio et al. 2000). Although the studies included in the aforementioned meta-analysis were not sufficiently large to draw unequivocal conclusions regarding an increased incidence of sudden death in CAN, recent evidence indicates the ANS plays an important role in triggering sudden death in both non-diabetic and diabetic subjects with low HRV.

Epidemiology

Although the impact of CAN is increasingly recognised, only little information exists concerning its frequency in representative diabetic populations. In the Oxford Community Diabetes Study the overall prevalence of abnormal results in ≥ 1 of 3 autonomic tests was 20.9 % in type 1 patients and 5.8 % in type 2 patients (Neil et al. 1989). In the clinic-based DiaCAN study we reported prevalence rates of borderline or definite CAN of 8.5 % or 16.8 % among 647 unselected type 1 diabetic patients and 12.2 % or 22.1 % in 524 type 2 diabetic patients attending clinical and outpatient diabetes centres (Ziegler et al. 1993). In the EURODIAB IDDM Complications Study, among the total of 3,250 patients studied, 19.3 % (range between centres: 7.8–51.8 %) had abnormal HRV and 5.9 % (0–14.5 %) had postural hypotension (Stephenson & Fuller 1994). In 130 newly diagnosed type 1 diabetic patients the prevalence of definite and borderline CAN was 7.7 % and 9.2 % respectively (Ziegler 1999). Thus, CAN cannot be generally regarded a late complication of diabetes.

The prevalence of CAN increases with age, duration of diabetes and poor glycaemic control, and in the presence of distal symmetric polyneuropathy, microangiopathy and macroangiopathy (Ziegler 1999). Recent data suggest a correlation between the components of the metabolic syndrome and reduced HRV. In the MONICA/KORA cohort we showed at the population level that age, diabetes, obesity and smoking should be regarded as primary risk factors of reduced HRV (Ziegler et al. 2004).

Clinical features

Heart rate changes

The hallmark and earliest indicator of, and the most frequent finding in, subclinical and symptomatic cardiac autonomic dysfunction is a reduced heart rate variability (HRV), i.e. the magnitude of heart rate fluctuations around the mean heart rate, which can be detected using various noninvasive autonomic reflex tests, described below. A fixed heart rate, defined as unresponsiveness to moderate exercise, stress or sleep, is an infrequent feature of CAN and indicates almost complete cardiac denervation (Ewing & Clarke 1986; Ziegler et al. 2004).

It has long been recognised that resting tachycardia and fixed heart rate are characteristic findings in diabetic patients with advanced CAN (Ewing & Clarke 1986). Resting heart rates of 90–100 beats/min and occasionally heart rate increments up to 130 beats/min have been observed in association with CAN. Group comparisons of diabetic patients and matched controls have shown an average increase of about 10 beats/min in the diabetic groups. The highest resting heart rates have been found in patients with parasympathetic damage, while those with evidence for combined vagal and sympathetic involvement showed lower rates. Thus, heart rate may decline with increasing severity of CAN and does not provide a reliable diagnostic criterion.

Postural hypotension

Postural hypotension is recognised as the clinical hallmark of CAN in diabetic patients (Ewing & Clarke 1986). It is characterised by weakness, faintness, dizziness, visual impairment and even syncope following the change from the lying to the standing posture. In some cases, this complication may become disabling, but the blood pressure fall may also be asymptomatic. It is generally agreed that postural hypotension is defined by a decrease in systolic blood pressure upon standing of 30 mm Hg or more (Figure 16.1). It is important to note that orthostatic symptoms can be misjudged as hypoglycaemia and be aggravated by a number of drugs including vasodilators, diuretics, phenothiazines, and in particular tricyclic antidepressants and insulin.

Exercise intolerance

In diabetic patients without evidence of heart disease, but with asymptomatic vagal CAN, exercise capacity (greatest tolerable workload and maximal oxygen uptake), heart rate, blood pressure, cardiac stroke volume and hepatosplanchnic vascular resistance are diminished.

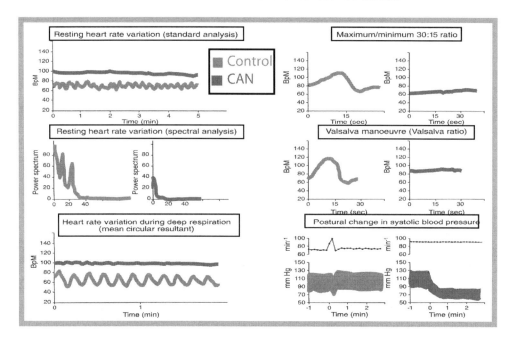

Figure 16.1 Test battery for the detection and characterisation of cardiovascular autonomic neuropathy (CAN).

A further decrease in exercise capacity and blood pressure is seen in patients with both vagal CAN and orthostatic hypotension. The severity of CAN correlates inversely with the increase in heart rate at any time during exercise and with the maximal increase in heart rate. Thus, CAN contributes to diminished exercise tolerance. Therefore, autonomic testing offers a useful tool for identifying patients with potentially poor exercise performance and for preventing hazard when they are introduced to exercise training programmes (Ziegler 1999).

Left ventricular dysfunction

CAN may be associated with abnormalities in left ventricular systolic and particularly diastolic function in the absence of cardiac disease in diabetic patients. Echocardiographic studies have shown a significant correlation between the severity of CAN and reduced peak diastolic filling rate and an augmented atrial contribution to diastolic filling, as assessed by Doppler echocardiography. However, it is difficult to judge whether CAN is an independent contributor to these abnormalities since other factors such as interstitial myocardial fibrosis, microangiopathic or metabolic changes, which are being discussed in the pathogenesis of diabetic heart muscle disease, may also be responsible for left ventricular dysfunction (Ziegler 1999).

Silent myocardial infarction and ischaemia

In view of the increased prevalence of coronary artery disease (CAD) in diabetic patients, it is difficult to differentiate between the impact of coronary ischemia and CAN on cardiac autonomic function. In other words, silent ischemia in diabetic patients may either result from CAN or from autonomic dysfunction due to CAD itself, or both. In the Framingham study, the rates of unrecognised myocardial infarctions were 39 % in diabetic subjects and 22 % in non-diabetic subjects, but the difference was not significant (Margolis et al. 1973). In a survey from the National Registry of Myocardial Infarction 2 (NRMI-2), of 434,877 patients with myocardial infarction, 33 % did not have chest pain on presentation. The rates of patients with diabetes were 32.6 % among those presenting without chest pain vs 25.4 % among those with (Canto et al. 2000). It has been suggested that features such as sympathovagal balance (see below), impaired fibrinolysis and altered hemostasis, which are commonly clustered together, may trigger coronary plaque disruption and superimposed thrombosis in diabetic patients in a more unpredictable manner than they would in the absence of diabetes (Nesto 1999).

A meta-analysis including 12 studies (n = 1,468) revealed an increased risk of silent myocardial ischemia (SMI) during exercise of 1.96 (1.53–2.51) in diabetic patients with CAN, compared to those without CAN (Maser et al. 2003; Maser & Lenhard 2005). CAN is a predictor of cardiovascular events in diabetic patients, the risk being highest in those who have both CAN and SMI (Valensi et al. 2005). The DIAD study showed that SMI is encountered in 22 % of asymptomatic type 2 diabetic patients and correlates more strongly with reduced HRV than with male sex and the duration of diabetes (Wackers et al. 2004). In diabetic patients with exertional chest pain, a prolonged anginal perceptual threshold, i.e. the time from onset of 0.1 mV ST depression to the onset of angina pectoris during exercise ECG, has been demonstrated. This delay was associated with the presence of CAN (Ambepityia et al. 1990). Hence, patients with CAN and CAD are jeopardised, because the longer threshold permits them to continue exercising despite increasing ischaemia (Figure 16.2).

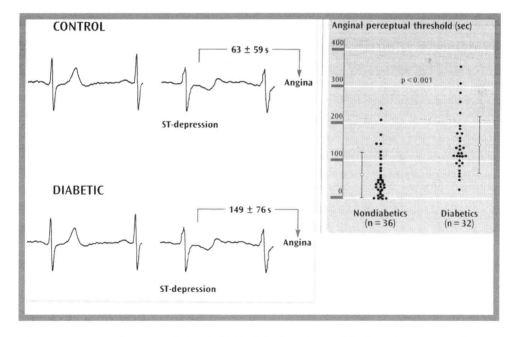

Figure 16.2 Anginal perceptual thresholds in diabetic and non-diabetic patients. Data points are the time from onset of 0.1 mV ST segment depression to onset of angina in individual patients during treadmill exercise.

Furthermore, it has been demonstrated that patients with silent ischaemia are more frequently diabetic, and impairment in several autonomic function tests including standard indices and 24-h HRV was not seen in the nondiabetic patients in the silent group but was confined to the diabetic patients with silent ischaemia (Marchant et al. 1993). These findings suggest CAN plays an important role in silent ischaemia in diabetic subjects. However, it has also been argued that the increased incidence of CAD in diabetes mainly reflects accelerated coronary atherosclerosis and that there is no convincing clinical and epidemiological evidence for CAN playing a major role in the lack of ischemic pain (Airaksinen 2001). Given the complex and controversial mechanisms of silent myocardial ischaemia even in the absence of diabetes, further studies are needed to clarify the exact role of CAN in this context.

A diagnostic algorithm for diabetic patients without ischemic symptoms published by Deutsche Diabetes-Gesellschaft (DDG) (Standl et al. 2001), according to the statements of the American Diabetes Association (ADA) (1998) and American Heart Association (AHA), (Grundy et al. 1999) is shown in Figure 16.3.

Perioperative instability

Perioperative cardiovascular morbidity and mortality is believed to be 2–3 fold increased in patients with diabetes. Heart rate and blood pressure in diabetic patients undergoing general anaesthesia may decline to a greater degree during induction of anaesthesia and increase to a lesser degree following tracheal intubation and extubation, as compared with nondiabetic subjects. However, some patients may also show hypertensive reactions during induction of anaesthesia. Diabetic patients who require intraoperative blood pressure support by vasopressor drugs have significantly greater impairment of autonomic function tests compared with those who do not need vasopressors (Burgos et al. 1989). Moreover, patients with diabetes and CAN experience more severe intraoperative hypothermia than those without CAN and may therefore fail to develop a normal core temperature plateau (Kitamura et al. 2000). Because of the increased risk of intraoperative cardiovascular instability, preoperative screening of cardiac autonomic function may be useful in identifying those patients who are at risk. This could help the anaesthetist in planning the anaesthetic management of patients with CAN (Ziegler 1999).

Diagnostic assessment

Cardiovascular autonomic reflex tests

It has been proposed that autonomic testing should be noninvasive, simple, easy to perform, related to known physiological function and suitable for longitudinal evaluation. It should be borne in mind that numerous factors may influence the test results: age, heart rate, respiratory rate, blood pressure, eating, drinking coffee, smoking, body position, volume status, mental stress, drugs, exercise and time of day (Genovely & Pfeifer 1988).

During the last quarter of the 20th century, several noninvasive cardiovascular reflex tests for computer-assisted assessment of abnormalities in HRV and blood pressure regulation were described. It is generally accepted that the diagnosis of CAN should be based on the results of a battery of autonomic tests rather than one single test (Ziegler 1999). HRV can be assessed either by calculation of indices based on statistical analysis of R-R

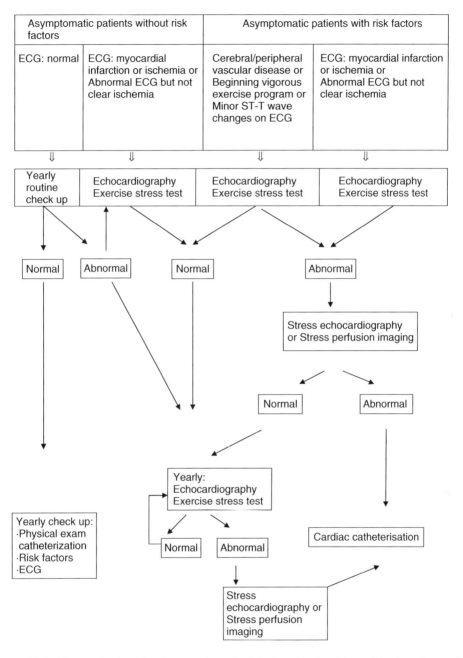

Figure 16.3 Diagnostic algorithm for asymptomatic diabetic patients with or without cardiovascular risk factors.

intervals (time domain analysis) or by spectral analysis (frequency domain analysis) of an array of R-R intervals (Figure 16.4). Spectral analysis involves decomposing the series of sequential R-R intervals into a sum of sinusoidal functions of different amplitudes and frequencies by several possible mathematical approaches such as fast Fourier transformation

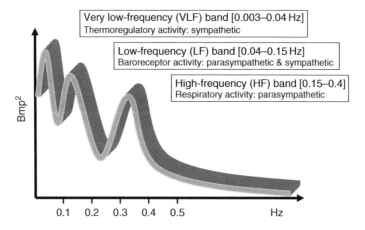

Figure 16.4 Spectral analysis of heart rate variability.

and autoregressive models. The result (power spectrum) can be displayed with the magnitude of variability as a function of frequency. In other words, the power spectrum reflects the amplitude of the heart rate fluctuations present at different oscillation frequencies. The power spectrum of HRV has been shown to consist of three major peaks: 1) very low-frequency component (below 0.05 Hz), which is related to fluctuations in vasomotor tone associated with thermoregulation; 2) low-frequency component (around 0.1 Hz), which represents the so-called 10 s rhythm (Mayer waves) associated with the baroreceptor reflex; and 3) high-frequency component (around 0.25 Hz), which is related to respiratory activity (Figure 16.4). The very low-frequency heart rate fluctuations are thought to be mediated primarily by the sympathetic system; the low-frequency fluctuations are predominantly under sympathetic control with vagal modulation; while the high-frequency fluctuations are under parasympathetic control. Since spectral analysis is carried out under resting conditions, it has the advantage that active cooperation of the patient is not required.

Commercially available computer programmes (e.g. VariaCardio TF5) are usually employed to assess autonomic nerve function, but conventional ECG equipment can also be used. We have validated a combination of autonomic function tests based on standard, spectral, and vector analysis of HRV. This test battery includes measurement of the following indices (Figure 16.1):

1) Coefficient of variation (CV) of R-R intervals or spectral power in the high-frequency band at rest; 2) spectral power in the very low-frequency band and 3) low-frequency band; 4) HRV during deep breathing, including mean circular resultant of vector analysis or expiration/inspiration (E/I) ratio; 5) maximum-minimum 30:15 ratio; 6) Valsalva ratio; and 7) postural change in systolic blood pressure. The age-related normal ranges of the seven indices included in this battery, which have been selected by specific criteria (different physiological basis, independence of heart rate and relatively high sensitivity and reproducibility), have been reported. We suggest that definite CAN be defined as the presence of ≥ 3 abnormalities in these seven parameters (specificity: 100 %). Borderline or incipient CAN is assumed when ≥ 2 abnormal findings are present (specificity: 98 %) (Ziegler et al. 1992a,b). If a computer system is not available, the last four parameters should be determined. In this case, definite CAN is diagnosed in the presence of ≥ 2 abnormal findings. Because of the

potential risk of inducing retinal or vitreous haemorrhage, the Valsalva manoeuvre should not be performed in patients with advanced diabetic retinopathy.

24 Hour heart rate variability

Evidence has accumulated indicating a circadian variation in the frequency of acute cardio-vascular events, with an increased incidence in the early morning hours. Neural activities represent typical examples of circadian rhythms, i.e. the day-night cycle, and it is well known that circulatory changes follow a similar circadian cycle. This highlights the importance of continuous 24-h monitoring of heart rate and blood pressure changes in studying the neural control of circulation in healthy and diabetic subjects. Using power spectral analysis of heart rate applied to 24-h ECG recordings, a circadian rhythm of sympathovagal balance has been observed in the general population. While the low-frequency (LF) power spectrum compo-nent is predominant at daytime, a prominent increase of the high-frequency (HF) component occurs during the night, resulting in a marked decrease in the LF/HF ratio from day to night (Figure 16.5). This can be explained by the dominance of sympathetic activity influencing the LF component during the day, which decreases during the night in coincidence with vagal arousal. Diabetic patients with CAN display an impairment in absolute values of both HF and LF oscillations. However, blunting in nocturnal increase in the HF component, which expresses vagal modulation of the heart, seems to be the earliest and most prominent event (Figure 16.5). This leads to a relative predominance of sympathetic activity during the night.

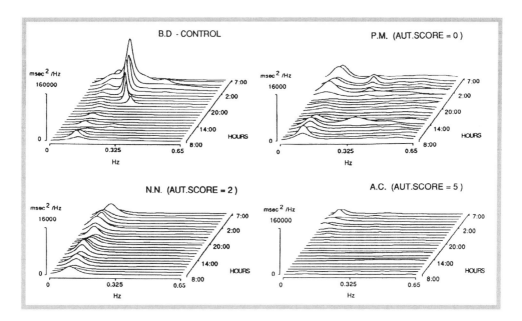

Figure 16.5 Examples of circadian patterns of low-frequency (LF) and high-frequency (HF) compo-nents of power spectrum over 24 hours. BD: normal pattern: predominance of LF during the day and of HF during the night; PM: attenuation of nocturnal HF increase in a patient without CAN; NN: blunted nocturnal HF increase with nocturnal LF predominance in a patient with early CAN; AC: only residual nocturnal LF activity left in a patient with definite CAN.

The abnormal circadian pattern of sympathovagal balance has been shown to be related to a similar abnormality in the BP pattern. These two abnormalities could be relevant to the excess cardiovascular mortality rates described in the diabetic population and in patients with CAN (Spallone et al. 1993).

During the last decade, registration of 24-h HRV using multichannel ECG recorders has been increasingly used, particularly for risk stratification after acute myocardial infarction and congestive heart failure. In 1996, the Task Force of the European Society of Cardiology and the North American Society of Pacing and Electrophysiology defined the standards of measurement and clinical use of HRV (Task Force of the European Society 1996). Several studies in diabetic patients suggest that assessment of 24-h HRV may be more sensitive in detecting CAN than standard autonomic reflex tests (Ziegler et al. 1998; Ziegler 1999).

Spontaneous baroreflex sensitivity

The development of a technique based on servoplethysmomanometry that measures blood pressure in the finger on a beat-to-beat basis (Peňáz et al. 1976) has expanded the diagnostic spectrum in diabetic patients with CAN. This method (Finapres) is increasingly becoming an integral constituent in the assessment of ANS function, allowing the assessment of neural modulation of the sinus node by arterial baroreceptors. In the past decades, the baroreceptor-cardiac reflex sensitivity (BRS) has been quantified by measuring the changes in R-R interval produced in reflex to acute pharmacologically induced changes in blood pressure. More recently, it has been shown that the analysis of spontaneous baroreflex sequences gives results equivalent to the pharmacological methods (James et al. 1998). Two analyses for spontaneous BRS have been proposed. The first consists of analysing recordings of simultaneous blood pressure (BP) and R-R intervals for sequences in which BP or R-R are either rising (+BP/+R-R) or falling (–BP/–R-R) in parallel for at least three beats. The second method involves spectral analysis, enabling the linkage or cross-spectrum between the BP and R-R interval signals to be quantified in terms of amplitude or gain, phase (the time shifts between two signals) and coherence. It has been suggested that coherence is acceptable in two frequency bands (LF 0.05–0.15 and HF 0.20–0.35) (James et al. 1998). Studies in diabetic patients with or without CAN indicate that both time and frequency domain measures of spontaneous BRS could allow earlier detection of CAN than AFTs (Weston et al. 1996; Frattola et al. 1997; Ziegler et al. 2001), but further studies providing information on normal ranges, reproducibility and sensitivity are required.

Non-linear measures

Non-linear analyses of HRV include methods derived from fractal geometry and chaos theory. The basic property of a fractal object is self-similarity or scale invariance, i.e. the details of the structure are similar when zooming at different resolutions. The fractal dimension measures the degree of irregularity (Mansier et al. 1996). Another non-linear measure is the Poincaré plot (scatterplot, return map), representing a diagram in which each R-R interval of a tachogram is plotted as a function of the previous R-R interval. The plot is graphically displayed as a pattern of points and lends itself to visual analysis more readily than statistical measures of HRV (Huikuri et al. 1996). Chaotic behaviour is characterised by sets of differential or difference equations describing the evolution of a system that can display solutions that are totally unpredictable in the long run, because of sensitive dependence on initial conditions (Mansier et al. 1996). Measures of chaos dynamics include the Lyapunov exponents, which allow the quantification of sensitive dependence on initial conditions (Mansier et al. 1996), and approximate entropy (ApEn), which represents the amount of regularity, with more regular activity indicating compromised health or aging and larger numbers indicating more irregularity (randomness, complexity) (Pincus & Goldberger 1994). Data in diabetic patients indicate weak correlations of time and frequency domain measures with ApEn or fractal dimension, suggesting that linear and non-linear measures of HRV reflect distinct aspects of autonomic regulation (Bernardi et al. 1996). The correlation dimension (CD) analysis of circadian rhythms of HRV (CDCR) was found to be unphysiologically rotated to the diurnal hours of the day in type 2 diabetic patients. The diurnal inversion of CDCR suggests that the chaotic component of HRV has an abnormal rhythmic pattern over the day-night period. The diurnal phase of shift in CDCR might be another potential indicator of asymptomatic CAN (Curione et al. 2005).

Cardiac radionuclide imaging

Radionuclide techniques for cardiac mapping have recently been used to directly quantify cardiac sympathetic innervation in various diseases including CAN (Figure 16.6). The non-metabolised norepinephrine analogue metaiodobenzylguanidine (MIBG) participates in norepinephrine uptake in postganglionic sympathetic neurons. Several studies have demonstrated decreased myocardial MIBG uptake in patients with CAN, as assessed by autonomic reflex tests. There is evidence to suggest that scintigraphic assessment using MIBG and single photon emission computed tomography (SPECT) is more sensitive in detecting CAN than indirect autonomic reflex testing, since MIBG uptake was reduced in patients with normal autonomic tests (Langen et al. 1997; Ziegler et al. 1998, 1999). The MIBG uptake defects were localised predominantly in the left ventricular posterior and inferior segments (Figure 16.6A). In advanced CAN, completely absent MIBG uptake may be observed (Figure 16.6B).

The norepinephrine analogue [^{11}C]hydroxyephedrine (HED) has also been employed to examine cardiac innervation defects. In diabetic patients, attenuated HED retention was related to the severity of CAN and was most pronounced in the inferior, apical and lateral segments (Stevens et al. 1998b). In severe CAN, the myocardial retention of HED was remarkably heterogenous, since as the extent of distal deficits increased, HED retention became paradoxically increased in the proximal myocardial segments, which showed the highest deficits in coronary blood flow reserve (Stevens et al. 1998a). Such a proximal hyperinnervation complicating distal denervation could result in potentially life-threatening myocardial electrical instability. Because the myocardial dysinnervation correlated with impairment in myocardial blood flow regulation, such as reduced blood flow reserve, it has been suggested that augmented cardiac sympathetic tone and impaired myocardial perfusion may contribute to myocardial injury in diabetes (Pop-Busui et al. 2004).

Cardiac radionuclide imaging provides a unique and sensitive tool for direct assessment of the pathophysiology and progression of early sympathetic innervation defects not accessible to indirect autonomic function testing. Additional studies using tracers of parasympathetic cardiac neurons will allow a more complete, direct quantitative characterisation of CAN in the near future.

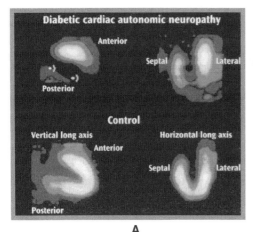
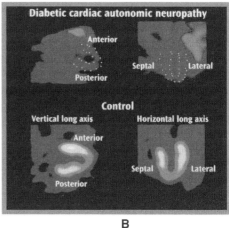

| A | B |

Figure 16.6 A) defects in MIBG uptake in the posterior and apical left ventricular segments in a patient with early CAN as compared with a healthy subject; B) complete absence of MIBG uptake in the left ventricle in a patient with severe CAN. This patient died from sudden death one year after this cardiac imaging was performed.

References

Airaksinen KEJ (2001) Silent coronary artery disease in diabetes: a feature of autonomic neuropathy or accelerated atherosclerosis? *Diabetologia* **44**, 259–66

Ambepityia G, Kopelman PG, Ingram D, Swash M, Mills PG, Timmis AD (1990) Exertional myocardial ischemia in diabetes: a quantitative analysis of anginal perceptual threshold and the influence of autonomic function *J Am Coll Cardiol* **15**, 72–77

American Diabetes Association (1998) Diagnosis of coronary heart disease in people with diabetes *Diabetes Care* **21**, 1551–9

Bernardi L, Spallone V, Ricordi L, Ferrari MR, Maiello MR, Vandea I et al. (1996) Comparison of linear (spectral analysis of heart rate variability) and non-linear methods (chaos theory) to detect cardiac autonomic neuropathy, Neurodiab VI Meeting, Baden, Austria (Abstract)

Burgos LG, Ebert TJ, Asiddao C, Turner LA, Pattison CZ, Wang-Cheng R et al. (1989) Increased intra-operative cardiovascular morbidity in diabetics with autonomic neuropathy *Anesthesiology* **70**, 591–7

Canto JG, Shlipak MG, Rogers WJ, Malmgren JA, Frederick PD, Lambrew CT et al. (2000) Prevalence, clinical characteristics, and mortality among patients with myocardial infarction presenting without chest pain *JAMA* **283**, 3223–9

Curione M, Cugini P, Cammarota C, Bernardini F, Cipriani D, De Rosa R et al. (2005) Analysis of the chaotic component of the sinusal R-R intervals as a tool for detecting a silent cardiac dysautonomia in type 2 diabetes mellitus *Clin Ter* **156**(4), 151–8

Ewing DJ, Clarke BF (1986) Diabetic autonomic neuropathy: present insights and future prospects *Diabetes Care* **9**, 648–65

Frattola A, Parati G, Gamba P, Paleari F, Mauri G, Di Rienzo M et al. (1997) Time and frequency domain estimates of spontaneous baroreflex sensitivity provide early detection of autonomic dysfunction in diabetes mellitus *Diabetologia* **40**, 1570–5

Genovely H, Pfeifer MA (1988) RR-variation: the autonomic test of choice in diabetes *Diabetes Metab Rev* 1988 **3**, 255–71

Grundy SM, Benjamin IJ, Burke GL, Chait A, Eckel RH, Howard BV et al. (1999) AHA Scientific Statement Diabetes and cardiovascular disease *Circulation* **100**, 1134–46

Huikuri HV, Seppänen T, Koistinen MJ, Airaksinen KEJ, Ikäheimo MJ, Castellanos A et al. (1996) Abnormalities in beat-to-beat dynamics of heart rate before the spontaneous onset of life-threatening ventricular tachyarrhythmias in patients with prior myocardial infarction *Circulation* **93**, 1836–44

James MA, Panerai RB, Potter JF (1998) Applicability of new techniques in the assessment of arterial baroreflex sensitivity in the elderly: a comparison with established pharmacological methods *Clin Sci* **94**, 245–53

Kitamura A, Hoshino T, Kon T, Ogawa R (2000) Patients with diabetic neuropathy are of risk of a greater intraoperative reduction in core temperature *Anesthesiology* **92**, 1311–18

Langen K-J, Ziegler D, Weise F, Piolot R, Boy C, Hübinger A et al. (1997) Evaluation of QT interval lenght, QT dispersion and myocardial m-iodobenzylguanidine uptake in insulin-dependent diabetic patients with and without autonomic neuropathy *Clin Sci* **92**, 325–33

Mansier P, Clairambault J, Charlotte N, Medigue C, Vermeiren C, LePape G et al. (1996) Linear and non-linear analyses of heart rate variability: a minireview *Cardiovasc Res* **31**, 371–9

Marchant B, Umachandran V, Stevenson R, Kopelman PG, Timmis AD (1993) Silent myocardial ischemia: role of subclinical neuropathy in patients with and without diabetes *J Am Coll Cardiol* **22**, 1433–7

Margolis JR, Kannel WB, Feinleib M, Dawber TR, McNamara PM (1973) Clinical features of unrecognized myocardial infarction – silent and symptomatic. Eighteen year follow-up: The Framingham Study *Am J Cardiol* **32**, 1–7

Maser RE, Lenhard MJ (2005) Cardiovascular autonomic neuropathy due to diabetes mellitus: clinical manifestations, consequences, and treatment *J Clin Endocrinol Metab* **90**, 5896–903

Maser RE, Mitchell BD, Vinik AI, Freeman R (2003) The association between cardiovascular autonomic neuropathy and mortality in individuals with diabetes: a meta-analysis *Diabetes Care* **26**(6), 1895–901

Neil HAW, Thompson AV, John S, McCarthy ST, Mann JI (1989) Diabetic autonomic neuropathy: the prevalence of impaired heart rate variability in a geographically defined population *Diabetic Med* **6**, 20–4

Nesto RW (1999) Screening for asymptomatic coronary artery disease in diabetes *Diabetes Care* **22**, 1393–5

Peňáz J, Voigt A, Teichmann W (1976) Beitrag zur fortlaufenden indirekten Blutdruckmessung *Z Ges Inn Med* **24**, 1030–3

Pincus SM, Goldberger AL (1994) Physiological time-series analysis: what does regularity quantify? *Am J Physiol* **266**, H1643–56

Pop-Busui R, Kirkwood I, Schmid H, Marinescu V, Schroeder J, Larkin D et al. (2004) Sympathetic dysfunction in type 1 diabetes: association with impaired myocardial blood flow reserve and diastolic dysfunction *J Am Coll Cardiol* **44**(12), 2368–74

Proceedings of a consensus development conference on standardized measures in diabetic neuropathy. Autonomic nervous system testing *Diabetes Care* **15**, Suppl 3, 1095–103

Rundles RW (1945) Diabetic neuropathy: General review with report of 125 cases *Medicine* (Baltimore) **24**, 111–60

San Antonio Conference (1988) Report and recommendations of the San Antonio conference on diabetic neuropathy *Diabetes Care* **11**, 592–97

Spallone V, Bernardi L, Ricordi L, Solda P, Maiello MR, Calciati A et al. (1993) Relationship between the circadian rhythms of blood pressure and sympathovagal balance in diabetic autonomic neuropathy *Diabetes* **42**, 1745–52

Standl E, Eckert S, Fuchs C, Horstkotte D, Janka HU, Lengeling H-G et al. (2001) Deutsche evidenz-basierte leitlinie (DDG) diabetes und herz diabetes und stoffwechsel **10**, 29–42

Stephenson J, Fuller JH, EURODIAB IDDM Complications Study Group (1994) Microvascular and acute complications in IDDM patients: the EURODIAB IDDM Complications Study *Diabetologia* **37**, 278–85

Stevens MJ, Dayanikli F, Raffel DM, Allman KC, Sandford T, Feldman EL et al. (1998a) Scintigraphic assessment of regionalized defects in myocardial sympathetic innervation and blood flow regulation in diabetic autonomic neuropathy *J Am Coll Cardiol* **31**, 1575–84

Stevens MJ, Raffel DM, Allman KC, Dayanikli F, Ficaro E, Sandford T et al. (1998b) Cardiac sympathetic dysinnervation in diabetes: Implications for cardiovascular risk *Circulation* **98**, 961–8

Task Force of the European Society of Cardiology and the North American Society of Pacing and Electrophysiology (1996) Heart rate variability, standards of measurement, physiological interpretation, and clinical use *Circulation* **93**, 1043–65

Valensi P, Paries J, Brulport-Cerisier V, Torremocha F, Sachs RN, Vanzetto G et al. (2005) Predictive value of silent myocardial ischemia for cardiac events in diabetic patients: Influence of age in a French multicenter study *Diabetes Care* **28**, 2722–7

Veglio M, Sivieri R, Chinaglia A, Scaglione L, Cavallo-Perin P (2000) QT interval prolongation and mortality in Type 1 diabetic patients: A 5-year cohort prospective study *Diabetes Care* **23**, 1381–3

Vinik AI, Maser RE, Mitchell BD, Freeman R (2003) Diabetic autonomic neuropathy *Diabetes Care* **26**, 1553–79

Wackers FJ, Young LH, Inzucchi SE, Chyun DA, Davey JA, Barrett EJ et al. (2004) Detection of silent myocardial ischemia in asymptomatic diabetic subjects: the DIAD study *Diabetes Care* **27**, 1954–61

Weston PJ, Panerai RB, McCullough A, McNally PG, James MA, Potter JF et al. (1996) Assessment of baroreceptor-cardiac reflex sensitivity using time domain analysis in patients with IDDM and the relation to left ventricular mass index *Diabetologia* **39**, 1385–91

Whitsel EA, Boyko EJ, Siscovick DS (2000) Reassessing the role of QTc in the diagnosis of autonomic failure among patients with diabetes: A meta-analysis *Diabetes Care* **23**, 241–7

Ziegler D (1999) Diabetic cardiovascular autonomic neuropathy: clinical manifestations and measurement *Diabetes Rev* **7**, 342–57

Ziegler D, Dannehl K, Mühlen H, Spüler M, Gries FA (1992a) Prevalence of cardiovascular autonomic dysfunction assessed by spectral analysis, vector analysis, and standard tests of heart rate variation and blood pressure responses at various stages of diabetic neuropathy *Diabetic Med* **9**, 806–14

Ziegler D, Gries FA, Mühlen H, Rathmann W, Spüler M, Lessmann F et al. (1993) Prevalence of cardiovascular autonomic and peripheral diabetic neuropathy in patients attending diabetes centers *Diab Metab* **19**, 143–51

Ziegler D, Langen KJ, Weise F (1999) Contribution de l'imagerie scintigraphique à l'étude de l'innervation sympathique In: Valensi P, Feuvray D, Sachs R-N (Eds) *Cur et Diabète* Éditions Frison-Roche, Paris, pp. 443–55

Ziegler D, Laude D, Akila F, Elghozi J-L (2001) Time- and frequency-domain estimation of early diabetic cardiovascular autonomic neuropathy *Clin Auton Res* **11**, 369–76

Ziegler D, Laux G, Dannehl K, Spüler M, Mühlen H, Mayer P et al. (1992b) Assessment of cardiovascular autonomic function: age-related normal ranges and reproducibility of spectral analysis, vector analysis, and standard tests of heart rate variation and blood pressure responses *Diabetic Med* **9**, 166–75

Ziegler D, Piolot R (1998) Evaluation of statistical, geometric, frequency domain, and nonlinear measures of 24-hour heart rate variability in diabetic patients with various degrees of cardiovascular autonomic neuropathy *Clinical Autonomic Research* **8**, 282–3

Ziegler D, Weise F, Langen K-J, Piolot R, Boy C, Hübinger A et al. (1998) Effect of glycaemic control on myocardial sympathetic innervation assessed by [123I]metaiodobenzylguanidine scintigraphy: a 4-year prospective study in IDDM patients *Diabetologia* **41**, 443–51

Ziegler D, Zentai C, Perz S, Rathmann W, Haastert B, Meisinger C et al. (2004) Diminished heart rate variability (HRV) and prolonged QTc interval, but not increased QT dispersion (QTD) are predictors of mortality in the diabetic population MONICA/KORA Augsburg Cohort Study 1989/90 *Diabetes* **53**, Suppl 2, A57

17

Nerve Function Testing

Haris M Rathur and **Andrew J M Boulton**

Introduction

The neuropathies are among the most common of the long-term complications of diabetes, affecting up to 50 % of patients. Their clinical features vary and may present to a wide spectrum of specialities in primary, secondary and tertiary care. Progressive loss of nerve fibres may affect both somatic and autonomic divisions, producing a range of symptoms and signs. The criteria for the diagnosis of diabetic polyneuropathy (DPN) have been highly debated. Complex algorithms have been advocated for diagnosis, including neurophysiology, quantitative sensory testing, quantitative autonomic testing and even occasionally sural nerve biopsy (Britland et al. 1990; Ochoa 1995). The diagnosis is formulated on the basis of abnormal results in a given number of these tests, or by summary scores derived from components of these tests. Although these diagnostic strategies are useful research tools, they are too complex for the clinical setting.

It is generally accepted that in clinical practice, the diagnosis of diabetic neuropathy is accomplished by a full neurological history and examination, supplemented by simple quantitative testing. This chapter will consider assessment of the somatic peripheral nervous system for both clinical and research purposes.

Clinical Assessment

Symptoms

Many patients have difficulty in describing the symptoms of neuropathy. Pain and paresthesiae are personal experiences, but there is marked variation in the description of symptoms between individuals with similar pathological lesions. This has important implications for the assessment of symptoms; Huskisson (1976) clearly stated that 'pain is a personal psychological experience and an external observer can play no part in its direct measurement.' When recording symptoms in clinical practice, physicians must therefore avoid the temptation to 'interpret' or 'translate' patient reports; instead, they should record the patient's description verbatim.

Clinical Diabetes Research: Methods and Techniques   Edited by Michael Roden
© 2007 John Wiley & Sons, Ltd   ISBN 978-0-470-01728-9

A number of simple symptom screening questionnaires are available to record symptom quality and severity. A simplified neuropathy symptom score (NSS), which was used in the European prevalence studies, could also be useful in clinical practice (Young et al. 1993; Cabezas-Cerrato 1998). With the NSS, patients are asked questions about their experience of pain and discomfort in their legs. A maximum score of 9 is possible. A symptom score of 3–4 implies mild symptoms, 5–6 moderate symptoms and 7–9 severe symptoms (Table 17.1).

The Michigan Neuropathy Screening Instrument (MNSI) is a brief 15-item questionnaire that can be administered to patients as a screening tool for neuropathy (Feldman et al. 1996).

Other similar symptom scoring systems, such as the Diabetic Neuropathy Symptom (DNS) Score, have also been described (Feldman et al. 1996). The DNS Score is a four-item symptom score, consisting of the following items: 1) unsteadiness in walking; 2) pain, burning or aching at legs or feet; 3) prickling sensation in the legs or feet; and 4) numbness in legs or feet. Presence is scored 1, absence 0, with a maximum score of 4 points.

Simple visual analogue or verbal descriptive scales [VAS/VDS] may be used to follow patients' responses to treatment of their neuropathic symptoms (Scott & Huskisson 1976; Meijer et al. 2002; Ziegler 2003). VAS is a straight line, the ends of which are defined as the extreme limits of the sensation or response to be measured. However, identification of neuropathic symptoms is not useful as a diagnostic or screening tool in the assessment of DPN, as shown by Franse et al. (2000). Up to 50 % of patients with significant neurological deficits may be asymptomatic.

It is well recognised that both symptoms and deficits may have an adverse effect on quality of life (QOL) in DPN (Vileikyte 1999). The NeuroQol, a recently developed and validated QOL instrument, also includes a symptom checklist and may be used as an outcome measure in future clinical studies (Vileikyte et al. 2003).

Table 17.1 The Neuropathy Symptom Score

Neuropathy Symptom Score (NSS)	Patient Response	Score
Have you, in the last 6 months, had any pain or discomfort in your legs and feet when you are not walking?	Burning, Numbness, Tingling = 2 Fatigue, Cramping, Aching = 1 Others = 0	
Is this pain & discomfort most felt in the:	Feet = 2 Calves = 1 Thighs = 0	
Are these symptoms at their worst during the:	Night = 2 Day/Night = 1 Day = 0	
Have these symptoms ever kept you awake at night?	Yes = 1 No = 0	
Is there anything that can improve the pain and/or discomfort?	Yes, Walk = 2 No or Stand = 1 Others = 0	

Total NSS out of 9

Signs

The use of composite scores to assess clinical signs was pioneered by Dyck and colleagues (Dyck et al. 1997; Dyck 2003), who first described the Neuropathy Disability Score (NDS) and later the Neuropathy Impairment Score (NIS). A modified NDS has been used in several large studies (Young et al. 1993; Cabezas-Cerrato 1998; Abbott et al. 2002) and can also be used in the community by a trained nonspecialist. It has been shown to be the best predictor of foot ulceration and the best neuropathic end point in a large prospective community study (Abbott et al. 2002). It is derived from examination of the ankle reflex, vibration, pin-prick and temperature sensation on the great toe. The sensory modalities are scored as either present = 0 or reduced/absent = 1 for each side; and reflexes are scored as normal = 0, present with reinforcement = 1 or absent = 2 per side. The total maximum abnormal score is 10. A score of 3–5 is regarded as a sign of mild neuropathy, 6–8 as moderate neuropathy and 9–10 as severe neuropathy (Figure 17.1).

Similarly, the Toronto group (Perkins et al. 2001) has described a number of simple screening tests for the diagnosis of neuropathy in outpatient clinics. It has recently validated a clinical scoring system (Toronto Clinical Scoring System – TCSS) (Bril & Perkins 2002) and concluded that it can be used to document and monitor neuropathy in the clinic. The patient is questioned about the presence or absence of pain (characteristic of neuropathic pain such as burning, stabbing or shock-like), numbness, tingling and weakness in the feet; the presence or absence of similar upper-limb symptoms; and the presence or absence of unsteadiness on ambulation. The outcome is a continuous variable ranging from a minimum of 0

NDS

		Right	Left
VPT 128 Hz tuning fork; apex of big toe: normal = can distinguish vibrating/not vibrating	Normal = 0; abnormal = 1		
Temperature perception on dorsum of the foot Use tuning fork with beaker of ice/warm water			
Pin prick Apply pin proximal to big toenail just enough to deform the skin; trial pair = sharp, blunt; normal = can distinguish sharp/not sharp			
Achilles reflex	Present = 0 Present with reinforcement = 1 Absent = 2		
	NDS total out of 10		

Figure 17.1 The Modified NDS.

(no neuropathy) to a maximum of 19 points. 6 points are derived from symptoms, 8 from lower-limb reflexes and 5 from sensory examination distally at the toes.

Looking to the future, Dyck et al. (2002) recently reported electronic case-report forms for the recording of symptoms and signs of neuropathy.

Clinical screening devices (not requiring external power source)

Because there is to date no pathogenetic treatment for DPN, most clinical screening devices have been employed to identify patients with moderate/severe deficits who are at risk of foot problems, rather than those with early neuropathy.

Although the simple handheld screening devices are less sensitive than Quantitative Sensory Testing (QST) devices, they have the advantage of being relatively inexpensive, easy to operate and easily portable; therefore, their use in clinical practice is increasing.

The most widely used device in clinical practice is the Semmes-Weinstein 10 g monofilament (SWM) (Valk et al. 1997; Mayfield & Sugarman 2000). The nylon filament assesses pressure perception when gentle pressure is applied to the handle. Although filaments of many different sizes are available, the one that exerts 10 g of pressure is that most commonly used to assess pressure sensation in the diabetic foot. It is also referred to as the 5.07 monofilament because it is calibrated to exert a force, measured in grams, that is 10 X log of the force exerted at the tip; hence, 5.07 exerts 10 g of force. A number of cross-sectional studies have assessed the ability of the SWM to identify feet at risk of ulceration. Sensitivities vary from 86 to 100 % (Kumar et al. 1991; Armstrong et al. 1998; Miranda-Palma et al. 2003), although there is no consensus as to how many sites should be tested (Figure 17.2).

Some centres use the graduated Rydel-Seiffer tuning fork for the assessment of neuropathy (Hilz et al. 1998; Shin et al. 2000). This fork uses an optical illusion to determine the intensity of residual vibration on a 0–8 scale at the point of threshold (disappearance of sensation). Results with this instrument correlated well with other QST measures (Hilz et al. 1998).

The tactile circumferential discriminator assesses the perception of calibrated change in the circumference of a probe. Vileikyte et al. (1997) reported 100 % sensitivity in the identification of patients at risk of foot ulceration. This device also demonstrated good agreement with other measures of QST.

Finally, the recently reported Neuropen is a clinical device that assesses pain using a Neurotip at one end and a 10 g monofilament at the other. This was shown to be a sensitive device for assessing nerve function when compared with the simplified NDS (Paisley et al. 2002).

However, all these instruments have limited ability to detect mild neuropathy and minimal change. They should not be used in clinical trials to determine treatment efficacy.

Vibration thresholds

The relationship between the elevated vibration perception threshold (VPT) and DPN has been documented for over 100 years. When tested in the 50–300 Hz range, VPT reflects the activation of mechanoreceptors (i.e. Pacinian and Meissner corpuscles), conduction in

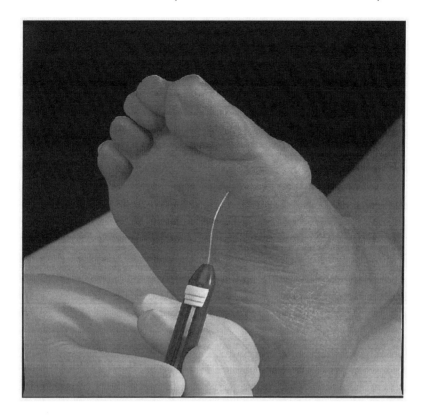

Figure 17.2   The Semmes-Weinstein 10 g Monofilament The filament is applied until it begins to buckle and is held in place for approximately 1.5 sec. Each site is tested three times.

large-diameter myelinated peripheral axons and transmission through the dorsal column spinal pathways.

Multiple studies have documented the relationship between loss of vibration sensation and the progression of a variety of indicators of DPN (Ziegler et al. 1988; Dyck et al. 1993). Dyck et al. (2000) used computer-assisted QST to evaluate three large cohorts and identified a 'strong and consistent correlation' between sensory loss and other markers of DN. These studies confirmed that vibration thresholds are especially sensitive to mild or subclinical neuropathy. Boulton et al. (1986) documented that vibration thresholds provide a strong indication of 'risk' for future ulceration across a wide range of ages and durations of diabetes.

The neurothesiometer is a hand held, rechargeable, battery operated, portable diagnostic instrument for assessing and determining VPT at selected sites on the surface of the body. It is placed on the tip of the big toe and vibrates on a linear voltage scale from 0 to 50 V. The vibration delivered increases as the voltage is increased. It is very similar to the biothesiometer (see below), except that it is battery powered (Abbott et al. 1998).

The NeuroQuick is an instrument for quantitative bedside testing of cold thermal perception (TPT) based on the wind chill factor, i.e. the effect that wind has on the perception of cold. This handheld, microprocessor-operated electronic device consists of a fan, designed to rotate at 10 different velocities (levels), and laser diodes, which ensure a constant distance from the skin (17 cm) is maintained (Ziegler et al. 2005).

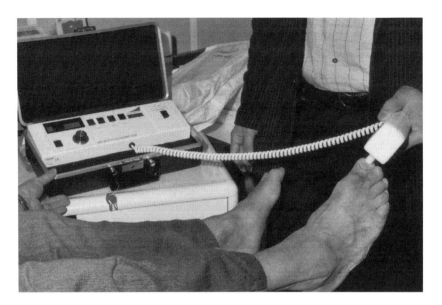

Figure 17.3 The Neurothesiometer The probe is placed over the hallux and vibrates on a linear voltage scale from 0 to 50 V to determine vibration sensitivity threshold. The patient should be asked to say when he first notices the vibration and a note of the value should be made.

Day to day clinical diagnosis of DPN can be made from history and examination, with exclusion of other causes. This may, on occasion, be supplemented by simple QST or electrophysiology.

For research purposes, it is generally recommended that these methods be supplemented with more complex assessments like QST, Nerve Conduction Velocity (NCV) and the Autonomic Function Test (see Chapter 16).

Quantitative sensory testing

QST consists of procedures requiring a power source, where the intensity and characteristics of the stimuli are well controlled and where the detection threshold is determined in parametric units that can be compared with established 'normal' values (Arezzo 2003). QST measures can be used to identify the sensory modalities affected and to estimate the magnitude of the deficit. QST measures of vibration, thermal and pain thresholds have proven valuable in identifying diabetic patients with subclinical neuropathy (Boulton et al. 2004), track progression (Bril 2003) and risk of foot ulceration (American Diabetes Association 1988). In addition, QST measures have played a key role as primary efficacy endpoints in a series of multicentre clinical trials evaluating the prevention or treatment of diabetic polyneuropathy (Okamoto et al. 2002; Ekberg et al. 2003).

The strengths of QST are well documented (Arezzo 2003) and include:

1. the accurate control of stimulus characteristics

2. the ability to assess multiple modalities

3. the use of well established psychophysical procedures to enhance sensitivity

4. the capacity to measure function over a wide dynamic range of intensities, thus supporting the evaluation of multiple degrees of neuropathy

5. the ability to measure sensation at multiple anatomical sites, enabling the exploration of a potential distal-to-proximal gradient of sensory loss

6. for most measures, the availability of data from large, age-matched, 'normal' comparison groups

The limitations of QST are also clear. No matter what the instrument or procedure used, QST is only a semiobjective measure, affected by the subject's attention, motivation and cooperation, as well as by anthropometric variables such as age, sex, body mass and history of smoking and alcohol consumption (Gerr & Letz 1994; Gelber et al. 1995). Expectancy and subject bias are additional factors that can exert a powerful influence on QST findings (Dyck et al. 1998). Further, QST is sensitive to changes in structure or function along the entire neuroaxis from nerve to cortex; it is not a specific measure of peripheral nerve function (Arezzo 2003).

QST testing for vibratory and cooling thresholds receives a class II rating as a diagnostic test. It is designated as safe, effective and established. Thus QST is accepted and commonly used in clinical trials of diabetic neuropathy.

The biothesiometer is a hand held electromagnetic vibrator with a stimulating probe (12 mm diameter) that vibrates at 100 Hz. The stimulating probe is placed on the site to be tested, usually the big toe or the finger, and rests on its own weight (300 g). In a four-year prospective study (Young et al. 1994), patients with baseline threshold elevated above a fixed value (i.e. 25 V with the biosthesiometer) were seven times more likely to develop foot ulcers. This observation is supported by a recent evaluation of 187 type 2 diabetic patients, which used multivariate logistic regression to document that an elevated VPT score was the strongest predictor of foot ulceration (i.e. relative risk of 25.40 (Kastenbauer et al. 2001)). The strength of the relationship between elevated VPT and foot ulceration is illustrated by the finding, in 1,035 type 1 and type 2 diabetic patients, that each 1 unit increase in vibration threshold (voltage scale) at baseline increased the hazard of foot ulceration by 5.6 % over a one year study period (Abbott et al. 1998).

Thermal thresholds

Although most mechanoreceptors and free nerve endings can be stimulated by thermal energy, true cutaneous thermoreceptors are orders of magnitude more sensitive to shifts in temperature. The sensation of pain can be driven by high-intensity stimulation of thermoreceptors, especially those sensitive to warming; this activation can be assessed by measuring heat-pain thresholds (Yaritsky et al. 1995).

As is the case with vibration, altered thermal thresholds have been well documented in patients with DPN defined by other criteria (Ziegler et al. 1988; Dyck et al. 2000; Abad et al. 2002) and their elevation has been associated with progression of neuropathy and ultimately with foot ulceration (Sosenko et al. 1990). Abnormal thermal thresholds have been reported in 75 % of subjects with moderate to severe DPN and elevated heat-pain thresholds were detected in 39 % of these subjects (Navarro & Kennedy 1991). Generally, there is a high correlation between elevated thermal and vibration thresholds, but these measures can be dissociated, suggesting a predominant small- or large-fibre neuropathy in individual patients.

The symptoms of neuropathic pain have been associated with altered thermal thresholds (Valk et al. 2000) but, as stated earlier, painful neuropathy likely involves both small- and large-diameter neurons (Otto et al. 2003). Lowered heat-pain thresholds have been reported in patients with DPN.

It is technically more challenging to measure thermal thresholds than vibration thresholds; the evaluation generally takes longer and the smallest detectable difference has been reported as approximately double that of vibration (Valk et al. 2000). Computer-assisted procedures (e.g. Computer Aided Sensory Evaluation IV (CASE IV; WR Medical Electronics, Stillwater, OH) or Computer Assisted Sensory Evaluator) may be especially valuable in examining thermal thresholds (Dyck et al. 1996). The CASE IV system is an automated diagnostic device for detecting and characterising sensory thresholds that have been altered by disease of sensory receptors, nerve fibres, central nervous system tracts and cerebral association areas. The system also detects improvement in sensory perception that results from medical treatment.

Despite the complexity of some devices, QST requires psychophysiological measures that rely on patient feedback; thus reproducibility is inferior to electrophysiology.

Electrophysiology

Whole nerve electrophysiological procedures (e.g. NCV, F-waves, sensory and/or motor amplitudes) have emerged as important methods for tracing the onset and progression of diabetic neuropathy (Bril 2003). Typically, neurophysiological studies show a reduction in the amplitude of sensory action potentials, which is most extreme in the lower limbs. Multiple consensus panels have recommended the inclusion of electrophysiology in the evaluation of DPN, as well as the use of these procedures as surrogate measures in multicentre clinical trials (American Diabetes Association 1988; Peripheral Nerve Society 1995). However, electrophysiology must be performed in triplicate samples and by trained individuals, as a recent study showed a six-fold difference in the ability to detect polyneuropathy (11.9 % by neurologists to 2.4 % by podiatrists) (Dillingham & Pezzin 2005). Furthermore, maximal nerve conduction velocity (NCV) only reflects a limited aspect of neural activity in a small subset of large diameter and heavy myelinated axons and is insensitive to early functional alterations, such as a reduction in Na/K ATPase activity (Hohman et al. 2000). Despite these limitations, multiple consensus panels have recommended the inclusion of whole nerve electrophysiology as a surrogate measure in clinical trials of human diabetic neuropathy (Peripheral Nerve Society 1995). A key role for electrophysiological assessment is to measure deficits or identify neuropathies (e.g. chronic inflammatory demyelinating polyneuropathy – CIDP) superimposed on DPN, which can often be problematic (Tamura et al. 2005; Wilson et al. 2005). Unilateral conditions, such as entrapments, are far more common in diabetic patients (Perkins et al. 2002). The symmetry of electrophysiological measures and the nature and magnitude of the deficits can help identify additional causes for neurological deficits and can be valuable in selecting appropriate subjects for clinical trials.

NCV

NCV is only gradually diminished by DPN, with estimates of a loss of $0.5 \, \mathrm{m/s^{-1}/year^{-1}}$ (Arezzo 1997). In a 10-year natural history study of 133 patients with newly diagnosed type

2 diabetes, NCV deteriorated in all six nerve segments evaluated, but the largest deficit was 3.9 m/s for the sural nerve; peroneal motor NCV was decreased by 3.0 m/s over the same period (Partanen 1995). A similar slow progression of change in NCV was detected in the diabetes control and complications trial (DCCT) (DCCT Research Group 1995), in which the sural and peroneal nerve velocities in the conventionally treated group diminished by 2.8 and 2.7 m/s respectively over the 5-year study period. It provides a sensitive but nonspecific index of the onset of DPN and can be valuable in detecting subclinical deficits. It can trace the progression of DPN and can provide a valuable measure of severity and 'quality of life related to peripheral nerve involvement' (Padua et al. 2002).

Changes in NCV are related to glycaemic control (Tkac & Bril 1998). In the DCCT, subjects who were 'free of confirmed neuropathy at baseline' had a 40.2 % incidence of abnormal NCV after five years in the conventionally treated group and only 16.5 % in the group receiving intensive therapy (DCCT Research Group 1995). A previous study in 45 type 1 diabetic patients utilised a regression analysis to document that a 1 % change in HbA_1 was associated with a 1.3 m/s change in maximal nerve conduction (Amthor et al. 1994).

Changes in NCV can reflect underlying structural pathology in large-diameter axons, including atrophy, demyelination and loss of fibre density (Arezzo & Zotova 2002).

NCV can improve with effective therapy (Airey et al. 2000) or with pancreas transplantation (Muller-Felber et al. 1993).

Amplitude

Peak amplitude of either the sensory nerve action potential (SNAP) or the compound muscle action potential (CMAP), driven by maximal stimulation, reflects the number of responding fibres and the synchrony of their activity. There is a strong correlation ($r = 0.74$; $P < 0.001$) between myelinated fibre density and whole nerve sural amplitude (Veves et al. 1991) in DPN. Russell et al. (1996) calculated that a change of $1.0\,\mu V$ in sural nerve SNAP amplitude is associated with a decrease of 150 fibres/mm^2, while a loss of 200 fibres/mm^2 is associated with an approximate 1.0 mV reduction in the mean amplitude of the CMAP from the ulnar, peroneal and tibial nerves. Longitudinal studies suggest an average loss of SNAP amplitude at a rate of 5 % per year in DPN over a 10 year period (Partanen et al. 1995). Measuring the total area of the SNAP and CMAP has been suggested as a means of assessing the contribution of slower conducting fibres, but these measures are severely limited by variability.

Sural/radial amplitude ratio (SRAR) is another sensitive, specific, age-independent electrodiagnostic test for mild DPN.

F-Waves

F-waves reflect the antidromic conduction of the compound neural volley to the ventral spinal cord, the activation of a subpopulation of spinal motor neurons, the orthodromic conduction of the newly established volley and the postsynaptic activation of a portion of the muscle fibres in the innervated muscle. Because of its 'long loop' nature, this measure is sensitive to factors that alter the speed of conduction, especially those widely distributed along the nerve.

F-wave procedures have been reported as a sensitive and reliable tool in patients with axonal polyneuropathy (Kohara et al. 2000). However, changes limited to the distal segment of the axon, including possible therapeutic benefits, may be poorly represented in F-wave measures. Minimal latency is the most frequent measure of F-wave activity.

Distribution of velocities

Several procedures have been developed to analyse the distribution of conduction velocities as a means of measuring activity in small-diameter axons (Wells & Gozan 1999). Using a computer assisted collision procedure with an assessment of velocities in slower conducting fibres, subclinical neuropathy was detected in 58 % of subjects, compared with only 11 % of subjects when using standard electrophysiology (Bertora et al. 1998).

Excitability

The magnitude and nature of the current necessary to establish the electrophysiologic response can be an important parameter in assessing neuropathy (Burke et al. 2001). Excitation studies have indicated that the diabetic nerve has less accommodation to hyperpolarisation (i.e. inward rectification), which may limit its ability to follow rapid stimulus trains (Yang et al. 2001).

Other methods of assessment

Axon reflex

Capillary dilatation due to an injury response can be captured as a red flare by arteriolar dilatation through a local axon reflex. A recent study has used heating of the skin to 44°C to evoke the flare (LDIflare) and assessed it using a laser Doppler imager to show that it demonstrates C-fibre dysfunction before it can be detected by CASE IV (Krishnan & Rayman 2004).

Sural nerve biopsy

Nerve biopsy, typically of the sural nerve, has been used for many years in the study of peripheral neuropathy, particularly if the etiology is unclear or in diabetic patients with atypical neuropathies (Thomas 1997). However, this is an invasive procedure with recognised sequelae that might include persistent pain at the biopsy site, allodynia and sensory deficits at the nerve distribution, particularly in diabetic patients (Dahlin et al. 1997). These prolonged sensory symptoms and sensory loss appear to occur more commonly in diabetic than in nondiabetic subjects (Dahlin et al. 1997). Thus, with the widespread availability of accurate QST and electrophsiological techniques, biopsies are rarely required for the routine diagnosis of DPN.

The Peripheral Nerve Society (PNS) consensus report on DPN in controlled clinical trials suggested that the use of biopsy findings in assessing response to therapy needs further validation (Peripheral Nerve Society 1995). The PNS also suggested that there is insufficient information on how well neuropathological measures predict the severity and course of neuropathy, and questioned the validity of assessments, such as as axonal atrophy and axo-glial dysjunction, which require electron microscopy.

In addition to assessing responses to therapy, nerve biopsies have been used to help determine the etiopathogenesis of neuropathy. Examples of this include studies of diabetic amyotrophy (Said et al. 1994) and the importance of glycaemic control in DPN (Perkins et al. 2001).

Skin biopsy

The significance and usefulness of immunohistochemically quantitated cutaneous nerves in the morphological assessment of DPN is increasingly being recognised (Hirai et al. 2000; Polydefkis et al. 2001). This technique, though still invasive, only requires a 3 mm skin biopsy and enables a direct study of small nerve fibres, which are difficult to assess electrophysiologically (Polydefkis et al. 2001). A number of neuronal markers, including neuron-specific enolase and somatostatin, have been used to immunostain for skin nerves, but protein gene product 9.5 (PGP-9.5) has proven to be the best cytoplasmic axonal marker. To define alterations in the most distal nerves, and thus those likely to sustain the earliest damage, $50\,\mu m$ formalin-fixed frozen sections have been used to visualise and quantify intraepidermal nerve fibre density in terms of number or length of epidermis idiopathic sensory neuropathy (Polydefkis et al. 2001; Smith et al. 2001). A recent study used a new morphometric modification to assess nerves per epidermal area that correlated highly with the accepted gold standard assessment of nerves per epidermal length (Koskinen et al. 2005). This method appears reproducible, diagnostically sensitive and less time consuming than intraepidermal nerve fibre counting, and may be adapted in any laboratory familiar with basic immunohistochemical methodology for PGP-9.5 staining (Koskinen et al. 2005). It has been proposed that the rate of epidermal nerve fibre regeneration before and after intervention could be used as an endpoint in clinical trials (Yaneda et al. 2003).

Non-invasive assessment

MRI

MRI has been used to assess involvement of the spinal cord in neuropathy. In an exploratory study, Eaton et al. (2001) used MRI of the cord and demonstrated that patients with DPN had a lower cross-sectional cord area than healthy control subjects in the cervical and thoracic regions, leading them to suggest that DPN is not simply a disease of the peripheral nerves. However, progression or regression of this abnormality has not been evaluated in prospective studies and, therefore, the potential for its use as an endpoint in clinical trials of human DPN is not established.

Corneal Confocal Microscopy (CCM)

The cornea is the most densely innervated part of the human body, containing $A\delta$-fibres and unmyelinated C-fibres. CCM permits sequential observations of the corneal subbasal nerve plexus comparable or even superior to those obtained with histopathological examination (Oliviera-Soto & Efron 2001). CCM detects significant alterations in corneal nerve fibre density, branching and tortuosity in patients with mild diabetic neuropathy, and these alterations relate to the severity of somatic neuropathy (Malik et al. 2003; Kallinikos et al. 2004).

Corneal nerve fibre density has recently been shown to improve with improved glycaemic control (Iqbal et al. 2005). Therefore, the ability of CCM to visualise and define the extent of nerve damage and repair occurring in diabetic patients is significant (Hossain et al. 2005). The noninvasive facility of CCM provides a means of expediting drug development programmes for therapies deemed to be beneficial in the treatment of diabetic peripheral neuropathy.

Conclusion

The diagnosis of DPN is important in instituting measures to slow disease progression to the end stage complications of foot ulceration and amputation. Simple, reliable and practical methods are available for use in the clinic. However, for research purposes, more complex and sophisticated tools are required. Noninvasive measures like corneal confocal microscopy hold great promise, particularly in the field of research.

References

Abad F, Diaz-Gomez NM, Rodriguez I, Perez R, Delgado JA (2002) Subclinical pain and thermal sensory dysfunction in children and adolescents with type 1 diabetes mellitus *Diabet Med* **19**, 827–31

Abbott CA, Carrington AL, Ashe H, Bath S, Every LC, Griffiths J et al. (2002) North-West Diabetes Foot Care Study: incidence of, and risk factors for, new diabetic foot ulceration in a community-based patient cohort *Diabet Med* **19**, 377–84

Abbott CA, Vileikyte L, Williamson S, Carrington AL, Boulton AJM (1998) Multicenter study of the incidence of and predictive risk factors for diabetic neuropathic foot ulceration *Diabetes Care* **7**, 1071–5

Airey M, Bennett C, Nicolucci A, Williams R (2000) Aldose reductase inhibitors for the prevention and treatment of diabetic peripheral neuropathy *Cochrane Database Syst Rev* **2**, CD002182

American Diabetes Association, American Academy of Neurology (1988) Report and recommendations of the San Antonio Conference on Diabetic Neuropathy (Consensus Statement) *Diabetes Care* **11**, 592–7

Amthor KF, Dahl-Jorgensen K, Berg TJ, Heier MS, Sandvik L, Aagenaes O et al. (1994) The effect of 8 years of strict glycaemia control on peripheral nerve function in IDDM patients: the Oslo Study *Diabetologia* **37**, 579–784

Arezzo JC (1997) The use of electrophysiology for the assessment of diabetic neuropathy *Neurosci Res Comm* **21**, 13–22

Arezzo JC (2003) Quantitative sensory testing In: Gris FA, Cameron NE, Low PA, Ziegler D (Eds) *Textbook of Diabetic Neuropathy*, Thieme, Stuttgart, pp. 184–9

Arezzo JC, Zotova E (2002) Electrophysiologic measures of diabetic neuropathy: mechanism and meaning *International Rev Neurobiol* **50**, 229–55

Armstrong DG, Lavery LA, Vela SA, Quebedeaux TC, Fleischli JG (1998) Choosing a practical screening instrument to identify patients at risk of diabetic foot ulceration *Arch Int Med* **153**, 289–92

Bertora P, Valla P, Dezuanni E (1998) Prevalence of subclinical neuropathy in diabetic patients: assessment by study of conduction velocity distribution within motor and sensory nerve fibres *J Neurol* **245**, 81–6

Bril V (2003) Electrophysiologic testing In: Gries FA, Cameron NE, Low PA, Ziegler D (Eds)*Textbook of Diabetic Neuropathy* Thieme, Stuttgart, pp. 177–84

Bril V, Perkins BA (2002) Validation of the Toronto clinical scoring system for diabetic polyneuropathy *Diabetes Care* **25**, 2048–52

Britland ST, Young RJ, Sharma AK, Clarke BF (1990) Association of painful and painless diabetic polyneuropathy with different patterns of nerve fibre degeneration and regeneration *Diabetes* **39**, 898–08

Boulton AJM, Kubrusly DB, Bowker JH, Skyler JS, Sosenko JM (1986) Impaired vibratory perception and diabetic foot ulceration *Diabet Med* **3**, 335–7

Boulton AJM, Malik RA, Arezzo JC, Sosenko JM (2004) Diabetic somatic neuropathies *Diabetes Care* **27**, 1458–86

Burke D, Kiernan MC, Bostock H (2001) Excitability of human axons *Clin Neurophysiol* **112**, 1,575–85

Cabezas-Cerrato J (1998) The prevalence of diabetic neuropathy in Spain: a study in primary care and hospital clinic groups *Diabetologia* **41**, 1263–9

Dahlin LB, Erikson KF, Sundkvist G (1997) Persistent postoperative complaints after whole nerve sural nerve giopsies in diabetic and non-diabetic subjects *Diabet Med* **14**, 353–6

DCCT Research Group (1995) The effect of intensive diabetes therapy on the development and progression of neuropathy *Ann Int Med* **122**, 561–8

Dillingham TR, Pezzin LE (2005) Under-recognition of polyneuropathy in persons with diabetes by non-physician electrodiagnostic service providers *Am J Phys Med Rehabil* **84**, 399–406

Dyck PJ (2003) Severity and staging of diabetic polyneuropathy In: Gries FA, Cameron NE, Low PA, Ziegler D (Eds)*Textbook of Diabetic Neuropathy* Thieme, Stuttgart, pp. 170–5

Dyck PJ, Dyck PJB, Velosa JA, Larson TS, O'Brien PC (2000) The Nerve Growth Factors Study Group: Patterns of quantitative sensation testing of hypoesthesia and hyperalgesia are predictive of diabetic polyneuropathy: a study of three cohorts *Diabetes Care* **23**, 510–17

Dyck PJ, Karnes J, O'Brien PC, Zimmerman IR (1993) Detection thresholds of cutaneous sensation in humans In: Dyck PJ, Thomas PK, Griffin JW, Low PA, Poduslo JF (Eds)*Peripheral Neuropathy* W B Saunders, Philadelphia, pp. 706–28

Dyck PJ, Kennedy WR, Kesserwani H, Melanson M, Ochoa J, Shy M et al. (1998) Limitations of quantitative sensory testing when patients are biased toward a bad outcome *Neurol* **50**, 1213

Dyck PJ, Melton LJ, O'Brien PC, Service FJ (1997) Approaches to improve epidemiological studies of diabetic neuropathy *Diabetes* **46**, Suppl. 2, S5–13

Dyck PJ, Turner DW, Davies JL, O'Brien PC, Dyck PJ, Rask CA (2002) Electronic case-report forms of symptoms and impairments of peripheral neuropathy *Can J Neurol Sci* **29**, 258–66

Dyck PJ, Zimmerman IR, Johnson DM, Gillen D, Hokanson JL, Kar JL et al. (1995) Diabetic polyneuropathy in controlled clinical trials: consensus report of the peripheral nerve society *Am Neurol* **38**, 478–82

Dyck PJ, Zimmerman IR, Johnson DM et al. (1996) A standard test of heat–pain response using case iv *J Neurol Sci* **136**, 54–63

Eaton SE, Harris ND, Rajbhandan SM, Greenwood P, Wilkinson ID, Ward JD et al. (2001) Spinal-cord involvement in diabetic peripheral neuropathy *Lancet* **358**, 35–6

Ekberg K, Brismar T, Johansson BL, Jonsson B, Lindstrom P, Wahren J (2003) Amelioration of sensory nerve dysfunction by C-peptide in patients with type 1 diabetes *Diabetes* **52**, 536–41

Feldman EL, Stevens MJ, Thomas PK, Brown MB, Canal N, Greene DA (1996) A practical two-step quantitative clinical and electrophysiological assessment for the diagnosis and staging of diabetic neuropathy *Diabetes Care* **17**, 1281–9

Franse LV, Valk GD, Dekker JH, Heine RJ, Van Eijk JTM (2000) 'Numbness of the feet' is a poor indicator for polyneuropathy in type 2 diabetic patients *Diabetes Care* **17**, 105–10

Gelber DA, Pfeifer MA, Broadstone VL (1995) Components of variance for vibratory and thermal thresholds testing in normal and diabetic subjects *J Diabetes Complications* **9**, 170–6

Gerr F, Letz R (1994) Covariates of human peripheral function: vibrotactile and thermal thresholds II *Neurotoxicol Teratol* **16**, 105–12

Hilz MJ, Axelrod FB, Hermann K, Haertl U, Duetsh M, Neundorfer B (1998) Normative values of vibratory perception in 530 children, juveniles and adults aged 3–79 years *J Neurol Sci* **159**, 219–25

Hirai A, Yasuda H, Joko M, Maeda T, Kikkawa R (2000) Evaluation of diabetic neuropathy through the quantitation of cutaneous nerves *J Neurolog Sci* **172**, 55–62

Hohman TC, Cotter MA, Cameron NE (2000) ATP sensitive K (+) channel effects on nerve function, Na (+), K (+) ATPase and glutathione in diabetic rats *Eur J Pharmacol* **397**, 335–41

Hossain P, Sachdev A, Malik RA (2005) Early detection of diabetic peripheral neuropathy with corneal confocal microscopy *Lancet* **366**, 1340–2

Huskisson EC (1976) Measurement of pain *Lancet* **2**, 1127–31

Iqbal I, Kallinikos P, Boulton AJM et al. (2005) Corneal nerve morphology: a surrogate marker for human diabetic neuropathy improves with improved glycaemic control *Diabetes* **54**, 871

Kallinikos P, Berhanu M, O'Donnell C et al. (2004) Corneal nerve totuosity in diabetic patients with neuropathy *Invest Ophthalmol Vis Sci* **45**, 418–22

Kastenbauer T, Sauseng S, Sokol G, Auinger M, Irsigler K (2001) A prospective study of predictors for foot ulceration in type 2 diabetes *J Am Podiatr Med Assoc* **91**, 343–50

Kohara N, Kimura J, Kaji R, Goto Y, Ishii J, Takiguchi M et al. (2000) F-wave latency serves as the most reproducible measure in nerve conduction studies of diabetic polyneuropathy: multicentre analysis in healthy subjects and patients with diabetic polyneuropathy *Diabetologia* **43**, 915–21

Koskinen M, Hietahraju A, Kylaniemi M et al. (2005) A quantitative method for the assessment of intraepidermal nerve fibres in small-fibre neuropathy *J Neurol* **252**, 789–94

Krishnan ST, Rayman G (2004) The LDIflare: a novel test of Cfibre function demonstrates early neuropathy in type 2 diabetes *Diabetes Care* **27**, 2930–5

Kumar S, Fernando DJS, Veves A, Knowles EA, Young MJ, Boulton AJM (1991) Semmes-Weinstein monofilaments: a simple effective and inexpensive screening device for identifying diabetic patients at risk of foot ulceration *Diabetes Res Clin Pract* **13**, 63–8

Malik RA, Kallinikos P, Abbott CA et al. (2003) Corneal confocal microscopy: a non-invasive surrogate of nerve fibre damage and repair in diabetic patients *Diabetalogia* **46**, 683–8

Mayfield JA, Sugarman JR (2000) The use of Semmes-Weinstein monofilament and other threshold tests for preventing foot ulceration and amputation in people with diabetes *J Fam Pract* **49**, Suppl., S517–29

Meijer JW, Smit AJ, Sondersen EV, Groothoff JW, Eisma WH, Links TP (2002) Symptom scoring systems to diagnose distal polyneuropathy in diabetes: the Diabetic Neuropathy Symptom Score *Diabet Med* **19**, 962–5

Miranda-Palma B, Basu S, Mizel MD, Sosenko JM, Boulton AJM (2003) The monofilament as the gold standard for foot ulcer risk screening: a reappraisal (Abstract) *Diabetes* **52**, Suppl. 1, A63

Muller-Felber W, Landgraf R, Scheuer R, Wagner S, Reimers CD, Nusser J et al. (1993) Diabetic neuropathy 3 years after successful pancreas and kidney transplantation *Diabetes* **42**, 1482–6

Navarro X, Kennedy WR (1991) Evaluation of thermal and pain sensitivity in type 1 diabetic patients *J Neurol Neurosurg Psychiat* **54**, 60–4

O'Brien PC (1996) A standard test of heat-pain responses using CASE IV *J Neurol Sci* **136**, 54–63

Ochoa JL (1995) Positive sensory symptoms in neuropathy: mechanisms and aspects of treatment In: *Peripheral Nerve Disorders II* Butterworth-Heinemann, Oxford, pp. 44–58

Okamoto T, Yamagishi SI, Inagaki Y, Amano S, Koga K, Abe R et al. (2002) Angiogenesis induced by advanced glycation end products and its prevention by cerivastatin *FASEB J* **16**, 1928–30

Oliviera-Soto L, Efron N (2001) Morphology of corneal nerves using confocal microscopy *Cornea* **21**, 246–8

Otto M, Bak S, Bach FW, Jensen TS, Sindrup SH (2003) Pain phenomena and possible mechanism in patients with painful polyneuropathy *Pain* **101**, 187–92

Padua L, Saponara C, Ghirlanda R, Padua R, Aprile I, Caliandro P et al. (2002) Lower limb nerve impairment in diabetic patients: multiperspective assessment *Eur J Neurol* **9**, 69–73

Paisley AN, Abbott CA, van Schie CHM, Boulton AJM (2002) A comparison of the Neuropen against standard quantitative sensory threshold measures for assessing peripheral nerve function *Diabet Med* **19**, 400–5

Partanen J, Niskanen L, Lehtinen J, Mervaala E, Siitonen O, Uusitupa M (1995) Natural history of peripheral neuropathy in patients with non-insulin dependent diabetes *New Engl J Med* **333**, 39–84

Perkins BA, Greene DA, Bril V (2001) Glycemic control is related to the morphological severity of diabetic sensorimotor polyneuropathy *Diabetes Care* **24**, 748–52

Perkins BA, Olaleye D, Bril V (2002) Carpal tunnel syndrome in patients with diabetic polyneuroapthy *Diabetes Care* **25**, 565–9

Perkins BA, Olaleye D, Zinman B, Bril V (2001) Simple screening tests for peripheral neuropathy in the diabetes clinic *Diabetes Care* **24**, 250–6

Polydefkis M, Hauer P, Griffin JW, McArthur JC (2001) Skin biopsy as a tool to assess distal small fiber innervation in diabetic neuropathy *Diabet Technol Ther* **3**, 23–8

Russell JW, Karnes JL, Dyck PJ (1996) Sural nerve myelinated fiber density differences associated with meaningful changes in clinical and electrophysiologic measurements *J Neurol Sci* **135**, 114–17

Said G, Goulon-Goeau C, Lacroix C, Moulonguet A (1994) Nerve biopsy findings in different patterns of proximal diabetic neuropathy *Ann Neurol* **35**, 559–69

Scott J, Huskisson EC (1976) Graphic representation of pain *Pain* **2**, 175–86

Shin JB, Seong YJ, Lee HJ, Kim SH, Park JR (2000) Foot screening technique in diabetic populations *J Korean Med Sci* **15**, 78–82

Smith AG, Ramachandran P, Tripp S, Singleton JR (2001) Epidermal nervinnervation in impaired glucose tolerance and diabetes-associated neuropathy *Neurology* **13**, 1701–4

Sosenko JM, Kato M, Soto R, Bild DE (1990) Comparison of quantitative sensory-threshold measures for their association with foot ulceration in diabetic patients *Diabetes Care* **13**, 1057–61

Tamura N, Kuwabara S, Misawa S, Mori M, Nakata M, Hattori T (2005) Superficial radial sensory nerve potentials in immune-mediated and diabetic neuropathies *Clinical Neurophysiology* **116**, 2330–3

Thomas PK (1997) Nerve biopsy *Diabet Med* **16**, 351–2

Tkac I, Bril V (1998) Glycemic control is related to the electrophysiologic severity of diabetic peripheral sensorimotor polyneuropathy *Diabetes Care* **21**, 1749–52

Valk GD, de Sonnaville JJ, van Houtum WH, Heine RJ, van Eijk JT, Bouter LM et al. (1997) The assessment of diabetic polyneuropathy in daily practice: reproducibility and validity of Semmes-Weinstein monofilaments and clinical neurological examination *Muscle Nerve* **20**, 116–18

Valk GD, Grootenhuis PA, van Eijk JT, Bouter LM, Bertelsmann FW (2000) Methods for assessing diabetic polyneuropathy: validity and reproducibility of the measurement of sensory symptom severity and nerve function tests *Diabetes Res Clin Pract* **47**, 87–95

Veves A, Malik RA, Lye, RH, Masson EA, Sharma AK, Schady W et al. (1991) The relationship between sural nerve morphometric findings and measures of peripheral nerve function in mild diabetic neuropathy *Diabet Med* **8**, 917–21

Vileikyte L (1999) Psychological aspects of diabetic peripheral neuropathy *Diabetes Rev* **7**, 387–94

Vileikyte L, Hutchings G, Hollis S, Boulton AJM (1997) The tactile circumferential discriminator: a new simple screening device to identify diabetic patients at risk of foot ulceration *Diabetes Care* **20**, 623–6

Vileikyte L, Peyrot M, Bundy C, Rubin PR, Leventhal H, Mora P et al. (2003) The development and validation of a neuropathy and foot ulcer specific quality of life rate *Diabetes Care* **26**, 2549–55

Wells MD, Gozan SN (1999) A method to improve the estimation of conduction velocity distribution over a short segment of nerve *IEEE Trans Biomed Eng* **46**, 1107–20

Wilson J, Chawla J, Fisher M (2005) Sensitivity and specificity of electrodiagnostic criteria for CIDP using ROC curves: comparison to patients with diabetic and MGUS associated neuropathies *Journal of the Neurophysiological Sciences* **231**, 19–28

Yaneda H, Tereda M, Maeda K et al. (2003) Diabetic neuropathy and nerve regeneration *Prog Neurobiol* **69**, 229–85

Yang Q, Kaji R, Takagi T, Kohara N, Murase N, Yamada Y et al. (2001) Abnormal axonal inward rectifier in streptozocin-induced experimental diabetic neuropathy *Brain* **124**, 1149–55

Yarnitsky D, Sprecher E, Zaslansky R, Hemli JA (1995) Heat pain thresholds: normative data and repeatability *Pain* **60**, 329–32

Young MJ, Boulton AJM, McLeod AF, Williams DRR, Sonksen PH (1993) A multicentre study of the prevalence of diabetic peripheral neuropathy in the UK hospital clinic population *Diabetologia* **36**, 150–6

Young MJ, Breddy JL, Veves A, Boulton AJM (1994) The prediction of diabetic foot ulceration using vibration perception thresholds: a prospective study *Diabetes Care* **17**, 557–60

Ziegler D (2003) Treatment of neuropathic pain In: Gris FA, Cameron NE, Low PA, Ziegler D (Eds) *Textbook of Diabetic Neuropathy* Thieme, Stuttgart, pp. 211–26

Ziegler D, Mayer P, Wiefels K, Gries FA (1988) Evaluation of thermal, pain, and vibration sensation thresholds in newly diagnosed type 1 diabetic patients *J Neurol Neurosurg Psychiatry* **11**, 1420–4

Ziegler D, Siekierka-Kleiser E, Meyer B, Schweers M (2005) Validation of a novel screening device (NeuroQuick) for quantitative assessment of small nerve fiber dysfunction as an early feature of diabetic polyneuropathy *Diabetes Care* **28**, 1169–74

18

Kidney Function

Sally M Marshall

Introduction

Abnormalities in kidney function can be found in the majority of people with diabetes if sufficiently detailed tests are performed. Many of these abnormalities do not appear to be deleterious to renal or patient survival, although our knowledge of their long-term effects is scanty. Only in a minority of diabetic patients do prognostically significant abnormalities arise, heralding a progressive decline in renal function and eventually endstage disease. Much research has focused on determining the causes of abnormalities and exploring interventions in the management of diabetic nephropathy. Research techniques have been directed mainly towards glomerular function but tubular processes have also been studied. Imaging techniques and quantitative histological analyses provide detailed information on renal structure.

This chapter will describe the main clinical research methods and techniques used in the investigation of renal function, renal haemodynamics, genetics and renal structure in diabetic nephropathy.

Glomerular function

Glomerular filtration

General principals

Accurate measurement of GFR necessitates measurement of clearance from the blood of a tracer substance that is non-toxic and inert, not bound to plasma proteins, not metabolised in the body, freely filtered across the glomerulus, not secreted nor reabsorbed by the tubule and excreted unmodified. Accurate measurements are obtained by administration of exogenous substances given either as a constant intravenous infusion, with or without a priming dose, or as a bolus.

Accuracy is critically dependent on the full dose of tracer being administered intravenously, and precise sampling timing. The procedure is time-consuming, taking 4–6 hours. The plasma decay curve is generally exponential, with a rapid fall as the tracer equilibrates with tissues,

Clinical Diabetes Research: Methods and Techniques   Edited by Michael Roden
© 2007 John Wiley & Sons, Ltd   ISBN 978-0-470-01728-9

and then, after steady state has been reached, a near-linear phase, generally from 2 h onwards, which reflects glomerular filtration. If GFR is very low, it may take 3 h to reach steady state. If the decay curve is analysed using a one-compartment model, blood samples are generally taken at 120, 180, 210 and 240 minutes after injection of tracer. However, a more accurate measure is obtained if a two-compartment model is used, particularly if there is hyperfiltration. Multiple blood samples are required, with more frequent sampling in the first hour.

Specific methods

The fructose polymer inulin is still regarded as the classic gold standard filtration marker (Hostetter & Meyer 2004), with GFR calculated by renal or plasma clearance (Earle & Berliner 1946; Berger et al. 1948; Hellerstein et al. 1993; Florijn et al. 1994; Van Acker et al. 1995; Orlando et al. 1998).

Filtration of radioactively labelled compounds, such as ^{51}Cr-EDTA, ^{131}I-iothalamate and ^{99}Tc-DPTA, gives a GFR value generally comparable to that of inulin clearance. The complex safety procedures and legislation governing the handling of such compounds has led to a decline in their use.

The contrast agents iohexol (Krutzen et al. 1984) and isothalamate (Gaspari et al. 1992; Isaka et al. 1992) are eliminated from plasma mainly by glomerular filtration and have an excellent correlation with the plasma clearance of ^{51}Cr-EDTA and inulin (Gaspari et al. 1995). Iohexol is more commonly used as it reportedly has lower allergenic potential. The most accurate estimate of GFR is obtained by sampling up to 600 min after injection, particularly in individuals with GFR <40 ml/min/1.73 m^2. However, the disappearance curve is linear after 120 min, so that in individuals with GFR >40 ml/min/1.73 m^2, sampling may be limited to only at 120, 150, 180, 210 and 240 min after injection.

Serum creatinine and endogenous creatinine clearance are inadequate reflections of GFR. However, in very large studies, the more detailed methods described above may be too time consuming and cumbersome. Mathematical equations – the so-called eGFR – have been developed whereby an approximate indication of GFR can be calculated from the patient's serum creatinine, age and gender, with or without factors for race and bodyweight. The most widely used equation, a variation of the modification of diet in renal disease (MDRD) formula, correlates well with GFR (Levey et al. 1999) and should prove useful in large, multi-centre studies.

Cystatin C is a naturally circulating, low molecular weight, basic protein which is freely filtered by the glomerulus and almost completely reabsorbed and catabolised by tubular cells. Serum levels are independent of age, sex and lean muscle mass. Although levels reflect trends in reduced GFR, particularly <40 ml/min/1.73 m^2, there is doubt about cystatin C's ability to detect changes in GFR before the serum creatinine has risen (Odoze et al. 2001; Laterza et al. 2002; Mussap et al. 2002; Tan et al. 2002; Buysschaert et al. 2003; Harmoinen et al. 2003; Christensson et al. 2004; Perkins et al. 2005). Also, measurement may be affected by non-renal factors (Harmoinen et al. 1999). Given this uncertainty, it seems premature to recommend the use of cystatin C as a marker of GFR.

GFR measurement in clinical studies and study endpoints

The advantages and disadvantages of the methods discussed above are summarised in Table 18.1. The proportion of participants in whom serum creatinine doubled, which has been used previously as an endpoint, should now be obsolete.

Table 18.1 Techniques for Measuring Glomerular Filtration Rate

Technique	Advantages	Disadvantages	Uses
Inulin clearance	Long-established Ideal filtration substance Can be repeated	Water loading Urinary clearance – bladder emptying IV continuous infusion Precise timing of sampling Laboratory measurement non-standard	Small, discrete studies
Radioactive tracer clearance	Urine collection not required Single IV bolus	Radioactivity – safety, cannot be repeated often Need for complete IV injection and accurate timing of sampling	Small, discrete studies
Iohexol	Single IV bolus Can be repeated Samples can be batched/shipped for analysis	Allergenic potential Laboratory technique non-standard Possible interference peaks on HPLC	Studies requiring repeated measurement of GFR
Serum creatinine	Very easy – one sample, standard laboratory technique	Very inaccurate	Not appropriate for research
eGFR	Very easy – one sample, standard laboratory technique Adjusted for age, bodyweight, gender and race	Not absolutely precise	Large, multi-centre studies requiring repeated measures of GFR
Serum cystatin C	Very easy – one sample, standard laboratory technique	May not relate closely to GFR	Not appropriate for research
Magnetic resonance imaging	Non-invasive	Requires IV contrast Expensive Complex	Currently being evaluated

Albumin excretion

The hallmark of diabetic nephropathy is the progressive rise in urinary protein excretion, which is primarily of glomerular origin. Our understanding of the natural history of diabetic nephropathy was revolutionised by the development of immunoassays specific for albumin and capable of detecting small (mg/l) amounts, so-called microalbuminuria (Keen & Chlou-verakis 1963). In clinical practice, urine albumin and creatinine are measured in a non-timed (preferably early morning) urine sample, and the urine albumin:creatinine ratio is calculated. However, for research purposes, collection of a timed urine sample with measurement of an albumin excretion rate (UAER) is preferable. Overnight collections are perhaps the easiest for the patient to perform but 24 h and short (several hours) collections are also used. Albumin excretion is extremely variable, with an intra-individual day to day coefficient of variation >40 %, so that multiple samples ($\geq$3) are required. If the albumin excretion rate is to be considered as a categorical variable (normo-, micro- or macroalbuminuria) then at least two of the three measurements at each time point should be within range. Recent data suggest

Table 18.2 Important Points in Measuring Urine Albumin Excretion for Clinical Research

- Use timed urine collections and calculate albumin excretion rate
- Make multiple measures (at least 3) over at least 6 months before study entry and ensure that at least 2 are within the appropriate range
- Make multiple measures (at least 3) at each time-point
- Store samples at room temperature or 4 °C for up to one week, or at −70 °C longer-term
- Avoid multiple freeze-thaw cycles
- Mix samples thoroughly after thawing and before assay
- Use change in albumin excretion rate as main study endpoint
- Use change in category of albumin excretion as secondary study endpoint
- Stratify normoalbuminuric groups into low and high levels (overnight UAER <10 or >10 μg/min)
- Stratify microalbuminuric groups into low and high levels (overnight UAER <100 or >100 μg/min)

that patients with low-level microalbuminuria may revert to normal albumin excretion, even after several years of microalbuminuria (Perkins et al. 2003), although subjects with UAER >100 μg/min persistently are unlikely to revert.

Urine albumin is stable at 4 and 20 °C for up to seven days (Collins et al. 1993) and is also stable stored frozen at −40 and −70 °C (Collins et al. 1993; Giampietro et al. 1993). At −20 °C, some authors suggest that short-term storage (up to six months) may be acceptable, but after longer periods the albumin concentration may be falsely low (Giampietro et al. 1993; Schultz et al. 2000). However, repeat thawing and freezing can lead to anomalous results if the urine is not adequately mixed before assay (Collins et al. 1993; Innanen et al. 1997).

The definitions of normo-, micro- and macroalbuminuria were agreed by consensus based on the evidence available in the late 1980s and considering primarily the risk of developing nephropathy. However, more recent data have demonstrated that the risk of developing proteinuria is increased at a level of albumin excretion much lower than the consensus lower limit of microalbuminuria of 20 μg/min in a timed overnight urine collection: several studies suggest that the risk is increased at ∼10 μg/min (Mathiesen et al. 1990; Microalbuminuria Collaborative Study Group 1999; Royal College of Physicians Edinburgh 2000). In addition, it is now well recognised that cardiovascular (CVD) risk increases with increasing albuminuria, the risk rising well below the lower limit of microalbuminuria of 20 μg/min (MacLeod et al. 1995).

The important implications for research studies of all these points are summarised in Table 18.2.

Total protein excretion

When UAER exceeds the microalbuminuric range, sensitive albumin assays are swamped and protein excretion is unselective. Total urine protein should therefore be measured. The same considerations as discussed above and in Table 18.2 for albumin excretion apply to total protein excretion.

Glomerular filtration barrier charge and size selectivity

Techniques that explore charge and size selectivity of the glomerular filtration barrier *in vivo* rely on examining the differential clearance of circulating proteins of varying charges and sizes or of neutral molecules of differing sizes. The clearance of albumin (Stokes-Einstein radius 36 Å, isoelectric point 4–5) is compared to that of IgG (radius 55 Å, isoelectric point 4–10) as an index of size selectivity, while the clearance of the most anionic species of albumin (glycated albumin) or IgG (IgG4) relative to those of less anionic or cationic species provides an indicator of charge selectivity. A selective increase in albumin compared to IgG indicates preservation of size selectivity, while an increase in fractional clearances of IgG4 and albumin (both anionic) represents a decrease in anionic pore charge (Deckert et al. 1988). An increase in the ratio of urinary IgG4/IgG also supports a decrease in charge selectivity (DiMario et al. 1989). An increase in excretion of glycated albumin, which is more anionic than native albumin, supports selective proteinuria (Ghiggeri et al. 1985; Kverneland et al. 1986).

Assessment of the pore size of the GBM *in vivo* is a much more demanding task. Neutral molecules of varying sizes, such as the neutral polymer dextran 40 (Nakamura & Myers 1988; Scandling & Myers 1992; Myers et al. 1995), are given by intravenous infusion, along with inulin. Dextran 40 is neither reabsorbed nor excreted by the tubule, so that the fractional clearance of a given dextran is the same as the ratio of its concentration in Bowman's Space fluid to plasma, i.e. its sieving coefficient. Clearance studies are performed and dextrans separated, usually by gel permeation chromatography, before quantification. The sieving coefficient is calculated as:

$$\text{Sieving coefficient} = \frac{(\text{urine concentration dextran} \div \text{plasma concentration dextran})}{(\text{urine concentration inulin} \div \text{plasma concentration inulin})}$$

Dextrans behave as random coils in solution but become uncoiled when subjected to shear stress. Thus their transport across the glomerulus is facilitated and effective pore size may be overestimated (Bohrer et al. 1984; Davidson & Deen 1988). Several groups have therefore used ficoll 70, which behaves as a rigid sphere during transglomerular permeation (Oliver et al. 1992; Blouch et al. 1997; Anderson et al. 2000). Tritiated ficoll 70, spanning a radius range of 10–90 Å, is infused along with inulin and para-aminohippurate (PAH). Ficoll fractions in urine and blood were separated by HPLC and the relative amounts in each fraction were determined by the radioactivity. Sieving coefficients for each discrete fraction are then calculated. Curves of sieving coefficients by size are constructed, assuming that the glomerular capillary wall is a heteroporous membrane perforated by a lower distribution of restrictive pores with a log-normal distribution and a parallel upper distribution of shunt-like pores (Blouch et al. 1997). A number of other assumptions must be made, including the glomerular transcapillary hydraulic pressure difference (ΔP).

Components of the glomerular filtration barrier

Urinary glycosaminoglycans (GAGs) have been isolated by ion-exchange chromatography and GAG composition determined by cellulose acetate electrophoresis and quantified by densitometry (McAuliffe et al. 1996; De Muro et al. 2002). Others have used antibodies specific for heparan sulphate chains (Yokoyama et al. 1999).

Tubular function

Tubular protein excretion

Evidence of tubular dysfunction has been sought by studying the urine excretion of the tubular lyzosomal enzyme N-acetyl glucosaminidase (NAG) and other tubular proteins such as retinol binding protein (RBP) and β_2-microglobulin. However, tubular protein excretion correlates with glucose control (Gibb et al. 1989; Ginevri et al. 1993) and decreases with improved glucose control (Ciavarella et al. 1982; Ginevri et al. 1993). One longitudinal study in children has demonstrated that tubular proteinuria in diabetic children with normal albumin excretion is not an early marker for microalbuminuria (Schultz et al. 2001). Thus elevated excretion of at least some tubular proteins may represent a temporary phenomenon induced by hyperglycaemia or glycosuria.

Tubular absorption and reabsorption functions

Micropuncture studies in animals have demonstrated that in health the flow of water and flux of sodium into the thin descending loop of Henle is kept constant over a wide range of GFR – the 'glomerular tubular balance'. This may be disrupted in diabetes. Studies to explore this in humans are based on the premise that plasma clearance of lithium (C_{Li}) is a good reflection of flow from the straight part of the proximal tubule into the thin descending limb of Henle (Thomsen et al. 1981). Tests require lithium (400 mg lithium carbonate on the night before the test) and water loading. From the simultaneous measurement of GFR, ERPF, mean blood pressure and clearance of lithium(C_{Li}) and sodium (C_{Na}), the following can be derived:

- Fractional proximal sodium reabsorption rate (FPR_{Na}): FPR_{Na} = 1-C_{Li} divided by GFR
- Fractional distal sodium reabsorption rate (FDR_{Na}): FDR_{Na}- 1-C_{Na} divided by C_{Li}
- Absolute proximal sodium reabsorption (ADR_{Na}): ADR_{Na} = (GFR$-C_{Li}$) multiplied by P_{Na}

where P_{Na} is the plasma sodium concentration.

- Absolute distal delivery (ADD): ADD = C_{Li}
- Fractional distal delivery (FDD): FDD = C_{Li} divided by GFR
- Absolute distal sodium reabsorption (ADR_{Na}): ADR_{Na} = (C_{Li} − C_{Na}) multiplied by P_{Na}
- Filtered load of sodium (FL_{Na}): FL_{Na} = GFR x P_{Na} x 10^3
- Fractional excretion of sodium (FE_{Na}): FE_{Na} = C_{Na} divided by GFR

Renal haemodynamics

Animal models of diabetes suggest that constriction of the efferent glomerular artery relative to the afferent artery, and thus increased intraglomerular pressure and renal resistance, are fundamental in the development of nephropathy. Catheterisation of the renal artery and vein and direct measurement of intraglomerular pressure are obviously inappropriate in human research, so indirect measures have been developed.

Renal blood flow

The effective renal plasma flow (ERPF) is derived directly from the clearance of hippuran, either as the renal clearance of para-amino-hippurate or as the plasma disappearance of ^{131}I-hippuran. Total renal blood flow (RBF) is then calculated as:

$$RBF = ERPF \text{ divided by } (1\text{-Hct})$$

where Hct is the haematocrit.

Renal vascular resistance

Estimates of the resistance to blood flow through the glomerulus can be derived from renal blood flow:

1) The filtration fraction is calculated as: filtration fraction = GFR divided by ERPF

An increased ratio suggests a higher GFR than would be expected for ERPF and suggests afferent: efferent arterial imbalance and raised intraglomerular pressure.

2) 'Renal vascular resistance' (RVR): RVR = MAP divided by RBF (Fioretto et al. 1990; Sambataro et al. 1996)

where MAP is the mean arterial pressure (SBP-DBP/3).
    Several groups have developed ultrasound methods to determine the 'renal resistive index' (Ishimura et al. 1997; Taniwaki et al. 1998; Matsumoto et al. 2000; Radermacher et al. 2003). Using intra-renal doppler ultrasound, signals are captured from 2–3 representative proximal segmental arteries. The peak systolic (v_{max}) and minimum diastolic (v_{min}) velocities are measured and the renal resistive index (RRI) calculated as:

$$RRI = (v_{max} - v_{min}) \text{ divided by } v_{max}$$

Obviously, this index is critically dependent on the observer and the selection of 'representative' arteries.

Renal structure

Renal imaging

Standard imaging techniques such as ultrasound, CT scanning and magnetic resonance imaging can be used to quantify total renal size and cortex and medullary volume. Very preliminary work suggests that magnetic resonance spectroscopy (MRS) may also be a useful tool (Katz-Brull et al. 2003).

Renal morphometry

Renal biopsy performed under ultrasound control with a preset biopsy gun is safe and several groups have performed biopsies for research purposes (Bilous et al. 1989; Østerby et al. 1990; White et al. 2002; Dalla Vestra et al. 2003; Steinke et al. 2005). Sufficient patients must be recruited to give the study adequate power. Histological analysis should be quantitative, using state of the art morphometric measurements at light and electron microscopy level. Such work is time consuming and requires a high degree of training and access to appropriate technology. The use of qualitative and semi-quantitative 'indices' is to be avoided as they are subject to bias. Tissue can also be examined by other techniques, including immunohistochemistry and in situ hybridisation.

Renal tissue obtained at biopsy can obviously be used in other ways, although the small amount of tissue available limits its use. Mesangial cells have been grown out from biopsy cores but more commonly, human renal endothelial, mesangial and epithelial cells are grown out from glomeruli isolated from whole human kidney or samples obtained at open biopsy (Denton et al. 1991; Mundel et al. 1997; Saleem et al. 2002; Bjornson et al. 2005). These cells in culture can then be used for a whole variety of laboratory-based experimentation, which is outwith the scope of this article.

Genetic studies

Many studies investigating genetic influences on the development of diabetic nephropathy have been marred by small sizes and inappropriate groups. Very large numbers of subjects are required and several DNA collections have now been established (Pettersson-Fernholm et al. 2004; Patel et al. 2005; Prevost et al. 2005). Care must be taken to ensure that probands actually have nephropathy: individuals must have proteinuria rather than microalbuminuria and also have retinopathy, so as to exclude non-diabetic renal disease. Selection of control subjects without nephropathy is more problematic as it is impossible to be sure that an individual will never develop diabetic kidney disease. A minimum duration of diabetes of 20 years is essential. Even then, there is a risk of microalbuminuria developing (Arun et al. 2003).

Provocation tests

Exercise

A standardised exercise test may unmask high rates of albumin excretion in individuals with normal UAER at rest, although the long-term significance of this is controversial (Bognetti et al. 1994; O'Brien et al. 1995).

Protein load

A protein load, given as a high-protein standard meal or infusion of amino acids, causes renal arteriolar vasodilatation, increased GFR and natriuresis (Brenner et al. 1982).

A number of groups have used protein loading ($100\,g$ of ground meat per $1.73\,m^2$ (Fioretto et al. 1990) or egg and meat (Chan et al. 1988)) in an attempt to clarify the haemodynamic abnormalities in diabetes.

Drug manipulation

Changes in kidney function after drug administration have helped our understanding of the haemodynamic abnormalities in diabetes. Angiotensin converting enzyme inhibitors, angiotensin II receptor 1 blockers and prostaglandin inhibitors have all been used.

Functional magnetic resonance imaging and spectroscopy

Functional magnetic resonance imaging (MRI) has great potential as a non-invasive tool for investigating glomerular filtration, tubular concentration and transit, blood volume and perfusion, diffusion and oxygenation (Grenier et al. 2003). Either endogenous (water protons for perfusion and diffusion, deoxyhaemoglobin for oxygenation) or exogenous (gadolinium for filtration and perfusion, iron oxide particles for perfusion) contrast agents are required. Limitations arise from the mobility of the kidney, difficulties in reproducibility and difficulties in determining the origin of the signal changes. Measurement of GFR, using a variety of mathematical models, has been reported but its precision is as yet unclear (Annet et al. 2004; Hermoye et al. 2004). Preliminary animal work suggests that MRI may provide a noninvasive method of measuring the sodium concentration gradient along the corticomedullary axis (Maril et al. 2004). Attempts have been made to determine renal blood flow using MRI with gadolinium contrast and the breath-holding technique (King et al. 2003; Di Cobelli et al. 2004; Zhang & Prince 2004) or ungated spiral phase-contrast MRI (Park et al. 2005). However, all these techniques require further evaluation. Figure 18.1 shows a 3D reconstruction of the aorta, renal arteries and kidneys following contrast agent administration. This dataset has a resolution of $0.8 \times 0.8 \times 1.5$ mm and was acquired in a single breath-hold. Figure 18.2 illustrates differentiation of cortex and medulla after contrast.

MRS and MRI may also provide details on renal metabolism (Kugel et al. 2000; Baverel et al. 2003; Tugnoli et al. 2003) and may be able to detect changes in content of metabolites, which can reflect disease states (Nurenberg et al. 2002; Economides et al. 2004; Hirayama et al. 2005; Serkova et al. 2005; Sonta et al. 2005). Quantification of urine GAGs and other proteins and enzymes by magnetic resonance spectroscopy has been attempted (Hauet et al. 2000). Changes in tissue oxygenation can be visualised with MRI via blood oxygen level-dependent (BOLD) contrast. Intrarenal R_2^* measurements are closely related to deoxyhaemoglobin concentration (Prasad et al. 1996, 1997; Mason 2006). Although R_2^* values cannot directly report on pO_2, dynamic changes after physiological or pharmacological intervention (Prasad & Epstein 1999; Hofmann et al. 2006; Tumkur et al. 2006) can identify abnormal kidney responses. Hyperglycaemia, decreased bioavailability of nitric oxide and increased oxidative stress may all contribute to increased oxygen consumption, exacerbating medullary hypoxia (Palm 2006). Medullary oxygen consumption during water diuresis does not increase in type 2 diabetic patients (Epstein et al. 2002; Economides et al. 2004).

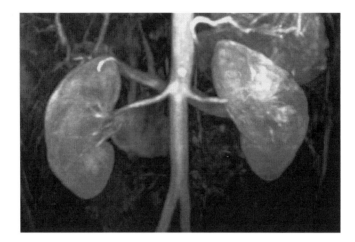

Figure 18.1 3D reconstruction of the aorta, renal arteries and kidneys following contrast agent administration. With kind permission of Dr P. Thelwell, University of Newcastle upon Tyne.

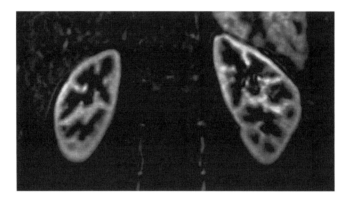

Figure 18.2 Differentiation of cortex and medulla after contrast. With kind permission of Dr P. Thelwell, University of Newcastle upon Tyne.

Conclusion

Many standard techniques are currently available for studying kidney function in diabetes, although they must be used in carefully selected and characterised clinical populations. The development and application of newer techniques may aid investigation and further our understanding.

References

Anderson S, Blouch K, Bialek J, Deckert M, Parving HH, Myers BD (2000) Glomerular permselectivity in early stages of overt diabetic nephropathy *Kidney Int* **58**, 2129–2137

Annet L, Hermoye L, Peeters F, Jamar F, Dehoux JP, Van beers BE (2004) Glomerular filtration rate, an assessment with dynamic contrast-enhanced MRI and a cortical-compartment model in the rabbit kidney *J Magn Reson Imaging* **20**, 843–849

Arun CS, Stoddart J, Mackin P, MacLeod JM, New JP, Marshall SM (2003) Significance of microal-buminuria in long-duration type 1 diabetes *Diabetes Care* **26**, 2144–2149

Baverel G, Conjard A, Chauvin MF, Vercoutere B, Vittorelli A, Dubourg L et al. (2003) Carbon 13NMR spectroscopy, a powerful tool for studying renal metabolism *Biochimie* **85**, 863–871

Berger EY, Farber SJ, Earle DP (1948) Comparison of the constant infusion and urine collection techniques for the measurement of renal function *J Clin Invest* **27**, 710–716

Bilous RW, Mauer SM, Sunderland DE, Steffes MW (1989) Mean glomerular volume and rate of development of diabetic nephropathy *Diabetes* **38**, 1142–1147

Bjornson A, Moses J, Ingemansson A, Haraldsson B, Sorensson J (2005) Primary human glomerular endothelial cells produce proteoglycans, and puromycin affects their posttranslational modification *Am J Physiol Renal Physiol* **288**, F748–756

Blouch K, Deen WM, Fauvel JP, Bialek J, Derby G, Myers BD (1997) Molecular configuration and glomerular size-selectivity in healthy and nephritic humans *Am J Physiol* **273**, F430–437

Bognetti E, Meschi F, Pattarini A, Zoja A, Chiumello G (1994) Post–exercise albuminuria does not predict microalbuminuria in type 1 diabetic patients *Diabetic Med* **11**, 850–855

Bohrer MP, Patterson GD, Carroll PJ (1984) Hindered diffusion of dextran and Ficoll in microporous membranes *Macromolecules* **17**, 1170–1173

Brenner BM, Meyer TW, Hostetter TH (1982) Dietary protein intake and the progression of kidney disease, the role of haemodynamically mediated glomerular injury and the pathogenesis of progressive glomerular sclerosis in aging, renal ablation and intrinsic renal disease *N Engl J Med* **307**, 652–659

Buysschaert M, Joudi I, Wallemacq P, Hermans MP (2003) Comparative performance of serum cystatin C versus serum creatinine in diabetic subjects *Diabetes Metab* **29**, 377–383

Chan AY, Cheng ML, Keil LC, Myers BD (1988) Functional response of healthy and diseased glomeruli to a large, protein-rich meal *J Clin Invest* **81**, 245–254

Christensson AG, Grubb AO, Nilsson JA, Norrgren K, Sterner G, Sundkvist G (2004) Serum cystatin C advantageous compared with serum creatinine in the detection of mild but not severe diabetic nephropathy *J Intern Med* **256**, 510–518

Ciavarella A, Flammini M, Stefoni S, Borgnino LC, Forlani G, Bacci L, Vannini P (1982) Kidney function after improved metabolic control in newly diagnosed diabetes and in diabetic patients with nephropathy *Diabetes Care* **5**, 624–629

Collins AC, Sethi M, MacDonald FA, Brown D, Viberti GC (1993) Storage temperature and differing methods of sample preparation in the measurement of microalbuminuria *Diabetologia* **36**, 993–997

Dalla Vestra M, Masiero A, Roiter AM, Saller A, Crepaldi G, Fioretto P (2003) Is podocyte injury relevant in diabetic nephropathy? Studies in patients with type 2 diabetes *Diabetes* **52**, 1031–1035

Davidson MG, Deen WM (1988) Hindered diffusion of water-soluble macromolecules in membranes *Macromolecules* **21**, 3474–3481

Deckert T, Feldt-Rasmussen B, Djurup R, Deckert M (1988) Glomerular size-and charge-selectivity in insulin–dependent diabetes mellitus *Kidney Int* **33**, 100–106

De Muro P, Fresu P, Formato M, Tonolo G, Mameli M, Maioli M, Sanna GM, Cherchi GM (2002) Urinary glycosaminoglycan and proteoglycan excretion in normoalbuminuric patients with type 1 diabetes mellitus *J Nephrol* **15**, 290–296

Denton MD, Marsden PA, Luscinskas FW, Brenner BM, Brady HR (1991) Cytokine-induced phagocyte adhesion to human mesangial cells, role of CD11/CD18 integrins and ICAM-1 *Am J Physiol* **261**, F1071–F1079

Di Cobelli F, Fiorina P, Perseghin G, Magnone M, Venturini M, Zerbini G et al. (2004) L-arginine-induced vasodilation of the renal vasculature is preserved in uremic type 1 diabetic patients after kidney and pancreas but no after kidney-alone transplant *Diabetes Care* **27**, 947–954

Di Mario U, Morano S, Cancelli A, Bacci S, Frontoni S, Pietravalle P, Gambardella S, Andreani D (1989) New parameters to monitor the progression of diabetic nephropathy *Am J Kidney Dis* **13**, 45–48

Earle DP, Berliner RW (1946) A simplified clinical procedure for measurement of glomerular filtration rate and renal plasma flow *Proc Soc Exp Biol Med* **62**, 262–264

Economides PA, Caselli A, Zuo CS et al. (2004) Kidney oxygenation during water diuresis and endothelial function in patients with type 2 diabetes and subjects at risk to develop diabetes *Metabolism* **53**, 222–227

Economides PA, Caselli A, Zuo CS, Sparks C, Khaodhiar L, Katsilambros N et al. (2004) Kidney oxygenation during water diuresis and endothelial function in patients with type 2 diabetes and subjects at risk to develop diabetes *Metabolism* **53**, 222–227

Epstein FH, Veves A, Prasad PV (2002) Effect of diabetes on renal medullary oxygenation during water diuresis *Diabetes Care* **25**, 575–578

Fioretto P, Trevisan R, Valerio A, Avogaro A, Borsato M, Doria A, Semplicini A, Sacerdoti D, Jones S, Bognetti E et al. (1990) Impaired renal response to a meat meal in insulin–dependent diabetes, role of glucagon and prostaglandins *Am J Physiol* **258**, F675–F683

Fioretto P, Trevisan R, Valerio A, Avogaro A, Borsato M, Rodia A et al. (1990) Impaired renal response to a meat meal in insulin-dependent diabetes, role of glucagon and prostaglandins *Am J Physiol* **258**, F675–F683

Florijn KW, Barendregt JNM, Lentjes EGWM et al. (1994) Glomeurlar filtration rate measurement by 'single shot' injection of inulin *Kidney Int* **45**, 252–259

Gaspari F, Mosconi L, Vigano G et al. (1992) Measurement of GFR with a single intravenous injection of nonradioactive iothalamate *Kidney Int* **41**, 1081–1084

Gaspari F, Perico N, Ruggenenti P, Mosconi L, Amuchastegui CS, Guerini E, Daina E, Remuzzi G (1995) Plasma clearance of nonradioactive iohexol as a measure of glomerular filtration rate *J Amer Soc Nephrol* **6**, 1–7

Ghiggeri GM, Candiano G, Delfino G, Queirolo C (1985) Electrical charge of serum and urinary albumin in normal and diabetic humans *Kidney Int* **28**, 168–177

Giampietro O, Penne G, Clerico A, Cruschelli L, Cecere M (1993) How and how long to store urine samples before albumin radioimmunoassay, a practical response *Clin Chem* **39**, 533–536

Gibb DM, Tomlinson PA, Dalton NR, Turner C, Shah V, Barratt TM (1989) Renal tubular proteinuria and microalbuminuria in diabetic patients *Arch Dis Child* **64**, 129–134

Ginevri F, Piccotti E, Alinovi R, DeToni T, Biagini C, Chiggeri GM, Gusmano R (1993) Reversible tubular proteinuria precedes microalbuminuria and correlates with the metabolic status in diabetic children *Pediatr Nephrol* **7**, 23–26

Grenier N, Basseau F, Reis M, Tyndal B, Jones R, Moonen C (2003) Functional MRI of the kidney *Abdom Imaging* **28**, 164–175

Harmoinen AP, Kouri TT, Wirta OR, Lehtimaki TJ, Rantalaiho V, Turjanmaa VM, Pasternack AI (1999) Evaluation of plasma cystatin C as a marker for glomerular filtration rate in patients with type 2 diabetes *Clin Nephrol* **52**, 363–370

Harmoinen A, Lehtimaki T, Korpela M, Turjanmaa V, Saha H (2003) Diagnostic accuracies of plasma creatinine, cystatin C and glomerular filtration rate calculated by the Cockcrof-Gault and Levy formulas *Cli Chem* **49**, 1223–1225

Hauet T, Gibelin H, Richer JP, Godart C, Eugene M, Carretier M (2000) Influence of retrieval conditions on renal medulla injury, evaluation by proton NMR spectroscopy in an isolated perfused pig kidney model *J Surg Res* **93**, 1–8

Hellerstein S, Berembom M, Alon U, Warady BA (1993) The renal clearance and infusion clearance of inulin are similar but not identical *Kidney Int* **44**, 1058–1061

Hermoye L, Annet L, Lemmerling P, Peeters F, Jamar F, Gianello P et al. (2004) Calculation of the renal perfusion and glomerular filtration rate from the renal impulse response obtained with MRI *Magn Reson Med* **51**, 1017–1025

Hirayama A, Nagase S, Ueda A, Oteki T, Takada K, Obara M et al. (2005) In vivo imaging of oxidative stress in ischaemia–reperfusion renal injury using electron paramagnetic resonance *Am J Physiol Renal Physiol* **288**, F597–603

Hofmann L, Simon–Zoula S, Nowak A et al. (2006) BOLD–MRI for the assessment of renal oxygenation in humans, acute effect of nephrotoxic xenobiotics *Kidney Int* **70**, 144–150

Hostetter TH, Meyer TW (2004) The development of clearance methods for measurement of glomerular filtration and tubular reabsorption *Am J Renal Physiol* **287**, F868–870

Innanen VT, Groom BM, de Campos FM (1992) Microalbumin and freezing *Clin Chem* **43**, 1093–1094

Isaka Y, Fujiwara Y, Yamamoto S et al. Modified plasma clearance technique using nonradioactive iothalamate for measuring GFR *Kidney Int* **42**, 1006–1011

Katz–Brull R, Rofsky NM, Lenkinski RE (2003) Breathhold abdominal and thoracic proton MR Spectroscopy at 3T *Magn Reson Med* **50**, 461–467

Keen H, Chlouverakis G (1963) An immunoassay method for urine albumin at low concentrations *Lancet* **186**, 913–914

King BF, Torres VE, Brummer ME, Chapman AB, Bae KT, Glockner JF et al. (2003) Magnetic resonance measurements of renal blood flow as a marker of disease severity in autosomal–dominant polycystic kidney disease *Kidney Int* **64**, 2214–2221

Krutzen E, Back SE, Nilsson-Ehle I, Nilsson-Ehle P (1984) Plasma clearance of a new contrast agent, iohexol, A method for the assessment of glomerular filtration rate *J Lab Clin Med* **104**, 955–961

Kugel H, Wittsack H-J, Wenzel F, Stippel D, Heindel W, Lackner K (2000) Non-invasive determination of metabolite concentrations in human transplanted kidney in vivo by 31P MR *Acta Radiol* **41**, 634–641

Kverneland A, Feldt-Rasmussen B, Vidal P, Welinder B, Bent-hansen L, Soegaard U, Deckert T (1986) Evidence of changes in renal charge selectivity in patients with type 1 (insulin-dependent) diabetes mellitus *Diabetologia* **29**, 634–639

Laterza OF, Price CP, Scott MG (2002) Cystatin C, an improved estimator of glomerular filtration rate? *Clin Chem* **48**, 699–707

Levey AS, Bosch JP, Lewis JB, Greene T, Rogers N, Roth D (1999) for the modification of Diet in renal disease Study Group A more accurate method to estimate glomerular filtration rate from serum creatinine, a new prediction equation *Ann Intern Med* **130**, 461–470

MacLeod JM, Lutale J, Marshall SM (1995) Albumin excretion and vascular deaths in type 2 diabetes *Diabetologia* **38**, 610–616

Maril N, Margalit R, Mispelter J, Degani H (2004) Functional sodium magnetic resonance imaging of the intact rat kidney *Kidney Int* **65**, 927–935

Mason RP (2006) Non-invasive assessment of kidney oxygenation, a role for BOLD MRI *Kidney Int* **70**, 10–11

Mathiesen ER, Ronn B, Jensen T, Storm B, Deckert T (1990) Relationship between blood pressure and urinary albumin excretion in development of microalbuminuria *Diabetes* **39**, 245–249

Matsumoto N, Ishimura E, Taniwaki H, Eoto M, Shoji T, Kawagishi T, Inaba M, Nishizawa Y (2000) Diabetes mellitus worsens intrarenal hemodynamic abnormalities in nondialyzed patients with chronic renal failure *Nephron* **86**, 44–51

McAuliffe AV, Fisher EJ, McLennan SV, Yue DK, Turtle JR (1996) Urinary glycosaminoglycan excretion in NIDDM subjects, its relationship to albuminuria *Diabetic Med* **13**, 758–763

Microalbuminuria Collaborative Study Group (1999) Predictors of the development of microalbuminuria in patients with type 1 diabetes mellitus, a seven year prospective study *Diabetic Med* **16**, 918 925

Mundel P, Reiser J, Kriz W (1997) Induction of differentiation in cultured rat and human podocytes *J Amer Soc Nephrol* **8**, 697–705

Mussap M, Dalla Vestra M, Fioretto P, Saller A, Varagnolo M, Nosadini R, Plebani M (2002) Cystatin C is a more sensitive marker than creatinine for the estimation of GFR in type 2 diabetic patients *Kidney Int* **61**, 1453–1461

Myers BD, Nelson RG, Blough K, Bennett PH, Knowler WC, Ming T, Beck G, Mitch WE (1995) Progression of overt nephropathy in non-insulin-dependent diabetes *Kidney Int* **47**, 1781–1789

Nakamura Y, Myers BD (1988) Charge-selectivity of proteinuria in diabetic glomerulopathy *Diabetes* **37**, 1202–1211

Nurenberg P, Sartoni-D'Ambrosia G, Szezepaniak LS (2002) Magnetic resonance spectroscopy of renal and other retroperitoneal tumours *Curr Opin Urol* **12**, 375–380

O'Brien SF, Watts GF, Powrie JK, Shaw KM (1995) Exercise testing as a long-term predictor of the development of microalbuminuria in normoalbuminuric IDDM patients *Diabetes Care* **18**, 1602–1605

Oddoze C, Morange S, Portugal H, Berland Y, Dussol B (2001) Cystatin C is not more sensitive than creatinine for detecting early renal impairment in patients with diabetes *Am J Kidney Dis* **38**, 310–316

Oliver JD, Anderson S, Troy JL, Brenner BM, Deen WM (1992) Determination of glomerular size-selectivity in the normal rat with Ficoll *J Am Soc Nephrol* **3**, 214–228

Orlando R, Floreani M, Padrini R, Palatini P (1998) Determination of inulin clearance by bolus intravenous injection in healthy subjects and ascitic patients, equivalence of systemic and renal clearances as glomerular filtration markers Br *J Clin Pharmacol* **46**, 605–609

Østerby R, Parving HH, Hommel E Jorgensen HE, Lokkegaard H (1990) Glomerular structure and function in diabetic nephropathy Early to advanced stages *Diabetes* **39**, 1057–1063

Palm F (2006) Intrarenal oxygen in diabetes and a possible link to diabetic nephropathy *Clin Exper Pharmacol Physiol* **33**, 997–1001

Park JB, Santos JM, Hargreaves BA, Nayak KS, Sommer G, Hu BS, Nishimura DG (2005) Rapid measurement of renal artery blood flow with ungated spiral phase-contrast MRI J *Magn Reson Imaging* **21**, 590–595

Patel A, Scott WR, Lympany PA, Rippin JD, Gill GV, Barnett AH, Bain SC (2005) Warren 3/UK GoKind Study Group The TGF-beta 1 gene codon 10 polymorphism contributes to the genetic predisposition to nephropathy in Type 1 diabetes *Diabetic Med* **22**, 69–73

Perkins BA, Ficociello LH, Silva KH, Finkelstein DM, Warram JH, Krolewski AS (2003) Regression of microalbuminuria in type 1 patients *N Engl J Med* **348**, 2285–2293

Perkins BA, Nelson RG, Ostrander BE, Blouch KL, Krolewski AS, Myers BD, Warram JH (2005) Detection of renal function decline in patients with diabetes and normal or elevated GFR by serial measurements of serum cystatin C concentration, results of a 4-year follow-up study *J Am Soc Nephrol* **16**, 1404–1412

Pettersson–Fernholm KJ, Forsblom CM, Perola M, Fagerudd JA, Groop PH' FinnDiane Study Group (2004) Dopamine D3 receptor gene polymorphisms, blood pressure and nephropathy in type 1 diabetic patients *Nephrol Dial Transplant* **19**, 1432–1436

Prasad PV, Chen Q, Goldfarb JW et al. (1997) Breath-hold R2* mapping with a multiple gradient–recalled echo sequence, application to the evaluation of intrarenal oxygenation *J Magn Reson Imaging* **7**, 1163–1165

Prasad PV, Edelmann RR, Epstein FH (1996) Noninvasive evaluation of intrarenal oxygenation with BOLD MRI *Circulation* **94**, 3271–3275

Prasad PV, Epstein FH (1999) Changes in renal medullary pO2 during water diuresis as evaluated by blood oxygenation level-dependent magnetic resonance imaging, effects of aging and cyclooxygenase inhibition *Kidney Int* **55**, 294–298

Prevost G, Fajardy I, Besmond C, Balkau B, Tichet J, Fontaine P et al. (2005) Polymorphisms of the receptor of advanced glycation endproducts (RAGE) and the development of nephropathy in type 1 diabetic patients *Diabetes Metab* **31**, 35–39

Radermacher J, Mengel M, Ellis S, Stuht S, Hiss M, Schwarz A, Eisenberger U, Burg M, Luft FC, Gwinner W, Haller H (2003) The renal arterial resistance index and renal allograft survival *N Engl J Med* **10**(349), 115–124

Royal College of Physicians of Edinburgh Diabetes Register Group (2000) Near-normal urinary albumin concentrations predict progression to diabetic nephropathy in type 1 diabetes mellitus *Diabetic Med* **17**, 782–791

Saleem MA, O'Hare MJ, Reiser J, Coward RJ, Inward CD, Farren T et al. (2002) A conditionally immortalised human podocyte cell line demonstrating nephrin and podocin expression *J Am Soc Nephrol* **13**, 630–638

Sambataro M, Thomaseth K, Pacini G, Robaudo C, Carraro A, Bruseghin M, Brocco E, Abaterusso C, DeFerrari G, Fioretto P, Maioli M, Tonolo GC, Crepaldi G, Nosadini R (1996) Plasma clearance rate of 51Cr-EDTA provides a precise and convenient technique for measurement of glomerular filtration rate in diabetic humans *J Am Soc Nephrol* **7**, 118–127

Scandling JD, Myers BD (1992) Glomerular size-selectivity and microalbuminuria in early diabetic glomerular disease *Kidney Int* **41**, 840–846

Schultz CJ, Dalton RN, Neil HA, Konopelska-Bahu T, Dunger DB, Oxford Regional Prospective Study Group (2001) Markers of renal tubular dysfunction measured annually do not predict risk of microalbuminuria in the first few years after diagnosis of Type 1 diabetes *Diabetologia* **44**, 224–229

Schultz CJ, Dalton RN, Turner C, Neil HA, Dunger DB (2000) Freezing method affects the concentration and variability of urine proteins and the interpretation of data on microalbuminuria: The Oxford Regional Prospective Study Group *Diabetic Med* **17**, 7–14

Serkova N, Fuller TF, Klawitter J, Freise CE, Niemann CU (2005) H-NMR-based metabolic signatures of mild and severe ischaemia/reperfusion injury in rat kidney transplants *Kidney Int* **67**, 1142–1151

Sonta T, Inoguchi T, Matsumoto S, Yasukawa K, Inuo M, Tsubouchi H et al. (2005) In vivo imaging of oxidative stress in the kidney of diabetic mice and its normalisation by angiotensin II type 1 receptor blocker *Biochem Biophys Res Commun* **330**, 415–422

Steinke JM, Sinaiko AR, Kramer MS, Suissa S, Chavers BM, Mauer M, International Diabetic Nephropathy Study Group (2005) The early natural history of nephropathy in Type 1 diabetes, III Predictors of 5-year urinary albumin excretion rate patterns in initially normoalbuminuric patients *Diabetes* **54**, 2164–2171

Tan GD, Lewis AV, James TJ, Altmann P, Taylor RP, Levy JC (2002) Clinical usefulness of cystatin C for the estimation of glomerular filtration rate in type 1 diabetes, reproducibility and accuracy compared with standard measures and iohexol clearance *Diabetes Care* **25**, 2004–2000

Taniwaki H, Nishizawa Y, Kawagishi T, Ishimura E, Emoto M, Okamura T, Okuno Y, Morii H (1998) Decrease in glomerular filtration rate in Japanese patients with type 2 diabetes is linked to atherosclerosis *Diabetes Care* **21**, 1848–1855

Thomsen K, Holstein-Rathlou NH, Leyssal PP (1981) Comparison of three measures of proximal tubular reabsorption, lithium clearance, occlusion time and micropuncture *Am J Physiol* **214**, F348–355

Tugnoli V, Bottura G, Fini G, Reggiani A, Tinti A, Trinchero A, Tosi MR (2003) 1H-NMR and 13C–NMR lipid profiles of human renal tissues *Biopolymers* **72**, 86–95

Tumkur SM, Vu AT, Li LP et al. (2006) Evaluation of intra-renal oxygenation during water diuresis *Kidney Int* **70**, 139–143

Van Acker B, Koomen GCM, Arisz L (1995) Drawbacks of the constant-infusion technique for measurement of renal function *Am J Physiol* **268**, F543–552

White KE, Bilous RW, Marshall SM, El Nahas M, Remuzzi G, Piras G et al. (2002) Podocyte number in normotensive type 1 diabetic patients with albuminuria *Diabetes* **51**, 3083–3089

Yokoyama H, Sato K, Okudaira M, Morita C, Takahashi C, Suzuki S, Sakai H, Iwamoto Y (1999) Serum and urinary concentrations of heparin sulphate in patients with diabetic nephropathy *Kidney Int* **56**, 650–658

Zhang H, Prince MR (2004) Renal MR angiography *Magn Reson Imaging Clin N Am* **12**, 487–503

19

Techniques for the Investigation of the Eye in Diabetes

Ayad Al-Bermani and **Roy Taylor**

Introduction

Diabetes mellitus exerts several damaging effects on the eye. It can cause cataract, optical nerve head swelling, extra ocular muscle palsies by occlusion of the microvascular circulation of relevant cranial nerves and diabetic retinopathy. Cataract can be successfully dealt with by surgery, diabetic papillitis and extraocular muscle palsies are usually self limiting, but diabetic retinopathy is a leading cause of blindness in the Western world (Klein 1988), even though this blindness can be prevented. Indeed, it is the commonest preventable cause of registered blindness in the UK amongst the working age population (Evans et al. 1996).

Screening for diabetic retinopathy is essential, as the Early Treatment Diabetic Retinopathy Study (ETDRS) has shown that the risk of severe visual loss may be reduced by 50–90 % when retinal photocoagulation is applied in patients with high-risk proliferative retinopathy and/or clinically significant macular oedema (ETDRS 1991a).

Cost-effective screening for diabetic retinopathy has become even more important as the incidence of type 1 and type 2 diabetes is increasing (Green et al. 1992, 1996; Amos et al. 1997). More advanced techniques for examining and investigating the eye in diabetes have been developed, to facilitate early and successful detection of sight-threatening changes due to diabetic retinopathy.

This chapter describes techniques used in research on the abnormalities which characterise the eye in diabetes.

Visual acuity

This is the simplest and most important measurement of visual function. In common with other simple measurements, it is simple to do it badly. Careful attention to detail is essential for accurate measurements. The test assesses the optics of the eye, the retina and the central nervous mechanism subserving the foveal region. It is determined by the smallest retinal

Clinical Diabetes Research: Methods and Techniques   Edited by Michael Roden
© 2007 John Wiley & Sons, Ltd   ISBN 978-0-470-01728-9

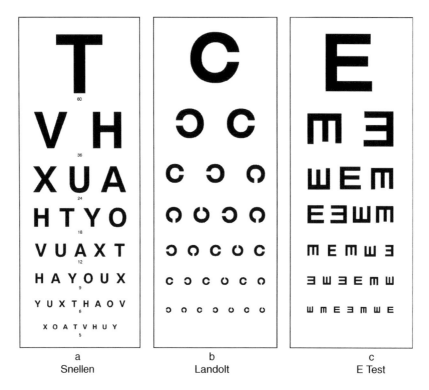

a	b	c
Snellen	Landolt	E Test

Figure 19.1 a) the Snellen chart; Reproduced with permission from Lueck CJ, Gilmour DF, McIlwaine GG (2004) Neuro-opthamology: examination and investigation, *J Neuro, Neurosurg Psych*, BMJ Publishing Group Ltd. b) & c) alternatives for individuals who would find it difficult to name letters.

image that can be appreciated and is measured as the smallest object seen clearly at a certain distance. In order to discriminate the form of an object, its parts must be differentiated. The most popular methods for testing visual acuity are:

The Snellen chart

This chart is named after a Dutch ophthalmologist (1834–1908). It consists of a series of letters of diminishing size as in Figure 19.1a. Each letter has an overall size five times the thickness of the lines composing the letter.

The results of the test are expressed as a fraction, in which the numerator is the testing distance (6 m) and the denominator is the distance at which a normal observer would be able to read the letter. Other test types, which are designed to be applicable to any nationality and to illiterate subjects, as in Figure 19.1b & c, follow the same principle.

The test types should be clearly printed, legible and uniformly illuminated. The patient should be sat at six metres, or at three metres using a reverse test type placed above the patient's head and observed as a reflection in a mirror hung on the opposite wall.

A new design of visual acuity chart has recently emerged: an example, the Bailey-Lovie chart (Bailey & Lovie 1976), is shown in Figure 19.2. This improved design has several advantages. First, the letters used are of approximately equal detectability, whereas earlier charts had some letters that were more legible than others. Second, each line has an equal

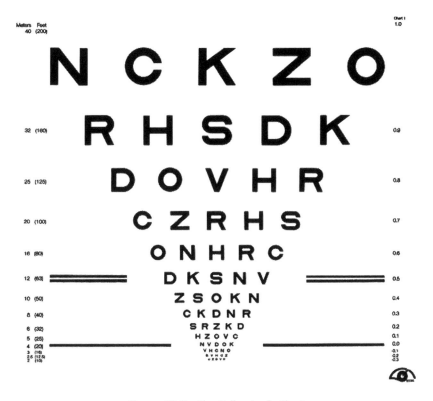

Figure 19.2 The Bailey-Lovie Chart

number of letters, as compared with earlier charts with only one or two letters for the 6/60 and 6/36 visual acuity lines, and a large number of letters for the 6/6 and smaller visual acuity lines. Third, the spacing between letters is proportional to the letter size, while the older acuity charts had unequal spacing between letters. Finally, the change in visual acuity from one line to another is in equal logarithmic steps, where there were very small changes for different lines at the small-letter end and rather large changes for the big-letter end of the older charts. This new eye chart permits more precise definition of visual acuity, especially at levels of diminished visual acuity. It is thus used in the current UK national study of photodynamic therapy in age related macular degeneration (TAP study group 1999; Bames et al. 2004). In addition, new methods of scoring responses to this type of visual acuity chart can provide greater sensitivity and reliability of measure. The ETDRS visual acuity chart is based on the design of this new eye chart.

One of the most important factors in testing visual acuity is the human interface. The tester must be competent at ensuring full and precise communication of what the subject can see. Patients should always be tested with their most updated glasses or with a pin hole.

Fluorescein angiography of the fundus

No other single technique has had more impact on retinal investigation than fundus photography with the dye fluorescein. It has contributed to the diagnosis and treatment of chorioretinal diseases, elucidated poorly understood retinal diseases and served as an indispensable research modality.

Sodium fluorescein is a yellow-red dye with a molecular weight of 376.67. It is used in 10 % or 25 % sterile aqueous solution. When injected, usually into the antecubital vein, 80 % of it is bound to plasma proteins, mainly albumin, and the remainder stays free. When subjected to blue light (wave length 465–490 nm) it absorbs photons. The molecule then emits green-yellow light (wave length 520–530 nm). This capability is called fluorescence. The fluoresein is eventually metabolised in the kidney and liver and eliminated in 24–36 hours.

A specially designed fundus camera with appropriate light filters is used. The pupil has to be dilated in order to obtain optimal images and the patient's cooperation is extremely important. The dye should be injected rapidly to maximise the contrast of the early filling phase, with precaution to avoid extravasation of the dye, which is very painful and may lead to tissue necrosis. The skin turns yellow for a few hours and the patient's urine may have an orange hue for a few days.

The dye first enters the short posterior ciliary arteries and is visualised in the choroid and optic nerve head 10–15 sec after the injection. The dye enters the choroidal lobules sequentially and appears initially patchy on the photograph, but as the choroidal filling completes, it gives rise to the choroidal flush. The retinal circulation begins 1–3 sec after the onset of choroidal filling, i.e. 11–18 sec after the injection. The dye does not cross the normal blood retina barrier. It does not cross Bruch's membrane, which separates the choroids from the retina; neither does it extravasate normal capillaries. The arterial filling is complete in one second. The early arteriovenous phase follows, with the dye in the central retinal artery, the precapillary arteriols and the capillaries; the late arteriovenous phase is characterised by the passage of the dye through the veins in a laminar pattern, as well as by maximal fluorescence in the arteries.

Maximal fluorescence is achieved in the juxtafoveal or perifoveal capillary network in 20–25 sec, as in Figure 19.3. This is called the peak phase.

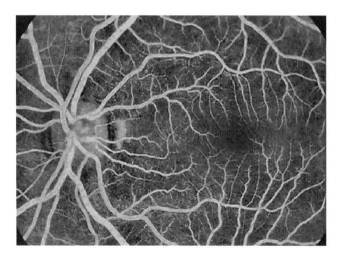

Figure 19.3 Peak phase at 25 Seconds

The normal capillary free zone is approximately 300–500 mu in diameter. The dark background to this zone in the macula is due to blockage of the choroidal fluorescence by the xanthophyll pigment and to the high density of the retinal pigment epithelial cells. The management of diabetic macular oedema requires an excellent peak phase series of images.

The first pass of fluorescein is complete at 30 sec and the dye recirculates giving rise to intermittent mild fluorescence. At 10 min the retinal and choroidal circulations are devoid of dye but the disc margins and the optic nerve head, Bruch's membrane, choroids and sclera remain stained.

Hypofluoresence is the term used whenever normal fluorescence is reduced either due to the masking effect of blood, exudate or any other retinal or choroidal pathology, such as chroidal naevus. It could also be due to vascular filling defect, as in retinal artery occlusion, or focal or extensive capillary drop out, as in proliferative diabetic retinopathy.

Hyperfluoresence is the term used whenever fluorescence is increased in an area either due to leakage, as in macular oedema, or due to a window defect that allows the choroidal fluorescence to show through an atrophic retina, as in macular degeneration. It can show as an area of pooling, as in pigment epithelial detachment (Rabb et al. 1978; Gass 1997).

In eyes with diabetes, fluorescein fundus angiography is particularly helpful in demonstrating leaking micro aneurysms, which helps in planning and carrying out laser treatment (Figure 19.4). It can demonstrate the status of the retinal vasculature, which may affect the decision for macula laser and pan retinal photocoagulation. From a research perspective, retinal circulation times, distribution of capillary filling and capillary permeability may each be quantified.

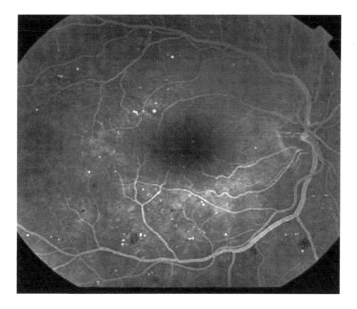

Figure 19.4 Background diabetic retinopathy demonstrating micro aneurysms. These leak in later sequences of the fluorescein angiography films. Other areas of vascular permeability are demonstrated on this film, especially below the fovea.

Optical coherence tomography (OCT)

This new technique for high-resolution cross-sectional imaging of various ocular structures was introduced in 1991. With an axial resolution of 10 mu, it provides the best resolution of retinal architecture of any imaging technique currently available. Information may be stored on computer disks and easily accessed in the future. This feature makes OCT particularly useful in the assessment, diagnosis and treatment of macular disease.

The limitations of OCT include the inability to obtain high-quality images through media opacities such as dense cataract or vitreous haemorrhage. The use of OCT is also limited to cooperative patients who are able to maintain fixation for the full acquisition time of 2.5 sec per section.

The operation of OCT is based on the principle of low coherence interferometry. In this technique, the sizes of and distances between structures in the eye are determined by measuring the 'echo' time for light to be backscattered from different structures at various axial distances. The imaging equipment can be attached to a standard slit-lamp or a specially designed fundus camera. Imaging is carried out without direct contact with the eye.

A light source projects a partially coherent light at a wavelength of 810 nm. For slit-lamp use, the light is focused with a standard mounted +78 diopter condensing lens and computer-operated scanning mirrors, onto the area of interest. The light beam is directed onto a partially reflective mirror (optical beam splitter). This mirror splits the light into two beams; one beam is directed into the patient's eye and is reflected from intraocular structures at various distances. This reflected beam consists of multiple echoes and provides information about the distance and thickness of various intraocular tissues. The second beam is reflected from a reference mirror at a known spatial location. This beam travels back to the beam splitter, where it combines with the optical beam reflected from the patient's eye. When the two light beams coincide, they produce a phenomenon known as interference, which is measured by a photodetector.

The beam of light reflected from the reference mirror coincides with the beam of light reflected from a given structure in a patient's eye only if both pulses arrive at the same time. This occurs when the distance that the light travels to and from the reference mirror equals the distance the light travels when it is reflected from a given intraocular structure. The position of the reference mirror can be adjusted so that the time delay of the reference light beam matches the time delay of the light echoes. Thus, the interferometer can precisely measure the echo delay of intraocular structures.

By measuring the echo delays of various intraocular structures, a translated axial image is produced. When successive axial measurements at different transverse points are combined, a tomographic or cross-sectional image of the tissue is obtained. OCT images are coloured to enhance differentiation of structures. Bright colours (red to white) correspond to tissues with high relative optical reflectivity, whereas darker colours (blue to black) correspond to areas of minimal or no optical reflectivity. Initial studies using postmortem eyes showed good correlation between OCT images and histological sections. Subsequent *in vivo* analyses demonstrated the ability of OCT to image the substructure of the retina. Figure 19.5 shows an OCT image of a normal fovea. The foveal centre demonstrates normal retinal thinning and has a characteristic pit to its contour. All retinal layers, choroid and sclera are well delineated.

The posterior aspect of the neurosensory retina is bounded in the OCT images by a highly reflective red layer about 70 mu thick that represents the choriocapillaris and retinal

OCT Image

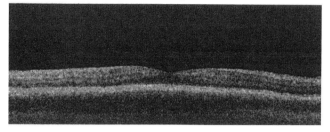

Figure 19.5 Normal Macula

pigment epithelium (RPE) layer. The high contrast between the choriocapillaris/RPE layer and the neural retina in OCT images provides a useful boundary for measurements of retinal thickness. The region just anterior to the choriocapillaris/RPE layer is typically weakly reflective and corresponds to the photoreceptor layer. The highly reflective yellow layer at the inner margin of the retina corresponds to the nerve fibre layer. Because retinal detail is so exquisitely imaged by OCT, this imaging modality can be applied to a large number of clinical entities. What is most interesting here is the assessment of macular oedema (Huang et al. 1991; Swanson et al. 1993; Hee et al. 1995), with potential for serial observation during any therapeutic intervention.

OCT in macular oedema

OCT can quantitatively demonstrate quantitative evaluations of retinal thickness, which is usually caused by accumulation of intraretinal fluid. This can be measured to within 10 mu and can be followed serially, as in Figure 19.5.

Macular oedema is the leading cause of decreased vision in patients with diabetic retinopathy. Although 'clinically significant macular oedema' continues to be a clinical diagnosis, OCT can provide the clinician with additional useful information (Figure 19.6). OCT images can quantitatively measure the amount of retinal thickening present and be correlated

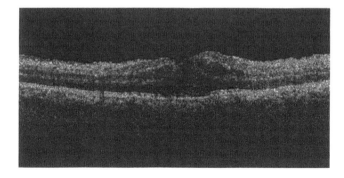

Figure 19.6 Macular Oedema The thickness is increased at the fovea.

with visual acuity. OCT can be used to follow the clinical response to focal laser treatment for clinically significant macular oedema.

A broad-bandwidth titanium sapphire laser has been used in preliminary studies to create cross-sectional images with a resolution of 3 mu and a reduced acquisition time of 2.5 seconds. Development of this technology would facilitate imaging of poorly cooperative patients.

Retinal imaging

In the ETDRS, assessment of diabeticretinopathy was based on seven field 30° stereo fundus photographs (ETDRS 1991b). Field 1 is centred on the optic disc, Field 2 is centred on the macula and Field 3 is just temporal to the macula. Fields 4–7 are tangential to horizontal lines passing through the upper and lower poles of the disc and to a vertical line passing through its centre (Figure 19.7).

This procedure may be unpleasant for the patient, time consuming and expensive for the community. It is therefore not ideal for large-scale screening programs. It has been shown that using two 45° fields per eye does not significantly alter the results but does reducing the cost, complexity and the time spent (Arun et al. 2003, In Press). Even single field 45° photography is highly effective in screening programmes (Taylor et al. 1990; Taylor 1996; Pandit & Taylor 2002; Arun et al. 2003).

The advent of digital computerised imaging has the potential to reduce the cost per patient and improve archiving and retrieval. Immediate reporting of images by trained technicians

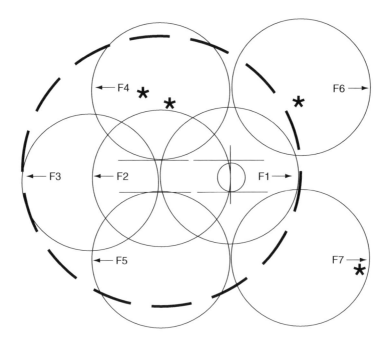

Figure 19.7 Seven standard fields (F1–F7) of the ETDRS protocol (shown for right eye) superimposed on one 60° fundus photograph (broken circle) centred on the macula. An asterisk indicates the location of each area of neovascularisation missed on the 60° photograph.

has been shown to be dramatically effective in screening for treatable sight-threatening diabetic retinopathy (Arun et al. 2006). Transfer of these images from screening to a referral centre can be achieved instantaneously if required. Delori et al. (1977) reported more accurate visualisation and documentation of the structures of the retina when using red-free green light than with the white light used to obtain colour photographs.

The efficacy of digital image acquisition, as compared to film-based acquisition, has been reported by several investigators. When comparing high-resolution stereoscopic digital fundus photography to contact lens biomicroscopy, Rudnisky et al. (2002) found a high level of agreement regarding the detection of clinically significant macular oedema in diabetic patients.

Scanlon et al. (2003) compared mydriatic and nonmydriatic photo screening programmes using dilated slit-lamp biomicroscopy as the reference standard. In the study of 3,611 patients, the sensitivity of mydriatic digital photography was 87.8 %, the specificity was 86.1 % and the technical failure rate was 3.7 %. Photography through an undilated pupil was found to provide a sensitivity of 86.0 %, a specificity of 76.6 % and a technical failure rate of 19.7 %. The authors concluded that while dilated digital photography is an effective method of screening for diabetic retinopathy, nonmydriatic photography has an unacceptable failure rate and low specificity.

For research purposes, sequential digital images can provide hard data on rates of change of retinopathy during any therapeutic intervention (Stratton et al. 2001; Arun et al. 2004, In Press; PKC-DRS Study Group 2005).

References

Amos AF, McCarty DJ, Zimmet P (1997) The rising global burden of diabetes and its complications: estimates and projections to year 2010 *Diabet Med* **14**, Suppl 5, S1–S85

Arun CS, Ngugi N, Lovelock L, Taylor R (2003) Effectiveness of screening in preventing blindness due to diabetic retinopathy *Diabet Med* **20**(3), 186–90

Arun CS, Pandit R, Taylor R (2004) Long term progression of retinopathy after initiation of insulin therapy in type 2 diabetes. *Diabetologia* **47**, 1380–84

Arun CS, Young D, Batey D, Shotton M, Mitchie D, Stannard K, Taylor R (2006) Establishing an ongoing quality assurance in retinal screening programme *Diabet Med* **23**, 629–634

Bailey IL, Lovie JE (1976) New design principles for visual acuity letter charts *Am J Optom Physiol Optics* **53**, 740–745

Barnes RM, Gee L, Taylor S, Briggs MC, Harding SP (2004) Outcomes in verteporfin photodynamic therapy for choroidal neovascularisation – 'beyond the TAP study' *Eye* **18**(8), 809–13

Delori FC, Gragoudas ES, Francisco R et al. (1977) Monochromatic ophthalmoscopy and fundus photography. The normal fundus *Arch Ophthalmol* **95**(5), 861–8

Early Treatment of Diabetic Retinopathy Study Group (1991a) Early photocoagulation for diabetic retinopathy: ETTRS report number 9 *Ophthalmology* **98**, 766–785

Early Treatment of Diabetic Retinopathy Study Group (1991b) Grading diabetic retinopathy from stereoscopic color fundus photographs – an extension of the modified Airlie House classification: ETDRS report number 10 *Ophthalmology* **98**, Suppl 5, 786–806

Evans J, Rooney C, Ashwood F, Dattani N, Wormald R (1996) Blindness and partial sight in England and Wales: April 1990 to March 1991 *Health Trends* **28**, 5–12

Gass JDM (1997) *Stereoscopic Atlas of Macular Diseases: Diagnosis and Treatment* 4Edn, Mosby-Year book, St Louise

Green A, Andersen PK, Svendsen AJ, Mortensen K (1992) Increasing incidence of early onset type 1 (insulin dependent) diabetes mellitus: a study of Danish male birth cohorts *Diabetologia* **35**, 178–82

Green A, Sjølie AK, Eshøj O (1996) Trends in the epidemiology of IDDM during 1970–2020 in Fyn County, Denmark *Diabetes Care* **19**, 801–6

Hee MR, Izatt JA, Swanson EA et al. (1995) Optical coherence tomography of the human retina *Arch Ophthalmol* **113**, 325

Huang D, Swanson EA, Lin CP et al. (1991) Optical coherence tomography *Science* **254**, 1,178

Klein R (1988) Recent developments in the understanding of diabetic retinopathy *Med Clin North Am* **72**, 1,415–33

Pandit RJ, Taylor R (2002) Quality assurance in screening for sight-threatening diabetic retinopathy *Diabet Med* **19**(4), 285–91

PKC-DRS Study Group (2005) The effect of ruboxistaurin on visual loss in patients with moderately severe to very severe nonproliferative diabetic retinopathy: initial results of the Protein Kinase C beta Inhibitor Diabetic Retinopathy Study (PKC-DRS) multicenter randomized clinical trial *Diabetes* **54**(7), 2,188–97

Rabb MF, Burton TC, Schatz H, Yannuzzi LA (1978) Fluorescein angiography of the fundus: a schematic approach to interpretation *Surv Ophthalmol* **22**, 387–403

Rudnisky CJ, Hinz BJ, Tennant MT et al. (2002) High-resolution stereoscopic digital fundus photography versus contact lens biomicroscopy for the detection of clinically significant macular edema *Ophthalmology* **109**(2), 267–74

Scanlon PH, Malhotra R, Thomas G et al. (2003) The effectiveness of screening for diabetic retinopathy by digital imaging photography and technician ophthalmoscopy *Diabet Med* **20**(6), 467–74

Stratton IM, Kohner EM, Aldington SJ, Turner RC, Holman RR, Manley SE et al. (2001) UKPDS 50: risk factors for incidence and progression of retinopathy in Type II diabetes over 6 years from diagnosis *Diabetologia* **44**(2), 156–63

Swanson EA, Izatt JA, Hee MR et al. (1993) In vivo retinal imaging by optical coherence tomography *Opt Lett* **18**, 1,864

TAP study group (1999) Photodynamic therapy of subfoveal choroidal neovascularisation in age-related macular degeneration with verteporfin. One-year results of 2 randomised clinical trials: TAP report 1 *Arch Ophthalmol* **117**, 1,329–45

Taylor R (1996) Practical community screening for diabetic retinopathy using the mobile retinal camera: report of a 12 centre study: British Diabetic Association Mobile Retinal Screening Group *Diabet Med* **13**(11), 946–52

Taylor R, Lovelock L, Tunbridge WM, Alberti KG, Brackenridge RG, Stephenson (1990) Comparison of non-mydriatic retinal photography with ophthalmoscopy in 2,159 patients: mobile retinal camera study *BMJ* **30**(6,763), 1,243–7

20

Basics of Molecular Genetics: Lessons from Type 2 Diabetes

Leif Groop and **Charlotte Ling**

Introduction

A disease can be inherited, acquired or both. While cystic fibrosis is an example of an inherited disease, most infectious diseases are acquired. But susceptibility to an infectious disease can be influenced by genetic factors. Heterozygous carriers of the mutation causing sickle cell anemia are resistant against malaria (Miller et al. 1975). A 32 basepair deletion in the gene encoding for the lymphoblastoid chemokine receptor (CCR5) was introduced into Europe by Yersina pestis during the plague in the fourteenth century (Stephens et al. 1998). Carriers of this deletion are today less susceptible to HIV infections.

Cystic fibrosis is caused by mutations in one gene, CTFR, and represents a monogenic disorder with early onset, usually from birth. The segregation of the disease follows a clear Mendelian recessive inheritance; in Europe one out of 2,000 children is affected. In contrast, a polygenic disease like type 2 diabetes is caused by 'mild' variations in several genes, shows a late onset and does not follow any clear Mendelian mode of inheritance. A polygenic disease is also referred to as 'complex' because of its complex inheritance pattern. A complex disease often appears to be acquired; the development of obesity and type 2 diabetes is triggered by environmental factors such as intake of dense caloric food and lack of exercise in genetically susceptible individuals. However, not all obese individuals develop diabetes; genetic susceptibility is a prerequisite. Given the complex interplay between genetic and environmental factors, a complex polygenic disease is also multifactorial.

Genetic risk

The relative genetic risk (λ_R) of an inherited disease is defined as the recurrence risk for a relative of an affected person divided by the risk for the general population; it can either be risk to a sibling (λ_S) or to an offspring (λ_O). The higher the λs, the easier is it to find (map) the genetic cause of the disease. The λs value for cystic fibrosis is approximately 500,

Clinical Diabetes Research: Methods and Techniques   Edited by Michael Roden
© 2007 John Wiley & Sons, Ltd   ISBN 978-0-470-01728-9

for type 1 diabetes, 15 and for type 2 diabetes, 3. It is therefore not surprising that cystic fibrosis was the first disease to be mapped by positional cloning or linkage analysis (Kerem et al. 1989), whereas success for type 2 diabetes has been limited (Florez et al. 2003). It may seem paradoxical that λ_S is higher for type 1 than for type 2 diabetes, as familial clustering (more than one affected member in a family) is stronger for type 2 than for type 1 diabetes (40 % vs 10 %). This is due to the much higher frequency of type 2 than of type 1 diabetes in the population. If several genetic factors contribute to the disease, it can be estimated how much of the λ_S value they each account for; in the case of type 1 diabetes, concordance at the HLA locus on the short arm of chromosome 6 explains about half of the λ_S value of 15. For type 2 diabetes, no genetic factor has been shown to explain more than 10–15 % of the λ_S value of 3.

The population attributable risk (PAR) is important from a public health perspective but it does not tell us anything about individual risk. It describes the fraction of a disease that would be eliminated if the genetic risk factor was removed from the population. The population attributable fraction (PAF) is high in monogenic rare disorders like cystic fibrosis (around 50) but low for rare alleles in complex diseases. If the disease-associated allele is common, PAF increases. This is illustrated by the role of the Apo ε4 allele in Alzheimer's disease and of the Pro12Ala polymorphism in the PPARγ gene in type 2 diabetes. The PAF for Apo ε4 in Alzheimer's disease is 20 % because of the high frequency of the Apo ε4 allele in the population (16 %). The PAF for the Pro12Ala polymorphism in the PPARγ gene is even higher, 25 %, as about 80 % of the general population carries the risk allele Pro.

Genetic variability

Mapping of an inherited disease requires identification of the genetic variability contributing to the disease. Such variability can take the form of deletions, insertions or changes in a single nucleotide in the genome (single nucleotide polymorphism – SNP). If a SNP results in a change in the amino acid sequence, it is called a non-synonymous SNP. There are about 10 million SNPs in the human 3 billion bp genome, which means one SNP at about 300 bp intervals. SNPs in coding sequences (exons) are seen at 1,250 bp intervals. Microsatellites are short tandem repeats of nucleotide sequences (e.g. CA) found at about 5,000 bp intervals. While SNPs are frequently bi-allelic, microsatellites have multiple alleles and are thus much more polymorphic than SNPs. Several public databases provide information on SNPs in different genes (e.g. www.ncbi.nlm.nig.gov/SNP). A SNP in a database is often referred to as dbSNP; at the moment (build 123), about 60 % of all SNPs are in public databases.

A SNP can either be the cause of a disease (causative SNP) or it can be a marker of a disease. The latter occurs when the disease susceptibility allele and the marker allele are so close to each other that they are inherited together, a situation called linkage disequilibrium (LD or allelic association). Such a combination of tightly linked alleles on a discrete chromosome is called a haplotype. While this region is characterised by little or no recombination (haplotype block), regions with high recombination rates usually separate haplotype blocks. LD thus describes the non-random correlation between alleles at a pair of SNPs; it is usually defined by D' or r^2 values. A D' value of 1 indicates that the two alleles are in complete LD, whereas values below 0.5 indicate low LD and a high recombination rate. LD extends over longer distances in isolated populations but is also seen more in European than in African populations. This is considered to reflect a population bottleneck at the time when humans first left Africa.

An international joint effort to create a genome-wide map of LD and haplotype blocks is called the HapMap project (http://www.hapmap.org/groups.html). The hope is that by knowing the haplotype block structure of the genome, one could capture the genetic variability of the genome by genotyping a much smaller number of SNPs that describe the haplotype block (haplotype tag or htg SNPs).

Mapping genetic variability

The aim of profiling genetic variation is to correlate biological variation (phenotype) with variation in DNA sequences (genotype). The ultimate goal of mapping genetic variability is to identify the SNP causing a monogenic disease or the SNPs increasing susceptibility to a polygenic disease. The most straightforward approach would be to sequence the whole genome in affected and unaffected individuals but this is for practical reasons not yet possible. Many indirect methods have been developed to achieve this goal, such as linkage and association approaches.

Linkage

The traditional way of mapping a disease gene has been to search for linkage between a chromosomal region and a disease by genotyping a large number (about 400–500) of polymorphic markers (microsatellites) in affected family members. If the affected family members share an allele more often than expected by non-random Mendelian inheritance, there is evidence of excess allele sharing. The most likely explanation for excess allele sharing is that a disease-causing gene is in close proximity to the genotyped marker. Ideally, such a genome-wide scan would be carried out in large pedigrees where mode of inheritance and penetrance are known. Since these parameters are not known and parents are rarely available in a complex disease with late onset, most genome-wide scans are performed in affected siblings, with no assumptions on mode of inheritance and penetrance (non-parametric linkage).

The LOD score defines the strength of linkage. This takes into account the recombination fraction (θ), which is the likelihood that a parent will produce a recombinant in an offspring. If the parental genotype is intact in the offspring, the recombination fraction is 0 (loci are linked); for completely unlinked loci it approaches 0.5. The probability test of linkage is called the LOD score (logarithm of odds). Two loci are considered linked when the probability of linkage as opposed to the probability against linkage is equal to or greater than the ratio of 1,000:1. A LOD score of 3 corresponds to an odds ratio of 1,000:1 ($p < 10^{-4}$). In a study of affected sibling pairs, a non-parametric LOD score (NPL) is presented. Although this threshold was developed for linkage mapping of monogenic disorders with complete information of genotype and phenotype, the situation for mapping complex disorders is much less straightforward. Lander & Kruglyak (1995) have proposed that the LOD threshold for significant genome-wide linkage should be raised to 3.6 ($p < 2 \times 10^{-5}$), while that for suggestive linkage (occurs one time at random in a genome-wide scan) can be set at 2.2 ($p < 7 \times 2^{-4}$). In addition, they suggest reporting all nominal p values <0.5 without any claim for linkage. In reality, each data set will have different thresholds based upon information on affection status, marker density, marker informativeness, etc. Therefore, these thresholds should be simulated with the existing data set before any claims of linkage are made.

Accuracy of genotyping and exclusion of Mendel errors are important for success, but so is the careful definition of affection status. This may not always be easy for diseases like asthma, schizophrenia or systematic lupus erythematosus (SLE). Even with diabetes, the definition is based upon artificial cut-offs of plasma glucose. Dichotomising variables may result in loss of power. One alternative is therefore to search for linkage to a qualitative trait, e.g. blood glucose, blood pressure or body mass index, instead of diabetes, hypertension and obesity. Heritability (h^2) is often used as a measure of the genetic component of a quantitative trait. The higher the heritability, the more likely it is a genetic cause of a trait will be found. Several statistical programmes have been developed to support genome-wide scans of quantitative trait loci (QTL), such as the variance component models SOLAR (www.sfbr.org/sfbr/public/software/solarR) and Merlin (www.sph.umich.edu/csg/abecasis/Merlin/tour). Linkage will only identify relatively large chromosomal regions (often >20 cM) with more than 100 genes. Fine mapping with additional markers can narrow the region further but eventually the causative SNP, or a SNP in LD with the causative SNP, has to be identified by an association study. Several approaches have been described to estimate whether an observed association can account for linkage (Li et al. 2004). Without functional support it is not always possible to know whether linkage and association represent the genetic cause of a disease. For many complex disorders, this can require a cumbersome sequence of *in vitro* and *in vivo* studies.

Calpain 10 and type 2 diabetes

In the first successful genome-wide scan of a complex disease like type 2 diabetes, Graeme Bell and co-workers reported significant linkage (LOD 4.1; $p < 10^{-4}$) between type 2 diabetes in Mexican American sib pairs and a locus on chromosome 2q37, called NIDDM1 (Hanis et al. 1996). Still, this region was quite large (12 cM), encompassing a large number of putative genes. A re-examination of the data suggested an interaction (epistasis) with another locus on chromosome 15 (with a nominal LOD of 1.5). This enabled the researchers to narrow the region down to 7 cM. Luckily, because it is telomeric with a high recombination rate, the 7 cM genetic map only represents 1.7 megabases of physical DNA. To clone the underlying gene, they genotyped 21 SNPs in this 7 cM interval and identified a three-marker haplotype that was nominally associated with type 2 diabetes. At the end, three intronic SNPs (43,44 and 63) in the gene encoding for calpain 10 (CAPN10) could explain most of the linkage (Horikawa et al. 2000). Calpain 10, a cystein protease with largely unknown functions in glucose metabolism, was not an obvious candidate gene for type 2 diabetes. Despite a number of subsequent negative studies, several meta-analyses have shown consistent association of SNPs 43 and 44 with type 2 diabetes (Parikh & Groop 2004). Neither was it easy to understand how intronic variation in this gene could increase risk for type 2 diabetes. Carriers of the G allele of SNP43 are associated with decreased expression of the gene in skeletal muscle and insulin resistance. How this translates into increased risk of type 2 diabetes is not known and will require functional studies.

Gene expression

Since genes are transcribed to RNA, RNA is translated into proteins, and defects in proteins cause disease, the ultimate goal would be to carry out a random search of expressed proteins in target tissues. This may not yet be completely feasible but the study of large-scale transcript profiles is. This approach has been successful in defining prognoses of cancers but for complex diseases affecting many target tissues it may not be that simple. Also, defining what is differentially expressed among more than 20,000 gene transcripts on a chip is a statistical challenge. Despite these problems, analysis of gene expression in skeletal muscle of patients with type 2 diabetes and prediabetes has provided new insights into the pathogenesis of the disease. It required, however, the analysis of coordinated gene expression in metabolic pathways rather than of individual genes. This is based upon the assumption that if one member of the pathway shows altered expression, this will be translated into the whole pathway. Genes regulating oxidative phosphorylation in mitochondria showed a 20 % coordinated down-regulation in muscle from prediabetic and diabetic individuals (Mootha et al. 2003; Patti et al. 2003). Furthermore, a similar down-regulation of the gene encoding for a master regulator of oxidative phosphorylation, the PPARγ co-activator PGC-1α, was observed. This pathway has thus emerged as central in the pathogenesis of type 2 diabetes and it appears that impaired mitochondrial function and impaired oxidation of fat may predispose to type 2 diabetes through a 'thrifty gene' mechanism (see below). By studying young and elderly twins we were able to demonstrate that elderly carriers of a Gly482Ser polymorphism in the PGC-1α gene had decreased expression of the PGC-1α gene in skeletal muscle, suggesting that genetic variants determine age-related decline in expression of key genes regulating oxidative phosphorylation (Ling et al. 2004) (Figure 20.1). This study gives an example of how genetic factors, in combination with non-genetic factors, can influence gene expression, which in turn affects glucose and fat metabolism (Figure 20.2).

Association studies

If there is already a strong candidate gene for a disease, the best approach is to search for associations between SNPs in the gene and the disease. This can either be a case control or nested cohort study. In a case-control study, the inclusion criteria for the cases are predefined and matched individual controls are searched for (or selected) in the same ethnic group as the cases. In a cohort study, affected and unaffected groups, not individuals, are matched. Ideally cohorts are population-based but often they represent consecutive patients from an outpatient clinic. It is preferable that controls are older than cases to exclude the possibility that they are still to develop the disease. The question of matching is crucial for the results; matching for a parameter influenced by the genetic variant (e.g. BMI) might influence its effect on a disease like type 2 diabetes.

If cases and controls are not drawn from the same ethnic group, a spurious association can be detected due to ethnic stratification. One way to circumvent this problem is to perform a family-based association study. Distorted transmission of alleles from parents to affected offspring would indicate that the allele showing excess transmission is associated with the disease. The untransmitted alleles serve as controls. This transmission disequilibrium test (TDT) represents the most unbiased association study approach but suffers from the drawback of low power; only transmissions from heterozygous parents are informative. The

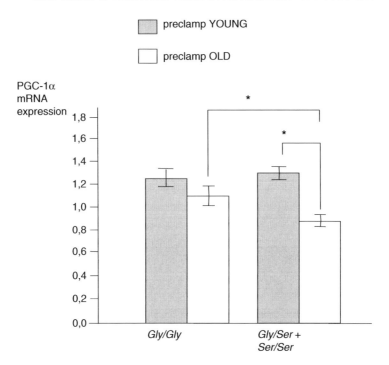

Figure 20.1 The effect of age on the association between skeletal muscle PGC-1α mRNA expression and the PGC-1α Gly482Ser polymorphism (Ling et al. 2004). Reproduced from Ling et al. (2004). Courtesy of the American Society of Clinical Investigation.

prerequisite of DNA from parents usually entails carrying out the test in individuals with an earlier onset of the disease.

Even screening only one gene for SNPs can represent a huge and expensive undertaking. The PPARγ gene on the short arm of chromosome 3 spans 83,000 nucleotides, with 231 SNPs in public databases, 7 of them coding SNPs. The gene encodes for a nuclear receptor, which is predominantly expressed in adipose tissue, where it regulates transcription of genes involved in adipogenesis. In the 5' untranslated end of the gene is an extra exon B, which contains a SNP changing a proline in position 12 of the protein to alanine. The rare Ala allele is seen in about 15 % of Europeans and was shown in an initial study to be associated with increased transcriptional activity, increased insulin sensitivity and protection against type 2 diabetes (Deeb et al. 1998). Subsequently there were a number of studies which could not replicate the initial finding. Using the TDT approach, we showed excess transmission of the Pro allele to the affected offspring (Altshuler et al. 2000). We thereafter performed a meta-analysis combining the results from all published studies showing a highly significant association with type 2 diabetes. The Pro12Ala polymorphism of the PPARγ2 gene is until now the best replicated gene for type 2 diabetes ($p < 2 \times 10^{-10}$) (Figure 20.3). The individual risk reduction conferred by the Ala allele is moderate, about 15 %, but since the risk allele Pro is so common, it translates into a population attributable risk of 25 %. There is also a strong interaction with nutritional factors and the protective effect of the Ala allele is enhanced with a high intake of unsaturated fat (Luan et al. 2001). This may not be too surprising as free fatty acids have been proposed as natural ligands for PPARγ.

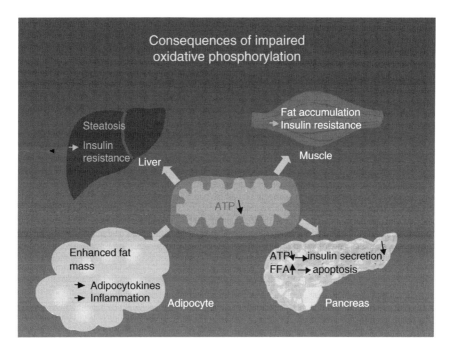

Figure 20.2 Schematic model demonstrating factors influencing the mRNA expression of PGC-1α in skeletal muscle, as well as the role of this transcriptional coactivator on glucose and lipid metabolism. (Ling et al. 2004). Reproduced from Ling et al. (2004). Courtesy of the American Society of Clinical Investigation.

If this information had not been available, we would have needed to genotype all SNPs in the gene, and even using information from public databases (dbSNPs) we might have missed some of the genetic variation unless we had sequenced the gene in cases and controls. One way of reducing the number of SNPs to be genotyped is to perform the initial screening in a reference panel, preferably parent-offspring trios, to make it easier to define which SNPs are polymorphic and thereby informative. This also allows us to create haplotypes and to identify which SNPs capture the genetic information encompassed within them. Several programmes for defining haplotypes and haplotype tag SNPs (htgSNPs) are publicly available, e.g. HaploView www.broad.mit.edu/mpg/haploview/index.php. These htgSNPs (which probably represent only 30 % of the initial SNPs) can be genotyped in the case-control test panel.

It is still debated whether common or rare variants are the cause of common complex diseases. The haplotype approach would work for common but not for rare variants. The common-variant common-disease hypothesis assumes that relatively ancient common variants increase susceptibility to common diseases like obesity, hypertension, type 2 diabetes etc. These variants would be enriched in the population as they have been associated with survival advantages during evolution; so-called thrifty genes (Veel 1962). Storage of surplus energy during periods of famine may have been beneficial for survival, while in Westernised society we rather need genetic variants which waste energy.

Why is it difficult to replicate the finding of an association with a complex disease? The literature on the genetics of complex diseases has been flooded with papers unable to replicate initial findings. There are several reasons for this. There is a clear tendency in first studies

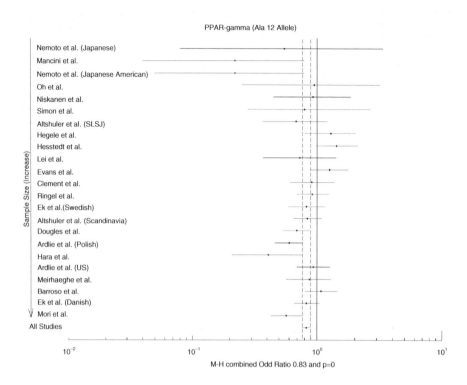

Figure 20.3 A meta-analysis demonstrating the strong risk of the Pro12Ala polymorphism in the PPARγ2 gene and type 2 diabetes.

to report the strongest association, as researchers and editors prefer strong positive findings ('winners' curse'). False positive findings are unfortunately common. In an analysis of 301 published studies covering 25 different reported associations, only half showed significant replication in a meta-analysis (Lohmueller et al. 2003). The most important reason is lack of power. The odds ratio for a complex disease is often below 1.5. The sample size is dependent not only upon the odds ratio but also on the frequency of the at-risk genetic variant. For an odds ratio of 1.3 and a frequency of the at-risk allele of 20%, at least 1,000 cases and controls are required. The Genetic Power Calculator is a useful tool for power calculations in genetic association studies (http://ibgwww.colorado.edu/~pshaun/gpc/) (Purcell et al. 2003).

Why don't linkage studies detect all associations?

Despite initial linkage, it has often been difficult to identify underlying genetic variations. This is particularly difficult if the disease-causing allele has a high frequency in the population. Under those circumstances, many individuals will be homozygous for the disease allele, in which case one will not observe linkage between the disease allele and an allele at a nearby locus because either of the homologous chromosomes can be transmitted to an affected offspring. This was the case for the Pro12Ala polymorphism in the PPARγ gene. No linkage has been observed between T2D and the region for PPARγ on chromosome 3p, since the Pro allele will typically be transmitted from both parents. A simulation indicated that 3 million sib pairs would be required to detect such a linkage (Deeb et al. 1998).

Future directions

The rapid improvement in high throughput technology for SNP genotyping and resulting decrease of cost per genotype (in 10 years the cost has decreased by a factor of 10) open new possibilities for both linkage and association studies. The use of DNA chips containing >11,000 SNPs instead of classic 450 microsatellites for genome-wide scans, detected additional regions and narrowed previous regions, yielding significantly higher LOD scores (Middleton et al. 2004).

Such high-density DNA chips may be useful for detecting rare genes with a strong effect in large pedigrees but for the detection of the genetic variation of complex diseases, association studies are needed. In the near future it will be possible to perform genome-wide association studies using SNPs. If the common-variant common-disease hypothesis holds, it may be possible to obtain an atlas of disease-associated genetic variants using 500,000–1,000,000 SNPs. This will not be a cheap undertaking and it is obvious that, while the tools are there, funding is the limiting factor for dissecting the genetics of complex diseases at the current time.

References

Altshuler D, Hirschhorn JN, Klannemark M, Lindgren CM, Vohl MC, Nemesh J et al. (2000) The common PPARgamma Pro12Ala polymorphism is associated with decreased risk of type 2 diabetes *Nat Genet* **26**, 76–80

Deeb SS, Fajas L, Nemoto M, Pihlajamaki J, Mykkanen L, Kuusisto J et al. (1998) A Pro12Ala substitution in PPARgamma2 associated with decreased receptor activity, lower body mass index and improved insulin sensitivity *Nat Genet* **20**, 284–7

Florez JC, Hirschhorn J, Altshuler D (2003) The inherited basis of diabetes mellitus Implications for the genetic analysis of complex traits *Annu Rev Genomics Hum Genet* **4**, 257–91

Hanis CL, Boerwinkle E, Chakraborty R, Ellsworth DL, Concannon P, Stirling B et al. (1996) A genome-wide search for human non-insulin-dependent (type 2) diabetes genes reveals a major susceptibility locus on chromosome 2 *Nat Genet* **13**, 161–6

Horikawa Y, Oda N, Cox NJ, Li X, Orho-Melander M, Hara M et al. (2000) Genetic variation in the gene encoding calpain-10 is associated with type 2 diabetes mellitus *Nat Genet* **26**, 163–75

Kerem B, Rommens JM, Buchanan JA, Markiewics D, Cox TK, Chakravati A et al (1989) Identification of the cystic fibrosis gene: genetic analysis *Science* **245**, 1073–80

Lander E, Kruglyak L (1995) Genetic dissection of complex traits: guidelines for interpreting and reporting linkage results *Nat Genet* **11**, 241–7

Li C, Scott LJ, Boehnke M (2004) Assessing whether an allele can account in part for a linkage signal: the genotype-IBD sharing test (GIST) *Am J Hum Genet* **74**, 418–31

Ling C, Poulsen P, Carlsson E, Ridderstråle M, Almgren P, Beck-Nielsen H et al. (2004) Multiple environmental and genetic factors influence skeletal muscle PGC-1α and PGC-1β gene expression in twins *J Clin Invest* **114**, 1518–26

Lohmueller KE, Pearce CL, Pike M, Lander ES, Hirschhorn JN (2003) Meta-analysis of genetic association studies supports a contribution of common variants to susceptibility to common disease *Nat Genet* **33**, 177–82

Luan J, Browne PO, Harding AH, Halsall DJ, O'Rahilly S, Chatterjee VK et al. (2001) Evidence for gene-nutrient interaction at the *PPAR*gamma locus *Diabetes* **50**, 686–9

Miller LH, Mason SJ, Dvorak JA, McGinniss MH, Rothman IK (1975) Erythrocyte receptors for (Plasmodium knowlesi) malaria Duffy blood group determinants *Science* **189**, 561–3

Mootha VK, Lindgren CM, Eriksson KF, Subramanian A, Sihag S, Lehar J et al. (2003) PGC-1alpha-responsive genes involved in oxidative phosphorylation are coordinately downregulated in human diabetes *Nat Genet* **34**, 267–73

Neel V (1962) Diabetes mellitus: a 'thrifty' genotype rendered detrimental by progress *Am J Hum Genet* **14**, 352–2

Middleton FA, Pato MT, Gentile KL, Morley CP, Zhao X, Eisener AF et al. (2004) Genomewide linkage analysis of bipolar disorder by use of a high-density single-nucleotide-polymorphism (SNP) genotyping assay: a comparison with microsatellite marker assays and finding of significant linkage to chromosome 6q22 *Am J Hum Genet* **74**, 886–97

Parikh H, Groop L (2004) Candidate genes for type 2 diabetes *Endocrine and Metabolic Disorders* **5**, 151–76

Patti ME, Butte AJ, Crunkhorn S, Cusi K, Berria R, Kashyap S et al. (2003) Coordinated reduction of genes of oxidative metabolism in humans with insulin resistance and diabetes: Potential role of PGC1 and NRF1 *Proc Natl Acad Sci* **100**, 8466–71

Purcell S, Cherny SS, Sham PC (2003) Genetic Power Calculator: design of linkage and association genetic mapping studies of complex traits *Bioinformatics* **19**, 149–50

Stephens JC, Reich DE, Goldstein DB, Shin HD, Smith MW, Carrington M et al (1998) Dating the origin of the CCR-5-Delta 32 AIDS resistance allele by the coalescence of haplotypes *Am J Hum Genet* **62**, 1507–15

21

Good Clinical Practice: Friend or Foe?

Christian Joukhadar and **Markus Müller**

Introduction

Clinical researchers frequently complain about the high demands imposed on them by the current regulatory legislation on the conduct of clinical trials. It is not surprising that the recent implementation of the European Union clinical trials directive (European Parliament Directive 2001) has led to an outcry among academic researchers in Europe, given the perceived inability of many clinical centers to adopt and comply with these new and still more demanding requirements (Grienenberger 2004).

Although this situation should raise concern, there can be no doubt about the valuable impact of the regulatory framework set up after World War II on the quality and methodology of clinical research. It is to a great extent due to these regulations that we have been able to establish an entirely new approach to our theory and practice of medicine, today frequently denoted 'evidence based medicine', a term coined by David Sackett (Sackett et al. 1997).

This concept represents a dramatic paradigm shift from a subjective, physician based philosophy of medicine towards an 'objectified' competition of prospectively formulated and falsifiable hypotheses. The roots of this ideological clash can be traced back to a philosophical clash, between the Romantic schools of philosophy represented paradigmatically by the German philosopher Hegel and a more experimental, Anglo-Saxon philosophical tradition represented by Sir Karl Popper. Some argue that the conflict can even be dated back to the ancient Greeks and the competing views of Plato and his more experimentally oriented pupil, Aristotle. Today, there can be no doubt that the Anglo-Saxon tradition and the Popperian and Aristotelian schools have had a dramatic impact on the concept of medicine. This is reflected by our current terminology, such as the entirely Popperian term 'hypothesis-testing study'.

Codices regulating medical practice date back to Hammurabi (1710 BC), but in the modern era, up until World War II, clinical trials were virtually unregulated. The historical steps which eventually led to the legal framework in place today started with the Nuremberg Codex in 1947 (Mitscherlich 1949; Vollmann & Winau 1996), which was amended, modified

Clinical Diabetes Research: Methods and Techniques   Edited by Michael Roden
© 2007 John Wiley & Sons, Ltd   ISBN 978-0-470-01728-9

and extended by the Declaration of Helsinki in 1964 (WMA 2000), the Belmont Report in 1979, the Note for Guidance on Good Clinical Practice in 1990 (CPMP 1990), the Council for International Organisations of Medical Sciences (CIOMS) and World Health Organisation (WHO) Guidelines on GCP in 1993 (International Ethical Guidelines 2002), the GCP International Conference of Harmonisation (ICH) guideline in 1996 (ICH-GCP 1997) and the EU directive 2001/20/EG in 2002 (European Parliament 2001), to name just a few notable milestones (Anhalt 1993).

   The details of current GCP regulations appear complex, but the core concept of GCP is to protect patients and participants in clinical trials. This concept relates to the key issues of 1) accountability, 2) responsibility and 3) reproducibility. GCP also provides ethical and scientific guidelines for planning and performing studies in humans and for interpreting and publishing data derived from such studies. In essence, every single step in the conduct of a trial needs to be meticulously documented so that the work is reproducible and key players are accountable, with clearly defined responsibilites. Accountability and reproducibility are terms that have become increasingly important in medical science, particularly in the last 10 years, as severe cases of scientific misconduct have been reported in the lay press.

Scientific misconduct

An issue that has long been overlooked, due to the high esteem in which scientists in general have been held in public opinion, is the credibility of the data gathering process in research. According to the literature, questionable credibility seems to be fairly prevalent in the scientific community. It is conservatively estimated that one severe case of documented fraud occurs per 100,000 scientists per year, and 1 in 10 audits have provided findings of major deviations (Marshall 2000; Steneck 2000). Cases of scientific misconduct that have led to impaired data credibility and false conclusions cover a broad spectrum, ranging from sloppiness and willful distortion of data to actual data fabrication (Kintisch 2005). The most notable cases of fraud – such as the data fabrication found in an article on high dose chemotherapy for breast cancer printed in a highly renowned medical journal (von Schilling & Herrmann 1995) – have probably led to a large number of casualties (Cooper-Mahkorn 1998). The reasons for this situation are manifold but it is indisputable that the introduction of GCP regulations has put a brake, albeit not a perfect one, on attempted or actual cases of scientific misconduct.

Publication bias

Medical drug treatment should rely on solid evidence, and it is now generally recognised that the standard basis for treatment guidelines relies on systematic literature reviews or meta-analyses of all randomised controlled trials. However, as meta-analyses are usually limited to publicly available data, several factors can lead to biased conclusions, including selection of studies submitted or accepted for publication but not yet published, inclusion of undetected duplicate publications and selective reporting (such as failure to report intention to treat results). Publication bias is a statistical tendency to produce erroneously significant results, arising from the fact that studies with negative results, no significant differences in results between groups or disappointing data do not find their way into the medical literature, even though they may have been well executed. Publication bias, therefore, dramatically skews our knowledge toward work with positive findings (Easterbrook et al. 1991). Several actors (editors, investigators and sponsors) affect whether and how scientific results reach the public domain. In clinical trials of drugs, the role of the sponsor is especially important (Melander et al. 2003). The sponsor usually has access to all data on his product but an obvious conflict of interest comes into play when he selects what to submit for publication.

Institutional review board/independent ethics committee

Every clinical trial in the US and Europe must be approved and monitored by an Institutional Review Board (IRB)/Independent Ethics Committee (IEC) to make sure that the risks conferred to volunteers or patients are as low as possible and are compensated for by the potential benefits. By federal regulation, and as stated in the GCP-ICH guidelines, all institutions that conduct or support biomedical research involving people must have an IRB/IEC that initially approves and periodically reviews the research. IRB/IECs aim at safeguarding the rights, safety and well-being of study subjects and pay particular attention to vulnerable subjects such as children, the elderly, comatose or cognitively impaired patients, students and employees, prisoners and anyone undergoing first-drug administration.

The approval of an IRB/IEC is increasingly being demanded by editors of high-standard medical journals, who will ask for a statement that ethical approval has been obtained before they consider a research report for publication. Thus, an IRB/IEC has high responsibility in pharmaceutical, medical and scientific affairs. In order to ensure proper decision making, the ideal committee should consist of several members who collectively have the qualifications and experience to review and evaluate the science, medicine and ethics of the proposed trial.

All health and community care research is subjected to rigorous pre-peer review by recognised IRB/IEC experts in the relevant fields, who are able to offer advice on project quality. This pre-peer review process offers the investigator the unique opportunity to receive an independent expert report on the clinical and statistical methodologies to be used in the study, as well as an assessment of the study's ethical viability. Adopting the advice of IRB/IEC experts is an important step in increasing the overall quality of clinical research and helps the investigator's chances of publication in a high-impact medical journal.

From this it follows that IRB/IECs play an eminent role in establishing high ethical and qualitative standards in medical research. This role is particularly eminent in those situations where a sponsor's interests are affected by overwhelming financial motivations and they run the risk of losing track of ethical considerations. IRB/IECs will help the investigator and scientist to adequately collect relevant data on the product under investigation and aid in the assessment of the risk-to-benefit ratio conferred to the subject by study procedures.

The term 'ethically acceptable' risk-to-benefit ratio will always be a matter of discussion and beliefs about what is ethically acceptable may differ substantially between IRB/IECs in one country and IRB/IECs in another. Recently, several astonishing clinical findings would never have been obtained without the brave decisions of some pioneer IRB/IECs (Horng & Miller 2002). For example, surgical intervention in osteoarthritis of the knee is considered the gold standard. The hypothesis that surgical intervention is not preferable to a placebo was being tested. The IRB/IEC decided to accept the withholding of a gold standard therapy in randomly selected patients, while still exposing them to the risks associated with surgery and anaesthesia. A total of 180 patients with osteoarthritis of the knee were assigned to receive arthroscopic debridement, arthroscopic lavage or placebo surgery (Moseley et al. 2002). Patients in the placebo group received skin incisions only and underwent a simulated debridement without insertion of the arthroscope. The outcomes after arthroscopic lavage or arthroscopic debridement were not better than those after a placebo procedure. Almost similar findings were obtained when another IRB/IEC allowed testing of the usefulness of right heart catheterisation in terms of survival, length of stay, intensity of care and cost of care in the intensive care unit (Dalen & Bone 1996; Connors 1997). The data from these studies debunked the rationale of long practiced interventional procedures and questioned incongruous actionism, particularly given the potential risks of surgical intervention, anaesthesia and insertion of a right heart catheter.

Usually IRB/IECs have to decide whether research related risks conferred to participants are acceptable in much less invasive studies. However, it is still a prerequisite that the benefits of a study clearly outweigh the risks to participants. It is unlikely any IRB/IEC would nowadays allow measurement of plasma glucose concentrations in healthy volunteers in normal conditions – plasma glucose concentrations are extensively documented in literature and, thus, no valuable additional information could be expected from such a study – even though the risk is limited to the needle puncture of fingers. The risk-to-benefit ratio nonetheless does not allow such a study. On the other hand, an IRB/IEC may decide that very invasive procedures such as biopsy of the liver or kidney are acceptable if fundamental information is expected from the investigation.

In an attempt to simplify decision-making and harmonise assessment of the risk-to-benefit ratio, so-called leading IRB/IECs have recently been given the power to vote for all other IRB/IECs in their respective countries.

Protocol and informed consent

According to GCP-ICH, every single step in an interventional trial has to adhere to a prospectively formulated protocol. (A noninterventional trial is one where the assignment of a patient to a therapeutic strategy is not influenced by the study and where no additional procedures are undertaken in that patient's treatment due to the study.)

Informed consent is the process of presenting enough information to a volunteer to allow them to intelligently decide whether or not to participate as a research subject. Ideally, the informed consent form describes the overall experience and explains the research activity, paying particular attention to any new drugs, extra tests, separate research records or nonstandard means of management, such as flipping a coin for random assignment, and any other design issues. Human subjects must be informed verbally and in writing about the foreseeable harms, discomforts, inconveniences and risks that may be associated with the research activity. Likewise, the benefits that subjects may reasonably expect to encounter should be reported, though they should be made aware that helping the public at large is the goal of the study. If payment is given to defray the incurred expense for participation, it must not be coercive in amount or method of distribution. The informed consent form should also describe any alternatives to participating in the research project. For example, in drug studies the medication(s) may be available through a family doctor or clinic without the need to volunteer for research activity.

Informed consent is a fundamental mechanism for ensuring respect for persons. The procedures used in obtaining informed consent should be designed to educate the subject population in terms that they can understand. Therefore, informed consent language, especially in explanation of the study's purpose, duration, experimental procedures, alternatives, risks and benefits, must be lay language. An example glossary of lay terms that may be used in preparing informed consent forms is provided at http://humansubjects.stanford.edu/medical/glossary.html.

Terms such as 'randomisation' are frequently used but are not commonly understandable to potential participants. Randomisation assigns research participants by chance, rather than by choice, to either the investigational group or the control group of a clinical trial. Each study participant has a fair and equal chance of receiving either the new intervention being studied or the existing or control intervention. This procedure must be clearly explained to volunteers. A randomised, controlled trial is considered the most reliable and impartial method of determining which medical interventions work the best. However, this approach also potentially withholds effective treatment from those allocated to the control group; a limitation that appears unavoidable in strengthening evidence in research.

If research-related injury (i.e. physical, psychological, social, financial or otherwise) that is more than 'minimal' risk is possible, an explanation must be given of whatever compensation and/or treatment will be provided. It is worth noting that a risk is considered 'minimal' when the probability and magnitude of harm or discomfort anticipated in the proposed research are not greater than those ordinarily encountered in daily life or during the performance of routine physical or psychological examinations or tests. The regulations do not limit injury to 'physical injury', which is a common misinterpretation. It is important not to overlook the need to point out that no penalty or loss of benefits will be incurred by subjects as a result of either not participating or withdrawing at any time. It is equally important to alert potential subjects to any foreseeable consequences to them should they unilaterally withdraw while dependent on some intervention to maintain normal function.

With few exceptions only, informed consent should be documented by the use of a written consent form approved by the IRB/IEC and signed by the subject or the subject's legally authorised representative. A signed informed consent form should thereby document that the voluntary subject has fully understood the purpose, the aim, the scope as well as the risks of their participation in the trial. The process of obtaining a patient's properly informed consent to take part in a clinical trial should not be seen as an exercise in bureaucratic form filling but as an essential part of the trial, requiring time, insight and communication skills. When patients refuse to give their consent, this is not a sign that the investigator has failed but rather an indication that the investigator was conscientious enough to ensure the patients were properly informed and made a free decision. If large proportions of patients refuse to enter a study, however, this may signify a problem with the study design.

Special populations

Waiver or alteration of informed consent procedure is sometimes necessary in order to perform studies in 'special populations'; these are prisoners, students or employees of the trial site, or persons who are legally incapable of giving informed consent, such as children and comatose, sedated or psychiatric patients. In addition, studies on women of childbearing age, alcohol or drug dependent individuals and individuals with a family history of drug or alcohol problems must be handled separately. An IRB/IEC may approve a consent procedure that does not include or alters some or all of the elements of informed consent set forth in the previous section, or else it may waive the requirement to obtain informed consent. This may only be done provided the IRB/IEC finds and documents that: 1) the research involves no more than 'minimal risk' to the subjects; 2) the waiver or alteration will not adversely affect the rights and welfare of the subjects; 3) the research could not practicably be carried out without the waiver or alteration; and 4) whenever appropriate, the subjects will be provided with additional pertinent information after participation. In such exceptional studies, investigators, nevertheless, must provide an appropriate explanation, seek the individual's assent, consider such persons' preferences and best interests, and obtain appropriate permission from a legally authorised person if such substitute consent is permitted or required by law.

Serious adverse event reporting

The purpose of documenting adverse events (AEs)/serious adverse events (SAEs) is to acquaint pharmacovigilant departments of pharmaceutical companies and regulatory authorities with data helping to identify, document and report on the safety and tolerability of pharmaceutical agents being tested in clinical studies. For that reason, the terms 'AE' and in particular 'SAE' have to be used in a very strict sense only. By definition, AEs are untoward clinical events experienced by a study participant while taking part in a clinical trial. Such events may be abnormal laboratory values, physical signs or symptoms. An AE becomes a SAE when it results in death; a life-threatening event; in-patient hospitalisation or prolongation of existing hospitalisation; persistent or significant disability/incapacity; a congenital anomaly/birth defect; or an important medical event that does not necessarily result in death, a life-threatening event or require hospitalisation though, based upon appropriate medical judgment, it may jeopardise the participant and require medical or surgical intervention to prevent one of the previously identified outcomes. It is important to note that the 'grade' of AE should be defined prior to the start of the trial. A representative and useful grading scheme may be found at http://ctep.info.nih.gov/reporting/CTC-3.html. Grade 3 events that fit the above criteria are treated as SAEs. Grade 4 events are in general considered SAEs.

In the interest of participants' safety in clinical studies and to fulfill regulatory requirements, all SAEs, *whether related to the study agent or not*, must be reported by the principal investigator or his delegates to the sponsor by contacting the medical monitor in writing within 24 hours of learning of the SAE. The sponsor itself must report to the local IRB/IEC and the federal ministry according to institutional guidelines.

In its role as investigational new drug (IND) sponsor, the sponsor is required to review and analyse all SAE reports for their impact on participant safety in a study. The medical monitor immediately reviews all SAEs to determine if the event is related to the study agent and is unexpected (suspected unexpected serious adverse event reaction – SUSAR). If the medical monitor judges that these criteria are met, regulatory authorities such as e.g. the US Food and Drug Administration (US-FDA) require the IND sponsor to file an expedited report to the authority within a period of less than 15 days. If the event is unexpected and fatal or life threatening and associated with the use of the study agent, then the authority must be notified within seven calendar days of the initial receipt of the information. This report, known as an IND safety report, must be circulated to all investigators participating in trials using the agent in case of multi-centre studies.

In line with this strategy, the European regulatory authority EMEA maintains a database in order to provide investigators with an overview of SUSARs linked to investigational medicinal products used in their studies. This database facilitates the review of safe use of these products in clinical trials and may be considered a superior watchdog system. The database also facilitates communication on this review and the safety of clinical trials between authorities. This process should enable an investigator and each of the member states involved to better oversee clinical trials and medicinal product development, and should provide for enhanced protection of clinical trial subjects and patients receiving medicinal products. The database is the clinical trial module of the EudraVigilance database. SUSARs are entered into a clinical trial module of the EudraVigilance database, thus creating a single overall database for European regulatory authorities, covering clinical trial safety reporting and post-marketing safety reporting.

Monitoring and inspection

Clinical research associates, project managers and team leaders were the first to receive the attention of monitors and auditors, but increasingly their influence has spread to pharmacovigilance personnel, data managers, statisticians, investigational medicinal product units and pharmaceutical physicians. Monitors and GCP-inspectors assess compliance with the requirements of applicable GCP regulations and guidelines by conducting inspections at the sites of pharmaceutical sponsor companies, contract research organisations, academic research organisations, investigational trial sites, clinical laboratories, GCP archives and other facilities involved in clinical trial research. As a rule, each clinical trial has to be monitored by a trained and predefined study monitor. However, inspection of clinical studies by GCP inspectors is much less complete and in the majority of cases, only one representative clinical trial is selected for examination as part of a 'systems' inspection. A fee is charged for these inspections in order to fund the activities of the GCP compliance unit.

Statutorily and voluntarily triggered inspections can be performed in response to a specific request, e.g. from other agencies, from assessors of licensing applications, etc. Sometimes inspections are conducted by foreign agencies, e.g. the US-FDA, the Japanese Ministry of Health and Welfare; normally these are shadowed by local inspectors. When a company or a trial site undergoes an inspection, the weeks before the arrival of the inspectors can be a period of intense activity and training. Internal and contract GCP auditors may be consulted and may indeed be invited to perform preparatory audits identifying areas requiring particular attention before the inspection. They may also be asked to prepare members of internal staff and investigational site staff for the inspectors' interviews.

Among the first things that inspectors and monitors may ask to see are the training records, curriculum vitaes and job descriptions of certain members of staff. Although it is a simple matter to check these documents prior to the monitors' or inspectors' visit, proper documentation is mostly lacking. It is advisable to ensure that CVs filed are up-to-date and not those which staff members submitted when they applied for their positions. The principal investigator and his team have to check that their CVs and training records include evidence that they are suitably qualified, trained and experienced. Inspectors may seek reassurance that investigators have received training in the most recent version of GCP and in standard operating procedures related to their duties. Such documentation is often absent and anecdotal accounts do not satisfy inspectors.

During preparation for trial site inspection, many small actions should be performed, e.g. tidying and ordering of files, cleaning of certain areas, interviewing investigational staff to clarify study-related matters and checking and completing inventories of investigational medicinal products. Most of these things happen without any record and without further implications. However, to maximise the benefits of the inspection, staff should be encouraged to document briefly all activities arising from the preparation and to analyse these records as carefully as possible post-inspection for quality systems improvement. Any study monitoring, data or report review should be performed according to standard procedures agreed in advance and should be carefully documented to provide an audit trail that indicates what has been done, when and by whom.

Conclusion

GCP-ICH regulations aim at maximising reproducibility and transparency in clinical data management and documentation while keeping the risks conferred to study participants as low as possible. Many of the GCP-ICH stipulations and guidelines are still regarded as highly bureaucratic by many investigators, and thus inspectors and monitors will have to work hard to establish an atmosphere of mutual trust and cooperation. The ultimate purpose of GCP-ICH is to protect the dignity, rights, safety and well-being of all actual or potential research participants and to help investigators conduct high-quality research. Thus, GCP-ICH provides the basis for an in depth knowledge and understanding of the principles of ethical research. Manuscripts that meet these criteria are more likely to be acceptable for publication and submission to health care authorities.

References

Anhalt E (1993) The development of good clinical practice in the EEC and in Germany *Methods Find Exp Clin Pharmacol* **15**(4), 217–22

Belmont Report (1979) http://www.crc.gov.my/clinicalTrial/documents/The%20Belmont%20Report.pdf

Cooper-Mahkorn D (1998) Many journals have not retracted 'fraudulent' research *BMJ* **316**(7148), 1850

Connors AF Jr (1997) Right heart catheterization: is it effective? *New Horiz* **5**(3), 195–200

CPMP Working Party on Efficacy of Medicinal Products note for guidance: good clinical practice for trials on medicinal products in the European Community (1990) CB-55-89-706-EN-C

Dalen JE, RC Bone (1996) Is it time to pull the pulmonary artery catheter? *Jama* **276**(11), 916–18

Easterbrook PJ et al. (1991) Publication bias in clinical research *Lancet* **337**(8,746), 867–72

European Parliament (2001) Directive 2001/20/EC of the European Parliament and Council of 4 April 2001 on the approximation of the laws, regulations and administrative provisions of the member states relating to the implemention of good clinical practice in the conduct of clinical trials on medicinal products for human use. *Official Journal of the European Communities* 2001(121), 34–44

Grienenberger A (2004) Establishing pan-European clinical trials: regulatory compliance and other practical considerations *J Biolaw Bus* **7**(4), 58–63

Horng S, Miller FG (2002) Is placebo surgery unethical? *N Engl J Med* **347**(2), 137–9

ICH-GCP (1997) http://www.emea.eu.int/pdfs/human/ich/013595en.pdf

International Ethical Guidelines for Biomedical Research Involving Human Subjects. Prepared by the Council for International Organizations of Medical Sciences (CIOMS) in collaboration with the World Health Organization (WHO) http://www.cioms.ch/frame_guidelines_nov_2002.htm

Kintisch E (2005) Scientific misconduct. Researcher faces prison for fraud in NIH grant applications and papers *Science* **307**(5717), 1851

Marshall E (2000) Scientific misconduct: how prevalent is fraud? That's a million-dollar question *Science* **290**(5497), 1662–3

Melander H et al. (2003) Evidence based medicine – selective reporting from studies sponsored by pharmaceutical industry: review of studies in new drug applications *BMJ* **326**(7400), 1171–3

Mitscherlich A (1949) The Nuremberg Code (1947) In: Schuman H *Doctors of Infamy: The story of the Nazi medical crimes*, xxiii–xxv

Moseley JB et al. (2002) A controlled trial of arthroscopic surgery for osteoarthritis of the knee *N Engl J Med* **347**(2), 81–8

Sackett D, Rosenberg W, Haynes RB (1997) *Evidence-Based Medicine: How to Practice and Teach EBM*, Churchill Livingstone, London

Steneck N (2000) Assessing the integrity of publicly funded research

Vollmann J, Winau R (1996) Informed consent in human experimentation before the Nuremberg code *BMJ* **313**(7070), 1445–9

von Schilling C, Herrmann F (1995) Dose-intensified treatment of breast cancer: current results *J Mol Med* **73**(12), 611–27

World Medical Association (WMA) (2000) Declaration of Helsinki, 52nd WMA General Assembly, Ethical Principles for Medical Research Involving Human Subjects, Edinburgh, Scotland http://www.wma.net/e/policy/b3.htm

22

Statistical Considerations in Diabetes Trials

Irene M Stratton and **Carole A Cull**

Introduction

Many excellent textbooks are available to aid and guide clinicians and scientists through the design and analysis of clinical trials and other kinds of clinical research (see References). However, these excellent books and others like them are far too often ignored (Stratton & Neil 2005). The general statistical techniques are well covered in these books and do not need to be described here, but items which are germane to diabetes research will be elucidated.

From the standpoint of the medical statistician, diabetes and its complications are a more complex challenge than those in most other fields of medicine. In other, acute conditions an intervention may be observed as 'kill or cure', and for some chronic conditions such as asthma a relatively short period of observation can be sufficient to assess the effect and tolerability of a new therapy. Diabetes has many forms, type 1 diabetes, type 2 diabetes, latent autoimmune diabetes of adults (LADA), maturity-onset diabetes of the young (MODY), gestational diabetes (GDM), and more are being identified by the geneticists almost weekly. Therapies used to control glycaemia need to do so without incurring hypoglycaemia or other unacceptable side effects such as oedema or weight gain, and some of these therapies can change blood pressure, lipid profiles and more. Treating one of these concomitant conditions may affect glycaemia, as is demonstrated by the worsening of glucose control in those allocated to beta blocker in the UKPDS hypertension study (UKPDS 1998b). The outcomes in trials in diabetes are not easily identified and quantified. In long term studies such as the UKPDS it is possible to assess therapeutic interventions using death, myocardial infarction or stroke, but in shorter term, smaller studies, surrogate endpoints often have to be used. Surrogates such as changes in digital retinal photographs need to be assessed by expert graders, and biochemical assays need to be quality controlled and assured to maintain comparability between centres and throughout a trial (Cull et al. 1997).

Clinical Diabetes Research: Methods and Techniques   Edited by Michael Roden
© 2007 John Wiley & Sons, Ltd   ISBN 978-0-470-01728-9

Requirements

The use of the CONSORT checklist and flowchart (Altman 1996, CONSORT No Date) is to be encouraged, and is now mandatory for submission to many journals. This ensures that the information needed to understand what has been done is presented in a standard way and, as well as allowing the reader to assess the validity of the conclusions of the current trial, allows comparison between different trials. Even if a journal does not require the CONSORT checklist to be submitted with a paper, its use by authors will always improve their work.

Study design and power calculations

Design of studies should take into consideration the need to ensure that the study population is truly representative of the patient population to whom the results will be applied. This is especially important where ethnic differences may influence patient characteristics. Few studies in diabetes report comprehensive power calculations or the considerations which led trialists to the design used. Power calculations can now be carried out using readily available software (Nquery, SAS proc power, Sample size) and should be presented in trial reports where appropriate.

Biochemical and clinical measurements

The required size of a study is influenced by the precision with which outcome measures can be measured, so it is essential to describe accurately all assays and measurement protocols. HbA_{1c} assays should be aligned to DCCT standards, and local normal ranges given, so that comparisons can be made between studies. In multi-centre studies it is essential that assays carried out in different centres are aligned and that protocols for obtaining samples are identical at all centres. Sample storage and transportation studies need to be undertaken if a multi-centre study is to use a central laboratory for any biochemical assays. If a study is to be carried out over years then it is important to maintain comparability over time and to check whether assay drift has occurred (Cull et al. 1997). Although these concerns may not appear to the researcher to be part of the brief of the statistician, such matters can require special consideration before statistical analyses are carried out.

Similarly, if measurements are to be made by different people in different centres or over a long period of time, steps should be taken to ensure that the procedures are comparable and do not change with time. For example, if outcome measures using grading of samples or photographs are used then training and comparability of graders is essential. In the UKPDS, a stratified sample of 100 sets of photographs was used to compare graders and grading outcome during the study, with Cohen's kappa statistics being reported as a measure of agreement between graders and between grading outcomes over years. Similarly, if blood pressure is being measured with automated machines, these will need to be checked regularly to ensure consistency of measurements, and if staff are measuring blood pressure with a standard sphygmomanometer, checks should be introduced to ensure that all such staff have similar standards for measurement (and that everybody can hear properly!) (UKPDS 1991).

Demographics

In most studies, the first table should describe the population under investigation. As diabetes is a heterogeneous collection of conditions, this should be comprehensive rather than minimalist to enable the clinician to see whether the results might be directly applicable to his patients and to assure the reader that the sample chosen for inclusion is truly representative of the populations that are being studied.

Table 22.1 shows the variables we recommend as a minimum. For studies in gestational diabetes, parity should be included. Other baseline variables may be reported when they are significant in the study design or choice of population, such as proportion with specified previous diabetic complications. Information about prior complications and surrogate disease markers such as albuminuria will be important in studies where the outcome is one or more diabetic complications.

Choice of inclusion/exclusion criteria should be clearly indicated in the text and, as required by CONSORT, numbers and characteristics of patients excluded as well as those included should be reported. The use of a CONSORT diagram or flowchart is recommended.

As longevity and the median age at diagnosis of type 2 diabetes increase, the justification for an upper age cut-off for inclusion in studies becomes less compelling. Although the inclusion of older patients is sometimes difficult because of concomitant age-related conditions, every effort should be made to ensure that there is no clearly defined sub-group of the relevant diabetic population that is excluded from a study simply on grounds of age, unless good reasons can be given.

Table 22.1 Variables that should be included in descriptions of patients with diabetes mellitus at commencement of the study (baseline measurements). Measure of central tendency and dispersion, or n and proportion

---

Type of diabetes
Gender: n and proportion male
Ethnicity: n and proportion for all ethnic groups $>1\%$ of total
Age at diagnosis or age at start of study
Time from diagnosis of diabetes
Height
Weight
Body mass index
Waist and hip measurement
Hypoglycaemia therapy: n and proportion
Measures of glycaemia (e.g. fasting plasma glucose, HbA_{1c})
Fasting plasma insulin and/or C-peptide
Blood pressure
Antihypertensive therapy: n and proportion
Lipid profile
Lipid lowering therapy: n and proportion
Family history of diabetes and its complications

Cross-over studies

In diabetes, as in other clinical disciplines, cross-over studies appear at first sight to be attractive, since, as each subject acts as his own control, fewer subjects (and hence fewer difficulties in recruiting and retaining them) are needed for a study of a given power.

However, in diabetes the use of cross-over studies is often fraught with difficulties. As it is a progressive disease, if the study period is long then the baseline glycaemia at the start of the second period may be higher than at the start of the first for reasons unconnected with the study, and therapies other than those under investigation may have changed. If HbA_{1c} is to be used as an outcome measure, it should be remembered that it is a measure of glycosylation over the last three months or so and therefore a wash-out period of at least 13 weeks is needed between study periods. Since retention of subjects within any study may be problematic, using a design that is at least twice as long as a parallel group study may not be feasible.

Long term studies

Since type 2 diabetes is a slowly progressive disease, long term studies may be necessary in order to collect sufficient information on many aspects of intervention. There are several complications associated with such studies that may well impinge on statistical analyses as they introduce sources of systematic error that need to be accounted for. Care needs to be taken to ensure that patients taking part in and completing long term studies are representative of the populations from which they are drawn so that 'survivor effects' can be eliminated.

Specialised trial designs

There are a number of trial designs, such as cluster randomised trials, case-control studies and factorial designs (to name but a few), that require specialist statistical expertise both during the design stage and during analysis. Unless the investigators are experts in these kinds of studies, or include among their number properly qualified and trained applied statisticians, they are well advised to seek professional help when considering such trials. Similar considerations apply when designing trials involving different methods of randomisation, such as minimisation, where the choice of criteria is critical. When projects involve the analysis of genetic data, specialist statistical geneticists should be consulted.

Reporting of study protocols

As in studies outside of diabetes, the reporting of study protocols in a clear manner is needed to ensure that the reader knows what has been done and to enable another investigator to repeat the study in another population.

Identification and measurement of outcome measures and surrogate outcome measures

It is critically important that outcome measures are properly defined in the context of the clinical situation that is being investigated. This is usually the role of the clinicians involved with the study, but discussion with the statistician is important to ensure that the defined outcomes are both measurable with the required precision and relevant to the condition under consideration. If combinations of outcomes are to be used as the primary or secondary endpoints for a study, these should be clearly defined prior to analysis and not overly heterogeneous. Certain complications of diabetes require special expertise in identifying the appropriate measures. Nephropathy, neuropathy and retinopathy are examples of complications of diabetes where there is substantial scope for variation in the definition and clarity is required. While it is the role of the clinician to decide on an appropriate index of neuropathy, training of those taking measurements and quality control should be in place to ensure consistency of reporting. For diabetic retinopathy, the gold standard remains ETDRS scores of seven field retinal photographs (National Eye Institute 1985).

Adjudicated endpoints

In clinical trials over long time periods, the endpoints will be death and major clinical events. It is critically important that the endpoints of a study are confirmed by a suitably qualified group of people who are not the same as those conducting the study. In the UKPDS, all potential endpoints were reported by each centre, all available evidence (including death certificates and clinical records) was assessed by two independent clinicians who were blind to the random allocation and current therapy, and all discrepancies were adjudicated by a three man committee (UKPDS 1998a). If consensus could not be obtained by this group, a further group of external experts was called upon to confirm the final adjudication.

Validation of data

If data is being collected on paper forms for entry into a computerised database it should be keyed in twice, by independent data entry staff, and compared, with differences being validated by a third person. Databases should be structured to include range checks and internal consistency, e.g. limits on height and blood pressures. These ranges may be obtained locally from earlier studies in a similar population, or if this is not possible, from published papers.

Other sources of bias and error

Many patients with diabetes have complications leading to reduced visual acuity, and this requires that the print size of self-administered questionnaires is larger than that used in other populations, to ensure that misreading biases are not introduced. Likewise, other sources of bias should be considered and eliminated, such as with tools designed to assess quality of life, where a relative or friend of the patient may fill in the form for them.

The prevalence of some forms of diabetes is high in certain ethnic groups; language difficulties can make recruitment and consent difficult in some populations. It will be important to consider cultural differences when translating patient information sheets and consent forms, and when dealing with individual patients. For instance, in some UK minority ethnic groups it is not appropriate to ask a young man to interpret for his mother regarding questions of an intimate nature.

Many of the biochemical measures in diabetes are not normally distributed. For instance, plasma insulin and triglyceride commonly follow a logarithmic distribution, while fasting plasma glucose at diagnosis has a lower limit by definition. To enable parametric statistical tests to be used, transformation of the data (usually by taking logarithms) may be needed. Geometric mean and the associated one standard deviation range should be reported; for variables where such a transformation is not possible, the median and 25th and 75th centiles provide measures of centrality and dispersion. Care should be taken to ensure that statistical tests are only used on data which conform to the underlying assumptions of those tests, and that suitable checks of distributions are made, before embarking on analysis. Particular care should be taken with data that consist of counts or ordered categorical scores.

In many cases, the reporting of family history of diabetes causes difficulties in interpretation. In order to assess the strength of these data it is important to know how many relatives a subject has in an age group by which diabetes might have been diagnosed when they die, and this could include the number of siblings. Consulting an expert geneticist is important when considering this kind of information.

Analysis

A few simple principles should be adhered to when analysing data:

- Follow the protocol. When analysing a clinical trial with a specified design, always analyse the data according to the design. Failure to do so leads to serious statistical errors and can result in drawing the wrong conclusions.

- Always inspect the data carefully to identify outliers or rogue items that need further checking. Decide what to do with outliers *before* proceeding to analysis, not in the light of what happens to the results if they are excluded. Be especially careful with protocol deviations.

- Look at the data first. One graph is worth a thousand calculations!

- Be sure that the methods of analysis are appropriate for the data. Do not use methods designed for categorical data on continuous data or vice versa. Be especially careful when analysing time-to-event data, and be sure to distinguish between incidence and prevalence.

- Always check for the constraints under which statistical methods may or may not work. For instance, do not use methods designed for normally distributed data on data with other distributions.

- Be sure you know what hypothesis is being tested.

- Give the reader enough information to make their own decisions about the validity of your conclusions. P-values should be presented to at least two significant digits, not rounded, nor using essentially arbitrary cut-off points such as <0.05.

- Be aware of the problems of multiple testing, of whether to test main effects and interactions, and whether to include subsidiary endpoints when primary endpoints do not provide conclusive proof of any hypothesis.

- Sub-group analyses should only be carried out if 1) pre-specified, 2) the primary analysis gives a significant result, and 3) there is sufficient power, or they are only to be used to generate further hypotheses for testing in another trial.

- The value and importance of consulting a well trained, experienced and qualified statistician before undertaking any clinical trial cannot be underestimated.

References

Altman DG (1990) *Practical Statistics for Medical Research*, Chapman & Hall/CRC

Altman DG (1996) Better reporting of randomised controlled trials: the CONSORT statement *BMJ* **313**, 570–1

Altman DG, Machin D, Bryant TN, Gardner MJ (Eds) (2000) *Statistics with Confidence*, BMJ Books

Armitage P, Matthews JNS, Berry G (2001) *Statistical Methods in Medical Research*, Blackwell Science, UK

Bland JM (2000) *An Introduction to Medical Statistics*, OUP

Campbell MJ (2006) *Medical Statistics: A Commonsense Approach for Health Professionals*, John Wiley & Sons

CONSORT statement http://www.consort-statement.org

Cull CA, Manley SE, Stratton IM, Holman RR, Turner RC, Matthews DR (1997) Approach to maintaining comparability of biochemical data during long-term clinical trials *Clinical Chemistry* **43**, 1913–18

National Eye Institute (1985) *Early Treatment Diabetic Retinopathy Study (ETDRS) Manual of Operations*, National Eye Institute, Bethesda, MD

Senn S (1997) *Statistical Issues in Drug Development*, John Wiley & Sons

Stratton I, Neil A (2005) How to ensure your paper is rejected by the statistical reviewer *Diabetic Medicine* **22**(4), 371–3

Tufte ER (2001) *The Visual Display of Quantitative Information*, Graphics Press, USA

UK Prospective Diabetes Study (UKPDS) Group (1991) UK Prospective Diabetes Study (UKPDS) VIII: Study design, progress and performance *Diabetologia* **34**, 877–90

UK Prospective Diabetes Study (UKPDS) Group (1998a) Intensive blood glucose control with sulphonylureas or insulin compared with conventional treatment and risk of complications in patients with type 2 diabetes: UKPDS 33 *Lancet* **352**, 837–53

UK Prospective Diabetes Study (UKPDS) Group (1998b) Tight blood pressure control and risk of macrovascular and microvascular complications in type 2 diabetes: UKPDS 38 *BMJ* **317**(7160), 703–13

Index

Note: page numbers in *italics* refer to figures and tables

Index compiled by Jill Halliday